Practice Management for the Veterinary Team

Front Office, Operations, and Development

Practice Management for the Veterinary Team
Front Office, Operations, and Development
Fourth Edition

Heather Prendergast, BS, AS, RVT, CVPM, SPHR

Certified Veterinary Practice Manager
Synergie Consulting
Las Cruces, New Mexico

ELSEVIER

Elsevier
3251 Riverport Lane
St. Louis, Missouri 63043

PRACTICE MANAGEMENT FOR THE VETERINARY TEAM: FRONT OFFICE, OPERATIONS, AND DEVELOPMENT, FOURTH EDITION

ISBN: 978-0-443-11708-4

Content Strategist: Melissa J. Rawe
Senior Content Development Manager: Somodatta Roy Choudhury
Senior Content Development Specialist: Priyadarshini Pandey
Publishing Services Manager: Deepthi Unni
Project Manager: Sheik Mohideen K
Design Direction: Ryan Cook

Printed in India

Last digit is the print number: 9 8 7 6 5 4 3 2 1

To my mother ~ the wind beneath my wings ~ who has guided and given me inspiration, motivation, and empowerment. You have been a truly amazing woman.
I miss you dearly.

PREFACE

Imagine having the ability to view the veterinary practice in a time machine: What did it look like before the year 2000? What were some of the challenges and wins of that century? How was that different from the years 2000–2019? Further, consider the challenges that practices faced from 2020–2022. And what will the practice of the future look like?

There is no doubt that the practices of today and the future are very different than veterinary practices prior to 2000. Thought processes around leadership, team leveraging, customer service, wages, benefits, and employment regulations have changed. Technology has evolved, thereby improving medical standards and the ability to enhance the client experience. But have businesses embraced the changes needed to get the practice to the next stage? "What got us here won't get us there" is a phrase that strongly applies to veterinary medicine.

The COVID years of 2020–2023 have changed the shape of veterinary medicine. Industry-identified issues include practice inefficiencies, poor client service, labor shortages, and the emotional well-being and satisfaction of employees; all must be the focus of every practice moving forward. There are many contributors to each of these topics, and all are addressed throughout this book.

Long-term solutions must be put into place and each role on the veterinary team contributes to that success. But it all starts with leadership; without the right leaders in place with the right skills, the team will struggle. Leaders must step up, focus on, and grow their most important asset to come out ahead in the long game.

The goal should be to do everything possible to make the practice the best place to work that no one wants to leave. When that can be achieved, the struggles of labor shortage and emotional well-being become less, and the focus can be on developing new efficiencies and implementing technology.

This textbook places a heavy focus on the role of leadership and creating a rock-solid culture. A team-centered environment is best served, and each chapter focuses on the management of the business, the people, and the clients.

FEATURES IN THIS TEXTBOOK

Critical Competencies

The Veterinary Hospital Managers Association (VHMA) created *Critical Competencies: A Guide for Veterinary Practice Management Professionals* as an overview of the skills needed to be an effective practice manager. The VHMA has identified five performance domains associated with the job of a veterinary practice manager: human resources, law and ethics, marketing and client relations, organization of the practice, and financial management. To be successful in each of the performance domains, certain knowledge requirements must be met, and a set of critical competencies must be achieved. The critical competencies that must be achieved to master each performance domain are listed at the beginning of the chapter along with the knowledge requirements for developing your career in each aspect of veterinary practice management. These critical competencies include decision making, integrity, critical and strategic thinking, planning and prioritizing, oral communication and comprehension, and writing and verbal skills. As you read the chapter, you will be reminded of these critical competencies when you see this icon. Read the description of a typical task that is required of a practice manager and think about which critical competency is needed to complete this task. When is it important to practice good decision making? What knowledge requirements would you need to conduct staff meetings or handle a client complaint? The goal of outlining these critical competencies and knowledge requirements within each job domain is to help you connect the dots among the skills required to be the best practice manager you can be and to show you how to practice these skills in the real world.

Other Features

Important Features Include the Following:

Learning Objectives and **Key Terms** at the beginning of each chapter guide you in your study and enable you to check your mastery of the content in each chapter.

Critical Competencies as described by the VHMA are listed throughout each chapter to indicate important skills as they relate to each job domain.

Leadership Points spotlight important tips for running a successful practice.

The Practice Managers Survival Checklist provides a checklist of "must dos" for the chapter.

Review Questions ensure that you have mastered complete comprehension of each chapter.

Recommended Readings provide additional sources of detailed information on important topics.

EVOLVE RESOURCES

The instructor Evolve site (for instructors only) includes:

A test bank including 500 multiple-choice questions with answer rationales

An image collection containing all the images from the book (over 400 images)

PowerPoint presentations for each chapter to assist with lecturing

The student and instructor Evolve site includes:

Interactive working forms allow students to practice. These forms include sample checks and deposit slips, and incident reports.

Practice quizzes

Comprehensive glossary

ACKNOWLEDGMENTS

The 2020–2022 pandemic years have been a whirlwind for the veterinary industry as a whole; it has changed the landscape of veterinary medicine for years to come. We learned how to navigate change and adapt daily, build resilience, and hold our teams up high, even in the face of adversity.

Being a leader in any organization takes dedication, most of all to the people we serve. When leaders place their team first and coach them to be the best they can be, then any adverse event can be weathered. Why? Because when a strong team is built to serve one another, then everyone has each other's back. This builds ***trust, integrity, respect, loyalty, and honesty***—the desired values that every team member would be honored to work with.

There are many colleagues that deserve recognition for the creation of this fourth edition. Not only did we teach and coach each other through adversity, but we also built each other up, leaned on one another, and came out with more knowledge than we had in 2020. Rebecca Metheny, Matt Peuser, Kimberly White, Brie Sleasman, Lu Olson, Amanda Edwards, Candiss Jacques, Cassie Mitliski, and Holly Daugherty, I am indebted to each of you for your valuable contributions, laughs, tears, honest conversations, and growth that we achieved together over the last 3 years. Each of you believes in, upholds, and demonstrates the values listed above. You are the true definition of leaders that develop leaders. Never let anyone or anything squish those values, nor the dreams each of you holds on to. I cherish the ride we have been on together and look forward to the future rides that are to come.

My husband, Clint Derk, has ridden this wild rollercoaster ride with me with pride and patience. I could not ask for a better man to stand by my side.

To each of my past, present, and future mentees and students: this career can be rewarding. Find a practice that allows you to shine, and that will shine the light on you. Or just build your own! ***Life is short. Chase your dreams. Do what makes you happy. Enjoy life while you can.***

CONTENTS

SECTION I Veterinary Practice Team and Development

SECTION II Veterinary Operations

SECTION I

Veterinary Practice Team and Development

1

The Heart of Veterinary Medicine

LEARNING OBJECTIVES

When you have completed this chapter, you should be able to:

- Compare and contrast the veterinary practices over the previous 20 years
- Identify issues facing the veterinary profession in 2023
- Define a sense of purpose
- Define the Frictionless Client Experience
- Define the Frictionless Employee Experience
- Provide solutions that overcome 2023 issues

OUTLINE

KEY TERMS

Maslow's hierarchy of needs
Purpose
Frictionless client experience
Frictionless employee experience
Emotional well-being and satisfaction

INTRODUCTION

Imagine having the ability to view the veterinary practice in a time machine; what did it look like before the year 2000? What were some of the challenges and wins of that century? How was it different from the years 2000–2019? Furthermore, consider the challenges that practices faced in 2020–2022. What will the practice of the future look like?

There is no doubt that the practices of today and that of the future are very different than veterinary practices prior to 2000. Thought processes around leadership, team leveraging, customer service, wages, benefits, and employment regulations have changed. Technology has evolved, thereby improving medical standards and the ability to enhance the client experience. However, have businesses embraced the changes needed to get the practice to the next stage? "What got us here won't get us there" is a phrase that strongly applies to veterinary medicine. To get us "there," we must understand what got us here.

TRADITIONAL VETERINARY PRACTICES

For clarity purposes, the word "traditional" can be defined in this context as the existence of veterinary practices and business standards prior to 2000. For comparison purposes, four topics will be considered: the client experience, team leveraging, work style, and change management.

Client Experience

In traditional veterinary practices, the client bonded only with the veterinarian. Veterinary team members were simply "helpers" who carried out tasks to help the veterinarian. Emergency and specialty practices were available, but not abundantly, so general practice veterinarians tended to urgent care and emergencies and worked up their cases daily. Cases that perplexed the veterinarian were the only cases sent to specialty during this time. Customer service and wait times were not a priority, as there was little to no competition in the veterinary space.

Team Leveraging

The veterinarian completed most patient care, including diagnostics, treatments, and triaging patients; the staff helped the veterinarian by answering phones, collecting payments, and restraining, cleaning, and feeding patients. In addition, the owner may have ordered inventory, reconciled deposits and books, and completed other business functions.

Work Style

Since veterinarians did most of the work, they worked 50–60 hours or more per week. The same was expected of team members. This led to highly productive and efficient practices that accommodated every patient. Afterall, patient care is what drove veterinarians into this business in the first place. They enjoyed the hard work and received joy from being able to care for "all." Business management was less of a priority over medicine, and financial goals and strategic planning were rarely completed.

Change Management

Although change management was a known concept prior to 2000, it was not a hot topic, nor was it a priority. Practices would settle into "what worked" and would maintain consistency around that model; challenging the status quo (or the way it had always been done) was unheard of.

PRACTICES OF THE YEARS 2000–2019

Effective business management and practice management started becoming hot topics in the early 2000s as the landscape of veterinary medicine started to change. There was more competition in veterinary communities as more veterinarians began to experience entrepreneurship. They wanted to have successful businesses and thus began putting protocols and standards of care into place. Business standards began to improve, as did revenues and successes of these new entrepreneurs.

Client Experience

The importance of client service became a part of successful business strategy, and there was a heightened sense of urgency to differentiate the practice. Clients came to the practice with higher expectations that they had discerned from other industries. Client concerns were addressed, and processes were put into place to ensure a consistent client experience.

Team Leveraging

Veterinary owners began hiring more credentialed veterinary technicians and delegating more tasks to team members, leveraging the team's skills, and considering their thoughts and opinions regarding business decisions. Practice managers became more integrated in business decisions, driving collaboration, and teamwork. Focus on inventory control, appointment management, safety in the practice, appropriate human resource protocols, professional development, and business profitability became priorities.

Work Style

Most owners of practices opened during this era worked longer hours to ensure business success. They were dedicated and truly enjoyed what they had developed. They still had high expectations of associate veterinarians; however, working 40 hours per week became the norm. Team members continued to work 40-hour work weeks with some overtime, depending on demographics and roles.

Change Management

Challenging the status quo and implementing change started evolving. To remain competitive, increase client capacity, and be profitable, smart business practices had to be implemented. While change management can be hard on an individual level, the overall scope of business practices evolved through successful change management.

PRACTICES OF THE YEARS 2020–2022

These years will forever be known as the years of the "COVID pandemic." Change management and pivoting in the moment to meet the needs of daily changes led to innovation, stress, and reevaluation of life. Team members' personal lives were impacted by the loss of loved ones, unavailable childcare or health care for themselves and their family, supply chain shortages, and uncertainty about the future.

Clients were impacted in the same manner; however, many were furloughed or lost their jobs completely, while others worked remotely. Clients were home with their pets 24 hours a day; these pets became children, sleeping in their "parents'" bed every night. Conditions or disease processes were observed by clients sooner than they had before, leading to dramatic increases in visits to the veterinary practice. People who had never adopted pets became first-time pet owners during the pandemic, leading to unprecedented demand on veterinary practices. Government subsidies contributed to client disposable income of every demographic. Restaurants were closed and vacations were canceled. Clients were spending more on their pets than ever before.

The increased demand of veterinary practices took a toll on veterinary team members. Practice efficiency decreased as curbside business models were put into place for safety purposes. Wearing masks in 100°+ heat or pouring rain, while trying to meet client expectations and seeing as many patients as possible, added stress and detracted from team communication, harmony, and overall teamwork.

Work-related stressors added to personal stressors and changed the shape of the veterinary environment. Team members of all generations evaluated "life and priorities," resulting in a significant impact to the labor market, practice efficiency, and the emotional well-being of team members and owners alike.

PRACTICES OF 2023 AND BEYOND

As stated earlier, it is important to understand what got the veterinary industry where it is today and the current issues that resulted. The next step is to identify ways to fix the current issues that will allow practices not only to thrive in the future but to succeed and exceed both client and team member expectations.

Industry identified issues include practice inefficiencies, poor team utilization, poor client service, labor shortages, and emotional well-being and satisfaction of employees; all must be the focus of every practice moving forward. There are many contributors to each of these topics, and all are addressed in subsequent chapters of this book. This section will summarize these topics as it ties to the ideal practice of the future. It is up to the practice manager and owner of the hospital to implement strategies to overcome these issues and lead a successful business while decreasing the stress felt by the team.

Practice Inefficiencies

Many practices are seeing less clients and patients per day than prior to the 2020 pandemic. It is important to acknowledge that 2020 and 2021 had the highest client demand ever. Practices did all they could to accommodate, but when the breaking point hit, practice owners/managers made the decision to stop accepting new clients and limit the number of patients they would see in a day. They went into survival mode. In reflection, this has likely led to a current anomaly in which practices now schedule team members to work when they "want to work," not when it best serves clients. Practices are also resistant to adapting to team member schedule flexibility (hiring more team members who work less hours) to provide the care that best serves clients. The result is a patient care barrier; pets are not getting the care they need because access is limited.

CRITICAL COMPETENCY: ADAPTABILITY

Practice managers must be open to change and flexible work methods and able to adapt behavior to changing conditions or new information.

In mid-2022, client and patient visits began normalizing, similar to 2019 key performance indicators (KPIs). However, what was adaptable in 2019 is a tall order in the current landscape.

Team members are still mentally exhausted from the daily stressors and changes made during the pandemic; exhaustion makes it harder to implement and learn new technologies. Dedication and loyalty to the practice are at an all-time low, resulting in practices experiencing a high employee turnover, all of which contribute to decreased efficiency. Team members lack purpose in their daily roles. In summary, leadership and practices are working harder, not smarter, and patients receiving care continues to be a barrier.

CRITICAL COMPETENCY: RESILIENCE

Practice managers must have the ability to cope effectively with pressure and setbacks. Additionally, PMs must be able to handle crisis situations effectively and remain undeterred by obstacles or failure.

The leadership team may exhibit inefficiencies, overall impacting the team. Everything starts at the "top," as team members watch the behaviors of their leaders and model what they see. When leadership is inefficient, so is the team. The behaviors that result in wasted time include failure to plan and budget time accordingly, interruptions, failure to follow through and complete tasks, slow decision making, unnecessary work, and failure to delegate. Efficient time management requires that leaders be organized, maintain a daily schedule, establish deadlines (and meet them), and organize workflow.

Leaders must be held to high standards and set admirable examples for the team. If leadership cannot complete tasks early or on time, the rest of the team cannot be expected to do any better.

Where does one start to evaluate efficiency? Consider daily tasks and processes and ask: How can we make this task/process simpler and easier for both the client and team? Let's begin formulating thoughts around two concepts: the frictionless client experience and the frictionless employee experience. A frictionless experience can be defined as a lack of impediments to a client or employee experience. From a client's perspective, friction may result when trying to schedule an appointment, not being able to get an appointment, overall customer service from the team, frustration with the digital experience (website, pet portal, practice app, etc.), or difficulty doing business with the practice. From the employee's perspective, friction can result from poor culture, lack of leadership, decreased empowerment and utilization/leveraging, decreased communication, a lack of a sense of belonging, and schedule inflexibility. Friction can be found anywhere in the veterinary practice, and the leadership team must consistently work to create a frictionless experience for the most important assets of the business.

CRITICAL COMPETENCY: CRITICAL AND STRATEGIC THINKING

Strategic thinking and planning are an essential part of financial forecasting, marketing plans, and long-term plans for growth of the practice. Managers must have the ability to identify questions, problems, and arguments relevant to these issues and to use logic and critical reasoning to identify the strengths and weaknesses of alternative solutions or approaches to problems.

So, how do frictionless client experiences and frictionless employee experiences relate to efficiency? Both encompass tasks and procedures used daily. If any portion of delivering a frictionless client experience is inefficient, team members are working harder (not smarter), resulting in the feeling of consistently being overwhelmed and understaffed (Fig. 1.1).

The Frictionless Client Experience

A practice management integrative software (PIMS; see Chapter 8) that integrates a robust client communication platform and digital experience is the key to creating a frictionless client experience (Chapter 11). This also leads to an improved frictionless employee experience, as they can become more efficient and provide better service to clients. Chapter 8 reviews the importance of practice integrations; if that is not an option, consider the use of third-party apps to help build the frictionless client experience.

Making appointments: Clients should be able to make appointments online and not have to call the practice to get an appointment scheduled. Active clients should have follow-up visits (medical progress, booster vaccines, biannual and annual exams) scheduled prior to the client leaving the practice. This will free up phone lines and the receptionist's time to handle the clients that are present. Chapter 8 covers solutions that allow clients to schedule their own appointments, and Chapter 10, Appointments, covers forward booking that should be completed before a client leaves the practice.

Reminder calls/call backs: Implement two-way text messaging to remind clients of upcoming appointments and call backs of normal lab results. Some practices "feel" their clients would prefer a phone call to a text (phone calls feel more personal). But how often do clients really call back with updates? Ask clients how they prefer to be contacted; don't rely on what "we think" the client wants. Consider this: Can your team members walk away from a client to accept a call from their dentist? Likely not, but they can respond to a text once they have finished with the client (Fig. 1.2).

Check-in and exam room procedures: Have clients fill out forms online prior to arriving for their appointment, thus reducing check-in time. When clients are taken to exam rooms, both the doctor and technician should be present, allowing the client to tell their story

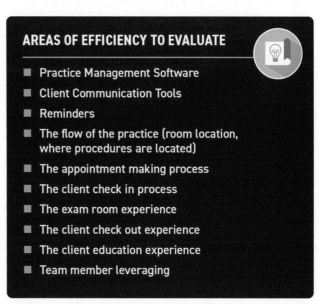

AREAS OF EFFICIENCY TO EVALUATE

- Practice Management Software
- Client Communication Tools
- Reminders
- The flow of the practice (room location, where procedures are located)
- The appointment making process
- The client check in process
- The exam room experience
- The client check out experience
- The client education experience
- Team member leveraging

Fig. 1.1 Team members that work harder (not smarter) consistently feel overwhelmed and understaffed.

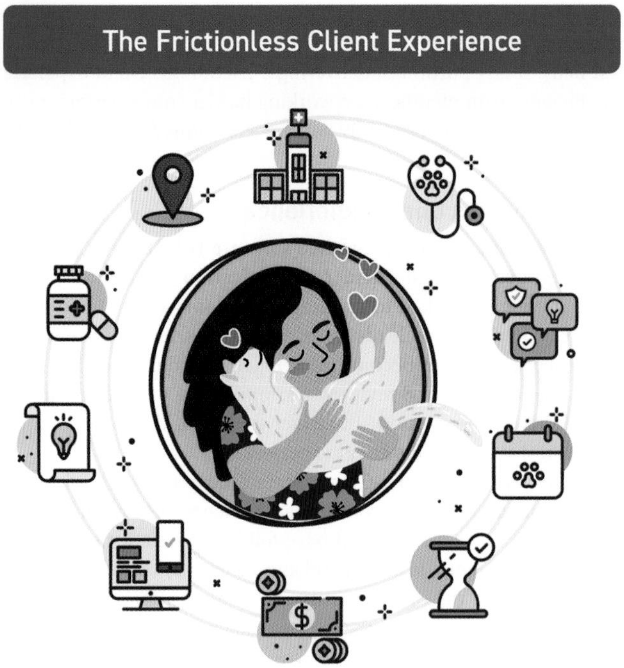

Fig. 1.2 Ensure the practice is "easy to do business with" by evaluating all facets of the client experience.

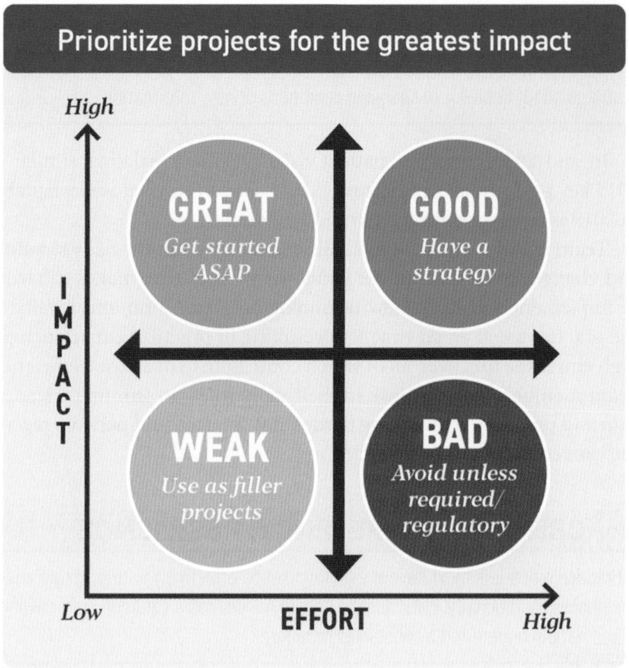

Fig. 1.3 Assess potential ideas based on the level of effort required to accomplish it and the potential impact when it is completed.

once, saving approximately 10 minutes. Vitals can be recorded at the same time. Rooms should be stocked with supplies needed for the top 20 diagnostic tests that can be completed in the exam rooms (complete as many diagnostic procedures as possible in the exam with the client to increase value). This eliminates the back-and-forth inefficiency.

Have a scribe in the exam room for the doctor to improve efficiency with paperless medical records. Templates should be set up allowing the scribe to add comments made by the doctor as they complete the medical exam. When the doctor communicates (out loud) normal and abnormal findings during the exam process, it increases the value perceived by the client (and the scribe documents the findings). The doctor then makes recommendations to the client and the scribe creates a treatment plan or makes labels for medications (whichever next step is most appropriate). If a treatment plan is indicated, the scribe/technician can review and obtain authorization from the client and start diagnostics. That same technician can carry the case from that point forward, allowing the doctor to move to the next patient.

Having standard operating protocols (SOPs) and standards of care (SOCs) in place agreed upon by all doctors allows the team to be efficient in making recommendations, diagnostic preparations, client education, reminders, and forward booking medical progress exams.

Consider surgical check-in procedures and protocols established. What efficiencies can be put in place? In an ideal practice, the technician team knows which drugs to administer, when to administer, and how much to administer, without having to be told what to do. This is another area in which SOPs and SOCs have a significant impact.

Checkout procedures: Checking clients out in the exam room with the same technician making follow-up appointments can expedite efficiency. Have credit card terminals (in each room) that integrate with the PIMS to eliminate manual entry errors, and a printer to print credit card receipts and client invoices.

Telemedicine: Practices already provide telemedicine (most without realizing it). Cases are triaged over the phone without visualizing the pet. This further increases the inefficiency of the team and does not meet client expectations. Millennial clients want to have professional veterinary opinions when they want it (on demand), and many practices are not meeting that need. Busy clients who either travel or see their own clients often don't have time to bring their pet in. Lastly, most practices are booked 3–6 weeks out. This creates a barrier to patient care, adding a further stressor to team happiness (their passion is to serve all patients, and they can't do that in the current model). Telehealth cases average 9 minutes and utilize a mix of credentialed veterinary technicians/nurses and doctors. Building this role into the practice meets client and patient needs, serves team member passions, and improves efficiency. Chapter 7, Telemedicine, covers all aspects of offering telehealth in the veterinary practice.

While these are only a few recommendations, saving five minutes per patient seen can add at least five more appointments per day, per veterinarian. In addition, working smarter and more efficiently contributes to team member well-being, and pets get the care they deserve. Every chapter in this book suggests solutions to improve practice efficiencies. Do not allow that to overwhelm you; rather, prioritize the options that have the most impact, and start there (Fig. 1.3).

The Frictionless Employee Experience

Labor Shortage

Post pandemic, self-evaluation and reflections made team members consider what was important to them. Working for the moment has become the priority, versus working for retirement. This has reduced the number of people in the workforce that want to work. According to the US Bureau of Labor Statistics, over 3.2 million people have chosen not to work post pandemic.[1] In addition, the baby boomer generation is beginning to retire. These decisions impact the ability to hire receptionists and veterinary assistants, roles that don't require previous experience. It has also impacted the ability to hire credentialed veterinary technicians and veterinarians.

In a 2022 Census of Veterinarians by the AVMA,[2] over 3000 veterinarians have chosen not to return to work. Of those working, a majority would like to work fewer hours for lower compensation. Additionally, 40% are considering leaving the profession,[3] and 54% of veterinarians younger than 35 years of age are barely getting by. This brings forth the question: Why are team members so unhappy?

To further the severity of the industry gap, nearly 41,000 veterinarians will be needed to serve the current estimated 75 million pets in 2030. However, veterinary schools estimate that they will only graduate 15,000 veterinarians by 2030, leaving the industry with a 15,000 doctor shortage. Additionally, it will take more than 30 years for veterinary technician/nurse graduates to meet the need for credentialed veterinary technicians/nurses.[4]

Not only is the veterinary industry facing a shortage of graduates to meet the growing demand; credentialed veterinary technicians/nurses and assistants are leaving practices for improved practice culture, optimal utilization, and higher wages. The average turnover rate of credentialed technicians/nurses is approximately 25%, more than 5% higher than that of registered nurses (RNs). The DVM turnover is over 15%, more than two times that of an MD.

CRITICAL COMPETENCY: PLANNING AND PRIORITIZING

Practice managers must be able to effectively manage time and workload to meet deadlines, thereby having the ability to organize work, set priorities, and establish plans to achieve goals.

Turnover costs the practice an average of 1.5 times that of the salary leaving, and whether that person can be adequately replaced is the bigger question. Turnover impacts revenue generation, client loyalty and retention, and client compliance. Increased turnover burns out existing team members who are already exhausted and have low levels of team morale and are tasked with effectively and repeatedly training new team members. This results in a less than subpar onboarding experience for the new team members (loyalty to the practice is established in the first 60 days of employment). Chapter 4, Human Resources, provides ideas to create an amazing employee onboarding experience.

As discussed, workload, clients, and salary are factors that contribute to unhappiness, but practices must determine what motivates their team. Motivation results from an individuals' passion and purpose. Credentialed technicians/nurses and veterinarians don't lack passion; in fact, most have wanted to be in this profession since they were kids. Therefore, purpose must be addressed. They struggle with a sense of belonging and may not feel they "fit" with the practice's culture and values. In fact, most are unaware of the practice's values and goals. Maslow's hierarchy of needs is covered in Chapter 2, Leadership, and must be addressed to start retaining team members.

CRITICAL COMPETENCY: LEADERSHIP

Practice managers must have the initiative to lead and take charge while simultaneously motivating and mobilizing others to achieve common goals.

The cost of not leveraging clearly impacts the satisfaction of team members, but it also has a significant impact on the revenue of the practice. In well-leveraged practices, DVMs diagnose, prescribe, and complete surgical procedures. Credentialed veterinary technicians/nurses complete all aspects of patient care, diagnostic tests, and most of the client education. Veterinary assistants restrain patients, provide patient care, and may also obtain samples for diagnostic tests, depending on skill and state regulation. They also significantly increase the efficiency of the credentialed technicalness/nurses and the doctors. If DVMs are performing any of these tasks for just 15 minutes per hour (reading UA's, fecal's, cytology's, etc.) versus seeing the next patient, they may be adding to the barrier of patient care by reducing availability by 8 appointments per day, or 40 appointments per week. This may reduce income by $10,000 per week or $500,000 per year (based on an average client transaction [ACT] of $250). This then negatively impacts the ability of the practice to be able to deliver a frictionless employee experience.

It is critical to commit to team member investment. When team members love their career (not a job), they are loyal and dedicated to achieving practice goals. What makes someone love their career? Culture, great leadership, professional development, inclusion, teamwork, collaboration, flexibility, leveraging, trust, and respect. One will notice that these are soft skills fostered by the leaders of the practice. Therefore, when turnover is high, leaders need take to take a close look at the impact they are having on the team; stop pointing fingers, accept blame, and fix the problem. Chapter 2, Leadership, and Chapter 4, Human Resources, outline all aspects needed to create a frictionless employee experience that results in dedicated and loyal team members.

Emotional Well-Being and Satisfaction

Loving a career and the impact on satisfaction were discussed above. Leadership plays a significant role in that, but emotional well-being is a weight carried by each person on the team. While poor culture and leadership have a heavy impact on emotional well-being, so do the hours worked, expectations by leadership, and the personal stressors outside of the practice (childcare, family, economics).

Every team member has a different level of well-being. While some may have external factors that also impact their sense of emotional well-being, others may be solely impacted by internal factors. Team members are not the same; treat each person as an individual and coach and grow each of them to be the best they can be. Coaching team members takes time, and as a leader, that is your responsibility. Not making time to do so is an irresponsibility on your part.

PREPARING FOR THE FUTURE

Some practices lack the basics needed to prepare for future business impactions. COVID was a reality check for many, and one that could have been disastrous to the veterinary industry. One must always consider "what could happen" and mitigate the risks associated with such disasters through analysis of strengths, weaknesses, opportunities, and threats (SWOT). Threats are external factors that could severely impact the business. While the leaders of the practice have no impact on the threats, they can reduce the risk associated with the threats. Take the events that occurred over 2020–2022 as learning experiences and use these as examples of what to prepare for:

- world events such as war that impact the supply chain and US economy;
- pandemics that may impact supply chain and the economy;
- natural disasters (fires, tornados, hurricanes, floods);
- inflation that will impact consumer spending and costs to the practice;
- recession that will impact consumer spending and costs to the practice; and
- large competitors opening new practice nearby.

CRITICAL COMPETENCY: CONTINUOUS LEARNING

Practice managers should have a curiosity for learning. Actively seeking out new information, technologies, and methods while keeping skills updated allows the application of new knowledge to the job.

When thinking of potential competition, consider the impact Uber had on the taxi industry. Uber made a conscious decision to "make it easy to do business" and ensure that service was available to anyone. While taxi service is still available, companies like Uber and Lyft have revolutionized the industry. This will happen to the veterinary industry as well; it is only a matter of when. What is your practice doing to be prepared for that threat? For more specifics on completing and implementing the results of a SWOT analysis, see Chapter 12, Marketing.

SOLUTIONS THAT MUST BE IMPLEMENTED

Practice management and medicine must be married (Fig. 1.4); you can't have one without the other. Medicine drives the revenue of the business while practice management cares for the business and the people that deliver medicine. Practice management encompasses all elements of the practice. Office procedures, operations, and development are interwoven; you can't have one without the others. People must be developed and they must have the tools (operations) to perform for leadership and to exceed client expectations. Every team member contributes to office procedures regardless of their role. Take medical records for example; it is not just the medical team that "touches" a medical record. The receptionist team must add new clients to the PIMS, check clients in and add notes, schedule future appointments, manage medication refill requests, etc. In addition to medical records, consider the client recommendations; every person on the team makes recommendations to clients, not just the medical team. The receptionists make recommendations on the phone and through client communication tools. Technicians and assistants may check clients out in the room. However, no team member can deliver any front office procedure items without having the protocols and technology implemented and integrating well together (operations).

CRITICAL COMPETENCY: DECISION MAKING

The practice manager must be able to make good decisions based on critical thinking and problem solving and make decisions that positively impact the practice. While many alternatives are available, the PM must be able to gather and effectively analyze relevant data and choose decisively.

Owners and practice managers have no choice but to modernize and step up to the plate. What worked in the past clearly will not move the practice or industry forward. Consider the following thoughts and use the remainder of this book to help advance initiatives that support these changes.

- Effective leadership that drives culture, a sense of purpose, belonging, teamwork, trust, flexibility, and collaboration.
- Ensure that team member communication is a top priority delivered through regularly scheduled meetings, daily huddles, an internal communication system (such as Slack or a feature that is integrated into the PIMS). Clearly communicate the practice goals (values, vision, mission, strategic plan) and update the team during meetings about progress to attaining goals, goal achievement, and the celebration of such wins. Additionally, tie the importance of each role to goal achievement in every meeting.
- Create a relationship-centered practice where the client bond is established with the team, not one doctor.
- Create a frictionless customer experience to serve as a differentiator.
- Ensure credentialed technicians/nurses are working at the highest level their license allows (review the state veterinary practice act).
- Leverage staff to work at their highest ability to increase practice efficiency and improve the employee experience.
- Increase wages and benefit options to help attract and retain the "right" team members.
- Reduce hours of team members to improve emotional and well-being balance.
- Implement technology that increases workflow efficiencies and client satisfaction.

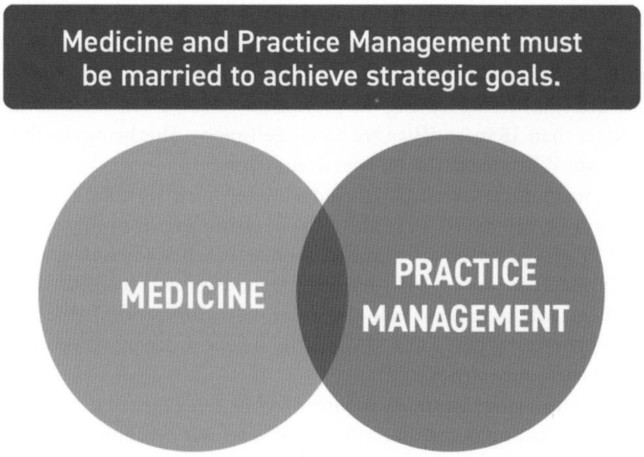

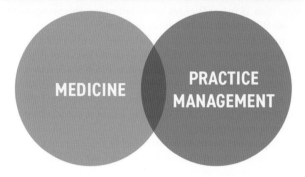

Fig. 1.4 Ensure medicine and management are synergistically aligned in the veterinary practice.

It is also important for practice managers and owners to fully understand the financial picture of the practice so that the frictionless client and employee experience can become a reality. These experiences cost money. But they also generate money when done well. Watch industry trends from the Veterinary Hospital Managers Association (VHMA), the American Veterinary Medical Association (AVMA), the American Animal Hospital Association (AAHA), and the Veterinary Management Group (VMG). Is your practice performing at the same level financially as the benchmarks produced by these organizations? How do you know what to look at? More importantly, how do you know what to fix and how to fix it? Don't worry; this book will help guide you through those answers. Here are few pointers to get started.

Mental Health and Emotional Well-Being

It was previously mentioned that each person has a different level of emotional well-being. Different levels result from past experiences obtained during childhood, school, or previous work experiences. To evaluate each team member fairly, set time aside and ask questions such as:

- "How are you doing?"
- "Do you feel well balanced?"
- "What stressors are in the workplace that could create an imbalance?"
- "How do you feel about your fellow team members, and their emotional well-being? Is there anyone that you are specifically concerned with?"

Teach team members to respect others for their level. Each person deals with past experiences differently, and a team that is willing to embrace the differences, adapt as needed, and support one another will be loyal to the practice.

Consider the flexibility of working hours and how that can positively impact the emotional well-being of the team. Perception has changed from "live to work" to "work to live," meaning that people prefer to take things one day at a time and appreciate the small things in life. It was mentioned previously that veterinarians want to work fewer hours for less compensation; could it be assumed staff would want the same? Forty-hour work weeks don't have to be the norm. To accommodate workforce shortages and enhance the well-being of team members, consider 30-hour work weeks as full-time status. Businesses that have implemented 30-hour work weeks have found team members to be more focused, be more creative and collaborative, and have less burnout.[5] The impact of shorter work week hours and more team members is the increased cost of benefits, but that is a smaller issue (that can be overcome) than a lack of loyal employees who produce revenue.

Payroll Evaluation

Average benchmarks for non-DVM employees are 19%–21% of gross revenue (total revenue produced without considering any tax expenses). The first question to ask is: Is my payroll higher or lower than industry average? If it is higher than average, that doesn't necessarily mean you should terminate team members so that your average can be close to benchmarks. Cutting people may also impact the customer experience. It is important to review employee overtime as that can increase your percentage, in addition to burning out team members. Before you dig into methods to further decrease costs associated with payroll, look at your revenue capture. Are you capturing all revenue possible? On average, veterinary practices miss at least 10% of annual revenue due to missed charge capture and discounts. Review Chapter 16, Finance, for more specifics. Next, look at team development. Are all team members trained appropriately to be able to deliver high-level recommendations to clients? What is the compliance rate of recommendations? How efficient is the team? Do they work well with each other and have each other's backs (resulting from practice culture)? Capturing all revenue is likely more of an issue than high payroll costs. In some instances, a practice may have too many team members, and too many team members can decrease efficiency. A practice may also have too many team members scheduled during slow times and not enough to support busy times. Average benchmarks indicate 3–4 team members per DVM as the norm (this includes receptionists, credentialed technicians/nurses, assistants, and kennel assistants).

If payroll is low, the practice may be a well-oiled machine that runs incredibly efficiently with the level of current staff. Or it may be low because the practice needs team members to help drive the frictionless client experience (thereby increasing revenue). The last factor to consider (if the payroll percentage is lower than benchmarks) are wages. Does the practice pay adequate wages for the demographic in which the practice resides? Wages in veterinary medicine are usually low. Review the VHMA benchmarks on wages by role and experience (Fig. 1.5).

Veterinarians may be paid a salary or a base salary plus a percent of production that is generated. The practice must determine what is right for their culture and whether veterinarians should be incentivized in addition to their base salary. Regardless of the method chosen, an easy evaluation when reviewing veterinary total compensation (year to date) is to ensure that each doctor is generating revue that is five times the total compensation.

CRITICAL COMPETENCY: ANALYTICAL SKILLS

The practice manager must have the ability to grasp complex information, analyze information, and use logic to address problems accurately, quickly, and efficiently.

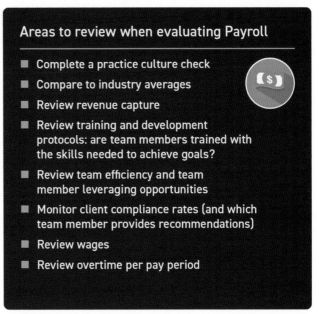

Areas to review when evaluating Payroll

- Complete a practice culture check
- Compare to industry averages
- Review revenue capture
- Review training and development protocols: are team members trained with the skills needed to achieve goals?
- Review team efficiency and team member leveraging opportunities
- Monitor client compliance rates (and which team member provides recommendations)
- Review wages
- Review overtime per pay period

Fig. 1.5 Payroll is not just about numbers; it is also the ability to identify inefficiencies in the veterinary practice.

Factors that impact DVM production

- What is the total compensation paid per doctor, and how are they paid?
- What is the ADT of each doctor?
- Compare number of exams by DVM to industry benchmarks, taking into consideration:
  - Number of hours worked
  - Team member competency
  - Culture, leveraging, and efficiency of the practice
  - Service and inventory pricing
  - Service mix (ratio of services and inventory)
  - The experience clients receive in the practice

Fig. 1.6 Veterinarians must have a well-leveraged and trained staff to reduce the barrier clients experience with access to patient care.

It is also important to look at the number of exams, the number of hours worked, and the average doctor transaction (ADT). Team member competency (efficiency, training, skills) is also important as it improves the doctor's ability to efficiently produce revenue. Poor culture and lack of customer service also impact the ability to produce revenue as clients will likely decline recommendations. Finally, inventory pricing impacts doctors that are paid on production. Obviously, low pricing models reduce production amounts. On the flip side, any price increase also gives doctors a pay raise. Chapter 16, Finance, reviews DVM production (Fig. 1.6).

Cost of Goods (COGs) Evaluation

COGs average 18%–20% of gross revenue with the implementation of online pharmacies. As with payroll, the percent is still impacted if full

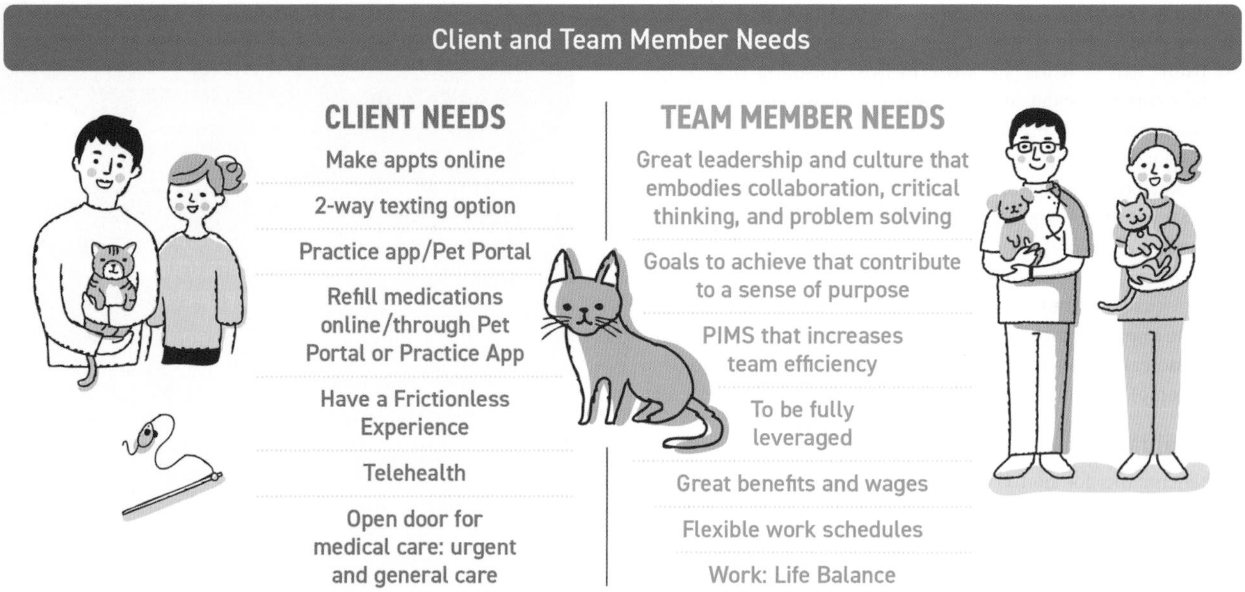

Fig. 1.7 Clients and team members have differing needs from the veterinary practice; both must be met to provide a frictionless client experience and a frictionless employee experience.

revenue is not being achieved; however, factors that impact COGs are more than just the price you pay for goods or how much is ordered. While getting the best price helps reduce the costs associated with obtaining the products, it is important to build in reorder points and reorder quantities that are based off seasonal and historical sales so that the right quantity of products is being ordered at the right time.

How the practice prices inventory is another large factor, and when product arrives at the practice and is put on the shelf, the price to clients must be increased to mirror the increase the practice most likely experienced. In addition, any service that utilizes goods to deliver diagnostics (slides, mineral oil, stain, syringes), surgery (suture, plates, screws, autoclave materials), anesthesia (gas, injectables, scavenger materials), dentistry (suture material, polish), or procedures in general (syringes, gauze, bandage material, catheters, tape) must also be increased. Utilize the service pricing tool in Chapter 16, Finance, to determine the base price for services the practice provides, including the current cost of inventory items used to produce those services. If veterinarians are paid a percent of inventory items as a production-based pay system, that too must be included in the price to the clients.

As a practice manger, diligence lies in completing cycle counts to ensure product is being sold (with charge capture) and not being given away or walking out the door with employees. Ensure that corrected cycle counts update the inventory numbers in the PIMS regularly and utilize the PIMS for maximal tracking of inventory products. Review Chapter 13, Inventory, for maximal inventory pricing and oversight.

P&L Evaluation

Practice managers and owners must review their profit and loss statement monthly. Unfortunately, many practice owners simply allow the CPA to produce year end P&Ls for tax purposes only, but this is not acceptable in running a successful business. Practice managers and owners must know where their money is coming from (what revenue centers), and where their money is going (expense centers). Reviewing both monthly will help identify if there has been an error made in entry of either revenue or expense, or if there is fraud or embezzlement occurring in the practice. Always compare the last month's P&L to previous months and look for large swings. Chapter 16 reviews the details of P&Ls, but do not allow being unfamiliar with how to read and interpret P&Ls as an excuse for not completing this monthly activity. Many resources are available through VHMA to increase the competency in this important are. In addition, Chapter 16 covers the specifics of P&Ls to get you started.

THE IDEAL PRACTICE

Many concepts have been discussed, but what does this look like in a real practice? It can no doubt seem daunting, but every practice has a little bit of everything already in the works. All concepts presented in this chapter are covered extensively throughout the book.

Always start with the goals of the practice. Every choice made must support the ability to achieve the goals established. Many ideas will come and go. The ones that "go" are those that did not support the goals. Those that "come" must be prioritized by the impact they will have on the practice goals. Those with greater impact have highest priority.

Establish practice goals with the vision, mission, and core values. Chapter 2 covers this in depth. Everything must tie to these goals. Leadership initiatives, strategic planning, financial budgets, marketing initiatives, training protocols, SOPs, SOCs, customer service initiatives, hiring team members, and team member feedback must all contribute to goal achievement.

The leader(s) of the practice must be influential, collaborative, and transformative, all leading the execution of the vision of the practice. A practice manager that leads through influence must be able to successfully execute the vision through innovative and strategic planning, all supported by the established core values.

In addition to the practice owner and practice manger, a leadership team must be developed to successfully lead and professionally develop the team for which they are responsible. These leaders help execute goals for each department (receptionists, technicians, groomers, kennel staff).

The ideal practice has regular team meetings and departmental meetings that review goals, collaboration of new protocols and procedures, team building, and the celebration of wins. Daily huddles or shift huddles are implemented to set a plan to get through the day or shift together, whether that is navigating challenging clients, cases, or team shortages. Communication and collaboration are essential to practice success.

The veterinary team is responsible for working up cases and being willing to see urgent care cases as they come. Working up cases is defined as suspecting a diagnosis and completing the diagnostics that confirm the diagnosis. Sending cases to a specialist to do the workup and determine a diagnosis is poor service and patient care. It also adds an unbalanced burden to the specialty practice. If a patient needs to be seen by a specialist, ensure that all diagnostics have been completed by the practice, and all attempts have been made to diagnose the case before sending. Urgent care is very similar; see cases that come to the practice daily and send true emergencies to ER practices after hours. DVMs and team members have been trained to handle emergency cases during business hours; when the work-life balance of team members are in check, they can handle these cases. If team members are resistant to both initiatives, it is the responsibility of leadership to determine why and implement immediate measures to repair accordingly. Review Chapter 2 on Leadership and Chapter 4 on Human Resources for culture cultivation and building a frictionless employee experience that embodies work-life balance and team scheduling that allows flexibility (Fig. 1.7).

SUMMARY

Use this book to put long-term solutions in place. Each role on the veterinary team has responsibilities in achieving the ideal practice and each chapter has examples and thoughts to consider to make it ideal. It all starts with leadership; without the right leaders in place with the right skills, the team will struggle. The team needs leaders to help them learn the skills needed to further achieve practice goals. Most importantly, it is a marathon, not a sprint, and the work never ends.

At the end of each chapter, a practice manager survival check list will provide guidance to responsibilities that need to be implemented or revisited based on the current landscape and challenges that practices are facing. Practice managers have a lot of responsibilities, but with the right team that can be empowered, many of the tasks become oversights, allowing the practice manager to focus on being the best influential leader possible.

The responsibility is yours. Step up and lead the practice the way it needs to be led. Do everything in your ability to make your practice the best place to work that no one wants to leave. When you can achieve that, you have achieved the ideal practice! Celebrate the success, and never take your eye off that goal.

Enjoy the journey, my friends. Loving what you do is just as important as why you do it. It is inspirational to others, and when combined with great business practices, the results are both intrinsically and extrinsically rewarding. At the end of the day, what do you want to be remembered for?

PRACTICE MANAGER SURVIVAL CHECK LIST

- ☐ Culture, Culture, Culture!
- ☐ Communication, Communication, Communication!
- ☐ Leadership!
- ☐ Provide a sense of purpose and a culture of belonging for team members.
- ☐ Build in team member schedule flexibility.
- ☐ Place work-life balance as a top priority for each person, including leaders.
- ☐ Rewards wins, even small ones.
- ☐ Customize expectations for each team member.
- ☐ Ensure strategic goal progression is communicated in every meeting; include how the values, vision, and mission contribute to goal achievement along with how each role achieves such goals.
- ☐ Ensure DVMs work up cases efficiently and effectively.
- ☐ Evaluate areas in which to increase practice efficiency.
- ☐ Ensure the team is leveraged to their fullest potential.
- ☐ Implement full house technology, NOW.
- ☐ Integrate Telehealth to the appointment schedule.

REFERENCES

1. Salois M. Weathering the Next Storm. Veterinary Hospital Managers Association (VHMA) Webinar. August 2022. http://vhma.mycrowdwisdom.com/diweb/catalog/item/id/10905877/q/n=2&c=444&o=-d
2. 2021 Economic State of the Profession. American Veterinary Medical Association. Accessed August 2022. https://www.avma.org/resources-tools/reports-statistics
3. Zak I. Why are veterinarians unhappy? dvm360. Accessed October 2022. https://www.dvm360.com/view/why-are-veterinarians-unhappy-
4. Welser J. We Must Unite as an Industry. Today's Veterinary Business. Accessed October 2022. https://todaysveterinarybusiness.com/workforce-shortage-innovation-station/
5. 30-Hour Workweek: Pros and Cons. Indeed. Accessed August 2022. https://www.indeed.com/career-advice/career-development/work-30-hours-a-week

2

The Leadership Team

LEARNING OBJECTIVES

When you have completed this chapter, you should be able to:

- Describe various leadership styles
- Define values, mission, and vision
- Define culture and give examples
- Define leveraging and empowerment, and describe the impact both have on employee engagement
- Describe Maslow's hierarchy
- Define psychological safety and provide an example of such an environment
- Discuss change management
- Implement effective conflict management techniques for team members
- Discuss the importance of time efficiency

OUTLINE

KEY TERMS

Change Management
Conflict Management
Culture
Employee Engagement
Empowerment
Intrinsic Motivation
Leadership
Leadership Fatigue
Maslow's Hierarchy
Mission
Psychological Safety
Situational Leadership
SMART goals
Transactional Leader
Transformational Leader
Values
Vision

INTRODUCTION

Anything and everything in the veterinary practice begins and ends with leadership. The owner and the practice manager are charged with setting the example, modeling the desired behaviors, framing the culture, setting goals, and delivering on promises made to the team. Leadership is a big deal. Own it and do it well.

The leadership team is referred to often throughout this book. While the owner and the practice manager set the example by modeling the behaviors, the leadership team extends to Associate DVMs, lead credentialed technicians/nurses, lead assistants, and lead receptionists. The associate veterinarians, whether they consider themselves leaders or not, are seen as leaders by the team; therefore, they must understand how they impact the team through behaviors, tone of voice, and interactions with one another. Lead technicians and receptionists must do the same as they are leading/influencing a team that reports to them. If a practice does not have a lead team in place, the owner and practice manager may consider appointing them to help empower each department to take "emotional ownership" of their area. Emotional ownership is considered taking ownership of their department and making decisions that are in the best interest of the practice, clients, and patients. While financial ownership involves money and is the owner's role, emotional ownership is what team members should have to elevate the practice to the next level. Having a team in place that the practice manager can effectively empower reduces the management load on the manager, allowing him/her to lead and execute practice goals. The caveat is that the practice manager and owner must teach the lead team how to demonstrate effective leadership behaviors and competencies while balancing their management duties.

There are also "silent" leaders in a practice, and while they may not carry a title or speak outwardly, they certainly influence the actions and behaviors of others. The hope is that they are influencing for the good through teaching best practices; however, bad leaders do exist and are toxic employees that destroy practice culture (and influence others to do so as well).

Positive and influential leadership in the veterinary practice is essential to business survival; great leadership builds a strong employee bond and creates a proactive environment that requires little management. Poor leadership yields high employee turnover, unsatisfied clientele, low client compliance, and high management/human resource responsibilities.

Leadership of a veterinary practice includes both organizational development and employee development. Organizational development is defined as the development, improvement, and effectiveness of an organization that includes its culture, values, systems, and behaviors. Employee development is defined as building team retention, motivation, engagement, and individual well-being. Both are intertwined and support one another and are covered in this chapter, as well as Chapters 4 (Human Resources) and 17 (Strategic Planning).

UNDERSTANDING LEADERSHIP

Leadership is influence; when leaders influence others, it motivates others into action, inspiring them to become the best they can be. Leadership is demonstrated through character, behaviors, and actions, and therefore leaders must self-reflect (often) and ask themselves if they are exhibiting the characteristics and behaviors that they are seeking from their team members. Additionally, effective leaders seek feedback from others (both peers, colleagues, and their team), always seeking ways to self-improve. Through actions, leaders can compel individuals to enthusiastically support the values, mission, and vision of the practice.

CRITICAL COMPETENCY: LEADERSHIP

Practice managers must have the initiative to lead and take charge while simultaneously motivating and mobilizing others to achieve common goals.

SUGGESTIONS FOR CREATING POSITIVE LEADERSHIP INTERACTIONS

- Help others be right, not wrong
- Have fun and celebrate the small stuff
- Smile!
- Be enthusiastic
- Seek ways for new ideas to work, not reasons why they won't
- Be courageous
- Make time to check in with the team
- Maintain a positive attitude
- Maintain confidentiality
- Verify information provided
- Do not gossip; teach others to stop the gossip
- Always speak positively of others
- Say "thank you" for kind gestures
- If you don't have something positive to say, don't say anything
- Work with the team on the floor; not above them from your desk

Fig. 2.1 Leading by example has a more profound effect on team members than telling them "how-to-do."

When the team's efficiency, professionalism, and standards are in question, practice managers and owners should first evaluate themselves and consider how their actions may be negatively contributing to the actions of the team. Leadership that delivers poor standards and professionalism negatively affects the team simply because team members are only as good as their leaders.

A leader's personal effectiveness directly influences a hospital's financial success. Leaders must hold themselves to a higher standard of patient care, customer service, performance, and personal behavior. Leading by example has a more profound effect on team members than leading by directive; therefore, showing team members how to deliver service is more impactful than simply telling them (Fig. 2.1).

Leadership skills can be broken into three areas: human, technical, and conceptual skills. Human skill is the ability to understand people and what motivates them. Effective leaders can direct team behavior through positive leadership. Not all team members respond to leadership, training, or education in the same manner. Characteristics such as shyness, lack of confidence, and poor communication skills make it more difficult to train some team members (but can easily be overcome). Domineering, independent, and strong-willed individuals may have a hard time accepting direction. Successful leaders can determine what motivates these various personality types and have a positive influence on each. When building teams, exceptional leaders attract the right people and place them into the right positions. They also integrate personal growth with practice growth by encouraging the career development of team members. Without fostering personal growth and development, the overall practice growth will be compromised (Fig. 2.2).

Technical skill is the ability to comprehend processes, procedures, equipment knowledge, and hospital policies successfully; then leaders must be able to provide team training (or effectively empower/delegate training) for successful implementation. A leader that teaches others the aforementioned skills normally has full comprehension, as "to teach is to learn twice over," a famous quote by Joseph Joubert.

Conceptual skill is the ability to understand the "big picture" by considering how all the roles within a practice work together, determining when and how change is needed, and assessing how best to solve problems in a positive, influential manner. Not all leadership

FUNDAMENTALS THAT BUILD EFFECTIVE LEADERSHIP

- **Trust:** Development of a trusting relationship with each team member facilitates open communication.
- **Accept change:** Effective leaders understand that disruptions occur and are willing to make and accept change to succeed.
- **Focus:** Leaders can achieve and direct their time and energy to achieve goals.
- **Commitment:** Effective leaders work continually to find new ideas to help make policies and procedures succeed. Accepting change helps promote commitment.
- **Compassion:** Leaders care about and desire to understand team members and their families.
- **Integrity:** Integrity demands that leaders seek to create quality assurance for their clients, patients, and team members and facilitate a positive relationship with all.
- **Endurance:** Leaders demonstrate courage, perseverance, and strength when situations, people, or the environment becomes chaotic or difficult

Fig. 2.2 "Walking the walk" vs. "talking the talk" is critical to building team culture and trust.

styles have a positive effect on team members and can prevent effective policy implementation. An effective leader deploys various leadership styles to achieve the desired outcome (see Leadership Commitment in the next section).

Effective leaders commit to their careers, their team members, and themselves. When leading by example, leaders must fulfill commitments, as team members depend on these commitments. Leaders who do not uphold commitments set a poor example and can expect the same lack of follow-through from team members. If team members are not upholding their commitments, leaders may need to evaluate their own actions to address the problem. Is leadership setting a good example for the team?

Leading with enthusiasm shows team members that their leaders are engaged and interested in the well-being of the practice. Enthusiasm is contagious (and free!) and should be a part of every practice culture. Enthusiastic team members are excited to come to work, enjoy sharing positive experiences with others, appreciate humor, and they enjoy supporting teamwork in their environment.

Everyone makes mistakes, including leaders, but effective leaders are vulnerable and admit mistakes. Great cultures create psychological safety, allowing mistakes to be made while creating a learning environment. Most mistakes that occur in the practice are non-life-threatening, and team members are willing to go above and beyond and challenge their skills when errors are not career-ending. If team members do not feel safe, they will not risk trying something new. This stalls innovation and creativity and should be avoided at all costs. Effective leaders help team members critically think through and learn from errors to prevent mistakes from occurring again. Allowing for mistakes does not encourage team members to complete tasks carelessly, but mistakes are addressed by creating learning opportunities.

LEADERSHIP POINT

"If you don't understand vulnerability, you cannot manage and lead people. If you're not showing up vulnerably as a leader, you can't expect anyone to follow you—period."

Dr. Brené Brown

Varying leadership and communication styles are essential in the management of people and businesses. A solid leader understands what motivates each individual and how he or she communicates and can direct an employee's behavior toward a desired outcome. Ultimately, leaders are responsible for positively influencing the behavior of others.

There are many schools of thought regarding leadership styles. The most successful concept is to lead the team with a style that most effectively influences others. Keep in mind that different situations require different leadership styles.

SITUATIONAL LEADERSHIP

In situational leadership, it is the responsibility of the leader to recognize and adapt to the situation, as well as the individual that he/she is leading. The team should be willing to change and adapt as well, which occurs through the positive influence of the leader.

Situational leadership is a flexible, adaptive style of leadership that determines whether a leader is more directive or supportive based on their team members' individualized needs.[1]

If a team member is highly skilled, the leader will provide more leadership support and ask questions to help the team member think critically and achieve a goal. The less skilled the team member is, the more direct the leader will be in helping the team member achieve the goal. *Direct* in this example is giving very specific directions and tasks the team member needs to complete to achieve the goal.

Team members may have "the will" to learn but have little skill in a specific area. The more willing and confident the team member is in their ability to achieve a goal, the more supportive a leader will be; the less confident a team member is, the more directive the leader will need to be.

Skill and will are also referred to as the "maturity" of the team. It is important to define maturity as the level of maturity concerning a specific task, not the team member's general maturity. A team member that is highly skilled and confident in one area may be unskilled and unconfident in another.[2]

Depending on how strong the skill and will of the entire team is, the balance between the directives given or the critical thinking coaching questions will vary. Figure 2.3 demonstrates the stages of a team based on maturity (forming, storming, norming, or performing), the amount of direction that must be given by the leader, the amount of conflict that may be seen, how many ideas are generated based, and who makes the decisions.

A forming team is comprised mostly of team members with less skill and will need full directives given by the leader. Conflict usually does not exist because the team has yet to develop the skills or competencies to challenge the status quo and simply do as they are told. As a result, the generation of ideas is nonexistent, and decisions are all made by the leader of the group.

The storming team is comprised of individuals who are learning and are able to ask questions as they begin to critically think and problem-solve on their own. The storming team will still need direction, and conflict will rise as some begin to challenge the status quo and idea generation evolves.

The norming team is one that is grasping the flow. They still need some direction from the leader, but they are doing a great job at leading themselves, generating ideas, and being able to come to a decision through a consensus. There may be some individuals who challenge the status quo, and as respect among the group develops, conflict decreases, therefore allowing a consensus to be achieved.

The performing team is the dream team for the practice manager and owner. The team needs very little direction and very little conflict exists among the group. They are able to solve problems and come to decisions via collaboration. The drawback of having a mature team is that they "are all on the same page" and often don't challenge the status quo, resulting in

Four Stages of Team Maturity				
Stage	**Direction Given by Leader**	**Conflict Among Team Members**	**Generation of Ideas**	**Decisions Made by**
Forming	All direction	Nonexistent	None	Leader
Storming	Mostly	Can become hostile	Starting	Leader
Norming	Moderate	Settle down	Moderate	Consensus
Performing	Very little	Only occasionally	All	Collaboration

Fig. 2.3 Leaders must be able to adapt and lead according to both the situation and the level of team maturity.

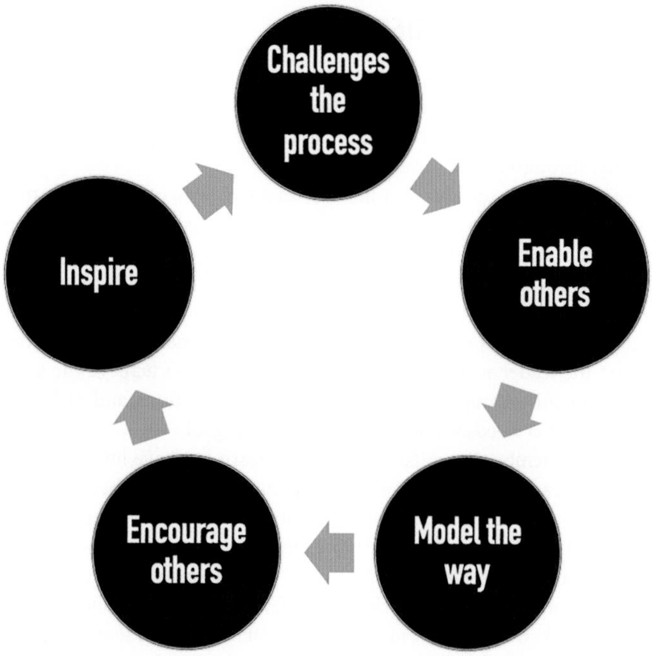

Fig. 2.4 Key leadership behaviors that are consistently modeled by successful leaders.

team members rarely thinking outside the box if an "idea could be better" with more critical thought. The performing team will need to be provided challenges by practice leadership to continue evolving.

The Leadership Challenge

The leadership challenge, founded by Kouzes and Posner, clarifies how success can be achieved when leaders evaluate each situation and utilize the strength of the team to produce results (Fig. 2.4). Great leadership:

Challenges the process: challenging the status quo leads to innovation when changes are needed.

Enables others to act: great leaders enable and empower collaboration among team members.

Models the way: leaders walk the walk, not just talk the talk.

Provides encouragement: leaders encourage team members through recognition and accomplishments.

Creates inspiration: leaders inspire a shared vision and create buy-in of the values and mission.

With exceptional leadership comes the need for management; there must be a blend of both leadership and management. You can't have one without the other, and they must support one another. Recall that leadership uses the process of influence to inspire others to achieve goals. The management portion focuses on planning, organizing, and executing processes or procedures to achieve the desired goal. Leaders need someone to execute the plans; managers need someone to maintain focus on the end goal and not allow distractions to stall the process (Fig. 2.5).

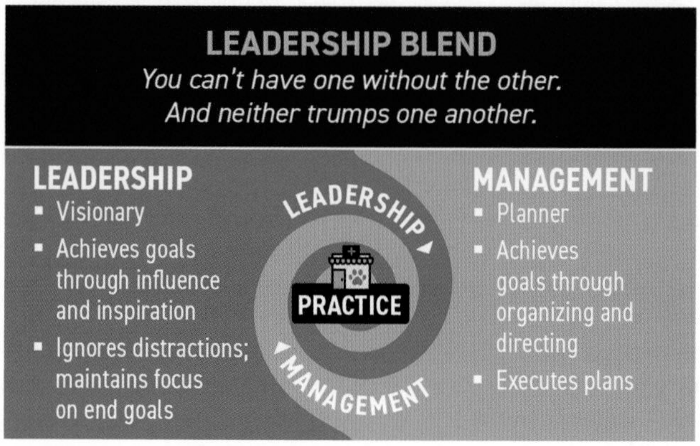

Fig. 2.5 Much like medicine and management, there must be a synergistic alignment to achieve practice goals.

VALUES, MISSION, AND VISION

The values, mission, and vision (VMVs) of a hospital are core concepts that must be integrated into every practice. VMVs provide structure by creating a positive culture and goals that help define team member expectations. Without VMVs, owners operate without a clearly defined path to success, managers struggle to implement policies and procedures that support unclear goals for the hospital, and team members lack the direction needed to be successful in their roles. The VMVs should be evaluated annually to ensure they continue to be in alignment with the beliefs of the owner(s) and still resonate with the team.

Values

Core values are words that describe desired behaviors that every team member should demonstrate, ultimately contributing to the culture of the practice. They are the guiding principles of the practice that should not be compromised; violation of core values could be considered grounds for immediate termination (if stated in the employee manual). Consider the acronym CARE (Compassion, Advocacy, Respect, and Empathy) and the impact it has on patients, their owners, and fellow team members (Fig. 2.6). To further the clarity of the core values, each word should have a description of the behavior(s) that are expected to be displayed by each team member. These values should then be tied into job descriptions, training programs, coaching, performance reviews, and if needed terminations.

> **CRITICAL COMPETENCY: INTEGRITY**
>
> Practice managers must adhere to ethical principles and values, and be seen as honest, trustworthy, and sincere professionals (demonstrated through behaviors and words).

How are core values developed that resonate with a majority of the team? Give each team member a pad of sticky notes and ask them to write down words that describe the desired behaviors they expect from their fellow team members (on individual notes). During this exercise, the practice manager should make clear to the team that these are desired behaviors that are expected to be displayed by everyone on the team. Future decisions, protocols, procedures, and expectations will be developed around the core values with the goal of creating a great place to work.

Take the individual sticky notes, place them on a wall, and organize them by similarity; there will likely be the same words repeated several times. Those are the words that will become the core values. Next, as a team, select no more than four values that best represent the team's beliefs, and define the expected behaviors that each team member will demonstrate daily.

Mission

The mission is defined as the purpose of the hospital and the fundamental reason that the practice exists. Mission statements should be concise and easy to remember while stating the overarching goal of the practice. For example, if the goals of ABC Veterinary Hospital are to provide superior medical services for patients, exceptional client care, and an excellent team environment, one might develop the following mission statement: *"To provide high-quality veterinary care with an emphasis on exceptional patient care and client service, while providing team members with a positive working environment."*

Once the mission statement has been developed, it should be implemented into job descriptions, training programs, coaching sessions, performance reviews, and strategic planning. It holds leadership accountable to the team members, team members accountable for their actions to both clients and fellow employees, and helps clients develop expectations of the practice. Team members should be able to recall the mission statement at any time, without even thinking about it. It should be woven into every decision made on behalf of clients, patients, and team members.

The development of the mission statement can also be a team activity but should heavily be led by the owner(s) of the practice; the team can help wordsmith an overly long mission statement into a more memorable phrase.

Vision

The vision statement describes the future of the practice. Where does the practice want to be (financially, medically, staffing, etc.) in 1 year, 5 years, or 10 years? As an example of a vision statement, Southwest Airlines wants to *"become the world's most loved, most flown, and most profitable airline."* The vision for a veterinary practice may be "to become the communities most trusted veterinary provider by providing exceptional customer service and medical care."

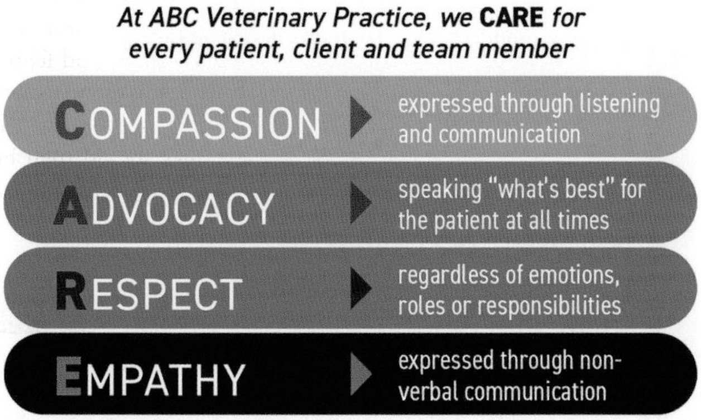
At ABC Veterinary Practice, we CARE for every patient, client and team member
COMPASSION
expressed through listening and communication
ADVOCACY
speaking "what's best" for the patient at all times
RESPECT
regardless of emotions, roles or responsibilities
EMPATHY
expressed through non-verbal communication

Fig. 2.6 Examples of Core Values.

The vision statement must support the mission and must be attainable. This then allows a gap analysis to be completed that identifies the current state and goal state. Questions can be asked when determining objectives to achieve the vision, such as *"Do the current procedures and/or policies support the vision? If not, what needs to be changed to reach this goal?"* Use the SWOT analysis, gap analysis, and SMART goals examples in Chapter 12, Marketing, to complete this activity.

Understanding the Goals of the Practice

Values, Mission, and Vision create guidelines that influence every decision (current and strategic). Often, practice managers try to implement policies and procedures without having VMVs in place resulting in team members resisting the policy or procedural changes because they do not understand the goal(s), or how a policy or procedure may support it.

> **LEADERSHIP POINT**
>
> A beautiful culture develops when leadership demonstrates the values and carries out the mission of the practice daily.

To implement guidelines for everyone to follow, the team must first understand the goals and why it is important to achieve the goal(s). Fig. 2.7 demonstrates how goals can fail when VMVs are not understood. The values are the building block; it is the strong base that supports everything else. Without a strong base and mission statement, the implementation of policies and procedures is harder to achieve. Another way to visualize the values and mission is to "see" how each goal supports the achievement of the mission (Fig. 2.8).

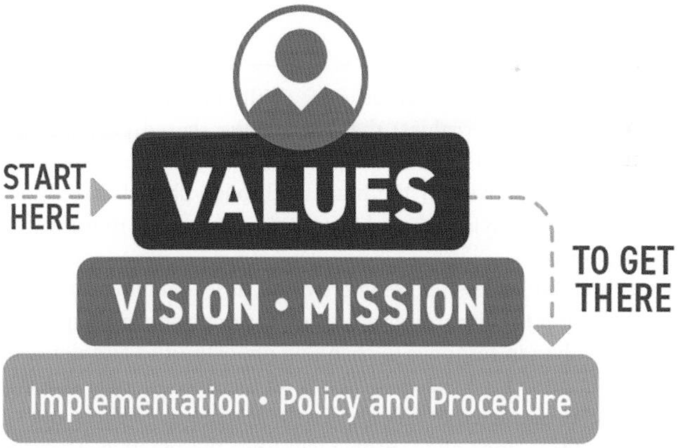
START HERE
VALUES
TO GET THERE
VISION • MISSION
Implementation • Policy and Procedure

Fig. 2.7 Team members must understand the Values, Mission, and Vision of the hospital before policies and procedures can be successfully implemented.

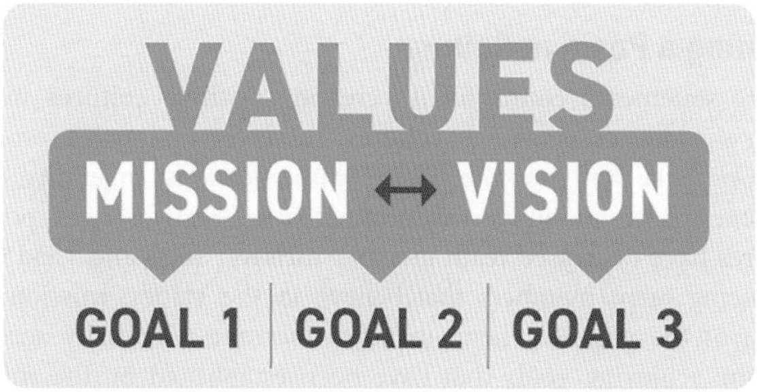
VALUES
MISSION ↔ VISION
GOAL 1
GOAL 2
GOAL 3

Fig. 2.8 Goals must support the mission and carried about through values.

Once VMVs have been clearly established, goals and objectives for the hospital can be set. The following is a short list (although not conclusive) of areas that VMVs affect:

Human resources: Practice managers can hire new employees knowing what direction the practice is headed and the desired behaviors that are expected. Consider the following questions:

- What type of team member is needed, and what skills are essential to help the practice attain the VMVs?
- If team members are not meeting the expectations created by the VMVs, can they be coached to improve, or should they be terminated?
- For high-producing team members, what continuing education is needed to retain them and help them continue contributing to the success of the practice and achieving the mission and vision?

Marketing: A marketing plan is much easier to create and implement with a mission and vision.

- Where is the practice going?
- What important messages should be relayed to clients? How will messages be relayed?
- Does the internal team understand the messaging?
- How will clients perceive the message? Does the message achieve the desired goals?

Finance: A strategic plan (Chapter 17, Strategic Planning) and practice budget (Chapter 16, Finance) can be developed with long-term goals in mind. Goals may incur expenses, which must be budgeted for. Strategic planning must have SMART goals developed, ensuring the vision is achieved in the stated timeline.

- What profit centers should be established and/or maintained to meet the goal(s) of the hospital?
- If the goal is to provide an exceptional level of care, does the existing equipment and technology support that standard of care?

CULTURE

Culture is defined as the social order of the practice. It shapes attitudes and behaviors (values) that achieve the shared purpose (mission) of the practice. Culture expresses goals through values and beliefs and guides the activity of the practice through shared assumptions and group norms.[3] It is anchored in unspoken behaviors, mindsets, and social patterns.

Culture and leadership are intertwined, as leadership sets the culture in motion that imprints values and assumptions in the practice. Culture evolves in response to changing opportunities and demands, and the success of the change depends on the strength of leadership.

People are attracted to cultures based on matching beliefs and values; when these don't align, people will leave the practice. Therefore, finding the right "fit" when interviewing potential employees is very important. See "Hiring the Perfect Team" in Chapter 4, Human Resources, to better understand best hiring practices that build in culture, diversity, and inclusion.

Creating a Positive Culture

VMVs statements contribute to creating positive cultures in veterinary practices. Positive cultures produce supportive working environments that promote open communications, ingenuity, independence, accountability, and productivity. Practices with positive cultures have decreased team member turnover rates and yield high-producing team members that believe in the values, mission, and vision of the practice. Team members become personally accountable for achieving goals that have been established by the mission and vision through the demonstration of behaviors that support the values.

> **LEADERSHIP POINT**
>
> "We need people to be braver, and we need to create a culture that allows for bravery."
>
> **Dr. Brené Brown**

Practices with negative cultures experience high turnover rates; individuals (versus teamwork) are less productive, lack passion, enthusiasm, integrity, and accountability. Negative cultures result in loss of clients, decreased client compliance, and poor patient care.

Every leader must evaluate the TRUE culture that exists in the practice: What is really going on in this hospital? What does it feel like when clients come into our practice? Leadership can become disconnected from the "real" culture as they wear multi-hats in the business. To evaluate, leaders should work the floor with the team and listen to how team members communicate with each other and clients. Implement anonymous team member surveys and focus groups or consider creating a culture committee to take the "pulse" of the practice. If the practice culture is not where it needs to be, changes must be instituted. Not working on improving culture every day is not an option.

Creating/evaluating/influencing a positive culture starts with the evaluation of the leaders and managers. Do leaders walk the walk (or just talk the talk)? Are the VMVs implemented into the "practice way of life"? Do the VMVs tie to job descriptions, training programs, coaching sessions, and performance reviews? Does leadership communicate well with the entire team? Is CE provided for all team members, regardless of their position? Does the practice have a safe environment that allows team members to be innovative, creative, try something new, or challenge the status quo without fear of retribution? When the leaders walk the walk, the team does as well.

Creating and maintaining a positive practice culture is one of the most important tasks a leader must accomplish. It is like cultivating a garden. Work on it never stops; it must be fertilized and watered frequently.

Changing the Current Culture

To make culture changes, the first step is to identify the current culture and what type of culture the practice would like to have (Fig. 2.9). In the second step, a gap analysis is completed, identifying the reasons

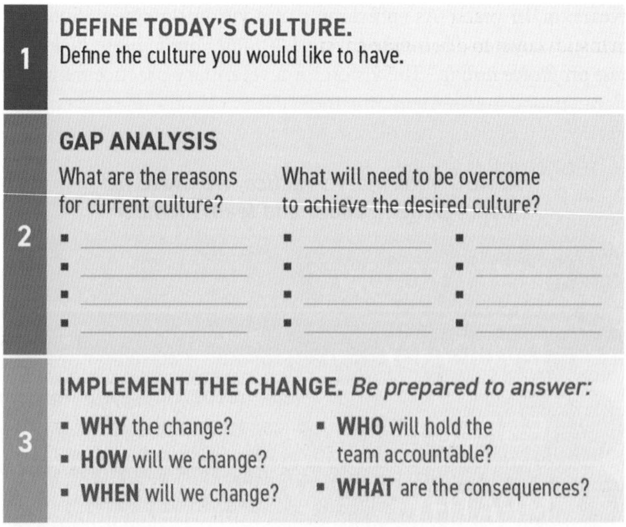

Fig. 2.9 A gap analysis helps provide leaders a clear direction when change needs to occur within the practice.

for the current culture, and addressing how to achieve the desired culture. The third step is incorporating the "how and why" of the culture change. This is often the most difficult step to overcome because some team members will be resistant to change. The fourth step is the implementation of the culture change plan.

Changing a practice culture is a marathon, not a sprint, and requires an ongoing effort. It is very easy to revert to the current comfort zone and the "way we have always done it," versus challenging the status quo for improvement. The influential leaders in the practice will need to coach team members daily to achieve the change desired. Some team members will be coached "up" to success while others may be coached "out" as their values no longer align. Changing habits can take 30 days to be effective; see the Change Management section in this chapter for more specifics.

The Positive Effects of a Team

A leader needs a team, and every team needs a leader. A veterinary practice is a team business in which a group of individuals with different skills and attributes contributes to the positive culture of the hospital. Effective leaders build teams that allow the business to succeed at all levels, including providing excellent patient and client care and maintaining a friendly and cohesive work environment. Leaders invite creative thinking from team members and integrate this creative thinking into daily conversations. Creative thinking fosters productive, problem-solving team members who are not afraid to think outside the box.

The leader of the team guides the group rather than micromanaging or dictating. They empower their team with resources and techniques to think critically and problem-solve instead of placing a Band-Aid on any issues that may arise. Teams openly discuss concerns and solutions and develop plans to implement new policies or procedures. An effective leader will help guide the team through the appropriate steps to achieve the solution. Recall the importance of situational leadership and the ability to adjust support and direction as needed based on team maturity. Support and direction are not micromanagement or dictation, but rather provide guidance in an influential manner.

The team should help with developing realistic and achievable goals. When each team member contributes to the development of goals, members will work harder to ensure they are achieved. This contributes to a sense of pride, accountability, and ownership of the practice. Team members with pride recognize the importance of disciplined work habits and ensure their behavior meets team standards. If team members need time off, they do everything in their power to have their shift covered or provide coverage for the team member who needs time off. Team members often understand one another's priorities and offer help or support when difficulties arise. This may occur in both the practice and in the team's personal lives.

New ideas and challenges can stimulate team members to become strong performers and encourage others to follow. Team members continually work together to improve their service to clients, patients, and each other, and all these team qualities make participation in a veterinary practice an excellent and rewarding career. A dedicated and proficient team that understands basic practice management is likely to achieve extraordinary goals and boost the practice's compliance rate. Team building is a continuous process that never ends; the trials and errors that are part of this process allow each team member to learn and grow from mistakes made along the way. Working in a supportive environment not only eases the burden of personal issues outside of work, but also allows team members to grow personally and professionally. This is the number one factor that will prevent burnout in employees. But none of this occurs without a strong culture that includes psychological safety.

Psychologically Safe Environments

The term psychological safety was developed by Harvard Business School professor Amy Edmondson as a shared belief that the team is safe for interpersonal risk-taking. It establishes a culture of safety that allows a space for people to speak up and share ideas without the fear of retribution. When psychological safety is present, it enhances employee engagement, inspiration, and creativity. When people are comfortable, they are more likely to collaborate to solve problems. It improves the mental health and well-being of team members, allowing them to continue performing at optimal levels and avoid stressors that induce anxiety. Safe environments reduce employee turnover, enhance overall team performance, and creates an opportunity for team members to "brag" about the practice.

Leaders must continuously work on creating/maintaining safe environments. Trust (a major component of a psychologically safe environment) can take years to build and moments to break down. Continuous leadership self-assessment is a requirement; consider having an accountability partner who can call you out for questionable behaviors in the moment.

While leaders should be modeling behaviors that create a safe environment, team members must also demonstrate the same behaviors and ensure fellow team members feel safe as well. In veterinary medicine, it is common to have a team member that everyone is afraid of (including management). Often, the behaviors of this team member are never addressed, and an unsafe environment is created. These team members have usually been in the practice "forever" and management will address the concern as "that is just the way they are." It is unacceptable for management to not address the issue and coach that behavior; the individual may be unaware of the impact they have on the remaining team or may display the behavior intentionally. Regardless, allowing one person to have a negative impact on the entire team undermines any leadership strategy that is put in place to create culture, trust, psychological safety, and long-term employee commitment to the practice. See Fig. 2.10 for behaviors that both leadership and team members can demonstrate to foster a safe environment in the practice, and Fig. 2.11 for behaviors demonstrated by a person who does or does not feel safe in their work environment. Fig. 2.12 provides examples of sentences or phrases that can be used when communicating with the team.

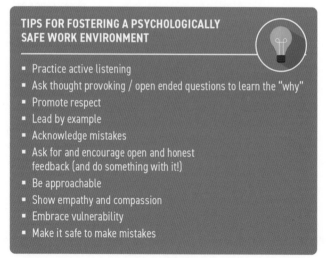

TIPS FOR FOSTERING A PSYCHOLOGICALLY SAFE WORK ENVIRONMENT

- Practice active listening
- Ask thought provoking / open ended questions to learn the "why"
- Promote respect
- Lead by example
- Acknowledge mistakes
- Ask for and encourage open and honest feedback (and do something with it!)
- Be approachable
- Show empathy and compassion
- Embrace vulnerability
- Make it safe to make mistakes

Fig. 2.10 All team members and leadership should demonstrate behaviors that contribute to a psychologically safe working environment.

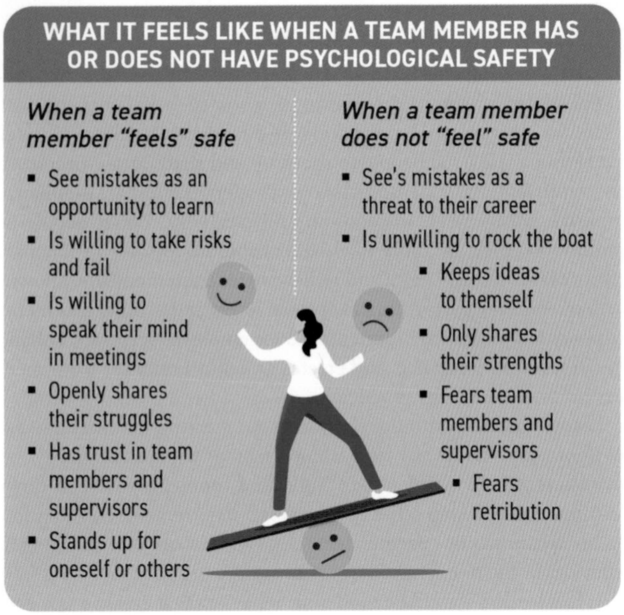
WHAT IT FEELS LIKE WHEN A TEAM MEMBER HAS OR DOES NOT HAVE PSYCHOLOGICAL SAFETY
When a team member "feels" safe
▪ See mistakes as an opportunity to learn
▪ Is willing to take risks and fail
▪ Is willing to speak their mind in meetings
▪ Openly shares their struggles
▪ Has trust in team members and supervisors
▪ Stands up for oneself or others
When a team member does not "feel" safe
▪ See's mistakes as a threat to their career
▪ Is unwilling to rock the boat
▪ Keeps ideas to themself
▪ Only shares their strengths
▪ Fears team members and supervisors
▪ Fears retribution

Fig. 2.11 Psychologically safe environments allow team members to thrive and try new things without fear of losing their job.

WHAT DO TEAM MEMBERS NEED?

Team members need excellent leaders that strive to make the practice a great place to work. Team members often spend more time at the practice than at home with family. Purpose, motivation, leveraging, empowerment, engagement, and continuing education are required to retain and attract team members. When the topics in the previous section have been implemented, the next section becomes a natural next step.

Team Member Purpose

Providing team members with a sense of purpose is essential with the ongoing workforce shortage. As identified in Chapter 1, workload, clients, and outside stressors are contributing factors to team members feeling burned out and mentally exhausted.

Burnout includes a sense of failure for reasons that are outside of one's control, which then turns into feelings of helplessness. This causes team members filling roles in the practice to be perceived as pointless; therefore, the people filling those roles lose a sense of meaning and purpose in their work. Loss of meaning is not tied to what the role is meant to accomplish, but rather to the feeling that one cannot accomplish it, no matter how hard one tries.

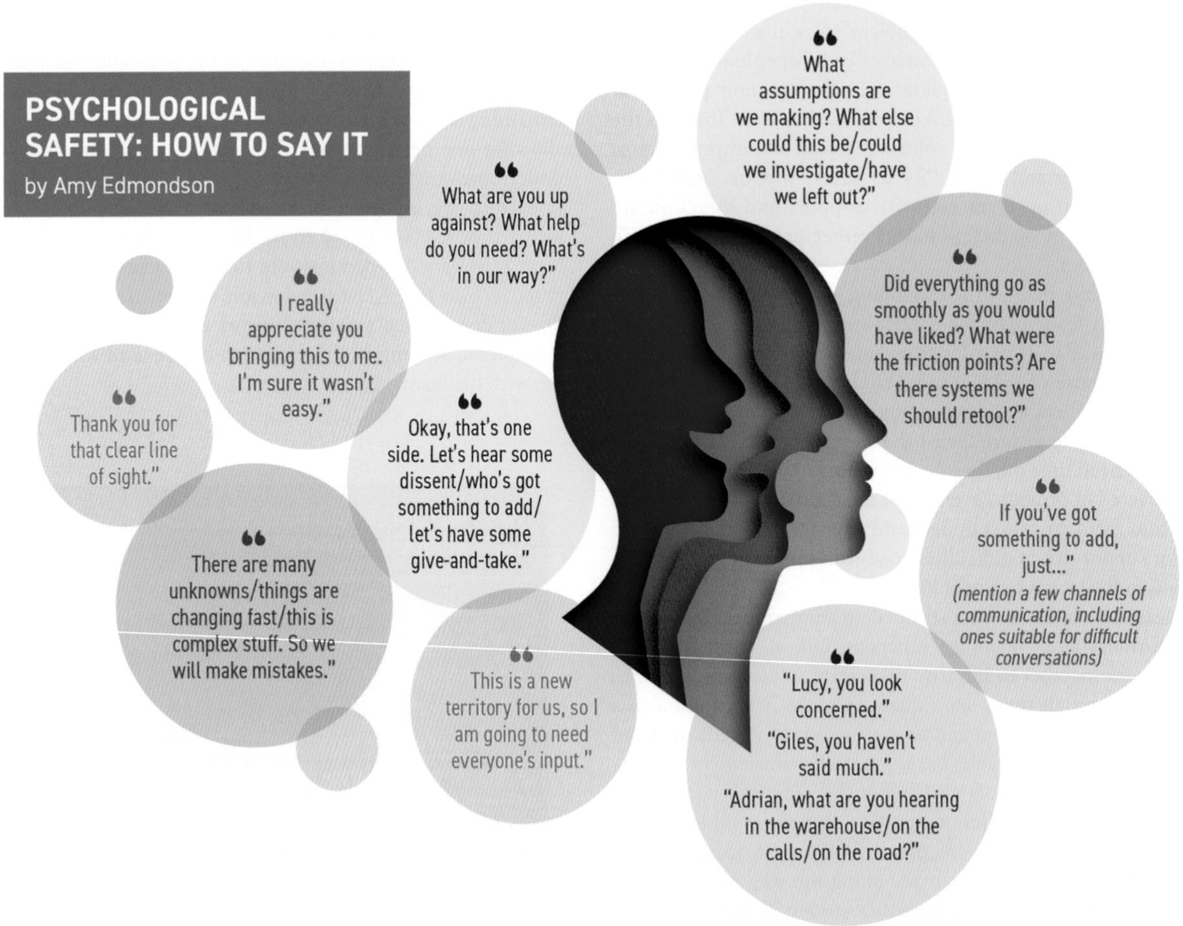

"What assumptions are we making? What else could this be/could we investigate/have we left out?"
"What are you up against? What help do you need? What's in our way?"
"I really appreciate you bringing this to me. I'm sure it wasn't easy."
"Thank you for that clear line of sight."
"Did everything go as smoothly as you would have liked? What were the friction points? Are there systems we should retool?"
"Okay, that's one side. Let's hear some dissent/who's got something to add/let's have some give-and-take."
"There are many unknowns/things are changing fast/this is complex stuff. So we will make mistakes."
"If you've got something to add, just..." (mention a few channels of communication, including ones suitable for difficult conversations)
"This is a new territory for us, so I am going to need everyone's input."
"Lucy, you look concerned."
"Giles, you haven't said much."
"Adrian, what are you hearing in the warehouse/on the calls/on the road?"

Fig. 2.12 Dr. Amy Edmondson provides excellent examples of how leaders can phrase topics that lead to a psychologically safe working environment.

Factors that cause burnout include a perceived lack of control, lack of fairness, values mismatch, workload, lack of reward or recognition, and poor work relationships.

Burnout in practice managers may result from the disconnect between wanting to make a difference for the team they lead, and not having the power or resources to do so. The feeling of inefficacy results in fatigue and a lack of empowerment.

Maslow's hierarchy of needs[4] states that the most basic level of needs must be met before higher levels can be achieved (Fig. 2.13). There are five levels to consider, broken down into three categories of basic, psychological, and self-fulfillment needs. This hierarchy is very applicable to the veterinary workplace.

Level one includes physiologic needs (food, shelter, and sleep) and safety and security needs (working conditions, wage rates). If team members are unstable in their personal life, motivation will be harder to achieve. If the practice pays low wages, the security and safety (both psychological and physical hazards) of the job are not being met, and team members will consistently look for better opportunities.

The second level is psychological well-being, which includes practice culture, purpose, inclusion, self-confidence, and self-esteem. When the practice culture is strong and goals (including vision, mission, and core values) are implemented into daily activities, inclusion and a sense of purpose naturally occur, therefore contributing to, and maintaining self-confidence and self-esteem. Don't forget, culture is like a garden. It must be continuously cared for; the work never stops. Great leaders deploy regular culture assessments and pivot to make changes as needed to continue growing the culture of their practice. Practice goals must be continuously developed around values, mission, and vision, and behavior exhibited supporting those goals should be rewarded, or coached out. Team member purpose further develops when they know why they come to work, love to come to work, and strive to achieve goals that directly serve their passion: being able to care for pets in the best way possible.

When level two is achieved, it directly supports level three: self-fulfillment. Level-three characteristics include team members that are highly motivated and seek opportunities for growth and development within the practice. This is also known as the "happiness" level. Self-actualization occurs through achieving one's fullest potential and reaching the peak of motivation. Team members that live in level three are excellent contributors, seek the next growth phase, are less likely to burn out, and feel mentally exhausted or leave the practice for better opportunities.

Chapter 1 addressed the labor shortage issue that practices are facing. Maslow's hierarchy provides insight into why veterinarians and credentialed technicians/nurses are leaving at alarming rates. The belief that doctors leave for higher salaries is likely disproven by a study conducted by the Center for Health and Well-being at Princeton University in New Jersey, indicating that although low-income correlates with unhappiness, emotional well-being does not progress beyond an annual income of $75,000. In other words, a veterinarian who makes $125,000 is unlikely to be happier than a veterinarian in similar circumstances who makes $100,000. Credentialed technicians/nurses, on the other hand, do have a wage barrier in the veterinary industry. Wages must increase for this sector, along with veterinary assistants, kennel assistants, and receptionists.

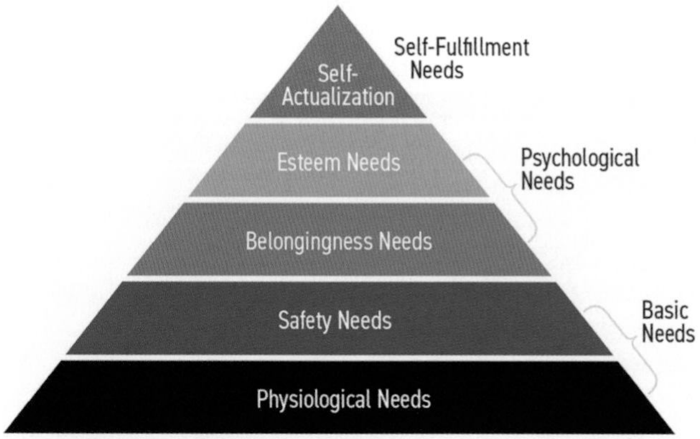

Fig. 2.13 Maslow's Hierarchy of Needs.

Further, a sense of belonging must be established by the practice. Relationships with friends and coworkers form a sense of tribe or people of similar values. People are naturally motivated by close relationships with their work family. Achievements, such as mastering new surgical techniques, are more exciting when shared, and a tribe mentality can make bad days more bearable. Without establishing inclusion and a tribe mentality in the veterinary practice, team members only have a "job" and will eventually leave the practice.

If a practice cultivates a culture of belonging, veterinarians and credential technicians/nurses will have their sense of belonging and purpose met, which develops reasonable happiness. Remember, however, that to cultivate culture, the vision, mission, and core values must be established, and built into daily routines, training, and communications. Leaders must demonstrate behaviors that support and attain the goals (actions speak louder than words) and set reasonable goals for each team member to achieve. Additionally, creating continuous feedback loops and having crucial conversations on the fly are required to help team members achieve a sense of growth, inclusion, and, ultimately, a sense of purpose.[5]

Further supporting purpose, best-selling author David Pink defines motivation as *"the desire to do things because they matter."* Three elements must exist for intrinsic (or internal) motivation to occur: autonomy, mastery, and purpose. Autonomy clarifies that people don't want to be micromanaged, and should a micromanaging situation occur, the team member would never be motivated. People want to master their skills (mastery), and when allowed to do so, are motivated to continue to improve. People want to have a purpose and make a difference (in patients' lives, team members' lives, etc.). When these three factors occur in tandem, intrinsic motivation occurs. Intrinsic motivation fosters increased performance, job satisfaction, decreased mental exhaustion and burnout, and team member engagement. What is your practice doing to drive autonomy, mastery, and purpose for each team member?

Leaders must ensure systems of fairness are in place, reinforced, and communicated. Team members must be empowered to achieve their purpose and have balanced workloads so that they can see a sense of accomplishment. They must also receive appropriate recognition and reward from practice leadership. The concept of reward and recognition does not equal a paycheck or a promotion, but rather reflects a sense of being valued and recognized as a valuable team member. Recognition and reward further reinforce the belief that one's work does make a difference, allowing a greater sense of purpose to be established.

Leveraging Team Members

Leveraging is an intangible asset, meaning it can be hard to place a dollar value on the subject. Effectively leveraged team members are more satisfied with their jobs.[6] Practices that effectively leverage have VMVs in place, strong positive cultures, and emotional buy-in from the team. Team members contribute to the best work environment, patient care, and team collaboration every day, resulting in dedicated, loyal team members with a sense of purpose and motivation.

To determine whether the practice is effectively leveraged, ask every team member, including doctors, to create a list of every task they do during a one-week period. Veterinarians should be doing medically specific tasks (diagnosing, prescribing, completing surgery). Credentialed veterinary technicians should be completing credentialed skill-level tasks, including surgical assisting, completing dental prophylaxis, obtaining laboratory samples, completing in-house diagnostics, treating patients, providing client education and any tasks that are outlined in the state veterinary practice act (to name a few). Veterinary assistants should be helping credentialed veterinary technicians and veterinarians become more efficient in restraint, sample preparation, getting equipment ready for the next procedure, etc. If the list of tasks completed by team members indicates veterinarians are doing credentialed technician tasks, and credentialed technicians are completing assistant tasks, effective leveraging is not occurring, and an improvement strategy must be put in place immediately. Keep in mind that each team member may need to help in other roles occasionally; the goal of the exercise is to ensure it is not happening as a normal event but under unordinary circumstances. Unleveraged team members are highly likely to leave the practice.

CRITICAL COMPETENCY RESOURCEFULNESS

The practice manager must have the ability to understand what it takes to complete the job by applying knowledge, skills, and expertise to perform tasks quickly and efficiently.

Many times, practices do not utilize credentialed veterinary technicians as they should, and often use veterinary assistants with no formal training instead. Leadership must effectively separate the duties of each and respect boundaries, especially when outlined by state veterinary practice acts. Having nontrained team members provide patient care can place the patient at higher risk for poor or inadequate care. Having formally trained veterinary technicians complete assistant duties devalues and demotivates these team members and will result in the loss of a skilled employee.

A practice would never hire a veterinarian and not allow them to diagnose cases as they were trained. In addition, a practice would never hire an unlicensed doctor to diagnose, prescribe, and complete surgery. Therefore, it makes no sense to hire a credentialed veterinary technician/nurse and not utilize them to their fullest potential, or to have a veterinary assistant complete tasks that should be completed by a formally trained and credentialed technician. The argument can be made that there are not enough credentialed veterinary technicians/nurses to supply the demand, and while that is true, there will never be enough credentialed technicians/nurses when practices are not willing to differentiate between assistant and credentialed duties and pay.

LEADERSHIP POINT

Great culture and leadership, alongside leveraging the team to their fullest potential, have a greater impact on employee retention than that of wage scales.

The tangible aspect of leveraging (or the monetary value) is just as important as the intangible benefits. Considering what it costs a practice to be open per minute, per hour, and per day (see Chapter 16, Pricing, based on practice financials), the most appropriate team member should be delivering services to best increase efficiency and efficacy and decrease costs as much as possible. For example, a credentialed veterinary technician should be drawing blood on a patient (not a veterinarian), while the veterinarian is examining the next patient. The veterinarian drives active income, which is further supported by passive income fulfilled by the credentialed veterinary technician and other team members.

CRITICAL COMPETENCY: DECISION MAKING

The ability to make good decisions, solve problems, and decide on important matters. The ability to gather and analyze relevant data and choose decisively among alternatives.

Empowering Team Members

Empower means to give someone official authority, permission, or freedom to complete tasks and objectives. Empowering is the concept of influencing, encouraging, and investing in employees to take initiative to improve operations, reduce costs, and improve the quality and quantity of service. Understanding the difference between empowering and delegation is critical; delegation is telling someone what to do and how to do it, versus giving the team member the expertise to make the right decision.

Exceptional leaders create an environment where team members are empowered to communicate openly, voice their concerns, and make changes where necessary to achieve the mission and vision. Employee empowerment is essential to the success of a veterinary practice.

Teams that are empowered are engaged in daily operations are proactive and strive for the highest quality of care for patients and clients while working to increase profits for the business. They understand the "why," "what," and overall practice goals. They model the behavior of leadership and take ownership of problems or issues. This incorporates personal accountability and creates followers among the leaders. The seven steps (Fig. 2.14) of problem-solving become much easier when team members are empowered to carry out goals.

Empowered employees are only as good as their expertise, and expertise comes from training and exceptional leadership. It is imperative to train team members on a continual basis. The strongest employees accept training to improve themselves and the practice. When employees take pride in their workplace and are given the autonomy to improve daily operations, they will exceed expectations. This emotional ownership of a practice (versus financial ownership) yields high returns. Training motivates team members to continuously improve their skills and helps retain the best employees while also preventing burnout (Fig. 2.15).

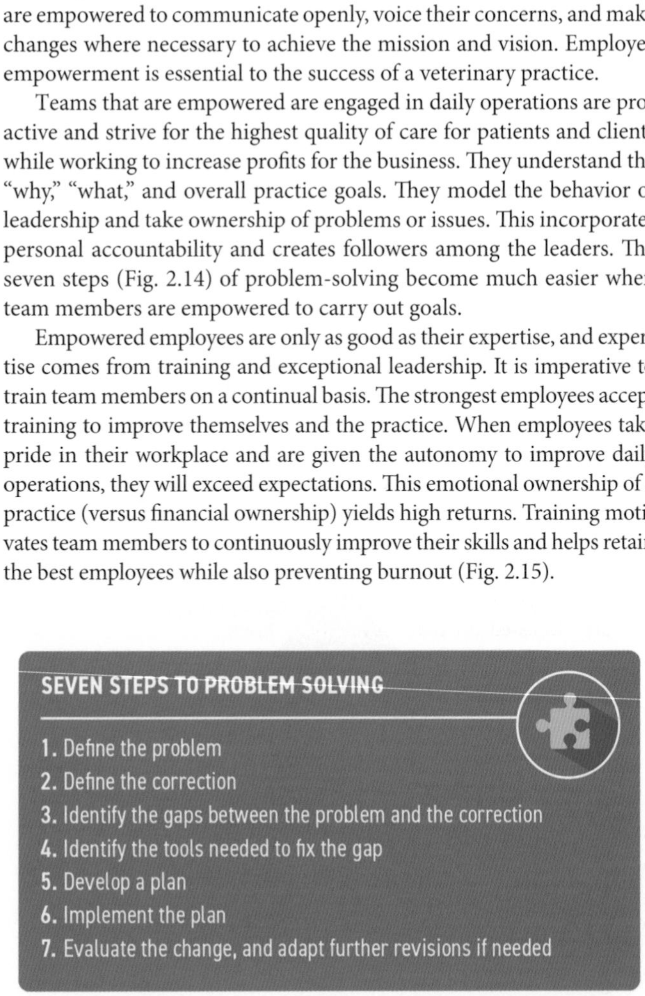
SEVEN STEPS TO PROBLEM SOLVING
1. Define the problem
2. Define the correction
3. Identify the gaps between the problem and the correction
4. Identify the tools needed to fix the gap
5. Develop a plan
6. Implement the plan
7. Evaluate the change, and adapt further revisions if needed

Fig. 2.14 Critical thinking and problem solving are demonstrated by team members that are empowered to achieve the practice goals.

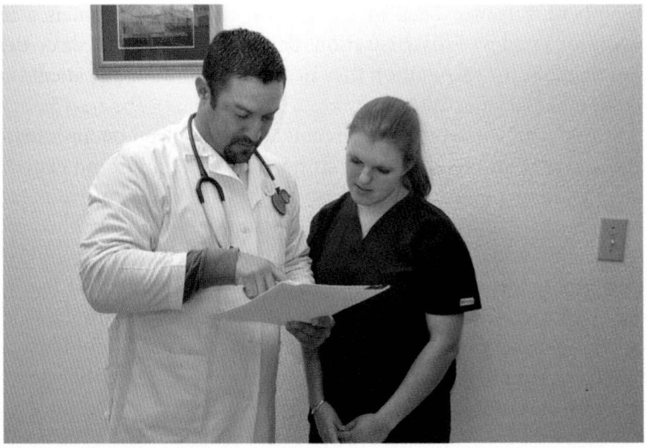

Fig. 2.15 Empowering and leveraging staff improves team morale.

Independent and strong-willed team members, practice managers, and leaders may find it hard to empower others (or delegate), often feeling that other team members will not complete tasks in the manner they would like. Some practice managers fear that by delegating tasks to others, they are admitting failure and the inability to complete those tasks. This is not the case. Empowerment (versus delegation) increases the efficiency of a leader while building a stronger, more responsible, and more productive team. One person cannot manage all the aspects of a veterinary practice. A veterinarian or practice manager cannot see and discharge patients, and manage accounts receivable, inventory, and accounts payable, while continuing to provide the best treatment possible for hospitalized patients. Empowerment is the key to a successful veterinary practice. It frees up time, reduces stress, allows work-life balance, and builds employee engagement and motivation. It also allows leaders to take vacations without receiving calls and text messages throughout the vacation and having a large workload upon return. The business must go on while leaders take time for themselves to recharge. Empowerment allows that to happen.

It is important to take small steps while learning to empower. One task should be empowered and completed, then the next. Often leaders give too many projects at once (sometimes without the detail needed for the employee to be successful) and receive negative results. The leader then stops the process (no one can do it better than them).

When empowering, it is essential for the team members involved in the process to be included in developing an action plan. This will help ensure a complete understanding of the project and the objectives required for success. Two-way conversations are encouraged (using open-ended questions), facilitating a complete understanding on both parts. Use SMART goals: this will ensure that all aspects and expectations of the task are addressed and that both parties agree with the expected results.

- **Specific:** Defines the specific goal that is to be achieved. Why is it being empowered, why is it important, and what are the expected outcomes?
- **Measurable:** Identifies how the success of the goal will be measured. How is this task going to be measured in terms of progress and completion?
- **Accountability:** Defines who will carry out the objectives of the goal.
- **Resources:** Identifies what resources will be needed to achieve and implement the goal successfully.
- **Time-bound:** Identifies when the goal will be achieved by and should also establish check-in points between the practice manager and the person accountable for achieving the set goal. Creating check-in points during the planning process prevents micromanagement and keeps the lines of communication open.

Additionally, situational leadership must be applied. What is the skill and will level of the team member being empowered, and what style form of leadership needs to be applied?

LEADERSHIP POINT

"I define a leader as anyone who takes responsibility for finding the potential in people and processes."

Dr. Brené Brown

To become efficient at empowerment, the leader must also be able to accept mistakes. When delegating tasks to team members, they will make mistakes, but they learn from their mistakes and are willing to try something new when a psychologically safe environment has been created. Great leaders encourage mistakes and discuss what the team member learned from these mistakes, and how they will overcome them.

When empowering duties, choose an employee who has interest in the task and the ability to accomplish it. Not all team members have the same strengths; therefore, choosing the right person for the task is essential for successful empowerment. Consider social media. It would be ineffective to give Facebook posts to a team member that does not use Facebook or understand the technology associated with the platform.

Along with learning how to empower effectively, it is also imperative that leaders learn to accept help graciously. Many leaders will not accept help from others because they believe it makes them appear ineffective or weak. Accepting help when needed is part of a positive, team-oriented culture, and models the behavior that leaders would expect of team members. Asking for help or empowering others builds a strong teamwork model and encourages members to ask for help when needed.

Team Member Engagement

Team members who are leveraged and empowered are more likely to be very engaged in the practice. Team member engagement is a critical factor in reducing turnover. However, those three factors don't drive employee engagement alone. Leadership must incorporate feedback from the team, which should come through open communication systems. However, some team members or new employees may be uncomfortable openly communicating concerns; therefore, anonymous surveys or employee suggestion systems should be implemented to encourage trust. Consider using an online platform for practice improvement suggestions, giving team members the opportunity to submit comments "safely."

The most important component of feedback is to address and implement or build on ideas that have been suggested. Asking for feedback and then doing nothing with the feedback sends a clear message to employees that their ideas or concerns don't matter.

Succession planning also plays a significant role in team member engagement. Succession planning is defined as identifying or developing new leaders who can replace current leaders should a leadership position become open. This helps maintain team member engagement, enhances the emotional buy-in of the practice, and creates long-term team members by providing career growth opportunities. Succession planning is discussed in Chapter 17, Strategic Planning.

Continuing Education

CE stimulates excitement, passion, and continuous improvement of team members. Employers benefit from providing CE in numerous ways including having highly skilled team members, developing future leaders, increasing productivity, and increasing employee retention. CE improves the self-image and self-confidence of team members while boosting morale and improving working relationships.

VHMA PERFORMANCE DOMAIN TASK

Practice managers implement continuing education and licensure/certification processes.

CE expenses should be built into the practice budget, allocating approximately 5% of gross revenue every year for team development. Every team member should be required to attend CE, not just veterinarians and credentialed veterinary technicians, but the reception team, veterinary assistants, and practice managers as well. In addition, more than just local CE events should be offered. A CE budget should include travel costs to attend national and regional events. If team members are expected to contribute ideas that support the mission and vision of the practice and achieve the goals associated with them, they must have the proper tools to be successful.

CE topics should be tied to the strategic goals of the hospital. If the practice is instituting rehabilitation as a profit center, CE would focus on the development of the center, learning techniques and equipment maintenance, client education, marketing/advertising opportunities, profit analysis, etc. Every team member's position contributes to the rehabilitation center's success; therefore, every team member should attend CE to support the new profit center.

Occasionally, leadership will encounter team members who do not value CE or do not feel it is necessary. Because team members typically welcome CE opportunities, this team member should be asked why they don't want to participate. Sometimes team members have attended CE in the past and never got to implement the learned information. They may have brought information back and heard "that's not the way we do it here." When responses of this nature occur, team members feel defeated and disengaged in taking courses that are perceived to have no benefit. In addition to poor past experiences, the team member themselves may be resistant to change. Tying team member engagement into the VMVs, coaching, and performance feedback can help leadership overcome these obstacles.

Retaining Team Members

Retaining team members is a leadership initiative that should be easy to achieve when purpose, motivation, goals, continuing education, engagement, and great culture are a part of daily practice life. But there's more. Identifying each team member's strengths, their wants and needs, and cultivating inclusion are important.

Every person has a unique set of strengths, things they are good at. When people are placed in the right seats on the right bus based on strengths, they will achieve greater results than when placed in seats that require skills they are weak in. Consider team members who are great at client communication. They are usually more extroverted than the analytic surgical technician/nurse that tends to be introverted but is amazing at analyzing data and patient care. Team members with great communication skills should be placed in a role that allows them to interact with clients most of the time. This allows the detail-oriented credentialed veterinary technician/nurse to focus on patient care in surgery (their greatest strength). Review CliftonStrengths results in Fig. 2.16 and see how identifying strengths in the team can excite and motivate existing team members and propel the practice forward in achieving goals. Consider these strengths, in addition to the communication styles found in Chapter 11, to put people in the right seats on your bus.

Good leaders understand the importance of positive reinforcement. It is essential for maintaining the team's enthusiasm and motivation. The simplest form of positive reinforcement comes through words and phrases that recognize an individual's hard work and dedication to the practice. Positive reinforcement is a tremendous incentive for strengthening teams. Lack of recognition and appreciation is a top reason for employee dissatisfaction. Seize the moment to show each team member the recognition they deserve; celebrating the small stuff (often) makes a large difference.

Consider how positive reinforcement can be given on an individual basis. A team member who has gone above and beyond expectations should be rewarded with something that is useful for that person (words of affirmation vs gifts). Words of affirmation are just that, calling out a job well done. If a person's love language[7] is receiving gifts, a leader would identify (as an example) that the team member has just purchased a new home and has previously discussed the need for new kitchen utensils. A simple reward of new pots and pans would be warranted. If a team member is remodeling a home, a gift certificate to a local hardware store may be appropriate. However, a gift certificate to Starbucks for a team member who does not drink coffee diminishes the positive reinforcement. Take the time to reward appropriately and the positive reinforcement will double in value.

Do team members have pride in the workplace? Is there a waiting list to be hired, or does the practice hire the first person that comes along? Do team members understand how the business is run? Consider factors that contribute to pride in the workplace, starting with the values, mission, and vision. When team members know the direction they are heading and the goals they need to achieve, pride is developed. Share goals, dreams, and monthly financials with everyone. Create an open books management system, maintaining business transparency. See Chapter 16, Open Books Management, for more details.

Losing team members not only impacts team morale, but also impacts client retention, satisfaction, and practice profitability. When team members need to continually train new team members and not grow themselves, the result is burnout. It costs the practice approximately 1.5 times the team member's salary (that is leaving for the year) to replace that team member, and that does not consider the impact on client satisfaction or the loss of revenue while an experienced team member is training (versus providing an efficient frictionless client experience).

Attracting Potential Team Members

Although attracting exceptional employees is covered in Chapter 4, it is important that leadership drives the initiative. Creating an employer brand and a strong practice culture is a leadership must. An employer brand is very similar to a practice brand (developed by the consistent, positive experiences that clients come to expect from the practice; see Chapter 12, Marketing). An employer brand is established by creating a strong positive culture that draws potential candidates to the practice seeking employment opportunities. If a poor culture exists, only mediocre candidates will accept an offer. Strong, positive cultures create a strong employer brand, resulting in a waiting list of potential team members wanting to be hired. Ensure the hospital is a place of employment that team members brag about. But don't stop there. What makes the practice great? Ask the team and consider how the examples in Fig. 2.17 make your hospital the practice of choice to be employed at.

What is leadership's responsibility in attracting talent? Developing and standing by the mission and vision of the practice, upholding the values through demonstrated behaviors, and taking care of the people that take care of the business.

It is also important to develop strong mentorship programs, especially for recent graduates. Many new graduates won't accept a position without a well-defined mentor program. Chapter 6, Professional Development, reviews the development of a program. Leadership must ensure it is a strong program that meets the needs of new team members and continues to attract team members; this ensures a long-term bond and loyalty to the practice.

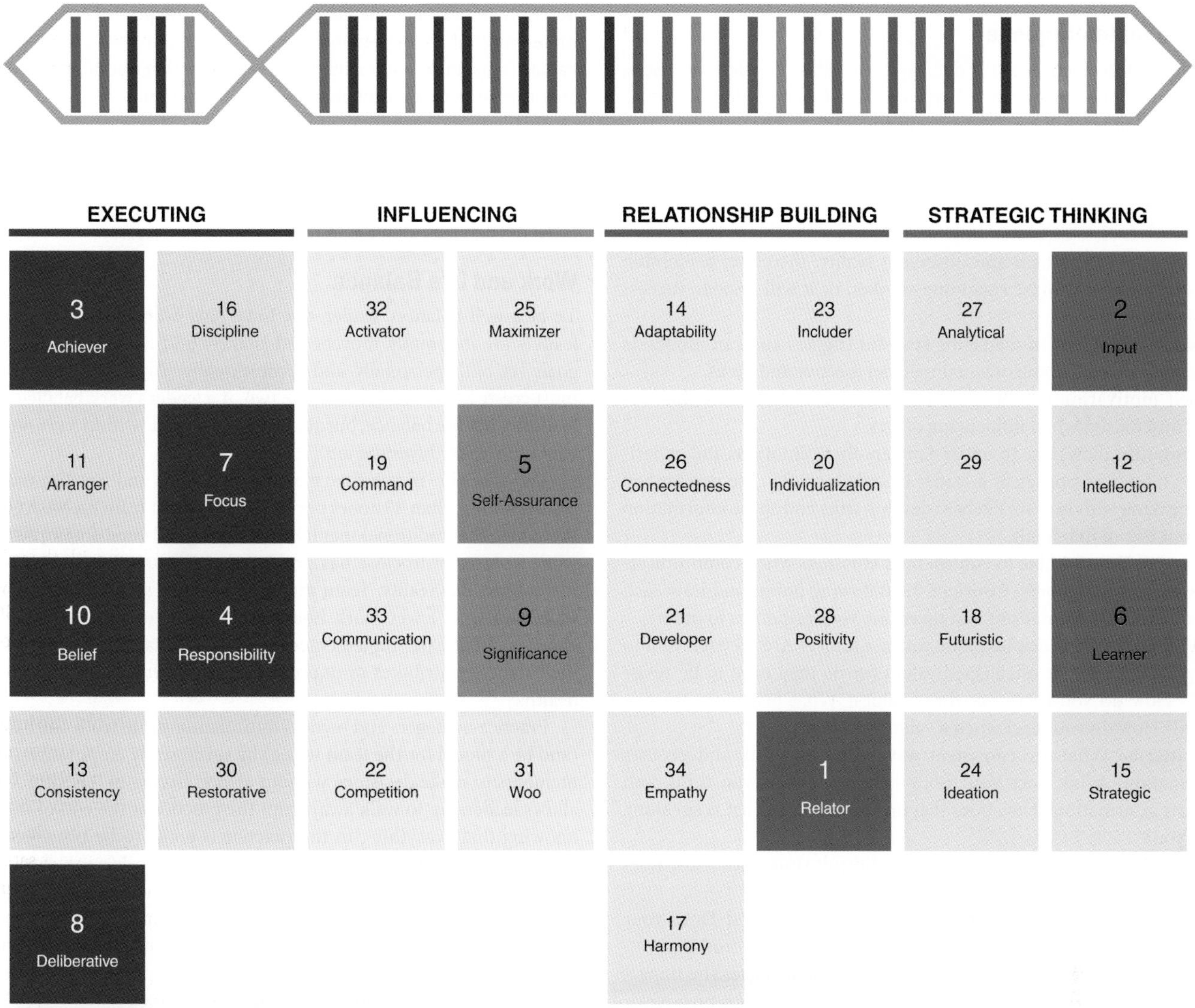

EXECUTING
INFLUENCING
RELATIONSHIP BUILDING
STRATEGIC THINKING
3 Achiever
16 Discipline
32 Activator
25 Maximizer
14 Adaptability
23 Includer
27 Analytical
2 Input
11 Arranger
7 Focus
19 Command
5 Self-Assurance
26 Connectedness
20 Individualization
29
12 Intellection
10 Belief
4 Responsibility
33 Communication
9 Significance
21 Developer
28 Positivity
18 Futuristic
6 Learner
13 Consistency
30 Restorative
22 Competition
31 Woo
34 Empathy
1 Relator
24 Ideation
15 Strategic
8 Deliberative
17 Harmony

Fig. 2.16 CliftonStrengths by Gallup® allows team members to be leveraged for their natural strengths.

WHAT MAKES A GREAT PLACE TO WORK?

- Trust, Honesty, Integrity, Transparency
- Goal achievement through collaboration
- A caring and psychologically safe environment
- A place where everyone has each other's back and there is no finger pointing

Fig. 2.17 Practice leaders that create a great place to work have higher retention rates, client compliance, and client bonding rates.

CHARACTERISTICS OF EFFECTIVE LEADERS

- Self-confident
- Sincere
- Enthusiastic
- Effective listener
- Effective communicator
- Accepting of diverse cultures
- Team player
- Problem solver
- Innovator and renovator
- Will admit mistakes

Fig. 2.18 Effective leaders demonstrate behaviors that are expected of others.

VHMA PERFORMANCE DOMAIN TASK

Practice Managers recruit, interview, and hire new employees.

BECOMING AN EFFECTIVE LEADER

Many topics have been discussed in this chapter to help leaders become the best they can be. Most of these topics grow over time; non can be neglected but recognize that they cannot happen overnight. Recall that this journey is a marathon, not a sprint. A little bit of cultivation each day will grow the ultimate team.

The previous section focused on what the team needs from the leaders. This section will focus on your personal development to become an effective leader.

Effective leaders utilize several tools, including leading by example, incorporating the values, mission, and vision, developing, and mastering emotional intelligence, cultivating inclusion, understanding diversity, implementing work-life balance, and overcoming communication barriers. Fig. 2.18, provides examples of characteristics of great leaders.

Emotional Intelligence

Emotional intelligence (EI) is defined as the ability to identify, assess, and control one's emotions. Characteristics of EI include self-awareness, self-control, self-motivation, and empathy.

Self-awareness involves the recognition of one's emotions and gives insight into the response that follows a trigger. The more self-emotions are understood, the easier it is to control ingrained responses. Self-awareness is also understanding how one impacts others. The perception of what others hear and observe is reality; therefore, perception and self-awareness must equal one another, or it will impede success as a leader.

Self-control aids in managing stressful triggers and can moderate anger responses, helping one maintain perspective and focus.

Self-motivation is contagious to others; leaders often use this tool (subconsciously) when influencing others.

Empathy allows one to understand another's emotions and experiences. If your responses as a leader include empathy, the person you are speaking with is more likely to develop trust and share information without fear of judgment.

Leaders must be able to control their emotions when communicating with team members. Consider the following points and how each impacts your own emotions and therefore, your responses to others:

Values: What principles guide you as a leader? Are they relevant to the practice's current established values (or do they need to be revisited)? How do you carry out those values? What behaviors are displayed? How do you react when a value is broken?

Patterns: What are consistent ways that you think and process information? What does your body language say as you think and process information? How does that impact someone that is speaking with you?

Reactions: How do you respond to difficult situations? How does that impact the team that surrounds you?

Overall impact: What effect do you have on others? Does your overall impact create a safe space for open, collaborative thinking?

Many resources are available on emotional intelligence. The impact you have on others will have a lasting effect; whether that is positive or negative is up to you. Think about how you want to be remembered, and let this help define your professional development journey.

Diversity and Inclusion

Leaders must be able to accept diverse ethnicities and cultivate inclusion to effectively manage a team. Diversity can include different races, ethnicity, ages, religions, and/ or experiences. A team member may have varying values, expectations, or goals associated with their diverse background. Diversity provides different insights that can be used to identify problems, solve problems, create solutions, or develop successful pathways to achieve goals. Diverse team members bring different strengths to the team, and those differences should be appreciated and built upon. When leadership incorporates all differences, inclusion occurs. Every team member can bring something to the table when leadership lets them. Don't squash innovation by scrapping inclusion.

Multiple generations coexist in today's workforce, and each brings different strengths and weaknesses to the team. Strong leaders understand and adapt to the generational traits of each age group.

Veterans, baby boomers, Generation X, Generation Y, and Generation Z all contribute to the workforce. People are living longer (and reduced retirement funds may force them into working longer), creating a unique situation in that five generations are found within the workplace. This unique situation creates new challenges for leaders because they must understand the different needs of each generation.

To really understand the generation gap, it's helpful to consider their underlying values, or personal lifestyle characteristics. Accepting these values/traits makes it easier to understand the resulting workplace characteristics that are attributed to each generation.

It is imperative to treat and respond to each generation differently (another example of situational leadership), enhancing the positive culture that each leader strives for. Further, understanding and incorporating the differences will contribute to offsetting the stressors identified in Chapter 1 that are impacting labor shortages.

Work and Life Balance

To be a well-balanced leader, one must have work-life balance. Many leaders are inherently movers and shakers and work hard to achieve goals set both personally and professionally. To be exceptional, one must create a balance between the two. If a leader's work balance overloads his/her life balance, burnout will likely occur within 5 years (even when the leader loves the job).

Traditionally, in veterinary medicine owners and practice managers work more than 40 hours per week and expect team members to do the same. The traditional mentality of having full-time employees who work from open to close has prevented many practices from accepting current-day reality. Team members are now seeking flexible work schedules with fewer work hours and more work-life balance, and changes should be implemented to accommodate this need. Work-life balance contributes to improved employee engagement and team health.

Practice managers and owners must demonstrate work-life balance (and be a model for the team to see) by successfully empowering team members to make decisions without always having to "check in." This allows leadership to walk away from the practice at the end of the day knowing that everything in the practice is going to be okay. Leaving work at the end of the day becomes exactly that: leaving work. The work brain can be turned off. This allows the home-life balance to kick in: making time for exercise, family time, reading a book, or seeing friends (and preventing burnout). Recall that burnout reduces enthusiasm, initiative, and productivity. When leaders experience burnout, the team follows (leaders lead by example!).

Review team member schedules, ensuring overtime is not accumulated on a regular basis. Help team members determine what lifestyle activities are important to them and help to make sure those activities are experienced after working hours. Tie these goals into coaching sessions and performance reviews.

COMMUNICATION

One of the most important leadership skills is to be an effective communicator; however, communication is a vast subject. There are many elements that contribute to effective communication. Keep in mind the end game; what needs to be communicated? How does one communicate that effectively? Who needs to hear the message? How does the message impact the listener? Was the message clear, concise, and understood?

CRITICAL COMPETENCY ORAL COMMUNICATION AND COMPREHENSION

The practice manager must have the ability to express thoughts verbally in a clear and understandable manner, and the ability to actively listen and address what others are saying.

Effective communicators think clearly, talk sparingly, and listen intently. Ask open-ended questions that solicit discussion (versus yes/no answers). Think through topics, seeking to understand all stakeholders' viewpoints before coming to a decision. Making a reactive decision could damage the trust and culture of the practice.

The tone of voice used to deliver the message is just as important as the words chosen. Positive, enthusiastic tones are much more effective than negative, authoritarian tones. Review the client communication section in Chapter 11, Client Experience, for more specifics on the impact of tone of voice.

Several barriers, including poor listening skills, preoccupation, impatience, and/or resistance to change or new ideas can contribute to leadership failure. Often, the behaviors associated with these barriers are demonstrated by leaders themselves, which are then demonstrated by team members.

An additional communication tool that is extremely helpful for leaders is the Pawsonality Assessment tool available from Patterson Veterinary University. Communicating with team members based on their communication style (versus your own) dramatically improves the understanding of the message conveyed, and, as a leader, allows you to better develop your team based on their natural styles. It can also decrease your frustration level as a leader when you feel your message has not been received by the listener, the way you intended it to be. See Understanding Client and Patient Needs in Chapter 11 to learn about driver, analytic, amiable, and expressive orientation communication styles.

Leaders have many duties, tasks, and responsibilities to complete, and are often annoyed when interrupted by team members. When interrupted, they appear preoccupied and do not listen to the team member with full intent. Leadership must stop what they are doing and make team member communication a top priority. If team members feel they have not been heard, or that the leader was preoccupied, they will follow the example being set for them.

Listening effectively is a lost skill in today's world. Listening is the ability to receive, attend to, interpret, and respond to words and body language. Poor listening skills can result in a misinterpretation of information and can lead to malpractice in the medical field. Poor listening and interpretation can cause a communication breakdown when a leader is trying to manage a practice effectively and lead team members in a positive manner.

Leaders that practice open and honest communication encourage ideas and opinions from team members, and team members should feel comfortable offering ideas and disagreeing with other team members from time to time. Strong teams are likely to have disagreements (which is a healthy part of communication); when disagreements are aired, all opinions can be discussed. Each team member is more likely to accept and understand others' thoughts and opinions and accept them with an open mind. With open communication, team members will resolve conflicts quickly and constructively, without the help of the leader. Open communication is a major component of successful practices.

Leadership teams feel they communicate very well with their team. However, most often, team surveys indicate there is a lack of communication, role clarity, and practice goal achievement from leadership. It is up to leadership to ensure that every channel of communication is used to keep the team on the same page. Superior communication is a driver of great practice culture, a sense of purpose, inclusion, and retention.

Team Meetings

Team meetings are used to increase communication within the practice. Practices that have intentful team meetings achieve higher than average practice benchmarks, have greater profitability, and improve client compliance with staff recommendations. Many practice owners argue that meetings cost money and lost revenue when the business is closed. However, practices cannot afford to NOT TO HAVE team meetings. Effective and efficient weekly meetings increase team member communications, problem-solving, and contribute to a positive culture (Fig. 2.19).

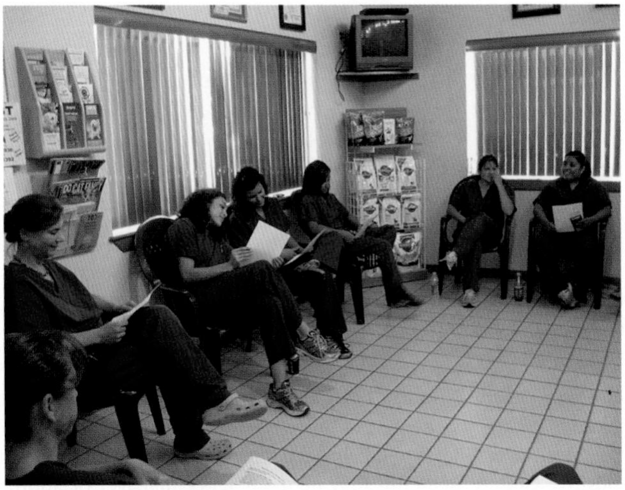

Fig. 2.19 Team meetings are critical for clear and open communication among all employees.

Employees must be paid for their time, and food may be provided for meetings. An hour-long meeting with 13 staff members and two veterinarians costs an average of $500 in wages. The accountability of team members and increased production from these meetings far outweigh the costs associated with hosting them. All veterinarians should be expected to attend every meeting; they are leaders in the practice and should be leading by example.

Some practices choose to have lunch meetings once a week (highly recommended); others close for half a day once a month to incorporate training sessions with the meetings. If meetings are held during the lunch break, team members should be allowed to eat lunch first, so they can decompress from morning activities.

It is highly recommended to have huddles to kick off every day, or when a new shift starts. Huddles are short (10 minutes) and can be used to cover tasks that don't need discussion ("fill the toilet paper roll when you use the last piece!"), creating plans for the day (who is on PTO, out sick, or needs to leave early), and clients and/or cases that are expected. Compare a daily practice huddle to that of the sports team: they are creating the plan for the next move, keeping everyone on the same page. They are not gripe sessions, but rather motivation to have an awesome team-driven day. Huddles allow staff meetings to remain positive and effective, as the daily issues get resolved in huddles or as issues rise.

VHMA PERFORMANCE DOMAIN TASK

Practice Managers host regular team meetings.

To expedite meeting processes and encourage collaboration, create an agenda with set goals that is distributed to the team prior. Team members will then know what topics are on the list and when to address ideas or concerns they may have. This keeps the meeting running on time and prevents getting off topic for lengthy amounts of time. Team members should be encouraged to contribute to the meeting topics. A note board can be placed in a central location where team members can add topics they feel need to be discussed. Topics may include anything team related such as further education on a specific procedure, policy clarification, or education regarding a disease. Some

MEETING FACILITATOR ROLES

- Agenda creation
- Start and end on time
- Set a maximum length of 45 minutes
- Follow agenda
- Facilitate positive discussion
- Include team participation
- Review accomplishments
- Create/distribute notes

Fig. 2.20 Meeting facilitators are charged with running a positive meeting that starts and ends on time.

items may get added to this list that can be covered in huddles, again, making meetings a better use of time.

A meeting facilitator will help keep meetings running on time with a positive vibe. A facilitator may be the practice manager or another team member and is responsible for keeping the meeting on schedule, controlling the agenda topics, and preventing negativity from overcoming the discussion (Fig. 2.20). Facilitating meetings does not necessarily come naturally; acquired skills may be needed to run meetings efficiently and with minimum stress.

Once the agenda has been created, the meeting facilitator should prioritize the topics. This ensures the most important topics are addressed first, allowing ample time for discussion. Other topics must also be addressed, if only briefly. If a topic is left off the agenda, team members may feel that their input was not important, and they may be reluctant to volunteer topics in the future.

It is vital that meetings start and end on time, and it is essential that the agenda be adhered to. Employees resent attending meetings that start late and run late, and the clinic appointment schedule is compromised. Meetings should begin when they are scheduled, regardless of who is present. Team members who arrive late must take responsibility to find out later what they missed. Topics should not be repeated for latecomers; this devalues the meeting for those who were on time.

The value of the meeting is also lost when team members lose interest. Meetings should not last for more than 45 minutes (unless training information is included). After 45 minutes of discussion, active participation in the meeting begins to drop. However, larger groups may require longer meetings so that each member can participate. If longer meetings are needed, breaks should always be factored in, and meetings should be held more frequently, allowing more productive meetings in a shorter time.

Team members should be asked to participate in meetings and should be held accountable for paying attention and actively listening. To help engage participation, team members can be asked open-ended questions or asked to present topics. This will help create important leadership skills and develops a sense of pride among the team, along with developing self-confidence and independence. To enhance the education being provided, team members may use learning games, videos, brochures, and/or develop handouts.

If one person dominates discussions, employees will lose interest in the meetings. The meeting facilitator is responsible for not letting this happen and must use tact when guiding discussions back to the agenda. If a heated discussion begins or emotions run high, it may be suggested (with empathy and compassion versus dismissive) that the topic be tabled, researched, and readdressed at the next meeting. This allows emotions to settle and team members are encouraged to bring solution options to the next meeting, rather than arguing about the problem. The next topic on the agenda can then be addressed. The same applies to topics that are taking an extensive amount of time. Team members can be asked to provide solutions at the next meeting and develop a list of pros and cons regarding the subject. The topic can then be added to the agenda for the next meeting, and the team can move on to the remainder of the current agenda.

Meetings should not be allowed to become gripe sessions, and it is important that the meeting facilitator prevent this from happening. If team members gripe, the leader must shift the conversation positively into a solution-seeking conversation. Positive energy trickles from the top down with team members taking nonverbal cues from the leadership team.

Always review accomplishments and successes before ending a meeting. Client compliments, employees' personal accomplishments, and successful change updates should all be addressed. Meetings ending on a positive note leave team members feeling confident and empowered, further establishing a sense of purpose and accomplishment.

A written or electronic summary of each meeting should be provided to team members after the meeting. Topics (and action plans), ideas, changes, or homework for the next meeting can easily be forgotten. Some team members may have been absent or were tardy for the meeting. Notes should be short and to the point listing the topic and the resolution that came from the discussion (with the goal that team members will review). Meeting notes also serve as proof of discussion for all team members when they "forget" a topic had been addressed and a solution was implemented. Notes from previous meetings can be pulled from the file and provided to employees who need a friendly reminder.

Other Forms of Internal Communication

Team members should be asked for their input on current apps they might like to facilitate easier team communications. Some practices use a private Facebook page created only for team members where internal messages can be posted and shared. Another popular tool is an app called *Slack*. Slack simplifies communication by bringing all the team's communication together, giving everyone a shared workspace for organized conversations. Slack builds a searchable archive of the team conversations making information easily accessible (http://www.slack.com). Some practices are also using Teams (available with Microsoft O365).

Regardless of the application used, going above and beyond to maintain open communication with all team members facilitates culture, inclusion, and practice transparency. Consider being able to share birthdays and special occasions (employment anniversaries, marriage, new babies), or events and CE that will occur in the coming months. Fun photos can be shared, as well as fun facts, employee spotlights, and awards/recognitions team members receive.

TEAM MEMBER FEEDBACK

All team members deserve regular feedback from their leaders. Poor leaders shy away from conflict or uncomfortable discussions; great leaders take conflict and uncomfortable discussions and turn them into opportunities for individual growth.

Feedback comes in both in-the-moment coaching opportunities and individual strategic planning sessions (Chapter 4) that are often done at the end of the year. Team members don't deserve to wait till the end of the year to get any feedback on their performance, but rather deserve to have coaching sessions throughout the year. Chapter 4 focuses on individual strategic planning sessions (ISPS), while coaching is focused on in this chapter as it is a leadership initiative.

LEADERSHIP POINT

"Giving feedback is incredibly vulnerable for this reason: If you're giving good feedback, you should not be able to script what's going to happen when you sit down with someone. You should be willing to be able to hear."

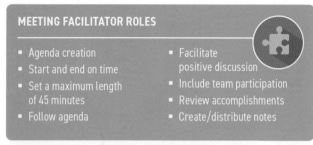

Dr. Brené Brown

Consider the role of a sports coach. They coach the football team up and are motivational, inspirational, and build the strengths of the winning team. Some football team members are exceptional at what they do while others need additional coaching; that is part of the coach's role. Ironically, that is also the role of leadership in the veterinary practice!

Every team member, including associate veterinarians, should have feedback on a weekly basis. Coaching can be informal, fun, and lighthearted. Coaching sessions can focus on positive results because of critical thinking, problem solving, or an amazing client experience delivered by that team member. Other times, leaders may ask for change, especially as it relates to behaviors that do not support the values, mission, or vision of the veterinary practice. It is okay to ask for change! When change is asked of a team member regarding a behavior that just occurred, the conversation can be lighthearted. Often team members don't realize the behavior they were exemplifying was even happening. Bringing it to their attention immediately will prevent it from happening again in the future. This is a positive coaching opportunity. Waiting to address the behavior until it has negatively impacted the remainder of the team will result in a negative conversation, one that is often avoided by leadership.

If several coaching opportunities around the same behavior or lack of accountability must be had, leadership should consider officially writing up the employee for documentation purposes. Write-ups become a more serious infraction for employees than a simple coaching session. But write-ups should be rare and let employees know that this is now the time to get serious about their improved performance. While Chapter 4 reviews write-up procedures, their use should be limited. Three write-ups should result in termination. Multiple write-ups with no termination decreases the team morale and trust/confidence in leadership and breaks the culture of the practice.

Set aside time to have informal conversations with team members just to do a check-in as well. Keep in mind that professional development, goal accomplishment, and ensuring a sense of purpose is being achieved are all coaching opportunities that help employees feel valued and included. Always provide positive feedback for skills or attributes that they deliver on a regular basis. This positive feedback drives a sense of purpose and accomplishment in the veterinary practice.

Coaching moments are "coaching up" or "coaching out." Coaching out must provide clear expectations and should a write-up or termination follow, the team member should not be surprised.

LEADERSHIP POINT

Take unofficial notes of your coaching sessions to help you remember what was discussed, with who, and when, allowing you to always present a professional and organized conversation with team members.

CONFLICT MANAGEMENT

Conflicts are normal among team members in the workplace. Some team members can effectively manage conflict by themselves while others need leadership to intervene and mediate (recall stages of team maturity). Conflicts should be viewed as an opportunity to solve problems. Confidential discussions between involved parties and leadership can help resolve issues before they become destructive. When conflict is properly handled, it can stimulate understanding of another viewpoint, improved self-awareness, and the impact of perception on others, while inviting a new way of thinking, progress, and growth. Unmanaged conflict divides team members and must be dealt with as soon as possible.

VHMA PERFORMANCE DOMAIN TASK

Mediate conflict between team members.

Practices without conflict can be just as harmful as those with conflict. Team members may be afraid to speak their opinions or may have been conditioned to simply complete orders given to them. This type of culture can be extremely detrimental; it prevents creative thinking, innovation, and change. It can also encourage passive resistance because opinions are not permitted. Employees are simply employees in environments such as this, not team members. When employees do not feel valued in their thoughts or opinions, they will likely become disgruntled and leave the practice seeking a more positive culture.

The top three issues that cause conflict in the workplace environment are lack of communication, lack of training, and gossip. Conflicts should be identified and confirmed with all parties involved. Improved communication, role clarity, and training protocols are a management responsibility; ensure those are in place along with a "no gossip" policy to harness a professional workplace environment.

When determining the extent of conflict, questions such as those listed in Fig. 2.21 can be asked. Open-ended questions stimulate discussion. Who, what, when, where, why, and how introduce open-ended questions. Many times, both parties in a conflict have underlying, unmet needs from the other party. If these needs can be determined, discussed, and understood by each other, positive conflict resolution can take place.

Once an issue has been confirmed, leaders should ensure all parties involved fully understand the issue(s) by repeating the problem to the presenting team member(s) and expressing empathy to both parties. If a simple misunderstanding has occurred, simply acknowledging, and explaining the other team member's opinion and view of the issue may solve the problem immediately. Both team members involved should be aware that leadership understands the problem and that each of their concerns is valid.

To help resolve conflict, specific facts should be used when discussing the problem (removing all emotions associated). As an example, "*Teresa did not clean cages today,*" is a statement that presents facts. "*Teresa did not clean cages today because she is lazy*" is a statement that includes emotion. Assuming one is lazy is an emotional response. Instead, explore why the perception of laziness exists. Perhaps the employee was asked to complete a different essential task by a manager or leader, or perhaps they were called away to assist with an emergency. These facts are needed to resolve conflict. Until the real problem is identified a resolution cannot be determined (Fig. 2.22).

Team members should not be told how to think or what to feel (this does not solve the problem). A caring and empathetic environment makes it easier for honesty and open communication (a normal part of practice culture), allowing conflicts to be resolved relatively easily.

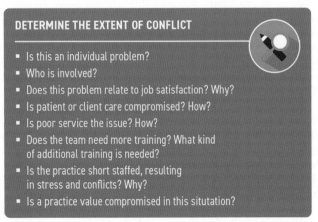

DETERMINE THE EXTENT OF CONFLICT

- Is this an individual problem?
- Who is involved?
- Does this problem relate to job satisfaction? Why?
- Is patient or client care compromised? How?
- Is poor service the issue? How?
- Does the team need more training? What kind of additional training is needed?
- Is the practice short staffed, resulting in stress and conflicts? Why?
- Is a practice value compromised in this situtation?

Fig. 2.21 Use a combination of open and closed-ended questions to determine the extent of the conflict.

GUIDELINES FOR CONFLICT RESOLUTION

- **Discuss the problem as soon as possible.** A delay in discussion may result in additional conflict or may be interpreted that management is not interested in the problem.
- **Listen to all the issues and keep an open mind.** Encourage team members to talk with open-ended questions.
- **Determine the real issue.** Frequently, a complaint is made about a superficial problem when a deeper problem exists. For example, a team member may have a workload complaint when a personality conflict is the real problem.
- **Exercise control and avoid arguments.** Everyone has opinions; let them be stated. Emotional outbursts lead nowhere.
- **Avoid a delay in decision-making.** Unresolved problems spread like wildfire and can add undue stress to the entire team.
- **Maintain records of the problem.** Document the conflict in case the same problem arises in the future. Recalling details later usually is impossible.

Fig. 2.22 Identifying the real issue of a conflict is key to finding an optimal resolution.

Some conflicts may involve leaders who can become defensive when confronted with a complaint. Just as with other team members, some will take complaints personally. Facts need to be listened to, internalized, and processed. Some points may be valid as team members often try to help the leader overcome weaknesses, just as the leader has helped team members in the past. Leaders accepting criticism sets the stage for how team members accept criticism. If a leader is reactive versus creating a learning experience from the conversation, the team will do the same.

If numerous complaints arise against one team member, a serious problem may exist. Regardless of the nature of the complaint, the details should be investigated, and a solution should be developed. Unmanaged conflicts can lead to unprofessional behavior and potential workplace violence. Should violence of any kind result, the practice owner(s) and practice manager may be responsible because they did not initiate any form of conflict resolution.

CHANGE MANAGEMENT

Implementing change is difficult, but without adapting and changing processes or procedures, detrimental results may occur. It's easy to stay with what's comfortable, and when challenging the status quo, a sense of chaos and discomfort is created. Many times, team members will use their energy voicing concerns about change versus problem solving and creating solutions. This is a common scenario, but leadership must be able to implement change to take the practice to the next level.

An adaptability quotient measures the ability to adapt and may include how they handle change, learn from mistakes, and overcome challenges; then adjust in real time. It's essentially rolling with the punches and working with change instead of against it. While practice leaders can't plan for the unknown, you can prepare for it. Building skills to adapt and embrace change will enhance future outcomes for both the practice and the team. The pandemic made the practice change daily protocols. It was exhausting, but teams learned how to problem solve, be flexible, allow innovation, and adopt new procedures and technology to survive. People and businesses are faced with change every day; adapting to it is the key to success.[8]

Four Steps to Managing Change

1	**DEFINE** the problem.
2	**PERFORM** a gap analysis.
3	**DEVELOP A PLAN** for change that includes defining objectives, creating a strategy, and implementation of the plan.
4	**EVALUATE** the change and tweak for improvements.

Fig. 2.23 Change management can be difficult to execute without a plan, and the results of the plan should be evaluated for future improvements.

CRITICAL COMPETENCY: ADAPTABILITY

Practice managers must be open to change and flexible work methods and can adapt behavior to changing conditions or new information.

The first step in managing change starts with defining the problem. The second step is gap analysis; leaders need to identify the gap between what is going on now, what the desired outcome should be (gap analysis), and be able to identify the causes of the gap (Fig. 2.23). The analysis should then be presented to the team (through team meetings, not individually) to ask for input and clarification. When team members are included and can offer their opinions on how a policy or procedure can be updated, they are more likely to accept and implement the change. Team members may have ideas or methods to better implement change that management had not considered. Consider these points of change resistance and how leadership can plan to overcome them with each change initiative:

Informational resistance is defined as team members not knowing why a problem exists, how it affects the business or organization, and where potential change could occur.

Personal resistance is a result of the loss of familiar patterns or relationships with fellow team members.

Cultural resistance is the opinion that change is not possible within the organization, or leadership is not capable of carrying out the change.

The third step in implementing change is designing a plan that includes clearly defined objectives, a strategy, and a course of action. Once the plan has been created, a summary of notes should be distributed to all team members. A follow-up discussion regarding the change (and the successes) should be on the agenda for the next meeting. It takes 30 days to change behaviors and habits and leaders must coach the team to greatness, keeping the plan moving forward and not letting the team procrastinate or regress back to the comfort zone.

The last step is evaluating the changes that have occurred, identifying both good and bad issues that may have risen because of the change, and pivoting or adapting as needed to achieve the originally desired outcome.

A failure to change is often the result of poor planning and communication, failure to act or follow through by leadership, and/or lack of leadership buy-in. Improve success rates by putting plans in writing with SMART goals (Chapter 12, Marketing). Ensure all leaders (owners, associate veterinarians, and managers) are on board with change plans; any reluctance or hesitation will be perceived by the staff as a lack of commitment (by leadership) to the change. Use a Change Planning Form (Fig. 2.24) to facilitate each step.

CHANGE PLANNING FORM

To effectively manage change within the hospital setting, the leader must understand what the change is, who it impacts, and what resources must be utilized for it to be successful.

What do you wish to change?

Why is this change important?

How will this change benefit CSRs?

How will this change benefit VAs and RVTs?

How will this change benefit DVM's?

How will this change benefit Management?

What systems or resources will need to be involved?

Anticipated cost of supplies and equipment

Outline your process.

Outline your training requirements.

Outline your execution and revision process.

Feedback from all stakeholders.

Optimized process outline.

Fig. 2.24 A detailed change planning form prevents the skipping of steps that could cause a plan to fail (courtesy, Rob Paisley).

PRACTICE MANAGER SURVIVAL CHECK LIST FOR THE LEADERSHIP TEAM

- ☐ Establish core values and the mission and vision statement. Implement and tie to the job descriptions, training programs, coaching, and feedback sessions.
- ☐ Develop/encourage continuing education for the team or make opportunities readily available.
- ☐ Ensure practice management software security is in place and monitored. Owners and practice managers should be the only team members allowed to delete, modify, or change prices, SOPs, or SOCs.
- ☐ Budget for team uniforms (initial order and to be replaced regularly), enhancing the professional perception by clients.
- ☐ Host weekly team meetings to advance communication.
- ☐ Post meeting agendas, take notes, and distribute notes within 24 hours of the meeting.
- ☐ Post the facility license and the city business license in public view.
- ☐ Ensure the team is leveraged appropriately and efficiency is implemented to prevent burnout.

CHAPTER REVIEW QUESTIONS

1. Define how great leadership can benefit the practice.
2. Define how poor leadership can negatively affect the practice.
3. Define organizational development.
4. Define employee development.
5. Name some ways effective leadership is shown.
6. Define situational leadership.
7. In the Leadership Challenge founded by Kouzes and Posner, name at least three components of great leadership.
8. Define a mission statement.
9. How can a lack of values, mission, and vision negatively impact the practice?
10. Name some areas in practice that VMVs can affect.
11. Explain some ways in which a diverse team can positively impact the practice.
12. Why is having a work-life balance important?
13. Name some effective methods for retaining team members.
14. Describe how an "employer brand" is established.
15. Define empowerment and why it's important to empower team members.

REFERENCES

1. Miller H. The Situational Leadership Model. September 2022. Leadership.com. Accessed December 2022. https://leaders.com/articles/leadership/situational-leadership/
2. Kenton W. Hersey-Blanchard Situational Leadership Model: How it Works. Investopedia.com. Accessed May 2023. https://www.investopedia.com/terms/h/hersey-and-blanchard-model.asp
3. Groysberg B, Lee J, Price J, Yo-Jud Cheng J. The Leader's Guide to Corporate Culture. *Harv Bus Rev*. Published January 1, 2018. Accessed August 2022. https://hbr.org/2018/01/the-leaders-guide-to-corporate-culture
4. Mcleod S. Maslow's Hierarchy of Needs Theory. Simply Psychology. Accessed October 2022. https://www.simplypsychology.org/maslow.html
5. Zack I. Why are veterinarians unhappy? DVM 360. Published June 15, 2021. Accessed October 2022. https://www.dvm360.com/view/why-are-veterinarians-unhappy-
6. NAVTA. NAVTA Demographics Survey. The NAVTA Journal. September/October 2016.
7. Chapman G. *The 5 Love Languages: The Secret to Love that Lasts*. Northfield Publishing; 2015.
8. Nwanne E. What is an Adaptability Quotient (AQ) and How to Improve your Adaptability. WorkPatterns.com. Published July 13, 2021. Accessed December 2022. https://www.workpatterns.com/articles/adaptability-quotient

RECOMMENDED READING

Goleman D. *Working with Emotional Intelligence*. Bantom Books; 2000.

Hersey P, Blanchard K. *Management of Organized Behavior*. 10th ed. Prentice Hall; 2012.

Kouzes J, Posner B. *The Leadership Challenge*. 4th ed. Gildan Media; 2008.

Pink D. *Drive: The Surprising Truth About What Motivates Us*. Riverhead Books; 2011.

Tropman J. *Making Meetings Work: Achieving High Quality Group Decisions*. 2nd ed. Sage Press; 2003.

Brown B. *Dare to Lead*. Random House; 2018.

Brown B. *Daring Greatly*. Avery; 2015.

3

The Veterinary Team and Front Office Procedures

LEARNING OBJECTIVES

When you have completed this chapter, you should be able to:

- Define various positions within a veterinary practice
- Describe job duties associated with each position in the hospital
- Define staff etiquette
- Differentiate forms used in the veterinary practice
- Identify veterinary health certificates
- List methods to accept payments on client accounts
- Explain how to reconcile the end-of-day transactions and totals
- Explain how to make daily deposits

OUTLINE

KEY TERMS

Active income
Client Patient Information Sheet
Debit Transactions
Deposit
End-of-Day Reconciliation
Etiquette
International Health Certificates
Master Problem List
Medical Records
Office Manager
Passive Income
Petty Cash
Practice Manager
Privacy Act
Rabies Certificates
Rabies-Neutralizing Antibody Titer
Receptionist
Species
Veterinarian
Veterinary Assistant
Veterinary Technician

VHMA PERFORMANCE DOMAINS

Veterinary Hospital Managers Association (VHMA) Performance Domains

Performance domains applicable to the veterinary team and office procedures include human resources, law and ethics, and marketing and client relations. The practice manager:

- Creates, reviews, and updates job descriptions
- Manages staff training and continuing education
- Ensures compliance with contract law as it applies to clients and patients
- Ensures compliance of confidentiality
- Manages client education

Application of VHMA Performance Domains for Practice Managers

Practice managers who develop a core team built on culture and values (respect, integrity, honesty, trust) provide leadership and growth opportunities for each, implement leveraging and empowerment, and will have a team that is not impacted by burnout, mental exhaustion, high employee turnover, or staffing issues.

INTRODUCTION

The veterinary practice is a highly structured environment that provides excellent career opportunities for all team members. The goal of every practice should be to provide superior medical care to patients and a frictionless client experience, while also providing a workplace that is friendly, efficient, and safe. Each team member contributes significantly to these goals, and even one team member not fulfilling their responsibilities impacts revenue and the client experience, while also lowering team morale.

Roles and responsibilities vary by practice and typically are defined in the job description section of the employment manual (Chapter 4, Human Resources). Team members working collaboratively improves job satisfaction and ultimately decreases burnout and mental fatigue. When outstanding teamwork is evident, clients notice and recommend the friendly, honest, and genuine service that a veterinary practice can provide. When a positive team environment is created, any role in the veterinary health care team is rewarding. Patients receive better care, clients receive better service, and employees enjoy coming to work. When team members enjoy their jobs, they are accountable, efficient, and strive to achieve higher goals both personally and professionally (Fig. 3.1).

Positive cultures generate a harmonious environment; team members respect one another, and clients build strong and loyal relationships. Strong client relationships result in an increase in client compliance, and pets get the care they need. When a negative culture exists, clients "feel" it when they enter the practice and easily read unhappy team members through poor body language and interpret negative comments that are made. Poor cultures lead to high employee turnover resulting in decreased client trust, bonding rates, and compliance. Chapter 2, Culture, provides specific examples of culture and the impact it has on the business, team members, and clients. Cultivating culture is a leadership responsibility, but team members must contribute through collaboration, trust, open communication, and personal accountability.

Team members may include, but are not limited to, students, groomers (Fig. 3.2), kennel assistants (Fig. 3.3), veterinary assistants, credentialed veterinary technicians and veterinary technologists, receptionists, veterinarians, office managers, and practice managers. Many practices also have specializations within each position. Having team leaders of the receptionist team and the technician/assistant team can significantly improve communications, efficiency, and accountability within each of those teams, enabling the leaders to achieve goals together.

Larger practices may have a structured hierarchy, with each team member having a specific role in the practice. Technicians may be limited to hospitalized patients, surgical recovery, or laboratory duties, whereas others may be assigned specifically to outpatient visits. Smaller practices have assistants and technicians assigned to all areas of the practice, many serving in cross-functional roles.

CHARACTERISTICS OF SUCCESSFUL TEAM ENVIRONMENTS

- Team members understand one another's priorities and difficulties and offer help when the opportunity arises
- Open communication exists among all employees, managers, and owners
- Problem solving occurs as a team
- The team is recognized for outstanding results, as are individuals for personal contributions
- The team has psychological safety and feel safe to make suggestions to improve workflow efficiencies, be innovative, and challenge the status quo
- Team members are encouraged to work outside their scope of work to continuously improve their knowledge, skills, and abilities
- Team members support one another and never finger point

Fig. 3.1 Teams that have a great working environment are more engaged and motivated to achieve practice goals.

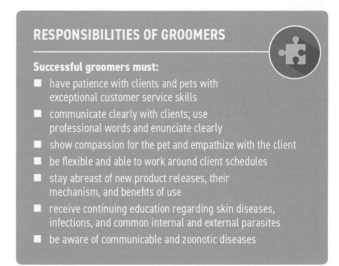

RESPONSIBILITIES OF GROOMERS

Successful groomers must:

- have patience with clients and pets with exceptional customer service skills
- communicate clearly with clients; use professional words and enunciate clearly
- show compassion for the pet and empathize with the client
- be flexible and able to work around client schedules
- stay abreast of new product releases, their mechanism, and benefits of use
- receive continuing education regarding skin diseases, infections, and common internal and external parasites
- be aware of communicable and zoonotic diseases

Fig. 3.2 Groomers are often the first to identify lumps or abnormalities that owners have yet to notice and bring it to the attention of the veterinary team.

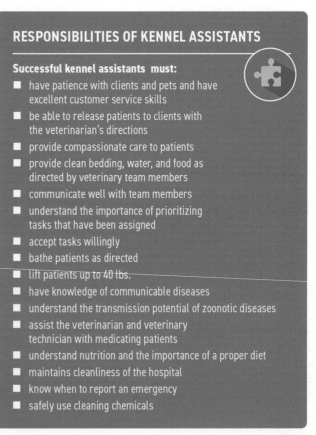

RESPONSIBILITIES OF KENNEL ASSISTANTS

Successful kennel assistants must:

- have patience with clients and pets and have excellent customer service skills
- be able to release patients to clients with the veterinarian's directions
- provide compassionate care to patients
- provide clean bedding, water, and food as directed by veterinary team members
- communicate well with team members
- understand the importance of prioritizing tasks that have been assigned
- accept tasks willingly
- bathe patients as directed
- lift patients up to 40 lbs.
- have knowledge of communicable diseases
- understand the transmission potential of zoonotic diseases
- assist the veterinarian and veterinary technician with medicating patients
- understand nutrition and the importance of a proper diet
- maintains cleanliness of the hospital
- know when to report an emergency
- safely use cleaning chemicals

Fig. 3.3 Kennel assistants are charged with providing exceptional patient care and alerting veterinary team members if they see any patient abnormalities.

COMMON QUESTIONS FOR NEW TEAM MEMBERS

- What are the common emergencies seen at the practice?
- Are emergencies accepted after hours? If not, where are clients advised to go?
- What species are seen by the practice?
- What are the common diseases seen in the practice's geographic area?
- What are local vaccination protocols?
- Which heartworm/flea/tick preventive is recommended?
- Which nutritional products and food are sold at the practice?
- What routine surgeries are performed in the practice?
- What postoperative pain protocols are available for each species?
- What specialty procedures are performed in the practice?
- Is the hospital accredited by the American Animal Hospital Association?
- Does the practice board animals? If not, who is recommended?
- Does the practice have a groomer? If not, who is recommended?
- At what age are pets recommended to be altered?

Fig. 3.4 New team members can become overwhelmed during their new hire period. Set them up for success by training the most common questions they will be expected to answer.

Effective and efficient team members take initiative to anticipate the needs of others (regardless of role) to achieve practice goals. For example, an assistant or veterinary technician/nurse should know exactly what the doctor will need for a patient in the examination room before the doctor reviews the medical record. A receptionist, assistant, or technician/nurse will anticipate what a client will need before they ask, or what a fellow technician will need to start an IV catheter. Kennel assistants may help a technician/nurse or assistant restrain a patient for laboratory work, and the medical team may need to clean kennels to make room for an incoming patient. Supportive teamwork leads to an environment where team members step up to help others before they are asked for help.

LEADERSHIP POINT

Leadership skills must be used to influence and develop an effective veterinary team. When done well, the practice manager position is a rewarding experience.

To support this type of environment, each new team member must become familiar with all roles within the practice during the onboarding process. Because practices use various products and equipment or perform procedures with different methods, a list of questions has been developed that each team member should be familiar with when starting a new position (Fig. 3.4). This list can serve as a starting example but must be tailored to the specific practice and added to, based on specific responsibilities. Chapter 4, Human Resources, covers the development of phase training programs for newly onboarding team members.

Cross-training team members in all areas of the practice is crucial, allowing backup should someone call out sick, take vacation, or just provide extra support on busy days. Cross training reduces the opportunity for only one person to "know how to do things," allowing the practice to resume normal activity when that team member is on PTO.

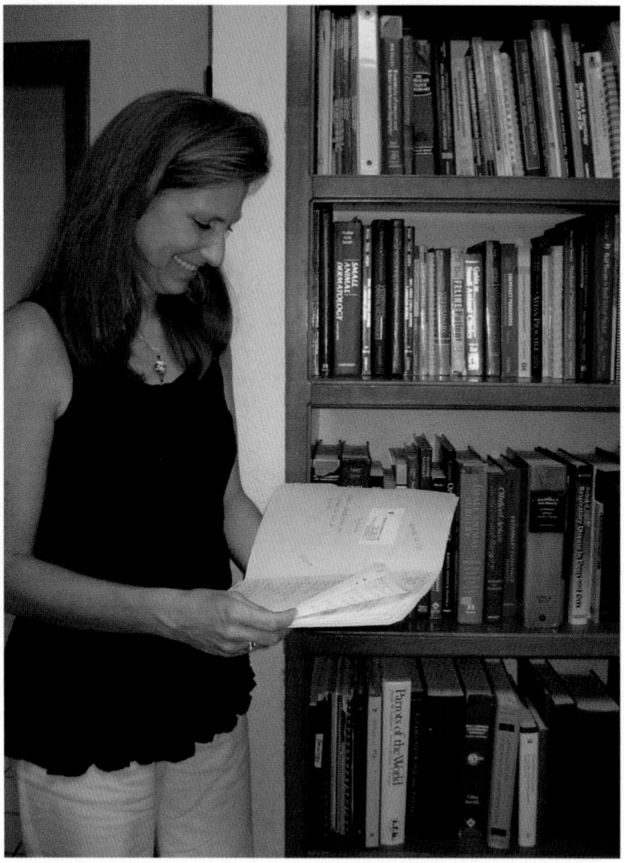

Fig. 3.5 Practice managers ensure the veterinary practice runs efficiently while demonstrating a professional and friendly attitude.

TEAM MEMBER RESPONSIBILITIES BY ROLE

Hospital Administrators

A hospital administrator may be a business manager from another industry, a technician, or an advanced practice manager, and generally has complete authority over the operation of the business and practice. Administrators are responsible for setting strategic goals, managing budgets, overseeing accounts payable, making purchasing decisions, performing financial, controlled substance, and inventory audits throughout the year, and creating an organizational structure (see Chapter 17, Strategic Planning). They oversee all the duties of the entire practice and, through organizational design, put leaders in roles that will achieve practice goals. Although a hospital administrator is not typically a veterinarian, this person should have general knowledge of quality assurance and performance in veterinary medicine and may act in an advisory role in helping establish and monitor protocols of the practice. A hospital administrator position is usually reserved for very large practices and serves in a visionary and strategic role and may report to the owner or shareholders (if multiple members own the practice).

Practice Managers

Practice managers may complete the same duties as a hospital administrator to a lesser degree, while also ensuring the entire team works together efficiently. PMs typically handle client and personnel issues (hiring, terminating), ensure team member training and safety protocols are established, review medical records for completeness, monitor invoices for missed charges, and ensure that standard operating protocols (SOPs) are followed correctly (Fig. 3.5). Some practice managers hold a bachelors or associates degree and report to the hospital administrator or owner of the practice.

RESPONSIBILITIES OF PRACTICE MANAGERS

Successful practice managers must:

- have patience
- lead the team in a positive manner
- address conflict immediately and provide consistent discipline to avoid discrimination claims
- oversee team schedules, maximizing use during busy times, and making alternative plans during slower times
- develop training protocols and performance evaluations and provide coaching for the entire team
- oversee building maintenance, including parking lot, lighting, and interior and exterior structures
- oversee inventory, controlled substance, and safety programs
- develop communication pieces for clients
- develop sales strategies to increase revenue
- hire, fire, and train in a legal manner
- develop and maintain employee benefits program
- determine efficient methods for completion of tasks and procedures for all positions in the practice
- develop and maintain budget for hospital, reconcile accounts, and track and measure income
- strategically plan and create goals for future purchases

Fig. 3.6 Practice managers wear many hats, but most notably they must be authentic leaders.

RESPONSIBILITIES OF OFFICE MANAGERS

In addition to the skills outlined for receptionists, successful office managers must:

- train and oversee duties of receptionists
- develop coping strategies to handle angry clients
- manage accounts receivable, statements, and collections
- review client satisfaction surveys

Fig. 3.7 Office managers are charged with leading a team that delivers a frictionless client experience.

A practice manager wears many hats while on the job: copier repair technician, computer technician, plumber, veterinary technician, kennel assistant, and counselor. PMs must have a positive, friendly attitude with an open-door policy for all team members resulting in a professional and successful atmosphere (Fig. 3.6). For more responsibilities, view the critical competencies and practice domains throughout this book as developed by the Veterinary Hospital Managers Association (VHMA)

Office Managers

The office manager is responsible for overseeing the front office staff as well as training receptionists to deliver a frictionless client experience (Fig. 3.7). An office manager's realm of authority and decision-making may be limited or quite broad, depending on the administrative needs and criteria established by the practice. Most office managers are responsible for accounts receivable, end-of-day reconciliation, and bank deposit preparation. An office manager must be courteous, friendly, and professional, as their demeanor (whether positive or negative) affects the entire team.

RESPONSIBILITIES OF VETERINARIANS

Successful veterinarians must:

- practice quality and current medicine with empathy and compassion
- communicate well with clients and team members
- educate clients and team members
- motivate team members, build and maintain team moral, and uphold core values of the practice
- attend continuing education seminars on a regular basis
- have patience and a positive attitude
- successfully delegate tasks
- diagnose, prescribe medication, and perform surgery
- accurately and legibly enter data into medical records in a timely manner

Fig. 3.8 Veterinarians diagnose, prescribe, and perform surgery. They are also charged with demonstrating leadership behaviors day in and day out.

Veterinarians

Veterinarians are the only members of the team allowed to diagnose, prescribe medications, and perform surgery on patients (Fig. 3.8). They have completed 4 years of a professional, AVMA-accredited school of veterinary medicine (after 3–4 years of undergraduate college). (Fig. 3.9). Veterinarians must be licensed in the state where they work and must pass both national and state examinations before receiving licensure. Veterinarians are required to complete a minimum number of hours in continuing education each year and may need to report their hours to the state veterinary board (varies by state). These requirements ensure veterinarians offer the best medical care available to patients and clients (Fig. 3.10).

It is important that team members keep the doctor team running efficiently. Appropriate tasks must be leveraged to credentialed veterinary technicians/nurses and assistants (see leveraging later in this chapter), allowing the veterinarian to continue seeing patients. Undue hardship on the veterinarians can occur when team members are undertrained, unleveraged, or unaccountable for their actions. Great team members can anticipate the needs of the veterinarian and have all equipment or supplies needed to complete diagnostics or procedures (before the veterinarian asks).

Veterinarians drive "active income" through diagnosing, prescribing, and performing surgeries. "Passive income" is produced by the remaining team members through leveraging duties and tasks such as making appointments, client education, nursing care of hospitalized patients, taking radiographs, and performing dental prophylaxis procedures (just to name a few). A well-managed practice with a strong performing team can produce passive revenue that exceeds 50% of the total revenue.

Veterinarians are responsible for establishing Standards of Care (SOC) (see Chapter 11, Standards of Care) ensuring that every patient gets the best recommendation every time they visit the practice. Often, veterinary team members prejudge a client's financial ability and offer substandard care based on what they think the client can afford, sometimes resulting in unintended patient neglect by the team. Every team member is responsible for educating clients and delivering SOCs established by the doctor team.

VETERINARY SCHOOLS

- **Auburn University College of Veterinary Medicine:** http://www.vetmed.auburn.edu
- **Colorado State University College of Veterinary Medicine and Biomedical Sciences:** http://www.cvmbs.colostate.edu
- **Cornell University College of Veterinary Medicine:** https://www2.vet.cornell.edu/
- **Cummings School of Veterinary Medicine at Tufts University:** http://www.tufts.edu/vet
- **Iowa State University College of Veterinary Medicine:** http://www.vetmed.iastate.edu
- **Kansas State University College of Veterinary Medicine:** http://www.vet.k-state.edu/
- **Lincoln Memorial University:** http://www.lmunet.edu
- **Long Island University:** https://liu.edu/vetmed
- **Louisiana State University School of Veterinary Medicine:** http://lsu.edu/vetmed/
- **Michigan State University College of Veterinary Medicine:** http://www.cvm.msu.edu
- **Midwestern University:** http://www.midwestern.edu
- **Mississippi State University College of Veterinary Medicine:** http://www.cvm.msstate.edu
- **North Carolina State University College of Veterinary Medicine:** http://www.cvm.ncsu.edu
- **Ohio State University College of Veterinary Medicine:** http://vet.osu.edu/
- **Oklahoma State University Center for Veterinary Health Sciences:** http://www.cvm.okstate.edu
- **Oregon State University College of Veterinary Medicine:** http://www.oregonstate.edu/vetmed
- **Purdue University School of Veterinary Medicine:** http://www.vet.purdue.edu
- **Texas A&M University College of Veterinary Medicine & Biomedical Sciences:** http://www.vetmed.tamu.edu/
- **Texas Tech University:** https://www.depts.ttu.edu/vetschool/
- **Tufts University School of Veterinary Medicine:** http://www.tufts.edu/vet
- **Tuskegee University College of Veterinary Medicine, Nursing & Allied Health:** http://www.tuskegee.edu
- **University of Arizona:** http://www.arizona.edu/
- **University of California School of Veterinary Medicine:** http://www.vetmed.ucdavis.edu
- **University of Florida College of Veterinary Medicine:** http://www.vetmed.ufl.edu
- **University of Georgia College of Veterinary Medicine:** http://www.vet.uga.edu
- **University of Illinois College of Veterinary Medicine:** http://www.vetmed.illinois.edu/
- **University of Minnesota College of Veterinary Medicine:** http://www.cvm.umn.edu
- **University of Missouri College of Veterinary Medicine:** http://www.cvm.missouri.edu
- **University of Pennsylvania School of Veterinary Medicine:** http://www.vet.upenn.edu
- **University of Tennessee College of Veterinary Medicine:** http://www.vet.utk.edu
- **University of Wisconsin-Madison School of Veterinary Medicine:** http://www.vetmed.wisc.edu
- **Virginia Tech Virginia-Maryland Regional College of Veterinary Medicine:** http://www.vetmed.vt.edu
- **Washington State University College of Veterinary Medicine:** http://www.vetmed.wsu.edu
- **Western University of Health Sciences College of Veterinary Medicine:** http://www.westernu.edu/veterinary

Fig. 3.9 Veterinary schools are being added every year. Visit the AVMA's website for the most current list of veterinary schools.

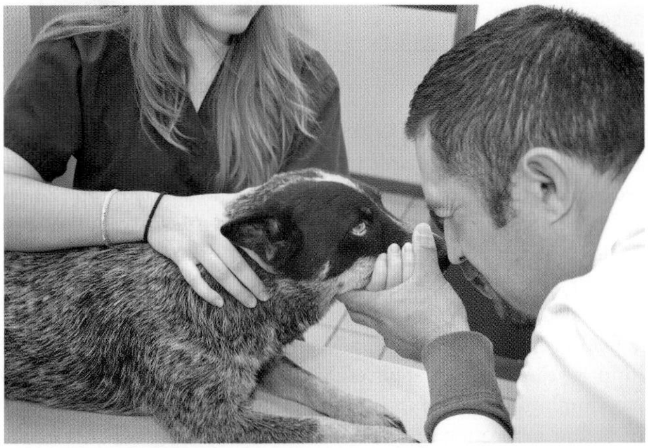

Fig. 3.10 Veterinarians who utilize and leverage their team well have higher job satisfaction than those who do not.

Veterinarians are either the owner(s) of the practice or associate veterinarians. Owners generally oversee both the business management and medical portion of the practice, while still seeing patients. Associate veterinarians may have suggestions for business improvements; however, their main goal is to see patients. Some practices may also have a veterinary medical director (usually a non-owner, but an associate that demonstrates the leadership of others) who is responsible for overseeing the medical aspect of the practice.

The Veterinary Technician Team

The role of the veterinary technician and assistant team is important and equal to that of the receptionist and doctor team. No role in the veterinary practice is better than another, as the entire team must work together and share knowledge, build trust with one another, and work toward achieving practice goals together.

The medical portion of this role is covered in many excellent veterinary technician books. What is covered here is how each of the roles contributes to the success of the practice, leading to goal increased efficiency, the emotional well-being of others, improved client and patient care, and the overall achievement of practice goals (Fig. 3.11).

When trust is established by both technicians and assistants, doctors are more likely to leverage tasks and duties without question. The goal for the team is to serve as a second set of eyes and ears for the doctor; credentialed technicians/nurses understand the why behind recommendations, diagnostics, medications, and procedures. Assistants are generally trained to carry out the skills of such recommendations (per state veterinary practice act regulation).

RESPONSIBILITIES OF CREDENTIALED VETERINARY TECHNICIANS/ NURSES AND TECHNOLOGISTS

In addition to the skills outlined for kennel and veterinary assistants, successful veterinary technicians and technologists must:

- perform physical assessments
- comprehend vaccines and vaccinations protocols and be able to explain vaccine recommendations to clients
- understand and teach clients the significance of disease prevention, nutrition, and preventative care
- provide treatments to patients, including SQ, IM, and IV injections
- comprehend the mechanism of action for drugs and their potential complications and side effects
- calculate dosage of drugs
- develop safety protocols for assistants
- perform common procedures and laboratory analyses
- become proficient at obtaining samples for laboratory analysis
- perform dental prophylaxis
- monitor patients perioperatively and postoperatively
- properly care for all surgical materials, sterilize packs, and maintain surgical facilities
- effectively place and secure IV catheters
- perform electrocardiograms
- any other duty as outlined by the state veterinary practice act

Fig. 3.11 While credentialed veterinary technicians/nurses and technologists are charged with carrying out the hard skills listed in this example, they must also demonstrate exemplary leadership skills that educate clients and fellow team members.

Credentialed veterinary technicians/nurses are responsible for contributing to the development of training protocols, onboarding new team members, attending team meetings (and contributing positive ideas that achieve practice goals), providing suggestions to increase team efficiency and leveraging, and seeking professional development opportunities that further enhance or build new skills.

Credentialed veterinary technicians/nurses have taken an oath to always be advocates for the patient and the client. They should understand the practice goals, core values, vision, and mission, and develop (and demonstrate) behaviors that support each. Technicians/nurses must also always be safety advocates, placing the safety of team members and patients as a top priority.

Any immediate concerns should be taken directly to the practice manager. Veterinary technicians/nurses should be advocates to stop gossip in the practice and cultivate a culture that creates a great place to work. Additionally, respect must be given to all other team members, regardless of their roles, by teaching and coaching veterinary assistants and receptionists to be the best that they can be (as both roles can be difficult without proper training).

VETERINARY TECHNICIAN SPECIALTIES

Credentialed veterinary technicians/nurses may decide to focus on a specific area of care that allows them to carry the designation Veterinary Technician Specialist (VTS). Currently, there are 14 specialty academies (Fig. 3.12) and credentialed technicians/nurses must meet rigorous standards to qualify to sit for the academy exam. Credentialed technicians/nurses who choose to specialize must accumulate a specific number of hours within a specialty during a set number of years. For example, The Academy of Internal Medicine for Veterinary Technicians requires a minimum of 3 years' experience as a credentialed veterinary technician/nurse, 6000 hours of experience in the field of internal medicine, and all experience must be completed within 5 years prior to application. Candidates are also expected to have a minimum of 40 hours of continuing education on internal medicine before application submission.

Some societies are also available to encourage professional development and consist of a group of individuals, veterinary technicians, hospital staff, and veterinarians interested in a specific discipline or area of veterinary medicine.

VETERINARY TECHNICIAN SPECIALTIES

- Academy of Laboratory Animal Veterinary Technicians and Nurses (ALAVTN): http://www.alavtn.org
- Academy of Veterinary Technicians in Anesthesia and Analgesia (AVTAA): http://www.avtaa-vts.org
- Academy of Veterinary Behavior Technicians (AVBT): http://www.avbt.net
- Academy of Veterinary Clinical Pathology Technicians (AVCPT): http://www.avcpt.net
- Academy of Veterinary Technicians in Clinical Practice (AVTCP): http://avtcp.org
- Academy of Veterinary Dental Technicians (AVDT): http://www.avdt.us
- Academy of Veterinary Technicians in Diagnostic Imaging: www.avtdi.org
- Academy of Dermatology Veterinary Technicians (ADVT): http://www.vetdermtech.com
- Academy of Veterinary Emergency and Critical Care Technicians (AVECCT): http://www.avecct.org
- Academy of Equine Veterinary Nursing Technicians (AEVNT): http://www.aaevt.org
- Academy of Internal Medicine for Veterinary Technicians (AIMVT): http://www.aimvt.com
- Academy of Physical Rehabilitation Technicians (APRVT): http://www.aprvt.com
- Academy of Veterinary Nutrition Technicians (AVNT): http://nutritiontechs.org
- Academy of Veterinary Ophthalmic Technicians (ACVO): http://www.avot-vts.org
- Academy of Veterinary Surgical Technicians (AVST): http://www.avst-vts.org
- Academy of Veterinary Zoological Medicine Technicians (AVZMT): http://www.azvt.org/AVZMT

Fig. 3.12 Veterinary technicians specialties allow credentialed technicians/nurses the ability to focus on a particular area that drives their passion.

Veterinary Assistants

Veterinary assistants are valuable assets to the hospital team that support veterinary technicians and veterinarians by providing patient

RESPONSIBILITIES OF VETERINARY ASSISTANTS

Successful veterinary assistants must:

- have patience with clients and pets and have excellent customer service skills
- maintain legible and accurate medical records
- provide compassionate care to patients
- provide clean bedding, water, and food as directed by veterinary team members
- prepare and maintain examination rooms and treatment areas
- communicate clearly with team members and clients
- accept tasks willingly
- bathe patients as directed
- have knowledge of communicable diseases and methods of prevention
- understand the transmission potential of zoonotic diseases
- assist the veterinarian and veterinary technician with medicating patients
- prepare and explain treatment plans for to clients
- understand nutrition and the importance of a proper diet
- release patients and clearly communicate directions provided by veterinarian
- maintain cleanliness of the hospital
- perform laboratory analysis on samples as instructed
- know when to report an emergency
- excel at animal restraint and be able to lift patients up to 40 lbs.
- effectively position patients for diagnostic radiographs
- understand common procedures performed in the practice
- have knowledge of common drugs used in the practice
- understand the importance of prioritizing tasks
- have initiative to learn and raise the practice to the next level of care

Fig. 3.13 Veterinary assistants are a critical component of an efficient veterinary team.

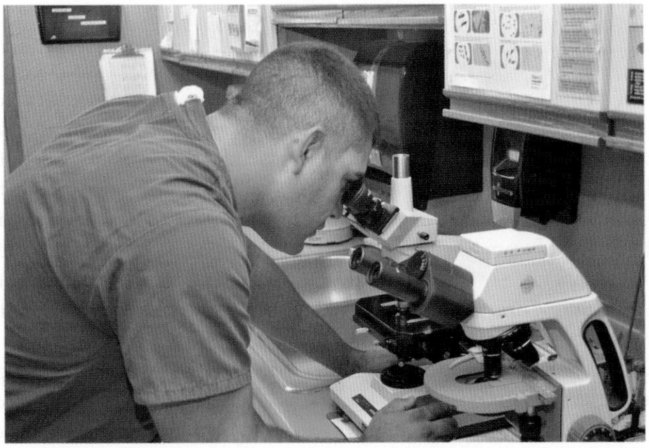

Fig. 3.14 A veterinary assistant plays a vital role in increasing the efficiency of veterinary technicians and veterinarians by preparing cytology tests to be read.

RESPONSIBILITIES OF RECEPTIONISTS

Successful receptionists must:

- have patience, empathy, and compassion for clients and patients
- communicate well with team members and clients in a professional, respectful manner
- provide exceptional service to every client by identifying their needs and wants
- answers phones efficiently with a positive tone of voice
- turn phone inquiries into appointments
- educate clients on basic animal care, parasites, and routine procedures
- listen to clients
- interpret patient medical records
- prepare client transactions, accept payment, and/or explain payment policy to clients
- minimize chaos at the front desk
- maintain an effective appointment system

Fig. 3.15 Receptionists are credited with having one of the hardest roles in the veterinary practice as they navigate client relationships.

restraint, laboratory skills, patient care, and client relations (Fig. 3.13). Veterinary assistants are key to practices that excel in the frictionless client experience and patient care. Kennel assistants may report to veterinary assistants, who in turn report critical patient information to either veterinary technicians or veterinarians (Fig. 3.14).

Veterinary assistants gain a wealth of on-the-job training in the veterinary practice, which is critical to the efficiency of the practice. Just as credentialed technicians/nurses, assistants must gain the trust of the team through work ethic, consistent skill application, and care of others, including staff, patients, and clients. Veterinary assistants help increase the efficiency of every role in the practice.

Assistants can be trained through veterinary assistant courses or on the job by credentialed veterinary technicians/nurses or practice managers and encouraged to become "approved veterinary assistants," receiving the designation of an AVA. The Approved Veterinary Assistant program is overseen by the National Association of Veterinary Technicians in America (NAVTA) and must qualify through the completion of an approved program and sit for an examination. Visit http://www.NAVTA.org for more information on becoming an AVA.

Credentialed veterinary technicians/nurses and veterinarians work more effectively when they have a trained assistant to aid them in the completion of their responsibilities. These valuable assistant-technician relationships enhance the client care experience, improve client bonding, and increase compliance rates.

The Receptionist Team

Receptionists are the "face" of the veterinary practice (Fig. 3.15) by providing immediate, consistent, dependable, and courteous service to the client. They play a significant role in the success of a practice and must be professional, polite, and caring. They listen to client stories, show empathy when needed, and be able to collect money from clients under difficult circumstances. They may (or may not) make a good first impression, succeed (or fail) at scheduling appointments, and enhance (or devalue) the client experience. This can be a difficult role, but with proper training and communication skills, this position can be very rewarding.

LEADERSHIP POINT

Set up the receptionist team for success by ensuring appropriate training programs are developed, efficient tools are available to serve client needs, and support/respect is given by all other roles in the practice.

Creating a positive first impression improves client retention, increases client referrals, and ultimately drives client compliance. Receptionists greet clients in a friendly manner as soon as they walk in the door and are the last members of the team to take care of the client. Making a lasting positive impression is a must. First and last impressions are what clients remember!

The reception team also supports quality client and patient care through effective communication with team members. Clients call throughout the day requesting updates on their pets, and the reception team is responsible for either relaying information to the owner or transferring the call to a knowledgeable team member.

The reception position in a veterinary practice is one of the hardest jobs on the team. They control the flow of chaos (to some degree) in the practice, and because receptionists have the first and last interactions with clients, they often receive the brunt of complaints. Additionally, there is often a "front staff" versus "back staff" mentality, and they are the "last to know" of changes that are made in the practice. Continuing education opportunities also tend to focus on the "back staff," so providing educational opportunities that impact this role is critical.

The reception team adds value and recognition to their positions by driving efficient processes while handling clients, kids, patients, and phones, all while being team players, and looking for opportunities to support the practice's vision, mission, and values. It is important that the reception team realizes they bring much more to the table than just a smiling face for clients. They are critical members of the team.

RESPONSIBILITIES OF ALL ROLES

Every team member is responsible for soft skills that impact clients, patients, and team members. Soft skills include a high level of work ethic, professionalism, respect for one another, working collaboratively, having initiative, and personal accountability for demonstrating behaviors that have been established by the core values (Chapter 2). Each of these skills can enhance or detract from the ability to deliver a frictionless client experience and client education, increasing efficiency so appointments run on time, exceeding expectations as outlined in SOPs and SOCs, and the ability for the practice to achieve goals that have been established by the vision and practice strategic plan.

CRITICAL COMPETENCY: CRITICAL AND STRATEGIC THINKING

Strategic thinking and planning are essential for long-term plans for growth of the practice. Managers must have the ability to identify questions, problems, and arguments relevant to these issues and to use logic and critical reasoning to identify the strengths and weaknesses of alternative solutions or approaches to problems.

Burnout, compassion fatigue, and mental exhaustion are issues impacting practices of 2023 (Chapter 1). And while it is leadership's responsibility to identify stressors and implement processes and tools to mitigate them (Chapter 2), it is also each team member's personal responsibility to utilize processes and tools and contribute to the cultivation of the practice culture. Each of the following areas is an example of how each role contributes to practice culture.

Trust: To increase trust with others (regardless of role), each team member must be honest, transparent, and communicate often. Communication involves the use of emotional intelligence, the ability to show empathy and compassion toward others, and seeking to understand the concerns of others, then addressing them professionally (Chapter 2). Help others grow by sharing knowledge and teaching the "why." Team members may feel they always need to have an answer for every question that is asked of them. That is not the case; it is okay to not know the answer, be vulnerable by admitting you don't have the answer, and acknowledge the will to find the answer (it is not okay to admit you don't know, then walk away and do nothing with it). Not knowing and being honest gains respect, having a positive impact on trust. Work ethic also contributes to the development of trust. Work ethic has historically been misperceived in the past and referred to as the number of hours worked (usually in excess). But work ethic is not about the hours worked; it is about always behaving professionally (dressing appropriately, arriving early, and being courteous to others), being organized in thoughts and actions resulting in a high level of efficiency, and teamwork and collaboration. Work ethic develops trust and respect from fellow team members, contributing to the great culture every workplace deserves.

Team members must understand their role in achieving the practice's strategic goals and vision. Without knowing how they each contribute; they simply have a job with no purpose.

Client education: Clients must hear the same message from every team member. While the words do not have to be exact, the meaning of the message must be consistent. The receptionist team may be asked *"what heartworm preventative should I give Fluffy?"* and *"How often am I supposed to test for heartworm disease"?* The receptionist must be able to give a specific product recommendation and testing protocol. If the receptionist responds that *"the doctor will make that recommendation,"* the client's trust in the receptionist team is eroded. The same is true of the veterinary technician/nurse or the assistant. Establishing SOCs and SOPs (Chapter 11 and Chapter 4, respectively) will ensure the entire team is on the same page, and clients will receive the same message, regardless of who is delivering the message. Additionally, clients need to hear the same consistent message three times to drive compliance (Chapter 11, Client Experience). Adding to the complexity of client education is how the message is delivered (verbal, para-verbal, and non-verbal communication), what learning styles (visual, verbal, tactile) should be applied for each individual client, and the type of communication preference the client may have (Chapter 11).

VHMA PERFORMANCE DOMAIN TASK

Practice managers develop and manage client education.

Frictionless Client Experience: Consider the entire process clients and patients experience when visiting the veterinary practice. The client experience is delivered by the entire team, and if the receptionist fails to deliver a frictionless experience, it sets the medical team up for failure. And if the doctor team provides an experience that is less than subpar, the rest of the team is set to fail. Every team member must work efficiently and collaboratively together to drive the client experience (Chapter 11).

Patient Care: Hospitalized patients require care from all team members during their stay. From kennel assistants to veterinarians, all team members are responsible for ensuring patient safety and comfort, regardless of their position in the practice. Any team member who sees a patient that needs care (dirty cage, needs food/water, showing signs of distress, etc.) must address the situation immediately. Patient care must be a primary focus.

Team Leveraging: Leveraging all team members to their highest potential contributes to increased employee retention, team member

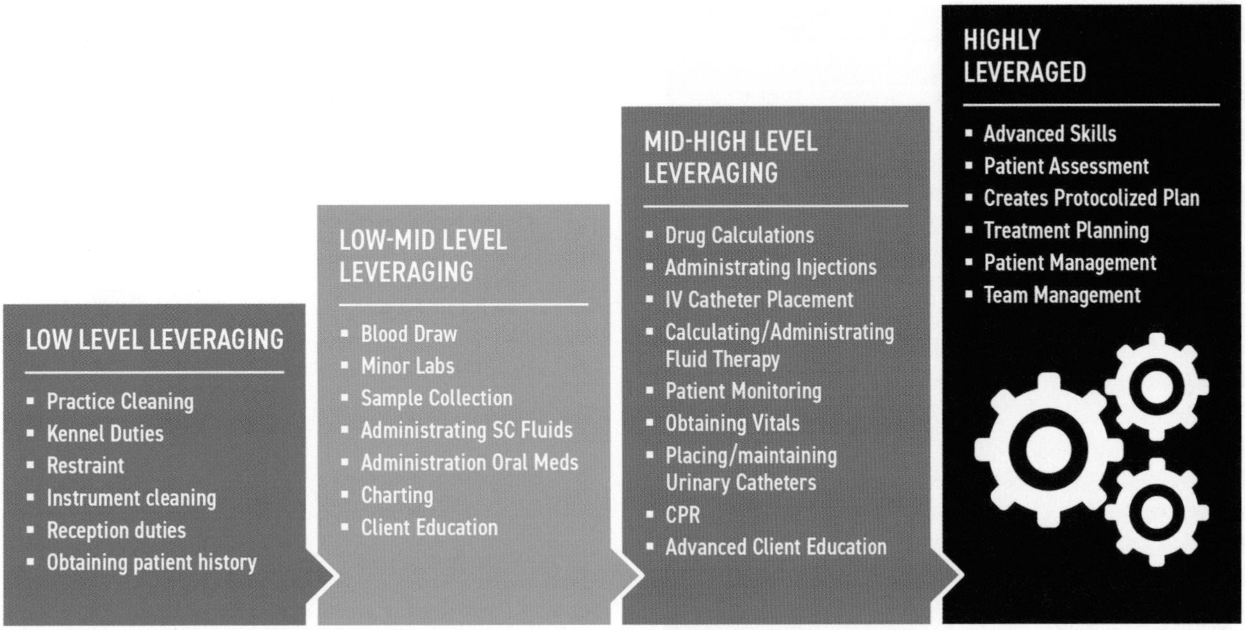

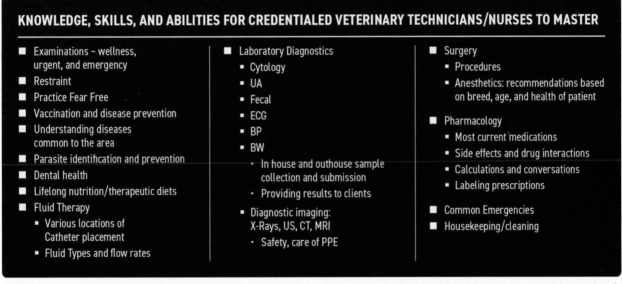

Fig. 3.16 Example of Levels of Leveraging. *Courtesy Kenichiro Yagi, MS, RVT, VTS (ECC) (SAIM).*

KNOWLEDGE, SKILLS, AND ABILITIES FOR CREDENTIALED VETERINARY TECHNICIANS/NURSES TO MASTER

- Examinations - wellness, urgent, and emergency
- Restraint
- Practice Fear Free
- Vaccination and disease prevention
- Understanding diseases common to the area
- Parasite identification and prevention
- Dental health
- Lifelong nutrition/therapeutic diets
- Fluid Therapy
  - Various locations of Catheter placement
  - Fluid Types and flow rates

- Laboratory Diagnostics
  - Cytology
  - UA
  - Fecal
  - ECG
  - BP
  - BW
    - In house and outhouse sample collection and submission
    - Providing results to clients
  - Diagnostic imaging: X-Rays, US, CT, MRI
    - Safety, care of PPE

- Surgery
  - Procedures
  - Anesthetics: recommendations based on breed, age, and health of patient
- Pharmacology
  - Most current medications
  - Side effects and drug interactions
  - Calculations and conversations
  - Labeling prescriptions
- Common Emergencies
- Housekeeping/cleaning

Fig. 3.17 Mastering medical skills is essential in building trust with veterinarians so that all things outside of diagnosing, prescribing, and performing surgery (veterinarians' role) can be leveraged to the technician team.

loyalty to the practice, and team member efficiency, and reduces the barrier to patient care. Veterinarians must empower the team to educate clients, deliver patient care recommendations to clients, perform diagnostics, and provide complete patient care. Fig. 3.16 lists skills that should be leveraged to appropriate team members (be sure to align with the state veterinary practice act). Skills may be leveraged depending on the experience of the individual team member for those that cannot complete all the skills listed, this provides a guideline of training that should be put in place to improve leverage. Mastery of medical skills is essential when building trust with doctors so that all things outside of surgery, diagnosing, and prescribing medications can be leveraged to technicians. Fig. 3.17 should be included in every onboarding training program, continuous training programs, the focus of continuing education, and Standard Operating Protocols (SOPs). Review Chapter 2, Leveraging, for more specific details.

CRITICAL COMPETENCY: CREATIVITY

Practice managers must have the ability to creatively think through situations and embrace new and different ways to see opportunities by using imagination and collaboration, resulting in innovative solutions.

Team Member Name Tags: Team members should always wear name tags to identify themselves; clients want to know who is caring for their pet(s). Veterinarians should also have a name tag, and if a technician is credentialed, the appropriate abbreviation should be included. Clients may assume a technician is treating their pet when, in fact, the veterinarian has entered the room. Identification can be in the form of a pin, a magnet, or an embroidered name on the team member's scrubs.

BEHAVIORS DEMONSTRATING STAFF ETIQUETTE

- Greet team members with a smile every morning. Happiness is contagious.
- Introduce team members when they are not acquainted with visitors and clients.
- Greet clients with a smile when they arrive; open doors for clients when they leave.
- Always say goodbye to both clients and team members as they leave the practice.
- Hold the door for the person behind you.
- Be on time.
- Be a team player.
- Dress and act professionally.
- Don't talk with your mouth full of food.
- Respect the personal space of others.
- Talk less; listen more.
- Keep your word.
- Avoid finishing the sentences of others.
- Treat others how you want to be treated
- Do not criticize. Take the opportunity to teach instead of reprimanding.
- Respect one another.
- Do not gossip.

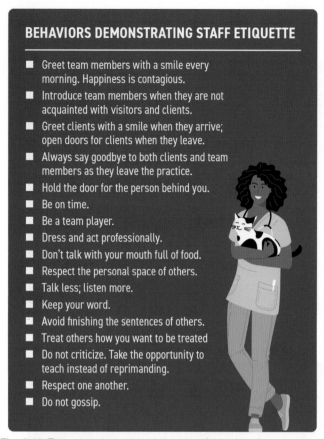

Fig. 3.18 Team members must be respectful and professional at all times to clients and team members to achieve practice goals.

Team Etiquette

Etiquette is the customary code of polite behaviors demonstrated among the members of a group. Team members must always behave professionally and treat others with kindness and respect. Clients and co-workers observe the behaviors and actions demonstrated by team members; it is easy to see a fractured dynamic, ultimately impacting practice growth when etiquette is not always displayed (Fig. 3.18).

> **LEADERSHIP POINT**
>
> Leaders must consistently observe the interactions between team members and if something seems "off," privately address it immediately.

Team etiquette obviously contributes to a positive team culture within the hospital. As mentioned previously, clients (as well as others) perceive (and feel) negative environments and cultures. Characteristics of a negative work culture include teams that do not work well together, employees who are not team players, and teams that gossip and form cliques. Negative cultures must be corrected and prevented to avoid creating a toxic workplace. Characteristics of a positive work culture include employees who take pride in tasks completed, ownership and accountability of the hospital's best interests, and provide client care that exceeds expectations (Fig. 3.19). When team members have respect for one another and practice etiquette accordingly, a positive culture is supported, clients return to the hospital, and they recommend the practice to friends and family. See Chapter 2 for more ideas on creating positive team environments.

Approaching Patients with Caution

Awareness of basic animal instinct is critical for all team members. New smells, sounds, pain, other animals, and unfamiliar people place animals on alert making them fearful and reactive. Even pets with wagging tails can nip or bite as a reaction to fear or stress. Team members must never place their faces close to the face of an animal or behave aggressively with trained police or narcotics dogs.

CHARACTERISTICS OF POSITIVE AND NEGATIVE TEAMS

POSITIVE TEAM CHARACTERISTICS	NEGATIVE TEAM CHARACTERISTICS
Teamwork	"I" statements: I need, I want...
Respect for one another	Disrespect
Strong rapport with each team member	Gossip
Accountability	Lack of accountability
Whole team wellness	Derogatory comments
Empowering/delegating/ leveraging	Spreading rumors
Model good behavior	Inappropriate behavior

Fig. 3.19 Positive teams create a great place to work. Every team member has the responsibility to contribute to a positive team.

Understanding Fear From a Pet's Perspective

Animals have two responses to fear: fight or flight. If they fight, the first response by the veterinary team is to hold them down. If they try to get away (flight), the veterinary team holds them down. Either way, they become frightened and have a horrific veterinary experience. Pets remember that experience, and the next time they come back to the veterinary practice, they remember the last experience and become more fearful. These events continuously build on each other until the owner stops bringing the pet to the practice. It is well known that patient visits are declining, and stress and anxiety associated with taking a pet to the veterinary practice is a contributor. Fear leads to trauma, and as a result, owners are seeking other options. Creating a safe environment for pets increases client comfort and compliance while decreasing the level of pet anxiety.

Creating a Fear-Free Environment

Creating a Fear-Free environment is essential for patient, client, and team safety (emotionally and physically) as well as team member emotional balance. Working in an environment in which patients return home in worse emotional condition than when they presented is damaging to team members and contributes to quicker burnout and compassion fatigue.

Recognizing and responding to patient fear is the number one step toward creating a "safe" environment. Think like a pet patient for one moment:

- Why do some pets love going to doggie daycare and the doggie spa? What creates that happy experience for them? It must be safe, fun, and relaxing.
- How can the veterinary team create that same experience for pets in the practice? Every activity performed in the practice (obtaining vitals, completing the physical examination, administrating medication) must be in the safe zone for the pet (Figs. 3.20 and 3.21).

Key concepts in implementing Fear Free® protocols while providing medical care include communication, considerate approach, gentle

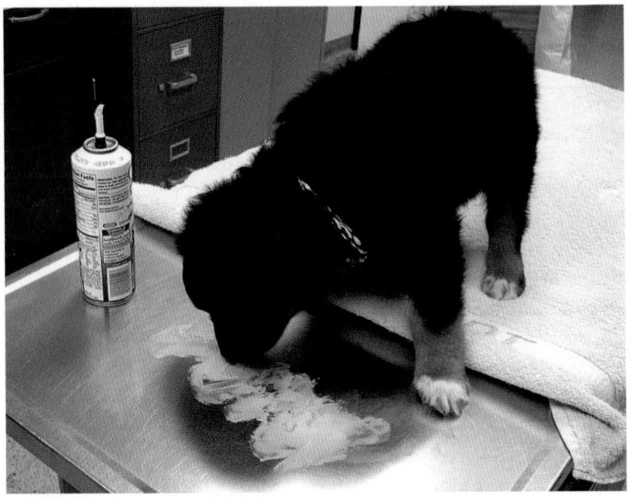

Fig. 3.20 Creating a Fear Free® experience involves providing treats the patient likes while obtaining vitals. This puppy is being distracted with cheese before a vaccination. (From Beaver BV. Canine behavior: insights and answers. 2nd ed. Saunders; 2009.)

control, and touch gradient. Creating a plan of action for each patient can be a quick process that saves time and creates a more pleasant experience for the veterinary healthcare team, the patient, and the client. Visit https://FearFreePets.com for more information.

CRITICAL COMPETENCY: CONTINUOUS LEARNING:

Practice managers should have a curiosity for learning. Actively seeking out new information, technologies, and methods while keeping skills updated allows the application of new knowledge to the job.

FRONT OFFICE PROCEDURES

In most practices, every team member contributes to or completes tasks that are associated with front-office procedures. In practices that cross train and develop team members to serve in several roles (veterinary assistant covering shifts as a receptionist or a credentialed technician/nurse serving as backup when the receptionists are busy), the delivery of each area listed below is critical. Additionally, in practices that check out clients in the exam room, the technician/assistant must master the following tasks to complete a frictionless client experience.

Managing the Reception Area

Many activities occur in the reception area: clients engage in conversation, pets may interact with one another, pets may arrive stressed and fearful, and children may be exploring the area, all of which come with risks.

Clients often attempt to share knowledge with each other, and on occasion, the information may not be accurate or appropriate. Team members should try to monitor conversations and may need to move a client into an examination room sooner than anticipated because of the topic being addressed. "Toxic" topics include a poor experience the client is having at the practice or has had in the past, incorrect information regarding diseases or treatments, and offensive topics and language. It is easier to isolate the offender and apologize to the victim than to remove the victim and let the offender repeat the conversation with another client arriving at the practice.

INITIAL STEPS IN CREATING A FEAR FREE® EXPERIENCE

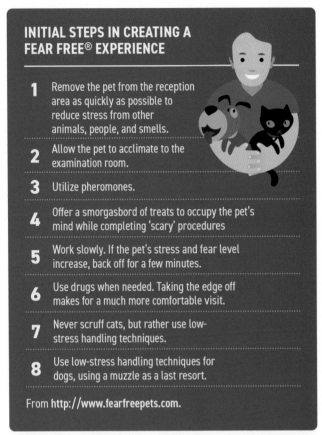

1 Remove the pet from the reception area as quickly as possible to reduce stress from other animals, people, and smells.

2 Allow the pet to acclimate to the examination room.

3 Utilize pheromones.

4 Offer a smorgasbord of treats to occupy the pet's mind while completing 'scary' procedures

5 Work slowly. If the pet's stress and fear level increase, back off for a few minutes.

6 Use drugs when needed. Taking the edge off makes for a much more comfortable visit.

7 Never scruff cats, but rather use low-stress handling techniques.

8 Use low-stress handling techniques for dogs, using a muzzle as a last resort.

From **http://www.fearfreepets.com.**

Fig. 3.21 Practices that encompass the Fear Free® have higher client compliance and retention rates than those that do not.

Monitoring Pet Behaviors

When clients are waiting for appointments, they may try and interact with other patients, clients, or children. Dogs may try to attack each other, and cats not in carriers could claw owners to escape. Team members should ensure that every dog is on a leash and provide one when necessary. If cats are not in a carrier, team members may offer to lend a carrier or place the cat in a kitty condo until a room is ready. Team members should make every effort to avoid accidents or injury in the reception area

Pets may arrive at the practice stressed and fearful, and most often, receptionists see these pets as they enter. Fig. 3.22 provides characteristics that stressed pets will display. Team members help reduce stress by:

- Getting patients into exam rooms as soon as possible to reduce interactions with other patients.
- Utilizing exam rooms with pheromones and explaining to clients that it is important that the pet have time to adjust and get comfortable before team members enter.
- Playing soft, classical music in the exam rooms to help pets and clients relax.
- Offering the pet a few treats to begin the calming process.
- Advising team members when a fearful or stressed patient has been placed in the exam room.
- Patients sometimes need medications to help reduce extreme stress levels. Relay this information to the medical team in case medications need to be administered before an exam occurs.

Monitoring Child Interactions

Children occasionally attempt to pet other animals in the waiting room which may be dangerous to the child or could facilitate the spread of contagious disease. Team members may need to remind parents of

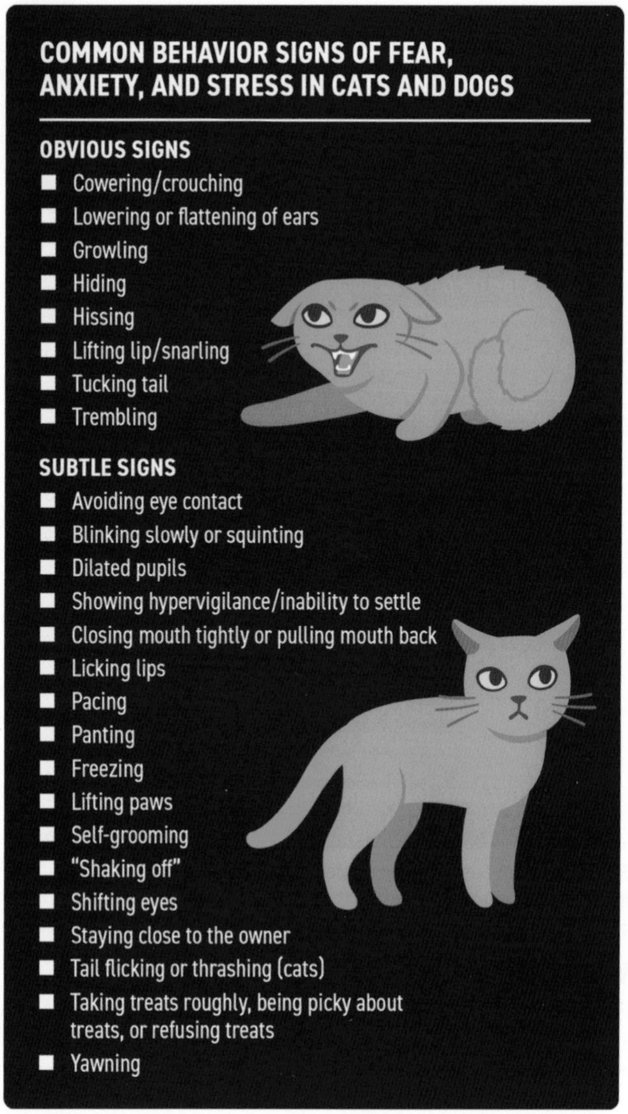

COMMON BEHAVIOR SIGNS OF FEAR, ANXIETY, AND STRESS IN CATS AND DOGS
OBVIOUS SIGNS
Cowering/crouching
Lowering or flattening of ears
Growling
Hiding
Hissing
Lifting lip/snarling
Tucking tail
Trembling
SUBTLE SIGNS
Avoiding eye contact
Blinking slowly or squinting
Dilated pupils
Showing hypervigilance/inability to settle
Closing mouth tightly or pulling mouth back
Licking lips
Pacing
Panting
Freezing
Lifting paws
Self-grooming
"Shaking off"
Shifting eyes
Staying close to the owner
Tail flicking or thrashing (cats)
Taking treats roughly, being picky about treats, or refusing treats
Yawning

Fig. 3.22 All team members must be trained on identifying FAS for the best patient experience.

these dangers while in the waiting room and be particularly observant of children; not all pets are fond of children.

> **LEADERSHIP POINT**
>
> Creating a child play area in the reception area can reduce attempted interactions with other patients.

Monitoring Lobby Cleanliness

Unfortunately, many clients do not inform veterinary team members when their pet has urinated in the waiting room or may not notice when they have urinated. Team members should scan the waiting room several times per hour for urine on the floor to prevent clients from slipping or falling and to prevent the odor from permeating the practice.

Scheduling Appointments

While all team members are responsible for creating appointments, the receptionist team likely creates the most. Appointment requests may come through phone calls, text messages, app notifications, or pet portals (Chapter 8, Practice Management Integrative Software). Medical team members may forward book medical progress exams, vaccine boosters, or biannual/annual exams, or ask the reception team to schedule them upon checkout. Chapter 10 provides details on the scheduling of appointments, but it is important to remember that the reception team can control the flow of chaos in the hospital by scheduling efficiently. It is helpful when sick appointments are interlaced with wellness exams, vaccines, or medical progress exams. This will allow the medical team to "catch up," even if it is just a few minutes of extra time. The reception team must also remind the medical team when appointments are running behind (and the medical team must identify how the delay happened to get back on track) and look for opportunities to increase efficiency by accepting drop-off patients. Cross training with the medical team helps receptionists better understand hospital flow, efficiency gaps, and collaborative opportunities for improvement.

Accepting Payment for Services

All team members contribute to the tasks that lead up to the client providing payment for services rendered, whether that is through the delivery of a patient treatment plan, for clients that are checked out in the exam room, or the receptionist accepting payment for a patient that is in the hospital and ready to be discharged.

When the medical team has appropriately presented a treatment plan to a client and the client agrees to the services recommended, presenting the invoice and accepting payment is easy. It is when this process is skipped that the receptionist becomes the target of an angry client. See Chapter 11 for treatment plan delivery and the reviewing of an invoice with a client prior to accepting payment to continue creating a frictionless client experience.

The most common forms of payment are by credit card (including debit card), check, or cash. The practice manager may choose which credit cards to accept (VISA, Mastercard, Discover, American Express, Care Credit). To increase efficiency and decrease manual errors, credit card terminals should be fully integrated with the PIMS (Chapter 8), and if client check out is provided in the exam room, each exam room should have a terminal.

> **CRITICAL COMPETENCY: CONTINUOUS LEARNING**
>
> Practice managers should have a curiosity for learning. Actively seeking out new information, technologies, and methods while keeping skills updated allows the application of new knowledge to the job.

Practices pay a percentage of the total credit card transaction through merchant fees; however, if a client uses their card as a debit transaction (versus credit), the practice pays less in fees. Therefore, team members are encouraged to ask clients if they would like to use their debit card for the transaction (if the practice accepts debit). Additionally, if a team member types in a card number versus swiping the card, the transaction fee paid by the practice is higher. If a practice does not currently accept debit cards and the team must type in the credit card number, practice managers should investigate alternative options. Industry benchmarks for credit card fees average 1.5% of gross revenue.

> **LEADERSHIP POINT**
>
> If the practice accepts debit cards as a form of payment, ask clients (when a card is presented for payment) if they would like to use debit.

CareCredit is a healthcare financing credit card that can be used for veterinary services (other divisions of CareCredit are available for human medical care). Clients can apply either online or while at the practice. A receptionist can enter client information online and approval can be received in as little as 10 minutes. CareCredit generally runs specials for first-time card users. Visit http://www.carecredit.com/vetmed for current information. In addition, many veterinary practices in the United States accept CareCredit, allowing clients to charge expenses related to veterinary care costs if their pet has an emergency after hours or is referred to a specialist for further care.

According to the Red Flags Rule established by the Federal Trade Commission, any credit card transaction should be verified with photo identification. The Red Flags Rule has been developed to help decrease fraud and the use of stolen credit cards. Visit the Federal Trade Commission website at http://www.ftc.gov/bcp/edu/microsites/redflagsrule/index.shtml for more information on Red Flags Rules.

Accepting cash has associated risks as cash can be counterfeit. Counterfeit money has no value, and detecting the passer can be difficult if they are not caught at the time of presenting the cash. Special pens can be used to mark bills that aid in counterfeit detection, and the practice's bank should be consulted for tips to share with the team to recognize counterfeit money.

EXAMPLE OF TRANSACTION TOTALS REPORT

ABC VETERINARY CLINIC

Transaction Totals	4/1/23
Total Invoices	$6,527.69
Total Cash	$1,009.65
Total Checks	$382.96
Total Credit Card	$4,105.08
Total Payment	$5,497.69
Total A/R	$1,030.00

Fig. 3.23 Receptionists are responsible for reconciling transactions at the end of the day. The total of payments received (cash, checks, and credit cards) must equal the total invoices from the practice management report.

Large amounts of cash should be kept in a separate locked safe, out of sight from clients. It only takes a second for a client or person off the street to reach over the counter and grab money from the drawer. Cash drawers should have a lock and be locked immediately after they are closed. Drawers should never be left unattended; one moment of inattention can result in the loss of hundreds of dollars.

When accepting checks, the receptionist must always make sure the check is signed, dated, and written for the correct amount. Check-processing machines benefit practices by being able to verify that funds are available in the client's account when a check is presented (thereby eliminating bounced checks). Checks are swiped through a terminal (much like a credit card), and when the transaction is approved, money is automatically withdrawn from the client's account and deposited into the practice's bank account. If the client has insufficient funds in the account, the transaction will be declined, and the client will need to provide another source of payment.

Daily Reconciliation

Reconciling forms of payment at the end of the day is a crucial task. Incomplete transactions, errors, missing money, credit card receipts, or checks must all be reconciled when balancing. It is much easier to find errors at the end of the day than to search for them the next day or the next week. Fig. 3.23 is an example of a transaction totals report, demonstrating the total dollar amount of closed invoices for the day, the total cash, checks, and credit cards that were collected (equals total payment,) and the total dollars for accounts receivable (clients that received a service, the invoice was closed, but they did not make a payment). It is important to recognize that total invoices may not equal total payment unless every client paid the full amount of their invoice that day.

Reconciliation is the process of matching and comparing figures from a transaction totals report (from the PIMS) with the actual receipts and funds accepted as payments. The balance of the transaction totals report must match the total funds. Practices may have different methods of ensuring reconciliation, but the goal is the same; the daily total transaction report must equal the total dollar amount of payments received. If they are not the same, the team must identify and correct the discrepancy.

The cash drawer or register may contain an "opening" amount of cash (various sizes of bills and coins) predetermined by the practice manager. It should be the same amount every day, comprised of a variety of bills to give change when needed. A recommendation may be $200, broken into one $20 bill, four $10 bills, eight $5 bills, 50 $1 bills, and $50 in quarters, dimes, nickels, and pennies. At the end of the day, the total amount in the cash drawer should be $200 plus any cash payments made by clients, (Fig. 3.24A) which must match the total cash amount on the daily total transaction sheet. If the remaining cash does not equal $200, the discrepancy must be found and corrected. Once

ABC ANIMAL CLINIC			TRANSACTION TOTALS	4/1/23	
Total Invoices	$6,527.69				
Total Cash	$1,009.65	(A)	Cash Counted	$1,209.65	(E)
Total Checks	$382.96	(B)	Checks Counted	$382.96	(F)
Total Credit Card	$4,105.08	(C)	Credit Card Slips Counted	$4,105.08	(G)
Total Payment	$5,497.69	(D)	Total Counted	$5,697.69	(H)
Total A/R	$1,030.00	(I)			

A = E + $200.00

B = F

C = G

D = H - $200.00 (starting cash balance)

Fig. 3.24 Transaction totals sheet with explanation.

the cash is balanced, the cash from client payments should be removed from the cash drawer and set aside for the daily deposit.

The checks must also be reconciled and compared against the check totals on the daily total transaction report (Fig. 3.24B). If a check machine is used, team members should "batch out" at the end of the day. The total on the check batch report must match the total of the checks as well as the daily transaction report. If they do not match, the discrepancy must be found and corrected. If a check machine is not used, checks must be totaled and compared with payment records; again, if a discrepancy exists, the discrepancy must be found and corrected.

Credit card slips must also be totaled and matched against the daily transaction total report (Fig. 3.24C). If there are any missing credit card slips or transactions, the discrepancy must be found and corrected. Credit card machines will also need to be batched out at the end of the day, and the total on the batch sheet must match the total of the credit card slips and the transaction report. Finally, the cash, checks, and credit cards must equal the total on the daily transaction report (Fig. 3.24D). If they do not match, the error must be found.

Credit card slips and checks deposited through an automatic check machine need to be stored in a safe and locked place. These documents should be kept for 7 years (depending on state law) for tax purposes and in the event of a client disputing charges.

As a last check (Fig. 3.24):

- A + B + C = D, and E + F + G = H.
- B = F and C = G.
- D = H − $200 (the starting cash balance).
- I = Accounts Receivable

If discrepancies exist, team members must be held accountable. Discrepancies must be identified and corrected before team members leave for the day.

Deposits

Deposits to the bank are recorded on a deposit slip; cash is entered on the cash line and checks are entered individually. If a check machine is used, the checks do not need to be deposited at the end of the day (because they have been electronically deposited). For practices without check machines, checks should be stamped "for deposit only, ABC Veterinary Clinic" on the back, including an account number. The cash and checks are totaled and entered at the bottom of the deposit slip. This total must match the cash and check total on the transaction sheet. Deposits should be made daily because it is unsafe to leave large amounts of cash in the office.

It is important to have a checks-and-balances system in place. All totals should match and must be double-checked. It is very important to eliminate errors as much as possible; double-checking a team member's work helps. The person checking the transactions as well as the team member double-checking the work should initial each transaction total.

Any adding machine tapes should be banded around receipts from checks and credit cards in case any questions arise regarding reconciliation. Deposit totals can be recorded in the practice checkbook or accounting software by the practice manager. The practice manager should always compare deposits from the bank statement to the transaction totals report.

Petty Cash

Petty cash is a term used to describe cash set aside in the practice to purchase items needed for the business when a check is not available. For example, the medical team may need some turkey meat for a patient that will not eat regular dog food. In this situation, a team member can take some money from the petty cash bag and purchase the meat. A receipt must be returned and placed in the bag for balancing and reconciliation purposes. The money should be counted at the end of every shift to ensure that money is not missing and that receipts account for any money spent.

The Medical Record

Practices may use paper medical records, be paperless, or be paper light. Paper medical records must be kept on 8½ × 11-inch sheets of paper (index cards are no longer acceptable) and each animal should have its own medical record as part of the overall client file. The medical record should be dated each time an entry is made, listing the presenting problems and the author's initials. Paperless and paper light practices will auto-date with each entry, and if the PIMS is set up appropriately, will include the initials of the team member logged into that computer at that time. Regardless of the type of medical records, every client conversation, consent form, laboratory report, consultation, physical examination, and medication administered and dispensed, must be documented in the medical record.

Paperless practices have the benefit of being more efficient (no need to search for lost medical records), saving space, and being able to access patient records, laboratory results, and radiographs from any computer station. See Chapter 9 for a complete medical records discussion.

FORMS COMMONLY USED IN VETERINARY PRACTICE

Clients may be asked to fill out various forms regarding their personal contact information their pet's information and history, or a variety of release forms. Team members need to be sure all forms are filled out completely when a new client enters information. Obviously, contact information is vital to reach the owner with updates regarding his or her pet's health. Address/email information must be current so that reminders may be mailed/emailed for vaccines, lab work, and/or medication refills. Any time a client returns to the practice, team members should verify that the contact information in the record is still current. It is also important that the client sign the bottom of the form, which should state that the client is responsible for any charges regarding the listed patients. It is also advised to ask the client (if they did not indicate already) if they have a spouse or significant other that they would like on the medical record. Only the owner(s) name(s) listed in the medical record can authorize treatment for the pet. In addition, when an account balance is due, the overdue invoice can only be discussed with those listed in the medical record.

The pet's information is an essential portion of the record. Details should include species, gender, date of birth, breed, color, and alteration status. Species refers to the classifications of dog, cat, bird, rabbit, reptile, and so forth (Fig. 3.25). Team members must learn about breeds within a species; owners can be easily offended when team members are unfamiliar with their pet's breed. Purebred animals are generally easy to classify; mixed breeds can be referred to by the breed they most resemble. Mixed-breed cats can be difficult to classify and are generally described by their hair coat. Domestic shorthair refers to a short-haired cat, domestic medium hair refers to a cat with medium-length hair, and domestic longhair refers to a long-haired cat. If a practice is paperless or paper light, this document should be scanned into, and become a part of the patient's medical record, especially if a signature is included indicating they agree to payment terms.

Consent Forms

Clients should always be asked to sign a consent form before treatments and/or procedures can be performed on their pets (Figs 3.26A and B). Every member of the team must be able to explain the meaning of any form a client is asked to sign. The forms are usually self-explanatory;

Species	Commonly Referred to as:	Abbreviation in PIMs
Canine	Dog	K-9 or Ca
Feline	Cat	Fe
Avian	Bird	Av
Iguanas, snakes, etc.	Reptile	Re
Lagomorph	Rabbit	Ra
Equine	Horse	Eq
Bovine	Cow	Bo

Fig. 3.25 Species identification chart.

however, team members must read the consent forms aloud to the client, ensuring the client understands what they are signing. The purpose of consent forms is to protect the veterinary health care team; if the form is documented in the record, it can be submitted if a court case arises. If the form or conversation is not documented, the assumption is that the risks, benefits, or information related to the procedure were never discussed or provided. All consent forms should contain the owner's and patient's names, the procedure the client is consenting to, along with the date and the initials of the team member explaining the forms to the client.

The information included on consent forms should include known risks, alternatives, prognosis, and possible complications. Anesthetic release forms clearly indicate that anesthesia could result in death. Vaccination release forms state the risks and benefits of vaccinating pets along with the possibility of an anaphylactic reaction, which may result in death. Euthanasia release forms state that the owner is presenting the pet for a painless, humane death. When reviewing any consent form, ensure that the person signing the documents is also listed on the medical record. If the person present is not listed on the medical record, they cannot consent to medical procedures.

Owners declining treatment or recommended diagnostic tests may also need to sign a release form based on practice policies. Owners can refuse pet vaccinations, heartworm preventatives, or tests for heartworm disease. In the best interest of the practice, the client should sign a release indicating that they do not hold the hospital, veterinarian, or any team member liable for any disease the client's pet may encounter when not accepting preventive measures recommended by the veterinarian and/or practice. When clients decline services of this nature, brochures and educational materials should be sent home with them. Sometimes, clients just need more information to decide. Always document literature that was sent home with the client in the medical record. This provides proof that additional information was given to the client, and if the client calls to ask about the handout, team members know which handout the client is referring to.

Patient History

A comprehensive patient medical history form helps collect information about new patients. Clients should fill out the form by answering questions regarding the pet's health history. This helps the veterinary team diagnostically if any problems arise. History forms can also include an area for the owner to sign that allows the practice to treat the patient and acknowledges that the owner agrees to pay for services rendered (on the day the service is provided). If the practice is paperless or paper light, this document must be scanned into the patient's medical record.

Master Problem List or Sheet

A master problem list/sheet is a summary of the patient's health status (Fig. 3.27) and is commonly used with both paperless and paper records. Vaccinations, laboratory tests, acute and chronic diseases, and current medications should be listed. Master problem lists increase efficiency when team members do not have to search through the entire record to find medication refill information, or when a pet is overdue for an examination, vaccinations, or laboratory work. Master problem lists should also include any vaccine, medication, or anesthetic reactions the pet may have had in the past.

Rabies Certificates

Rabies certificates are generated by the PIMS. The team member must enter the rabies tag number, lot number, and manufacturer of the vaccine. Lot numbers or serial numbers of vaccines are critical information that must be entered in the event of a recall. The PIMS will automatically populate client and patient information, and, depending on the software, the veterinary signature and license numbers. All are required for the printed certificate that the client receives.

If a rabies vaccine book (handwritten versus computer generated) is used, the correct owner and patient information must be legible. The date, of vaccination owner's name, address, phone number, patient's name, age, breed, and gender are required. The rabies tag number and lot number are then entered, along with the veterinarian's signature and license number. The rabies tag number helps identifies lost animals; therefore, it is important to ensure the information has been added correctly and legibly.

LEADERSHIP POINT

Rabies certificates and spay or neuter certificates should be made available to clients to automatically download from their pet portal or the practice app.

Spay or Neuter Certificates

Spay or neuter certificates are generated when a pet has been altered. This provides the owner with proof that the pet was altered if such proof is ever needed. This certificate may also be required when ordinances require pets to be registered with a city or county. Many city and county agencies require pets to be licensed, capping the number of pets allowed per household. All pets may be required to be licensed, including dogs, cats, rabbits, and ferrets, as well as some exotic species. Practices should be familiar with local laws regarding pet licensing. Local chapters of the Humane Society of the United States and animal shelters are excellent sources of information regarding laws and ordinances pertaining to pets.

Health Certificates

Health certificates are required by airlines and some state and federal agencies when traveling with pets. Airlines want to ensure the pet is in healthy condition before accepting it for transport and states want to ensure the pet is not importing any diseases. Both federal and state agencies are responsible for the prevention of disease and have various regulations regarding the entry of animals. Interstate health certificates are usually good for 10 days before shipment (Figs. 3.28A and B).

The pet must be fully examined by a USDA-accredited veterinarian before the certificate can be issued, and most states require submission of a copy of each health certificate that is issued. International health certificates are issued for pets traveling out of the United States and are usually good for 30 days (depending on the international

ABC Veterinary Clinic

Surgery/Anesthesia Consent Form

Client Name ______________________________ Date ______________

Pet's Name ______________________________

Your pet has been scheduled for a procedure requiring sedation or anesthesia. By signing this form, you authorize ABC Veterinary Clinic and its agents to administer tranquilizers, anesthetics, and/or analgesics that are deemed appropriate for your pet. Please be aware that all drugs have the potential for adverse side effects in any particular animal. The chances of such occurrence are extremely low.

I am aware that staff is not on premises after hours, and I agree to indemnify ABC Veterinary Clinic and its agents harmless from and against any and all liability arising from the care that is provided.

In an effort to ensure your pet's safety and to anticipate any problems before they may occur, we have available preanesthetic electrocardiogram and blood testing capabilities to detect hidden heart, liver, kidney, or other problems that may increase the risk to your pet. This testing is available for an additional charge. If abnormalities are detected, we will attempt to notify you, and the anesthetic procedure may be delayed or modified. Please verify the procedures being performed and indicate your wishes concerning the option of preanesthetic testing. If you have any questions, please ask BEFORE signing this form.

Procedures scheduled: ______________________________

Routine surgical procedures are painful. We recommend postoperative pain medication for each procedure. Pain medication is automatically dispensed for each patient. If you **decline postoperative pain medication, please sign here:** ______________________________

How may we contact you **today?** ______________________________

Home phone ______________ Work phone ______________

Cell phone/pager ______________ Client signature ______________

A

Pre-Anesthetic Blood Work Options

Please initial all options you are accepting.

______ Heartworm/Ehrlichia/Lymes test..$45.52
If not on prevention or tested recently

______ Feline Leukemia/FIV test..$44.87
If never tested and/or unknown history

______ CBC (Complete Blood Count)..$34.26
To check for anemia, clotting abilities, and infection
Recommended for all ages and all surgeries

______ Chemistry Profile Prep II..$48.76
To check liver and kidney function
Recommended for animals 6 years and younger for all anesthesia

______ Chemistry Profile Complete..$66.95
Full 12 chemistry profile
Recommended for animals 6 years and older for all anesthesia

______ CBC and Chemistry Profile Prep II..$73.51

______ CBC and Chemistry Profile Complete..$92.75

______ IV Catheter..$40.91
Open line for emergency medications and/or fluids
Recommended for all geriatric animals or patients with ongoing health risks

______ IV Catheter + Fluids..$63.68
To maintain blood pressure and hydration and for rapid recovery
Recommended for all geriatric animals or patients with ongoing health risks

______ HomeAgain Microchip..$38.81

______ E-Collar..$7 to $30

______ I have been advised of the importance of these options and have declined all blood work.

Signature ______________________________ Date ______________

B

Fig. 3.26 Example of an informed surgery/anesthesia consent form.

Master Problem List

Client name ______________________ Telephone number ______________________
Address ________________________________ Client number ____________________
Pet name _______________ Breed _______________ Color _______________________
Sex ___________ Altered ___________ DOB ____________ Age _________________

	Date received	Date received	Date received	Date received
DHLPP				
FVRCP				
FeLP				
Rabies				
HWT				
FeLV/FIV				

Chronic diseases/date of onset: ______________________________________

Current modifications and direction: ______________________________________

Fig. 3.27 Example of Master Problem List.

country's requirements) and require the signature of the examining USDA-accredited veterinarian, as well as the signature of the state veterinarian. Both forms of health certificates require the owner's name, address, and phone number along with the name, address, and phone number of the person who will be accepting and taking responsibility for the pet. All the animal's identifying information must be included, including age, breed, gender, and microchip or tattoo number. The animal's vaccines must be current, and all vaccination information (name of vaccine, manufacturer, and date administered) must be clearly stated on the form. Small animal and large animal health certificates differ; large animal certificates must indicate tests that have been completed (along with results). Before shipment to any state or country, regulations must be verified as some counties, states, or international countries have strict regulations regarding the importation of animals.

Some countries require a series of rabies vaccines and a rabies titer to import animals. The rabies-neutralizing antibody titer test (RNATT) is a general term for the methods that measure rabies virus-neutralizing antibody (RVNA) titers. Other countries may require a microchip before importation, along with deworming and the application of flea and tick preventive immediately before shipment. Visit the US Department of Agriculture at http://www.aphis.usda.gov/regulations/vs/iregs/animals/ for the most current information regarding animal importation procedures.

Medical Records Release Form

A signed consent form to release medical records may be required by some states. It is important to understand the Privacy Act and not release any records without the client's authorization. The Privacy Act of 1974 states, in part:

> "No agency shall disclose any record, which is contained in a system of records by any means of communication to any person, or to another agency, except pursuant to a written request by, or with the prior written consent of, the individual to whom the record pertains."

A medical records release should give an estimated time of when records will be available for pickup or will be emailed, and if there is a fee for the service (not recommended), that must be included. Keep in mind that clients should sign a medical records release before releasing records to boarding facilities or groomers.

Boarding Consent Form

It is common for boarding consent forms to be similar to other consent forms presented to clients, including a statement that releases the practice from liability should something happen to the pet, as well as authorizing the practice to treat any injuries that should occur while the pet is in the practice. They may also list services that are available that a client may elect (nail trims, anal gland expression, bathing, dental, annual exam, vaccines, fecal) (Fig. 3.29). When admitting a pet for boarding, it is important to document the names and dosages of medication(s) the pet will be receiving, what kind of food the animal eats (including at what frequency and times), what blankets and toys were brought by the owner, and emergency contact information in case of an emergency.

Many PIMS include consent forms that can be modified. When these consent forms are chosen by a team member, the client and carrier for transportation in commerce, unless accompanied by a health certificate executed and issued by a licensed veterinarian (7 USC 2143: 9 CFR, Subchapter A, Part 2).

(See reverse for additional OMB statement)

FORM APPROVED
OMB NO. 0579-0036)

U.S. DEPARTMENT OF AGRICULTURE
ANIMAL AND PLANT HEALTH INSPECTION SERVICE

UNITED STATES INTERSTATE AND INTERNATIONAL CERTIFICATE OF HEALTH EXAMINATION FOR SMALL ANIMALS

WARNING: Anyone who makes a false, fictitious, or fraudulent statement on this document, or uses such document knowing it to be false, fictitious or fraudulent may be subject to a fine of not more than $10,000 or imprisonment of not more than 5 years or both (18 U.S.C 1001).

1. TYPE OF ANIMAL SHIPPED
☐ Dog ☐ Cat ☐ Other
☐ Nonhuman Primate

CERTIFICATE NUMBER
P132195

2. TOTAL NUMBER OF ANIMALS

PAGE

3. NAME, ADDRESS AND TELEPHONE NUMBER OF OWNER/CONSIGNOR

USDA License/or Registration No. if applicable Telephone:

4. NAME, ADDRESS AND TELEPHONE NUMBER OF CONSIGNEE

USDA License/or Registration No. if applicable Telephone:

5. ANIMAL IDENTIFICATION *(To be completed by owner/consignor)*

6. VACCINATION HISTORY *(To be completed by veterinarian)* *attach original signature rabies certificate here*

COMPLETE USDA TAG COLLAR AND/OR TATTOO NUMBER	BREED - COMMON OR SCIENTIFIC NAME	AGE	SEX	COLOR OR DISTINCTIVE MARKS	RABIES ☐ Killed Virus ☐ Live Virus		D-H-L		OTHER VACCINATIONS, TESTS OR TREATMENT	
					Date	Product	Date	Product	Date	Type/Result
(1)										
(2)										
(3)										
(4)										
(5)										
(6)										
(7)										
(8)										
(9)										
(10)										

"X" applicable statements

☐ OWNER/CONSIGNOR CERTIFICATION: I certify that the information concerning the animals described above in Item 5 is true and correct, and that I am the owner/consignor of such described animals and that I have physical and legal custody of such animal (s).

☐ I hereby certify that the animal(s) in this shipment is (are), to the best of my knowledge acclimated to air temperatures lower than 7.2º c, (45º f).

SIGNATURE DATE

VETERINARY CERTIFICATION: I certify that the animal (s) described in item 5 have been examined by me this date, that the information provided in item 6 is true and accurate to the best of my knowledge, and that the following findings have been made "X" applicable statements.

☐ I certify that the animal (s) described and on continuation sheet(s) if applicable, have been inspected by me this date and appear to be free of any infectious or contagious diseases and to the best of my knowledge, exposure there to, which would endanger the animal or other animals or would endanger public health.

☐ I certify that the animal (s) described above, and on continuation sheet(s) if applicable, have been inspected by me this date and appear to be free of physical abnormalities which would endanger the animal.

☐ To my knowledge the animal (s) described above, and on continuation sheet(s) if applicable, originated from an area not quarantined for rabies and have not been exposed to rabies.

ENDORSEMENT FOR INTERNATIONAL EXPORT (WARNING: International Shipments require certification by an accredited veterinarian. States may also require such certification).

Apply USDA Seal or Stamp here

SIGNATURE OF USDA VETERINARIAN DATE

NAME, ADDRESS AND TELEPHONE NUMBER

Telephone:

LICENSE NO.

Accredited ☐ Yes ☐ No

LICENSING STATE

SIGNATURE DATE

APHIS FORM 7001 (AUG 2001) Replaces edition of (Aug 94) which may be used This certificate is valid for 30 days after issuance

PART 1 - TO ACCOMPANY SHIPMENT

A

No.

INTERSTATE ☐
EXHIBITION ☐
SALE ☐

OFFICIAL HEALTH CERTIFICATE
(COVERING CANINE, FELINE AND OTHER SMALL ANIMALS ONLY)

OWNER OR CONSIGNOR ____________ CONSIGNEE ____________

ADDRESS ____________ DESTINATION ____________
STREET STREET

CITY STATE CITY STATE

DESCRIPTION OF ANIMALS

SPECIES	BREED	SEX	AGE	COLOR AND MARKINGS	VACCINATION TAG NO.

IMMUNIZATION DATA

RABIES VACCINATION TYPE USED ____________ DATE ____________

DISTEMPER IMMUNIZATION (PERMANENT OR ANTI-SERUM) TYPE USED ____________ DATE ____________

HEPATITIS IMMUNIZATION (PERMANENT OR ANTI-SERUM) ____________ TYPE USED ____________ DATE ____________

I hereby certify that I have examined the above described animals and find same to be free from symptoms of contagious or infectious disease, and to the best of my knowledge and belief the above animals have not been exposed to infectious or contagious disease. I also certify that I am licensed by the State of New Mexico and accredited by the New Mexico Livestock Board and U.S. Department of Agriculture for the issuance of Health Certificates for interstate and international shipments. NOTE: Subject to requirements of state of destination.

CLINIC NAME DATE ISSUED SIGNATURE ACCREDITED VETERINARIAN

FORM NO. 15 4/04

B

Fig. 3.28 Example of (A) International health certificate and (B) interstate health certificate.

Arroyo Vista Animal Clinic

2303 Inspiration Lane, Anywhere, USA

Dr. Larsen, Dr. Cooke and Dr. Thompson

Boarding Admission Form

Owner____________________ Date__________

Address____________________ Phone__________

City__________ In case of Emergency, please call __________

Pets Name__________ Breed__________ Sex______ Age______ Color_____

Date of last vaccine:__________ Please circle which vaccine: DHPP FVRCP FeLV

Date of last Rabies __________ Date of last Bordetella__________

Medications while boarding____________________

Belongings____________________

Pets Name__________ Breed__________ Sex______ Age______ Color_____

Date of last vaccine:__________ Please circle which vaccine: DHPP FVRCP FeLV

Date of last Rabies __________ Date of last Bordetella__________

Medications while boarding ____________________

Belongings____________________

Pets Name__________ Breed__________ Sex______ Age______ Color_____

Date of last vaccine:__________ Please circle which vaccine: DHPP FVRCP FeLV

Date of last Rabies __________ Date of last Bordetella__________

Medications while boarding____________________

Belongings ____________________

While boarding, please perform the following procedures:

Physical Exam________ Vaccinations____________________

Heartworm Test__________ Bath __________ Dip______ Nail Trim_______

Other: 1: ____________________

2: ____________________

3: ____________________

4: ____________________

All animals entering the hospital must be up to date on vaccination and free of external parasites (Fleas, ticks) or they will be treated upon admission at the owners' expense.

I authorize Arroyo Vista Animal Clinic to treat my pet(s) in case an emergency situation should arise.

Pets are released only during the regular office hours. It is my responsibility to inform the hospital if I will be delayed in picking up my pets; I will assume all costs associated with an extended stay.

Owners signature____________________ Date__________

Fig. 3.29 Sample boarding form.

patient information is automatically populated; the form can then be printed and reviewed with the owner or provided in an electronic format that the client can sign on a signature pad.

CREATING THE EXCEPTIONAL FINALE IN THE FRICTIONLESS CLIENT EXPERIENCE AS A TEAM EVENT

Chapter 11, The Client Experience, provides specific detail that allows a practice to provide a frictionless client experience every time the client visits the practice. Each team member has a significant role in creating that experience, starting with leadership to implement tools that increase efficiency and make it easy for the client to do business with the practice. Chapter 8, Practice Integrative Management Software, details technologies that are available to achieve this goal.

The team must be fully on board with utilizing technologies while also recommending them to clients. Making appointments online, requesting medication refills, two-way texting, practice apps, and practice portals allow a seamless client experience, but the team must recommend them to the clients to increase awareness. When the team is enthusiastic about technology, the client will immediately embrace it, especially if they have heard about it from several team members (remember, clients need to "hear" a recommendation three times to fully grasp the concept).

> **CRITICAL COMPETENCY: PERSUASION**
>
> The practice manager must possess the ability to change the attitudes and opinions of others, persuade them to accept recommendations, and encourage behaviors that support practice goals.

Consider the very last interaction the client and patient have with the practice. It is the first and last impressions that stick in the memory of clients. How can the practice make the check-out experience the most memorable, exceptional experience? Whether clients are checked out in the exam room or the reception desk, the process is relatively the same.

- Review the medical recommendations made by the medical team and ask if there are questions, deliver medications, review dosage instructions if applicable, forward book upcoming appointments (Chapter 10), and review the invoice and services provided (Chapter 11).

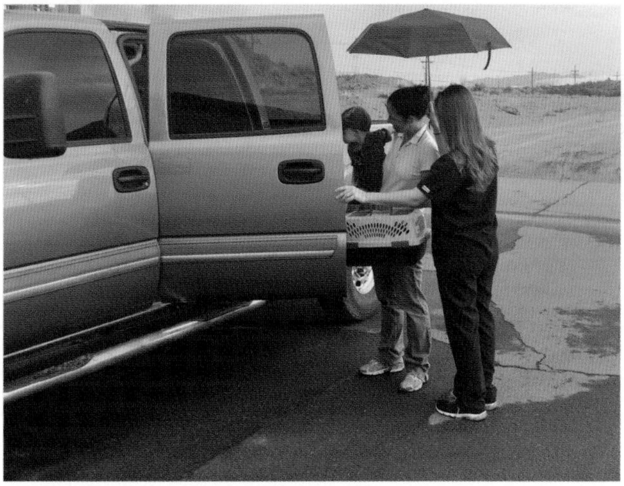

Fig. 3.30 A team member provides extra service by holding an umbrella for a client as they get into their car.

- Once the transaction is complete (the interaction is not done yet), help the client get to their car (don't ask if help is needed, just do it!). Carry food, pet carriers, or medication for the owner. If it is raining outside, provide umbrella service; walk the client out holding the umbrella over their head, keeping them dry getting into their car (Fig. 3.30). These thoughtful acts build long-lasting client bonds. These actions are the foundation of providing exceptional customer service.
- Follow up with every client, every time. When to follow up depends on what service was provided. If a puppy or kitten received vaccinations, call the client that night, making sure the pet handled the vaccinations without any side effects. This can be a great time to readdress the characteristics associated with mild vaccine reactions, or perhaps answer questions the client has since the visit earlier. If a pet had surgery or was released from the hospital that day, call the client that night (clients are most concerned about their pet the first night at home, so make the time to call and check on the patient). Last but not least, ask clients how their service experience was. They may tell you their wait time was too long, which gives you an opportunity to apologize. Or they might compliment your service, which you can gladly share with the members. Additionally, develop a follow-up survey that clients can submit to the practice anonymously (see Chapter 11 for more details and ideas).

Mediocre service may sustain a practice for years; however, outstanding service builds the client and practice bond, develops pride in team members, adds value to the practice's reputation, and increases profitability.

LEADERSHIP ROLE IN THE VETERINARY TEAM

The practice manager and owner set the expectations for team members to work as a team, develop trust with one another, and establish a culture of accountability. Highly cohesive teams drive higher client compliance rates, lower employee turnover rates, and achievement of strategic goals. Keep in mind, creating this environment is not a one-and-done process; it is an ongoing daily activity.

For the veterinary team to deliver a frictionless client experience, the leadership team must put into place all the tools needed by the team to achieve that goal. How can you, as a leader, make it easy for the team to do their job, and love what they do?

Make sure trust is established between all roles, reducing the variability of gossip and cliques. Ensure team members are trained and expectations are clear, allowing them to be utilized to their highest potential. And watch for behaviors that demonstrate respect (or lack of) for one another. No role, or person, is more important than the others. This is 100% the role of the leadership team.

PRACTICE MANAGER SURVIVAL CHECKLIST FOR SUPPORTING THE VETERINARY TEAM

- ☐ Develop a list of common questions new team members should be trained on during the onboarding process.
- ☐ Develop daily opening procedures (cash is accounted for and balanced).
- ☐ Develop daily closing procedures (cash, check, and credit card balances with daily reconciliation and deposit slips).
- ☐ Develop and implement a schedule to back up the computer data and check the backup to ensure it is retrievable.

REVIEW QUESTIONS

1. Provide some behaviors that demonstrate etiquette to fellow team members.
2. Why is the end-of-day reconciliation important to complete before the team leaves for the evening?
3. Define work ethic.
4. When should receptionists reconcile the transactions to ensure they are all correct?
   a. Daily, at the end of the day
   b. Weekly
   c. Daily, at the beginning of the following day
   d. On an as-needed basis
5. What is the purpose of requiring owners to sign consent forms?
   a. To ensure the owner understands why they are leaving their pet
   b. To protect the veterinary practice and team members from any issues that may arise and may need to be submitted in the case of a lawsuit
   c. To satisfy state law
   d. All the above
6. Which of the following is a requirement for becoming a credentialed Veterinary Technician?
   a. Passing only the state licensing examination
   b. Graduating from a 2-year veterinary technology program approved by the AVMA
   c. Obtaining at least 5 years of experience in the related field and then passing licensure examination
   d. None of the above
7. Which of the following is a responsibility of a veterinary assistant?
   a. Restraint of animals
   b. Client satisfaction
   c. Laboratory sample preparation
   d. All the above
   e. Both A and C

8. What does NAVTA stand for?
   a. Nationally Accredited Veterinary Technologist of America
   b. National Association of Veterinary Teams of America
   c. National Association of Veterinary Technicians in America
   d. None of the above
9. Which of the following are responsibilities of a Practice Manager?
   a. Overseeing only the front office staff
   b. Managing only the finances of the practice
   c. Ensuring the correct staff members are hired for team management
   d. Having multiple responsibilities covering all employees, client relations, finances, and overall maintenance of the practice
10. Which of the following are required of a veterinarian?
   a. Obtaining continuing education requirements each year
   b. Passing both national and state licensing examinations
   c. Graduating from an AVMA-accredited school of veterinary medicine
   d. All the above

RECOMMENDED READING

Wilson JF. *Legal consent forms for the veterinary practice*. 4th ed. Priority Press; 2006.

Martin D. Fear Free^{SM} and the veterinary nurses' role. *The NAVTA Journal*. December/January 2018:15–21.

Bassert JA. *McCurnin's clinical textbook for veterinary technicians*. 10th ed. Saunders Elsevier; 2021.

Fanning J, Shepherd AJ. Contribution of veterinary technicians to veterinary business revenue. *JAVMA*. 2010:236–846.

Fear Free Grooming Certification Program overview. Fear Free Pets. Published October 3, 2018. Accessed August 1, 2022. https://fearfreepets.com/fear-free-groomer-certification-course-overview/

4

Human Resources in the Veterinary Practice

LEARNING OBJECTIVES

When you have completed this chapter, you should be able to:

- Discuss specific laws associated with human resources
- Identify required posters
- Develop an employee personnel manual
- Develop Standard Operating Protocols
- Develop a wage scale for each role in the veterinary practice.
- Describe how to maintain payroll files
- Develop team training protocols
- Compare and review resumes
- Discuss methods used to interview candidates effectively
- List questions that can legally be asked of candidates
- List methods used to effectively terminate team members

OUTLINE

KEY TERMS

401(k)
1099-MISC
Benefits
COBRA
Direct Deposit
Employee Manual
Employee Polygraph Protection Act
Equal Employment Opportunity
Exempt Team member
ERISA
Fair Credit Reporting Act
FLSA
FMLA
FUTA
Independent Contractor
IRCA
Noncompete Agreement
Nonexempt Team member

Organizational Behavior
OSHA
Psychological harassment
Resume
SEPs
sIRA
Standard Operating Protocols
USERRA
W-2
W-4
Workers' Compensation Insurance

VHMA PERFORMANCE DOMAINS

Veterinary Hospital Managers Association (VHMA) Performance Domains

The Human Resource Performance domain is applicable to this chapter. The veterinary practice manager plans, directs, and coordinates the human resource management activities of the organization. Work activities include recruiting and hiring staff, providing guidance and direction to subordinates, setting performance standards and monitoring performance, and scheduling the work of others. Tasks also include:

- Manage personnel training and development programs
- Develop work schedules for staff and manage daily work assignments
- Conduct staff meetings
- Provide employee performance reviews
- Mediate internal disputes between team members
- Discipline and discharge team members
- Manage employee benefits programs
- Maintain confidential employee records
- Create, review, and update job descriptions and manuals
- Manage staff continuing education and licensure/certification

Application of VHMA Performance Domains for Practice Managers

The human resource performance domain requires knowledge of principles and procedures for recruitment, selection, training, and evaluation of personnel; leadership and management principles involve strategic planning, compensation, and scheduling.

INTRODUCTION

Human resource responsibilities are numerous within the practice with functions including (but not limited to) recruiting and hiring staff, providing guidance and direction to team members, setting performance standards, coaching and monitoring performance, and creating a team schedule. Typically, the veterinary practice manager plans, directs, and coordinates the human resource management activities for the practice. If the practice is owned by a corporate entity, some HR functions may be centralized at the home office; however, practice leaders continue to lead the culture, train and develop the team, manage conflict, coach people to greatness, and serve as an advocate for team members.

ORGANIZATIONAL BEHAVIOR

Basic management of a veterinary practice includes organizational development and team member development. Organizational development is the development, improvement, and effectiveness of an organization and includes the culture, values, system, and behaviors of such practice. Team member development contributes to the strategic goal achievement, culture, empowerment, learning, and problem-solving abilities of team members.

The vision of a practice is built by the owner and shared by the team. All team members should know what the vision of the practice is and contribute to it daily. With vision comes structure, practice culture, norms, codes of conduct, and core values. The culture created should be positive and provide an open communication policy for all team members. A code of conduct should be established and written in the employee manual so that all team members know what is expected of them. Review Chapter 2, Leadership, on the formation and implementation of core values, the mission and vision statements of the practice.

Team development is essential to the success of a practice. Creating the perfect team takes time and begins before team members are hired. It then continues with effective hiring procedures. Job descriptions must be detailed, and job responsibilities should be clear. Retaining the perfect team is of the utmost importance and must be a top priority for the practice. Encouraging teamwork and motivation will help ensure high team member retention rates, as does positive feedback, daily coaching, and feedback. Effective organizations have teams, not individuals.

LEADERSHIP POINT

Exceptional leadership is required to have effective human resource policies.

Leadership establishes the strategy and goals of the practice, but the implementation of such goals must be a collaborative effort with the team. Each team member needs to know and understand how their role contributes to goals and how they should strive to achieve those goals. Regularly scheduled team meetings should always review goals and how the team is helping to achieve them.

VHMA PRACTICE DOMAIN TASK

Practice managers conduct effective staff meetings.

The development of employee and procedure manuals (Standard Operating Protocols) takes time but greatly increases the efficiency and communication of a practice. By allowing the team to contribute to the development of manuals, fewer duties and descriptions are forgotten and more topics can be included. Manuals can help hold the team together and allow greater leadership in all areas of the practice. When a team creates manuals together, implementing and using them is achieved with greater success.

CRITICAL COMPETENCY: COMPLIANCE

Practice managers must be reliable, thorough, and conscientious in carrying out work assignments while having an appreciation for the importance of organizational rules and policies.

LAWS THAT REQUIRE FAMILIARITY

Before the team member manual can be developed, practice managers should have a clear understanding of laws and how they affect the veterinary practice. Laws and regulations change on a regular basis at both the federal and state levels. Every practice manager should be familiar with changes that occur, update the team with changes, and add to or modify the team member manual as needed. Membership in the Society for Human Resource Management (https://www.shrm.org)

can be extremely advantageous and provides a resource for practice managers to stay abreast of current federal and state changes.

VHMA PERFORMANCE DOMAIN TASK

Veterinary practice managers must understand and comply with employment and labor laws.

Required Posters

Posters informing team members of their rights regarding labor and employment laws are required and must be displayed in a location visible to all team members. Posters can be picked up at any local or state labor department free of charge and do not have to be purchased from solicitors (Fig. 4.1). Some states require more than these federally mandated posters. Visit the state department of labor for updated requirements.

Fair Labor and Standards Act

The Fair Labor and Standards Act (FLSA) was created to establish minimum wage and overtime pay standards, regulate the employment of minors, and define exempt and nonexempt team members (Fig. 4.2). Exempt team members are those that are salaried, and applies to any individual involved in executive, administrative, or professional duties. In the case of a professional team member, at least 80% of the duties must require knowledge of an advanced type of science or learning, artistic work, or teaching. Veterinarians and most practice managers qualify as exempt. Veterinary technicians/nurses, assistants, and receptionists are nonexempt team members and must be paid hourly, with overtime as applicable. Practices will receive large fines from the Department of Labor for not paying appropriate team member overtime.

The state, county, or city minimum wage may be higher or lower than the federal minimum wage. Whichever is higher supersedes the other. Minimum wage changes periodically, and managers should be aware of changes. Any team member working more than 40 hours in any workweek must be paid overtime at 1.5 times the regular rate of pay. The FLSA defines a work week as 7 consecutive 24-hour periods, a total of 168 hours. Some states have rules that supersede these federal guidelines, requiring overtime to be paid when work exceeds 8 hours in 1 day.

Veterinary team members are generally loyal and dedicated, and often work long hours; however, it is imperative that the practice manager monitor overtime hours. Working excess hours leads to burnout and mental exhaustion, ultimately causing team members to leave the practice.

Team members must be at least 16 years of age to work in non-farm-related jobs; youths who are 14 or 15 years old may be allowed to work outside school hours with a work permit. They can work only 3 hours per day during school days, and 8 hours per day on non-school days. Work cannot begin before 7 a.m. and cannot continue after 7 p.m. During the summer, hours are extended until 9 p.m. Work permits can usually be obtained from the youth's school district. Again, state regulations may supersede this federal law. Checking with the state department of labor is advised.

According to federal guidelines, employers are required to keep records on wages and hours for a minimum of 3 years after the termination of the team member. Some states require longer record retention.

- Family and Medical Leave Act
- Uniformed Services Employment and Reemployment Rights Act
- Fair Labor and Standards Act
- Equal Employment Opportunity
- Occupational Safety and Health Administration
- Immigration Reform and Control Act
- Employee Polygraph Protection Act

Fig. 4.1 Posters must be displayed for all employees to see, or businesses can receive a fine from the Department of Labor.

VHMA PRACTICE DOMAIN TASK

Practice managers understand and ensure compliance with regulatory agencies at the federal, state, and local levels.

The Family and Medical Leave Act (FMLA) was established in 1993 to protect and preserve the integrity of the family. FMLA applies to organizations with more than 50 team members; an organization with fewer team members is exempt from the act. It was designed to benefit team members without adversely affecting employers (Fig. 4.3), allowing team members to take as much as 12 weeks of unpaid leave for:

- Incapacity as a result of pregnancy, prenatal medical care, or childbirth;
- To care for the team member's child after birth, or arrange placement for adoption or foster care;
- To care for the team member's spouse, son, daughter, or parent who has a serious health condition; and
- A serious health condition that makes the team member unable to perform their job.

Military Family Leave Entitlements

Eligible team members whose spouse, son, daughter, or parent is on covered active duty, or call to covered active-duty status, may use their 12-week leave entitlement to address certain qualifying exigencies. Qualifying exigencies may include attending certain military events, arranging for alternative childcare, addressing certain financial and legal arrangements, attending certain counseling sessions, and attending post-deployment reintegration briefings.

The team member is guaranteed their job, or an equivalent one, upon return to work. Team members must have worked for the organization for at least 12 months, with at least 1250 hours acquired during those 12 months. The team member must give the employer at least 30 days' notice before leaving regarding when the period will begin and end. If these requirements are not met, the employer can deny the leave.

Uniformed Services Employment and Reemployment Rights Act

The Uniformed Services Employment and Reemployment Rights Act (USERRA) was created to protect individuals who are enrolled in any branch of military service. USERRA protects the rights of team members who voluntarily or involuntarily leave an employment position to undertake any military service. Employers cannot discriminate against past, present, and potential team members who are uniformed service members. Team members have the right to return to the employment position they had before leaving as well as any benefits that are or were available at that time (Fig. 4.4).

Immigration Reform and Control Act

The Immigration Reform and Control Act prohibits employment discrimination against any team member or potential team member because of national origin. Form I-9 should be filled out by new hires to confirm that they can legally work in the United States (Fig. 4.5). Form I-9 is required to be completed by employers and states that the

EMPLOYEE RIGHTS

UNDER THE FAIR LABOR STANDARDS ACT

FEDERAL MINIMUM WAGE

$7.25 PER HOUR

BEGINNING JULY 24, 2009

The law requires employers to display this poster where employees can readily see it.

OVERTIME PAY At least 1½ times the regular rate of pay for all hours worked over 40 in a workweek.

CHILD LABOR An employee must be at least 16 years old to work in most non-farm jobs and at least 18 to work in non-farm jobs declared hazardous by the Secretary of Labor. Youths 14 and 15 years old may work outside school hours in various non-manufacturing, non-mining, non-hazardous jobs with certain work hours restrictions. Different rules apply in agricultural employment.

TIP CREDIT Employers of "tipped employees" who meet certain conditions may claim a partial wage credit based on tips received by their employees. Employers must pay tipped employees a cash wage of at least $2.13 per hour if they claim a tip credit against their minimum wage obligation. If an employee's tips combined with the employer's cash wage of at least $2.13 per hour do not equal the minimum hourly wage, the employer must make up the difference.

NURSING MOTHERS The FLSA requires employers to provide reasonable break time for a nursing mother employee who is subject to the FLSA's overtime requirements in order for the employee to express breast milk for her nursing child for one year after the child's birth each time such employee has a need to express breast milk. Employers are also required to provide a place, other than a bathroom, that is shielded from view and free from intrusion from coworkers and the public, which may be used by the employee to express breast milk.

ENFORCEMENT The Department has authority to recover back wages and an equal amount in liquidated damages in instances of minimum wage, overtime, and other violations. The Department may litigate and/or recommend criminal prosecution. Employers may be assessed civil money penalties for each willful or repeated violation of the minimum wage or overtime pay provisions of the law. Civil money penalties may also be assessed for violations of the FLSA's child labor provisions. Heightened civil money penalties may be assessed for each child labor violation that results in the death or serious injury of any minor employee, and such assessments may be doubled when the violations are determined to be willful or repeated. The law also prohibits retaliating against or discharging workers who file a complaint or participate in any proceeding under the FLSA.

ADDITIONAL INFORMATION

- Certain occupations and establishments are exempt from the minimum wage, and/or overtime pay provisions.
- Special provisions apply to workers in American Samoa, the Commonwealth of the Northern Mariana Islands, and the Commonwealth of Puerto Rico.
- Some state laws provide greater employee protections; employers must comply with both.
- Some employers incorrectly classify workers as "independent contractors" when they are actually employees under the FLSA. It is important to know the difference between the two because employees (unless exempt) are entitled to the FLSA's minimum wage and overtime pay protections and correctly classified independent contractors are not.
- Certain full-time students, student learners, apprentices, and workers with disabilities may be paid less than the minimum wage under special certificates issued by the Department of Labor.

WHD WAGE AND HOUR DIVISION
UNITED STATES DEPARTMENT OF LABOR

1-866-487-9243
TTY: 1-877-889-5627
www.dol.gov/whd

WH1088 REV 07/16

Fig. 4.2 Fair Labor Standards Act.

employer has examined the required documents verifying employment eligibility. Verification documents include a birth or naturalization certificate, a U.S. passport, a valid foreign exchange passport authorizing employment in the United States, a resident alien card (green card), a Social Security card, and a driver's license or state identification card (Fig. 4.6).

Form I-9 should not be filled out until the first day of employment, and verification documents do not have to be copied. Managers must ensure the document is filled out entirely and correctly. Form I-9 can be inspected at any time, and violations for incomplete or incorrect forms can add up. Form I-9 must be kept for 3 years from the date of hire, or 1 year after termination, whichever is longer.

Employee Polygraph Protection Act

The Employee Polygraph Protection Act prohibits most employers from using lie detector tests for either preemployment screening or during employment. Employers cannot discriminate against team members who refuse to take a lie detector test. An exemption does apply to a veterinary practice that prescribes and dispenses controlled substances. It is advised to review this law further for additional information as it applies to veterinary medicine (Fig. 4.7).

Equal Employment Opportunity

Equal Employment Opportunity policy prohibits discrimination against team members based on race, color, sex, religion, or national origin. Employers cannot deny a promotion, terminate, or not hire a potential team member for any of those reasons. Equal Employment Opportunity also prevents discrimination against those with disabilities who can perform the job as described in the job duties (Fig. 4.8). The law also requires that organizations provide qualified applicants and team members with disabilities with reasonable accommodations that do not impose undue hardship on the employer. The Age Discrimination in Employment Act of 1967 protects applicants and current team members over the age of 40 years from discrimination based on age in hiring, promotion, discharge, and compensation. Title VII of the Civil Rights Act of 1964 prohibits sex discrimination in the payment of wages to men and women performing substantially equal work in the same establishment.

Occupational Safety and Health Administration

The Occupational Safety and Health Administration (OSHA) has set safety standards to protect team members. Employers must provide a safe work environment and comply with OSHA's safety (see Chapter 15 for more information). OSHA has the authority to inspect workplace environments without giving notice to the employer. Safety hazard plans should be in place to help protect team members from dangers and must be enforced by the employer daily (Fig. 4.9).

Pregnancy and Maternity Leave

State labor boards or commissions should be contacted to determine the most recent regulations regarding pregnancy and maternity leave. Some states/city ordinances require leave; others do not. Pregnancy is a protected class; mothers cannot be discriminated against. Team members can decide if they wish to continue working as their job description indicates. They can also ask for accommodations to help them carry out their job duties. If accommodations are requested, it is up to the employer to fulfill the request if it is within reasonable guidelines.

It is advised to state in the employee manual that team members inform management as soon as they are aware of the pregnancy so that all precautions can be addressed. A pregnant team member must decide what she can and cannot do. Safety issues can be addressed by leadership, such as radiation exposure, anesthesia, and heavy lifting; however, the team member must decide their own safety level. Her role cannot be reassigned unless she requests it.

> **LEADERSHIP POINT**
>
> DO NOT discriminate against an employee who is pregnant and remove them from their current position; allow them to decide if they should be moved to a temporary different role.

Sexual Harassment

Every team member must be protected from sexual harassment by both management and other team members. Sexual harassment is the uninvited and unwelcome verbal or physical behavior of a sexual nature, especially by a person in authority toward a subordinate. It can occur when unwelcomed sexual conduct has the purpose or effect of interfering with an individual's work performance or creating an offensive work environment. It can also occur when a supervisor conditions the granting of an employment benefit upon the receipt of sexual favors. Unwelcomed sexual conduct can be in the form of jokes, suggestive comments, insults, threats, suggestive noises, whistles, catcalls, touching, pinching, brushing against someone, assault, or coerced sexual intercourse. Policies must be developed, stated, and followed to protect the practice from a potential lawsuit. Promotion, demotion, or pay based on sexual innuendo cannot be allowed and must be clearly stated. The manual should also indicate with whom the team member should discuss possible sexual harassment violations and indicate that the discussion will occur without the possibility of retaliation. Practices must have a zero-tolerance policy when it comes to sexual harassment.

Psychological Harassment

Psychological harassment is just as important as sexual harassment. Bullying, gossiping, and creating a hostile work environment through behaviors that are not sexually related characterize psychological harassment. Psychological harassment can come from managers, leaders, or other coworkers. If a practice manager does not stop or prevent psychological harassment from a coworker, the manager can be charged with negligence. A zero-tolerance policy for both sexual and psychological harassment must be included in the team member manual.

> **LEADERSHIP POINT**
>
> Managers must handle any harassment claims immediately. The longer the claim is left unaddressed, the higher the risk of liability.

PERSONNEL FILES

A file of confidential information should be kept on each team member in locked filing cabinets that only the owner and practice manager can access. All information regarding a team member should be well organized for easy retrieval. Personnel files are broken into two main categories: personnel files and medical files. The personal file will contain the team member's application/resume, interview documents, employment verification, background checks, copies of credentials, offer letter, performance appraisals, training and development schedule, benefits, wages salary schedule, and any termination documents. The medical file will contain health and life insurance documents, any medical leave requests, accident reports, or workers' compensation claims.

> **VHMA PERFORMANCE DOMAIN TASK**
>
> Veterinary practice managers maintain confidential team member records.

EMPLOYEE RIGHTS

UNDER THE FAMILY AND MEDICAL LEAVE ACT

THE UNITED STATES DEPARTMENT OF LABOR WAGE AND HOUR DIVISION

LEAVE ENTITLEMENTS

Eligible employees who work for a covered employer can take up to 12 weeks of unpaid, job-protected leave in a 12-month period for the following reasons:

- The birth of a child or placement of a child for adoption or foster care;
- To bond with a child (leave must be taken within one year of the child's birth or placement);
- To care for the employee's spouse, child, or parent who has a qualifying serious health condition;
- For the employee's own qualifying serious health condition that makes the employee unable to perform the employee's job;
- For qualifying exigencies related to the foreign deployment of a military member who is the employee's spouse, child, or parent.

An eligible employee who is a covered servicemember's spouse, child, parent, or next of kin may also take up to 26 weeks of FMLA leave in a single 12-month period to care for the servicemember with a serious injury or illness.

An employee does not need to use leave in one block. When it is medically necessary or otherwise permitted, employees may take leave intermittently or on a reduced schedule.

Employees may choose, or an employer may require, use of accrued paid leave while taking FMLA leave. If an employee substitutes accrued paid leave for FMLA leave, the employee must comply with the employer's normal paid leave policies.

BENEFITS & PROTECTIONS

While employees are on FMLA leave, employers must continue health insurance coverage as if the employees were not on leave.

Upon return from FMLA leave, most employees must be restored to the same job or one nearly identical to it with equivalent pay, benefits, and other employment terms and conditions.

An employer may not interfere with an individual's FMLA rights or retaliate against someone for using or trying to use FMLA leave, opposing any practice made unlawful by the FMLA, or being involved in any proceeding under or related to the FMLA.

ELIGIBILITY REQUIREMENTS

An employee who works for a covered employer must meet three criteria in order to be eligible for FMLA leave. The employee must:

- Have worked for the employer for at least 12 months;
- Have at least 1,250 hours of service in the 12 months before taking leave;* and
- Work at a location where the employer has at least 50 employees within 75 miles of the employee's worksite.

*Special "hours of service" requirements apply to airline flight crew employees.

REQUESTING LEAVE

Generally, employees must give 30-days' advance notice of the need for FMLA leave. If it is not possible to give 30-days' notice, an employee must notify the employer as soon as possible and, generally, follow the employer's usual procedures.

Employees do not have to share a medical diagnosis, but must provide enough information to the employer so it can determine if the leave qualifies for FMLA protection. Sufficient information could include informing an employer that the employee is or will be unable to perform his or her job functions, that a family member cannot perform daily activities, or that hospitalization or continuing medical treatment is necessary. Employees must inform the employer if the need for leave is for a reason for which FMLA leave was previously taken or certified.

Employers can require a certification or periodic recertification supporting the need for leave. If the employer determines that the certification is incomplete, it must provide a written notice indicating what additional information is required.

EMPLOYER RESPONSIBILITIES

Once an employer becomes aware that an employee's need for leave is for a reason that may qualify under the FMLA, the employer must notify the employee if he or she is eligible for FMLA leave and, if eligible, must also provide a notice of rights and responsibilities under the FMLA. If the employee is not eligible, the employer must provide a reason for ineligibility.

Employers must notify its employees if leave will be designated as FMLA leave, and if so, how much leave will be designated as FMLA leave.

ENFORCEMENT

Employees may file a complaint with the U.S. Department of Labor, Wage and Hour Division, or may bring a private lawsuit against an employer.

The FMLA does not affect any federal or state law prohibiting discrimination or supersede any state or local law or collective bargaining agreement that provides greater family or medical leave rights.

For additional information or to file a complaint:

1-866-4-USWAGE

(1-866-487-9243) TTY: 1-877-889-5627

www.dol.gov/whd

U.S. Department of Labor | Wage and Hour Division

WHD WAGE AND HOUR DIVISION

WH1420 REV 04/16

Fig. 4.3 Family Medical Leave Act.

YOUR RIGHTS UNDER USERRA

THE UNIFORMED SERVICES EMPLOYMENT AND REEMPLOYMENT RIGHTS ACT

USERRA protects the job rights of individuals who voluntarily or involuntarily leave employment positions to undertake military service or certain types of service in the National Disaster Medical System. USERRA also prohibits employers from discriminating against past and present members of the uniformed services, and applicants to the uniformed services.

REEMPLOYMENT RIGHTS

You have the right to be reemployed in your civilian job if you leave that job to perform service in the uniformed service and:

☆ you ensure that your employer receives advance written or verbal notice of your service;
☆ you have five years or less of cumulative service in the uniformed services while with that particular employer;
☆ you return to work or apply for reemployment in a timely manner after conclusion of service; and
☆ you have not been separated from service with a disqualifying discharge or under other than honorable conditions.

If you are eligible to be reemployed, you must be restored to the job and benefits you would have attained if you had not been absent due to military service or, in some cases, a comparable job.

RIGHT TO BE FREE FROM DISCRIMINATION AND RETALIATION

If you:

☆ are a past or present member of the uniformed service;
☆ have applied for membership in the uniformed service; or
☆ are obligated to serve in the uniformed service;

then an employer may not deny you:

☆ initial employment;
☆ reemployment;
☆ retention in employment;
☆ promotion; or
☆ any benefit of employment

because of this status.

In addition, an employer may not retaliate against anyone assisting in the enforcement of USERRA rights, including testifying or making a statement in connection with a proceeding under USERRA, even if that person has no service connection.

HEALTH INSURANCE PROTECTION

☆ If you leave your job to perform military service, you have the right to elect to continue your existing employer-based health plan coverage for you and your dependents for up to 24 months while in the military.

☆ Even if you don't elect to continue coverage during your military service, you have the right to be reinstated in your employer's health plan when you are reemployed, generally without any waiting periods or exclusions (e.g., pre-existing condition exclusions) except for service-connected illnesses or injuries.

ENFORCEMENT

☆ The U.S. Department of Labor, Veterans Employment and Training Service (VETS) is authorized to investigate and resolve complaints of USERRA violations.

☆ For assistance in filing a complaint, or for any other information on USERRA, contact VETS at **1-866-4-USA-DOL** or visit its website at https://www.dol.gov/agencies/vets/. An interactive online USERRA Advisor can be viewed at https://webapps.dol.gov/elaws/vets/userra

☆ If you file a complaint with VETS and VETS is unable to resolve it, you may request that your case be referred to the Department of Justice or the Office of Special Counsel, as applicable, for representation.

☆ You may also bypass the VETS process and bring a civil action against an employer for violations of USERRA.

The rights listed here may vary depending on the circumstances. The text of this notice was prepared by VETS, and may be viewed on the internet at this address: https://www.dol.gov/agencies/vets/programs/userra/poster Federal law requires employers to notify employees of their rights under USERRA, and employers may meet this requirement by displaying the text of this notice where they customarily place notices for employees.

U.S. Department of Labor
1-866-487-2365

U.S. Department of Justice

Office of Special Counsel

1-800-336-4590

Publication Date — May 2022

Fig. 4.4 Uniformed Services Employment and Reemployment Act.

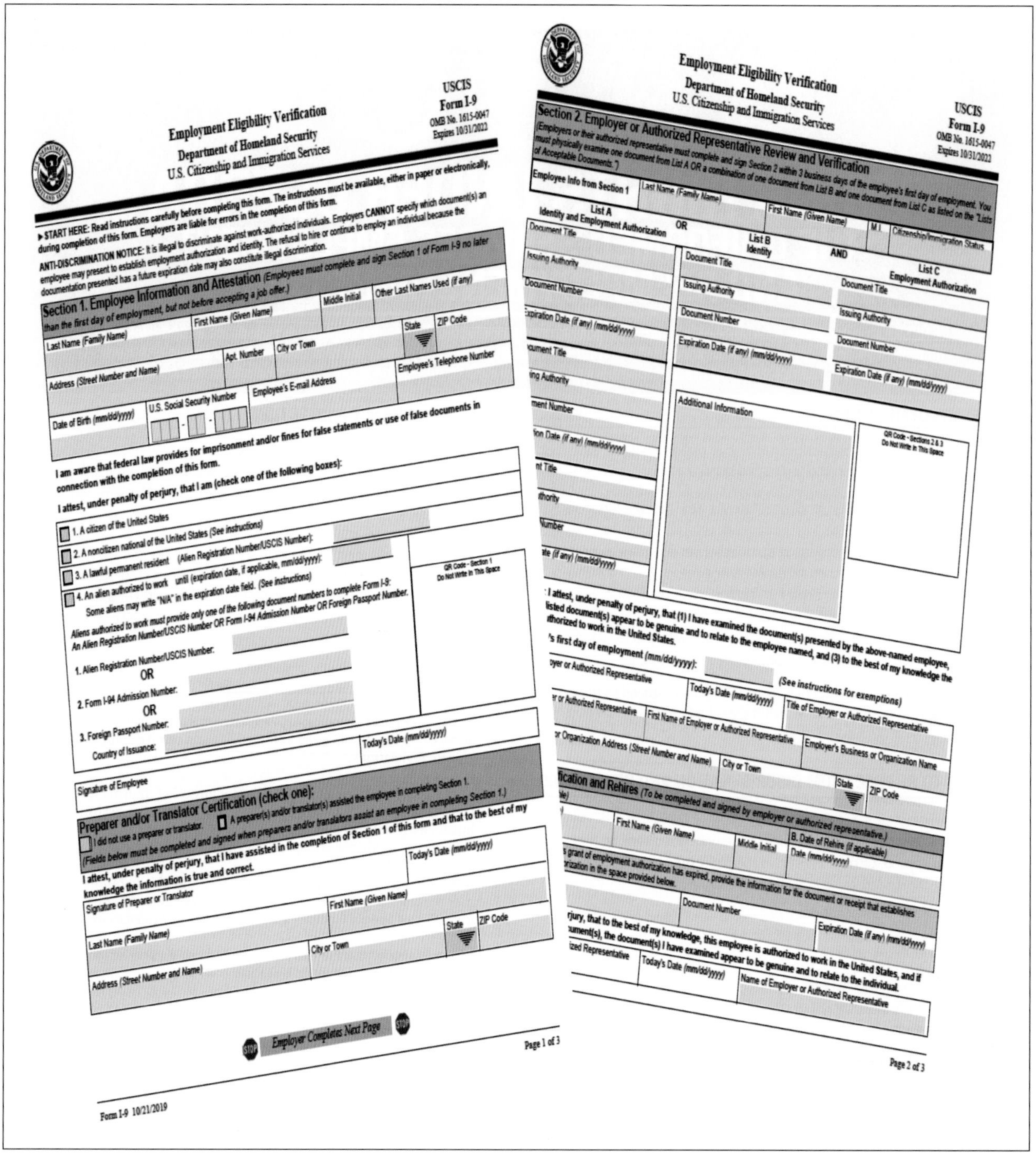
Employment Eligibility Verification
Department of Homeland Security
U.S. Citizenship and Immigration Services

USCIS
Form I-9
OMB No. 1615-0047
Expires 10/31/2022

▶START HERE: Read instructions carefully before completing this form. The instructions must be available, either in paper or electronically, during completion of this form. Employers are liable for errors in the completion of this form.

ANTI-DISCRIMINATION NOTICE: It is illegal to discriminate against work-authorized individuals. Employers CANNOT specify which document(s) an employee may present to establish employment authorization and identity. The refusal to hire or continue to employ an individual because the documentation presented has a future expiration date may also constitute illegal discrimination.

Section 1. Employee Information and Attestation (Employees must complete and sign Section 1 of Form I-9 no later than the first day of employment, but not before accepting a job offer.)

Last Name (Family Name) | First Name (Given Name) | Middle Initial | Other Last Names Used (if any)
Address (Street Number and Name) | Apt. Number | City or Town | State | ZIP Code
Date of Birth (mm/dd/yyyy) | U.S. Social Security Number | Employee's E-mail Address | Employee's Telephone Number

I am aware that federal law provides for imprisonment and/or fines for false statements or use of false documents in connection with the completion of this form.

I attest, under penalty of perjury, that I am (check one of the following boxes):

1. A citizen of the United States
2. A noncitizen national of the United States (See instructions)
3. A lawful permanent resident (Alien Registration Number/USCIS Number):
4. An alien authorized to work until (expiration date, if applicable, mm/dd/yyyy):
Some aliens may write "N/A" in the expiration date field. (See instructions)

Aliens authorized to work must provide only one of the following document numbers to complete Form I-9: An Alien Registration Number/USCIS Number OR Form I-94 Admission Number OR Foreign Passport Number.

1. Alien Registration Number/USCIS Number:
OR
2. Form I-94 Admission Number:
OR
3. Foreign Passport Number:
Country of Issuance:

QR Code - Section 1
Do Not Write In This Space

Signature of Employee | Today's Date (mm/dd/yyyy)

Preparer and/or Translator Certification (check one):
I did not use a preparer or translator. A preparer(s) and/or translator(s) assisted the employee in completing Section 1.
(Fields below must be completed and signed when preparers and/or translators assist an employee in completing Section 1.)

I attest, under penalty of perjury, that I have assisted in the completion of Section 1 of this form and that to the best of my knowledge the information is true and correct.

Signature of Preparer or Translator | Today's Date (mm/dd/yyyy)
Last Name (Family Name) | First Name (Given Name)
Address (Street Number and Name) | City or Town | State | ZIP Code

STOP Employer Completes Next Page STOP

Page 1 of 3

Form I-9 10/21/2019

Employment Eligibility Verification
Department of Homeland Security
U.S. Citizenship and Immigration Services

USCIS
Form I-9
OMB No. 1615-0047
Expires 10/31/2022

Section 2. Employer or Authorized Representative Review and Verification
(Employers or their authorized representative must complete and sign Section 2 within 3 business days of the employee's first day of employment. You must physically examine one document from List A OR a combination of one document from List B and one document from List C as listed on the "Lists of Acceptable Documents.")

Employee Info from Section 1 | Last Name (Family Name) | First Name (Given Name) | M.I. | Citizenship/Immigration Status

List A Identity and Employment Authorization | OR | List B Identity | AND | List C Employment Authorization
Document Title | Document Title | Document Title
Issuing Authority | Issuing Authority | Issuing Authority
Document Number | Document Number | Document Number
Expiration Date (if any) (mm/dd/yyyy) | Expiration Date (if any) (mm/dd/yyyy) | Expiration Date (if any) (mm/dd/yyyy)

Additional Information

QR Code - Sections 2 & 3
Do Not Write In This Space

I attest, under penalty of perjury, that (1) I have examined the document(s) presented by the above-named employee, (2) the above-listed document(s) appear to be genuine and to relate to the employee named, and (3) to the best of my knowledge the employee is authorized to work in the United States.

The employee's first day of employment (mm/dd/yyyy): (See instructions for exemptions)

Signature of Employer or Authorized Representative | Today's Date (mm/dd/yyyy) | Title of Employer or Authorized Representative
Last Name of Employer or Authorized Representative | First Name of Employer or Authorized Representative | Employer's Business or Organization Name
Employer's Business or Organization Address (Street Number and Name) | City or Town | State | ZIP Code

Section 3. Reverification and Rehires (To be completed and signed by employer or authorized representative.)
First Name (Given Name) | Middle Initial | B. Date of Rehire (if applicable) Date (mm/dd/yyyy)
If the employee's previous grant of employment authorization has expired, provide the information for the document or receipt that establishes continuing employment authorization in the space provided below.
Document Number | Expiration Date (if any) (mm/dd/yyyy)
I attest, under penalty of perjury, that to the best of my knowledge, this employee is authorized to work in the United States, and if the employee presented document(s), the document(s) I have examined appear to be genuine and to relate to the individual.
Today's Date (mm/dd/yyyy) | Name of Employer or Authorized Representative

Page 2 of 3

Fig. 4.5 I-9 Form.

Record retention for personal files differs by state and by document. Visit the state Department of Labor for the most up-to-date regulations. The retention average is 3 to 7 years. Tax audits can occur up to 7 years after the transaction has occurred. Job-related illnesses could present themselves up to 30 years later.

EMPLOYEE MANUAL

Before hiring can begin, a successful employment plan must be implemented. An employee manual, job descriptions, and expectations must be developed. Many practices are quick to hire and slow to fire, thereby creating a toxic work environment. Leaders often choose not to deal with issues that should be addressed immediately, because there is no structure in place to support a disciplinary decision. Creating an employee manual, job descriptions, and performance expectations before hiring will create a structure that every veterinary practice needs.

An employee manual provides a guide for team members and acts as a quick resource when a personnel issue arises. A manual can solve workplace problems quickly and fairly as policies have already been established. Employee manuals also hold practice managers and leaders accountable. If it is stated in the manual, then the procedure must

LISTS OF ACCEPTABLE DOCUMENTS
All documents must be UNEXPIRED

Employees may present one selection from List A
or a combination of one selection from List B and one selection from List C.

LIST A **Documents that Establish Both Identity and Employment Authorization** **OR**	**LIST B** **Documents that Establish Identity** **AND**	**LIST C** **Documents that Establish Employment Authorization**
1. U.S. Passport or U.S. Passport Card	1. Driver's license or ID card issued by a State or outlying possession of the United States provided it contains a photograph or information such as name, date of birth, gender, height, eye color, and address	1. A Social Security Account Number card, unless the card includes one of the following restrictions: (1) NOT VALID FOR EMPLOYMENT (2) VALID FOR WORK ONLY WITH INS AUTHORIZATION (3) VALID FOR WORK ONLY WITH DHS AUTHORIZATION
2. Permanent Resident Card or Alien Registration Receipt Card (Form 1-551)	2. ID card issued by federal, state or local government agencies or entities. provided it contains a photograph or information such as name, date of birth. gender. height. eye color, and address	2. Certification of report of birth issued by the Department of State (Forms DS-1350. FS-545. FS-240)
3. Foreign passport that contains a temporary I-551 stamp or temporary I-551 printed notation on a machine-readable immigrant visa	3. School ID card with a photograph	3. Original or certified copy of birth certificate issued by a State. county. municipal authority, or territory of the United States bearing an official seal
4. Employment Authorization Document that contains a photograph (Form I-766)	4. Voter's registration card	4. Native American tribal document
5. For a nonimmigrant alien authorized to work for a specific employer because of his or her status: a. Foreign passport: and b. Form 1-94 or Form 1-94A that has the following: (1) The same name as the passport; and (2) An endorsement of the alien's nonimmigrant status as long as that period of endorsement has not yet expired and the proposed employment is not in conflict with any restrictions or limitations identified on the form.	5. U.S. Military card or draft record	5. U.S. Citizen ID Card (Form 1-197)
(6) Passport from the Federated States of Micronesia (FSM) or the Republic of the Marshall Islands (RMI) with Form 1-94 or Form I-94A indicating nonimmigrant admission under the Compact of Free Association Between the United States and the FSM or RMI	6. Military dependent's ID card	6. Identification Card for Use of Resident Citizen in the United States (Form 1-179)
	7. U.S. Coast Guard Merchant Mariner Card	7. Employment authorization document issued by the Department of Homeland Security
	8. Native American tribal document	
	9. Driver's license issued by a Canadian government authority	
	For persons under age 18 who are unable to present a document listed above:	
	10. School record or report card	
	11. Clinic, doctor, or hospital record	
	12. Day-care or nursery school record	

Fig. 4.6 I-9 document requirements.

be followed (harassment, coaching, termination, etc.). If practice managers do not follow the guidelines that have been established, potential lawsuits from previous or disgruntled team members could result. In addition, poor culture will result (if leaders and managers don't follow the rules, why should team members?).

If an employer manual has not been developed, it is important to take the time to establish one. It is advised to have the practice attorney review the manual before distribution to ensure the practice is legally protected in every way possible (in addition, state laws differ regarding employment laws). Violations of the terms of the manual can be seen as a breach of contract; therefore, it is important to state in the front of the manual that it is not a contract and that the manual can be changed and updated at any time. New team members should read the manual, sign a document stating that they have received it, and understand that it is not a contract, but simply a guide to team member policy.

Employment and labor laws change frequently, and policies and manuals must be updated to reflect these changes. Practices should reserve the right to update and modify employee manuals at any time. It is important to remain flexible, and team members should be made aware of changes as they occur; it is important that they sign a form acknowledging any updates. When changes are implemented, save the file under a new name on the computer (indicating the date the changes were made). For example, the first version of an employee manual may be titled "Employee Manual.V1.6.10.22." The title indicates that the

EMPLOYEE RIGHTS

EMPLOYEE POLYGRAPH PROTECTION ACT

The Employee Polygraph Protection Act prohibits most private employers from using lie detector tests either for pre-employment screening or during the course of employment.

PROHIBITIONS Employers are generally prohibited from requiring or requesting any employee or job applicant to take a lie detector test, and from discharging, disciplining, or discriminating against an employee or prospective employee for refusing to take a test or for exercising other rights under the Act.

EXEMPTIONS Federal, State and local governments are not affected by the law. Also, the law does not apply to tests given by the Federal Government to certain private individuals engaged in national security-related activities.

The Act permits polygraph (a kind of lie detector) tests to be administered in the private sector, subject to restrictions, to certain prospective employees of security service firms (armored car, alarm, and guard), and of pharmaceutical manufacturers, distributors and dispensers.

The Act also permits polygraph testing, subject to restrictions, of certain employees of private firms who are reasonably suspected of involvement in a workplace incident (theft, embezzlement, etc.) that resulted in economic loss to the employer.

The law does not preempt any provision of any State or local law or any collective bargaining agreement which is more restrictive with respect to lie detector tests.

EXAMINEE RIGHTS Where polygraph tests are permitted, they are subject to numerous strict standards concerning the conduct and length of the test. Examinees have a number of specific rights, including the right to a written notice before testing, the right to refuse or discontinue a test, and the right not to have test results disclosed to unauthorized persons.

ENFORCEMENT The Secretary of Labor may bring court actions to restrain violations and assess civil penalties against violators. Employees or job applicants may also bring their own court actions.

THE LAW REQUIRES EMPLOYERS TO DISPLAY THIS POSTER WHERE EMPLOYEES AND JOB APPLICANTS CAN READILY SEE IT.

WHD
WAGE AND HOUR DIVISION
UNITED STATES DEPARTMENT OF LABOR

1-866-487-9243
TTY: 1-877-889-5627
www.dol.gov/whd

WH1462 REV 07/16

Fig. 4.7 Employee Polygraph Protection Act.

Equal Employment Opportunity is THE LAW

Private Employers, State and Local Governments, Educational Institutions, Employment Agencies and Labor Organizations

Applicants to and employees of most private employers, state and local governments, educational institutions, employment agencies and labor organizations are protected under Federal law from discrimination on the following bases:

RACE, COLOR, RELIGION, SEX, NATIONAL ORIGIN
Title VII of the Civil Rights Act of 1964, as amended, protects applicants and employees from discrimination in hiring, promotion, discharge, pay, fringe benefits, job training, classification, referral, and other aspects of employment, on the basis of race, color, religion, sex (including pregnancy), or national origin. Religious discrimination includes failing to reasonably accommodate an employee's religious practices where the accommodation does not impose undue hardship.

DISABILITY
Title I and Title V of the Americans with Disabilities Act of 1990, as amended, protect qualified individuals from discrimination on the basis of disability in hiring, promotion, discharge, pay, fringe benefits, job training, classification, referral, and other aspects of employment. Disability discrimination includes not making reasonable accommodation to the known physical or mental limitations of an otherwise qualified individual with a disability who is an applicant or employee, barring undue hardship.

AGE
The Age Discrimination in Employment Act of 1967, as amended, protects applicants and employees 40 years of age or older from discrimination based on age in hiring, promotion, discharge, pay, fringe benefits, job training, classification, referral, and other aspects of employment.

SEX (WAGES)
In addition to sex discrimination prohibited by Title VII of the Civil Rights Act, as amended, the Equal Pay Act of 1963, as amended, prohibits sex discrimination in the payment of wages to women and men performing substantially equal work, in jobs that require equal skill, effort, and responsibility, under similar working conditions, in the same establishment.

GENETICS
Title II of the Genetic Information Nondiscrimination Act of 2008 protects applicants and employees from discrimination based on genetic information in hiring, promotion, discharge, pay, fringe benefits, job training, classification, referral, and other aspects of employment. GINA also restricts employers' acquisition of genetic information and strictly limits disclosure of genetic information. Genetic information includes information about genetic tests of applicants, employees, or their family members; the manifestation of diseases or disorders in family members (family medical history); and requests for or receipt of genetic services by applicants, employees, or their family members.

RETALIATION
All of these Federal laws prohibit covered entities from retaliating against a person who files a charge of discrimination, participates in a discrimination proceeding, or otherwise opposes an unlawful employment practice.

WHAT TO DO IF YOU BELIEVE DISCRIMINATION HAS OCCURRED
There are strict time limits for filing charges of employment discrimination. To preserve the ability of EEOC to act on your behalf and to protect your right to file a private lawsuit, should you ultimately need to, you should contact EEOC promptly when discrimination is suspected:
The U.S. Equal Employment Opportunity Commission (EEOC), 1-800-669-4000 (toll-free) or 1-800-669-6820 (toll-free TTY number for individuals with hearing impairments). EEOC field office information is available at www.eeoc.gov or in most telephone directories in the U.S. Government or Federal Government section. Additional information about EEOC, including information about charge filing, is available at www.eeoc.gov.

Employers Holding Federal Contracts or Subcontracts

Applicants to and employees of companies with a Federal government contract or subcontract are protected under Federal law from discrimination on the following bases:

RACE, COLOR, RELIGION, SEX, NATIONAL ORIGIN
Executive Order 11246, as amended, prohibits job discrimination on the basis of race, color, religion, sex or national origin, and requires affirmative action to ensure equality of opportunity in all aspects of employment.

INDIVIDUALS WITH DISABILITIES
Section 503 of the Rehabilitation Act of 1973, as amended, protects qualified individuals from discrimination on the basis of disability in hiring, promotion, discharge, pay, fringe benefits, job training, classification, referral, and other aspects of employment. Disability discrimination includes not making reasonable accommodation to the known physical or mental limitations of an otherwise qualified individual with a disability who is an applicant or employee, barring undue hardship. Section 503 also requires that Federal contractors take affirmative action to employ and advance in employment qualified individuals with disabilities at all levels of employment, including the executive level.

DISABLED, RECENTLY SEPARATED, OTHER PROTECTED, AND ARMED FORCES SERVICE MEDAL VETERANS
The Vietnam Era Veterans' Readjustment Assistance Act of 1974, as amended, 38 U.S.C. 4212, prohibits job discrimination and requires affirmative action to employ and advance in employment disabled veterans, recently separated veterans (within three years of discharge or release from active duty), other protected veterans (veterans who served during a war or in a campaign or expedition for which a campaign badge has been authorized), and Armed Forces service medal veterans (veterans who, while on active duty, participated in a U.S. military operation for which an Armed Forces service medal was awarded).

RETALIATION
Retaliation is prohibited against a person who files a complaint of discrimination, participates in an OFCCP proceeding, or otherwise opposes discrimination under these Federal laws.

Any person who believes a contractor has violated its nondiscrimination or affirmative action obligations under the authorities above should contact immediately:

The Office of Federal Contract Compliance Programs (OFCCP), U.S. Department of Labor, 200 Constitution Avenue, N.W., Washington, D.C. 20210, 1-800-397-6251 (toll-free) or (202) 693-1337 (TTY). OFCCP may also be contacted by e-mail at OFCCP-Public@dol.gov, or by calling an OFCCP regional or district office, listed in most telephone directories under U.S. Government, Department of Labor.

Programs or Activities Receiving Federal Financial Assistance

RACE, COLOR, NATIONAL ORIGIN, SEX
In addition to the protections of Title VII of the Civil Rights Act of 1964, as amended, Title VI of the Civil Rights Act of 1964, as amended, prohibits discrimination on the basis of race, color or national origin in programs or activities receiving Federal financial assistance. Employment discrimination is covered by Title VI if the primary objective of the financial assistance is provision of employment, or where employment discrimination causes or may cause discrimination in providing services under such programs. Title IX of the Education Amendments of 1972 prohibits employment discrimination on the basis of sex in educational programs or activities which receive Federal financial assistance.

INDIVIDUALS WITH DISABILITIES
Section 504 of the Rehabilitation Act of 1973, as amended, prohibits employment discrimination on the basis of disability in any program or activity which receives Federal financial assistance. Discrimination is prohibited in all aspects of employment against persons with disabilities who, with or without reasonable accommodation, can perform the essential functions of the job.

If you believe you have been discriminated against in a program of any institution which receives Federal financial assistance, you should immediately contact the Federal agency providing such assistance.

EEOC 9/02 and OFCCP 8/08 Versions Useable With 11/09 Supplement *EEOC-P/E-1 (Revised 11/09)*

Fig. 4.8 Equal Employment Opportunity.

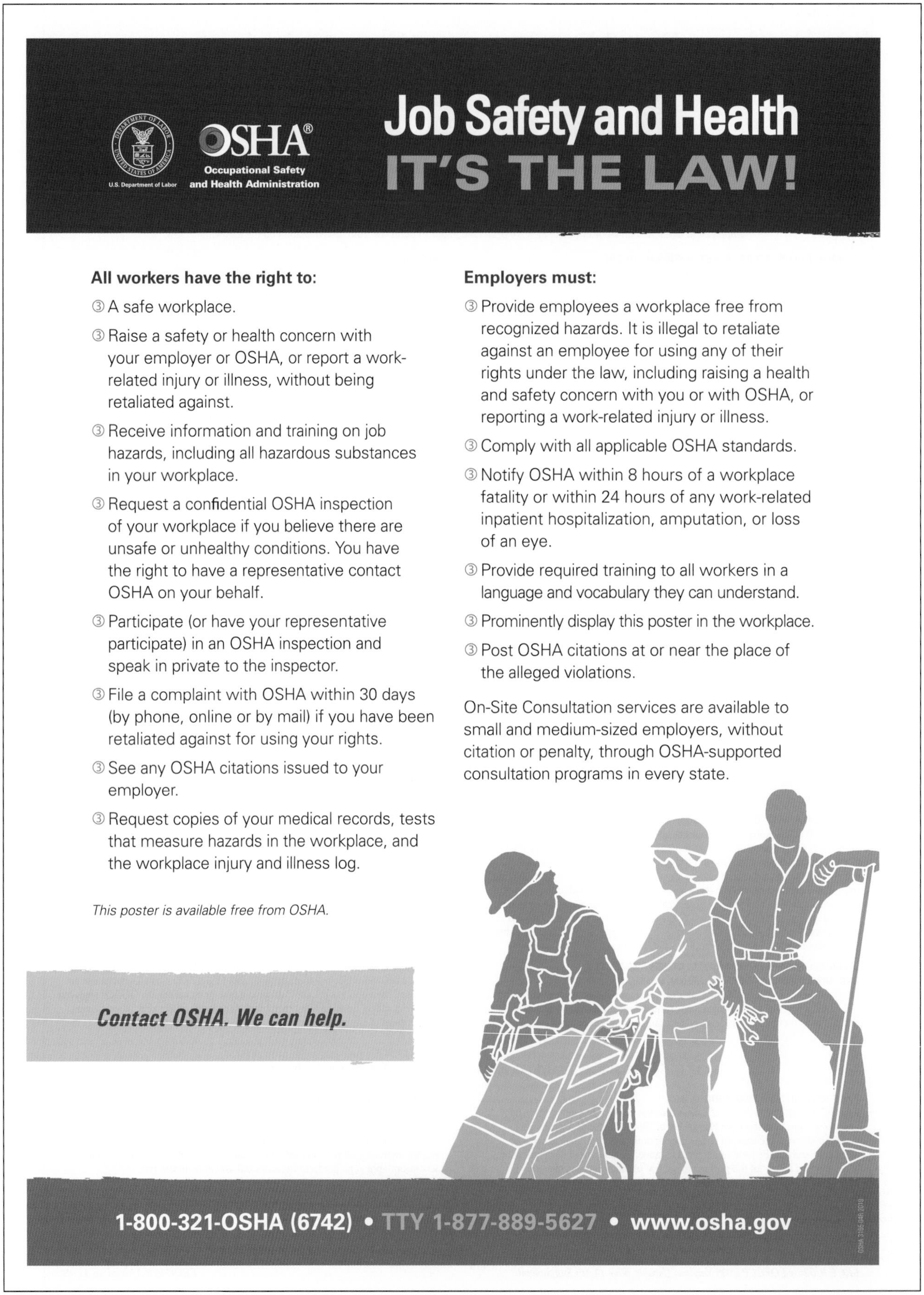

U.S. Department of Labor

OSHA®
Occupational Safety and Health Administration

Job Safety and Health
IT'S THE LAW!

All workers have the right to:

③ A safe workplace.

③ Raise a safety or health concern with your employer or OSHA, or report a work-related injury or illness, without being retaliated against.

③ Receive information and training on job hazards, including all hazardous substances in your workplace.

③ Request a confidential OSHA inspection of your workplace if you believe there are unsafe or unhealthy conditions. You have the right to have a representative contact OSHA on your behalf.

③ Participate (or have your representative participate) in an OSHA inspection and speak in private to the inspector.

③ File a complaint with OSHA within 30 days (by phone, online or by mail) if you have been retaliated against for using your rights.

③ See any OSHA citations issued to your employer.

③ Request copies of your medical records, tests that measure hazards in the workplace, and the workplace injury and illness log.

This poster is available free from OSHA.

Employers must:

③ Provide employees a workplace free from recognized hazards. It is illegal to retaliate against an employee for using any of their rights under the law, including raising a health and safety concern with you or with OSHA, or reporting a work-related injury or illness.

③ Comply with all applicable OSHA standards.

③ Notify OSHA within 8 hours of a workplace fatality or within 24 hours of any work-related inpatient hospitalization, amputation, or loss of an eye.

③ Provide required training to all workers in a language and vocabulary they can understand.

③ Prominently display this poster in the workplace.

③ Post OSHA citations at or near the place of the alleged violations.

On-Site Consultation services are available to small and medium-sized employers, without citation or penalty, through OSHA-supported consultation programs in every state.

Contact OSHA. We can help.

1-800-321-OSHA (6742) • TTY 1-877-889-5627 • www.osha.gov

Fig. 4.9 OSHA.

first version of the manual took effect on June 10, 2022. A subsequent update would be titled "Employee Manual.V2. 8.30.23," indicating the second version took effect in August of 2023. Keep copies of all documents in case changes ever come into question.

Developing an Employee Manual and Topics to Include

Employee manuals should maintain a positive tone, avoiding any authoritarian manner when possible. The purpose is to create a positive work environment, prevent problems before they arise, and allow communication to occur freely. Creating an atmosphere of open communication between team members and management can minimize issues related to human resources.

Many topics are addressed in employee manuals, including the philosophy or mission of the practice. Benefits are generally offered by all practices; however, the extent of the benefits can vary. Benefits packages can play a large role in attracting and retaining team members. Each benefit that is offered should be defined, and there should be clear statements about which team members qualify for them. If seasonal team members are employed, the length of employment and eligibility for benefits should be outlined. Also included are work schedule policies, codes of conduct, social media policies, and safety procedures. The following topics are covered in summary; review Fig. 4.10 for topics that may be included.

CRITICAL COMPETENCY: WRITING AND VERBAL SKILLS

The practice manager must have the ability to comprehend written material easily and accurately, as well as the ability to express thoughts clearly and succinctly in writing.

Philosophy and Mission Statements: The practice mission may be the same as a purpose statement: the fundamental reason for the organization to exist. What is the purpose? What services are provided? Why are they important? These are just a few questions that can be answered when developing the practice mission. A vision may include goals the practice wishes to achieve and how they will be achieved. The statement should be measurable and simple, and all team members should be able to contribute to achieving the vision, mission, and core values) of the practice (see Chapter 2).

Full-Time and Part-Time Employment: Full-time and part-time employment must be defined. Each practice can determine the number of hours per week required for a full-time position. Some practices may choose 40 hours per week, others may only require 34 hours. Overtime must be paid for any team member who works more than 40 hours per week (or as indicated by state law). Those in violation can be penalized severely (see Laws That Require Familiarity, FLSA).

As mentioned in Chapter 1, practice managers and owners should consider decreasing the number of hours required for full-time employment to help attract and retain loyal members. Potential team members are looking for practices that can provide flexible work schedules with decreased full-time hours.

Seasonal Team Members: Some practices are extremely busy during specific months and hire seasonal team members for coverage during these busy times. Job descriptions, duties, and dates of employment should be established to prevent any miscommunication. Seasonal team members should also sign that they have received, read, and understand the employee manual. Benefits are generally not offered to seasonal team members; however, this is at the discretion of the practice.

Benefits: Once the status of full-time and part-time team members has been established, the benefits each position receives should be defined. Many benefit plans are included in full-time employment; however, it is up to the practice to decide what to offer. Offering benefits is not required by law but offering them can help in recruiting and retaining team members. Review the section on health insurance and the

SAMPLE TABLE OF CONTENTS FOR EMPLOYEE MANUAL

- Statement or purpose of manual
- Philosophy and/or mission statement
- Laws of importance
- Americans with Disabilities Act
- Confidentiality
- Equal employment opportunity
- Family Medical Leave Act
- Pregnancy safety
- Sexual harassment policy

EMPLOYMENT POLICIES

- Appearance, dress code, uniforms
- Attendance, work schedule policy
- Code of Conduct
- Drug and alcohol abuse policy
- Drug-free workplace
- Employment on an at-will basis
- Employment statuses
- Hours of operation
- Probationary period
- Punctuality
- Romantic relationships
- Social media policy
- Violence in the workplace

BENEFITS

- Continuing education
- Disability
- Dues and license fees
- Holiday's recognized/ holiday pay
- Insurance
- Disability, health, liability
- Retirement
- Sick leave
- Vacation
- Veterinary services
- Workers' compensation benefits
- Jury duty
- Training procedures
- Probationary period

COMPENSATION

- Compensation schedule
- Overtime
- Personnel records

SAFETY

- OSHA/Safety Data Sheets
- Reporting an accident
- Security
- Termination procedures
- Resignation
- Dismissals
- Immediate dismissals

SIGNATURE PAGE

Each state has different laws regarding team member manuals and laws that must be covered. It is advisable to contact an attorney for review. Employment and labor laws change frequently, and policies and manuals must be updated to reflect the changes. Practices should reserve the right to update and modify team member manuals at any time. It is important to remain flexible, and team members should be made aware of changes as they occur and sign a form acknowledging the update.

Fig. 4.10 Since state laws vary, it is highly recommended that employee manuals be reviewed by an attorney familiar with the state's labor regulations.

Patient Protection and Affordable Care Act. It is highly recommended to offer as many benefits as possible to all team members (Fig. 4.11). Practice owners may wish to consider offering benefits that provide team members to choose which benefits they want. Not all team members need health insurance when a spouse has that coverage. But they should not be denied another benefit that may contribute to increased mental health and loyalty to the practice. Happy team members stay long term.

Team member salary and benefits statements should be provided to team members on an annual basis. Team members generally only see the monetary compensation they have received as shown on their year-end W-2. Annual statements show team members the value of the benefits they receive in addition to their compensation (Fig. 4.12).

Benefit statements should run for the entire fiscal year, giving a clear picture to the team member of how much the employer has paid in the previous year including benefits. Pretax compensation should be listed, along with Medicare and Social Security contributions made by the employer (team members do not realize the practice contributes to these funds). Insurance, vacation, continuing education, uniforms, sick days, holidays, pet health care, and any other benefits should be listed individually because each team member's benefit summary will be different. It should not take an excessive amount of time to prepare the statements, as all the information should be easily retrievable through the accounting software (i.e., QuickBooks).

Discuss the benefits statement with team members instead of handing them out without comment, allowing them to comprehend the full compensation and benefits plan. Historically, team members only consider their paycheck as compensation and forget that benefits are a real cost provided by the employer.

VHMA PRACTICE DOMAIN TASK

Practice managers develop, implement, and manage employee benefits programs.

Vacation: The amount of vacation that may be taken is determined by the practice and is generally built up over time. Vacation pay should be offered, and team members should be encouraged to take it. Without a vacation, stress, fatigue, irritability, and decreased production results.

Factors to consider when determining a vacation policy for the practice include the length of employment required before vacation can be used, time allotment, eligibility, accrual rate, schedule approval, whether unused vacation rolls over to the next year (and if does, how much), or if unused vacation is paid at the time of termination or resignation. As a general guideline, practices may allow 1 week per year for the first year, then increase 1 week per year to a maximum of 3 weeks. Many practices state that vacation should be used within the fiscal year, and do not allow rollover to the next year (this is the choice of a practice). Practices should review state law regarding paid time off (PTO). Some states have mandated accrual PTO, whereas others have not. Team members should be asked to give sufficient notice to use vacation time, allowing schedules to be adjusted accordingly. Overtime is not paid when PTO is used within the same week.

Another method of vacation determination is to base the time accrued on the number of hours worked per week. A long-term team member may receive 8 hours of vacation for every 100 hours of work.

Sick Leave: Just as with vacation, the amount of sick leave offered may accumulate based on years of service. Allowing one team member time off when they are sick is better than having multiple people sick at once. Trying to prevent the spread of a virus is more economically advantageous!

Factors to account for when determining the rules for sick leave include how long a person must be employed before receiving paid sick leave, accrual, whether the practice will allow it to accrue year to year, and whether it is paid on termination or resignation. Overtime is not paid when using sick leave. As with vacation, review state, county, and city laws regarding sick leave or PTO accumulation; some municipalities and states require a specified accrual rate.

Some practices may apply the broad term Paid Time Off (PTO) instead of breaking out vacation and sick leave. Generous PTO policies that define (in the employee manual) what time can be used for personal leave (whether vacation or sick leave) often meet the requirements of states, cities, and counties.

Liability insurance for veterinarians is generally paid for by the practice. It is imperative that liability insurance be high enough to cover any accident that may occur within the practice. This includes any animal-related injury, client injury, or accusation of malpractice. Managers must ensure these premiums are paid annually.

Health insurance can and should be available for full-time team members. It is generally cheaper for a business to offer health insurance than for individuals to purchase their own policies. Practices may offer to pay 100% of the monthly payment, or less if they choose. The team member is then responsible for the remaining percentage if the employer does not cover the entire premium. It is considered a pretax benefit, and the team member's portion is automatically deducted from their check.

Health insurance policies should be reviewed on an annual basis because premiums and coverage change frequently. When deciding which insurance plan to choose, practice managers should review both health maintenance organization (HMO) and preferred provider organization (PPO) plans because they can differ greatly in the doctors and laboratories covered as well as in copayments and annual deductibles. HMOs are usually well managed and usually cover all medical expenses if patients use the doctors and laboratories within the approved network. PPOs offer a network of physicians and laboratories and encourage patients to use them; this is not required, but team members receive a lower amount of coverage if they choose a doctor that is out of network.

The Patient Protection and Affordable Care Act applies to businesses with 50 full-time team members or more. At the time of publication, practices with less than 50 team members are not required to provide health insurance. Visit https://www.shrm.org for up-to-date information. It is important to consider that even if the practice does not offer health insurance as a benefit, every team member must have insurance, or will be fined by the government. Practices must keep this in mind and pay team members enough to cover their cost of healthcare.

Disability insurance is a benefit that some employers offer. Disability insurance is maintained to protect the team member against

EXAMPLES OF EMPLOYEE BENEFITS

- Health insurance
- Dental/vision insurance
- Continuing education
- Vacation
- Sick leave
- Holiday pay
- Professional liability insurance
- Disability insurance
- Life insurance
- Retirement plans
- Dues and licenses
- Veterinary care
- Gym membership
- Child care

Fig. 4.11 Employee benefits can differentiate a practice and attract talent. Consider thinking outside of the above examples to differentiate your practice.

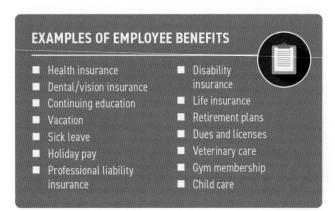

EXAMPLE OF TEAM MEMBER TOTAL COMPENSATION/ BENEFITS STATEMENT

Name of team member:	D. J. Stover
Period covered:	January 1, 2022 to December 31, 2022
Date of hire:	April 15, 2018
Salary or hourly wage:	$45,768.98 = $22/hour
Emergency compensation:	$0
Bonus:	$2,500
Social Security and Medicare contribution:	$2,837.68 + $663.63 = $3,501.31
Health insurance:	$309.87/month (pay 100%) = $3,718.44
Liability insurance:	$1,200
Disability insurance:	$102/month = $1,224
Holiday pay:	8 paid days; $22/hour x 8 hours/day = $176 x 8 days = $1,408
Vacation:	3 weeks, 40 hours/week; $22 x 40 = $880/week x 3 = $2,640
Sick time:	1 week (40 hours) = $22 x 40 = $880
Retirement:	3% of matching contribution = $3,042/year
Uniforms:	New uniforms twice yearly = $180
Continuing education:	$2,500 to be used at your discretion
Dues:	City and state veterinary medical associations, American Veterinary Medical Association = $350
Licenses:	State, controlled substances = $325
Pet medical care:	Total discounted services this year = $1,650.89
Miscellaneous:	Lunches, social events = $167.89/team member
Total benefits:	$25,287.53
Total salary and benefits:	$71,056.51
Benefits as a percentage of salary:	64%

Fig. 4.12 Employee total compensation and benefits statements help team members see all benefits they receive from the practice, beyond the paycheck.

injury that results in the inability to perform tasks needed to complete the job. Back injuries, bite wounds that result in permanent damage, and carpal tunnel syndrome are just a few conditions that may prevent a team member from working to their full capacity. Three forms of disability insurance are available. Own occupation disability insurance covers any disability that does not allow a team member to return to that line of work. For example, if a veterinarian could no longer perform surgery because of a permanent hand injury but could see patients in a limited way, he would receive a small disability pension. Any occupation disability insurance covers any disability that does not allow the team member to return to any occupation. Residual coverage is important to professionals who become partially disabled and incur a loss of income from reduced duties. Residual benefits are based on the percentage of income lost. Team members need coverage in case they are permanently injured, especially if they are the main income producer of the family.

Workers' compensation insurance is required in nearly all states. It is regulated by each state, and requirements vary significantly from state to state. The Workers' Compensation Act was developed to protect the employer against any accident or injury that occurs on the job site. This type of compensation is detailed later in this chapter.

Insurance agents are excellent at helping small businesses find the right insurance plan at all levels. Ask clients and other local practices for referrals of reputable and reliable agents who provide courteous service. They can maximize the benefits for both the employer and team member while finding the most economically feasible policy.

Retirement Funds: A great benefit to offer team members is a retirement fund. Retirement funds are a growing trend in veterinary medicine and complement the benefits package well. The most common form of a retirement fund in general veterinary practice is a SIMPLE IRA (sIRA). SIMPLE is the abbreviation for Savings Incentive Match Plan for Team members, and IRA is short for Individual Retirement Account. sIRA plans are established by employers who want to allow eligible team members to set aside part of their pretax compensation as a part of their retirement savings plan. The employer must contribute either dollar for dollar or a percentage to all eligible team members. The team member can either contribute a set dollar amount per pay period or a percentage of the total pretax compensation. 401(k) plans are another common form of retirement fund in which employers are not required to contribute to the team member's account but can if they wish. Team members determine how much they wish to contribute monthly to their 401(k) (the IRS determines maximum annual contributions).

Practices may also create a profit-sharing plan for team members in which they receive an annual share of the practice's profits. Profit sharing gives team members a sense of ownership in the company. This plan generally requires a plan administrator, and management determines the percentage of profits. Simplified Team member Pension plans (SEPs) are like profit-sharing plans and are appropriate for small organizations. They are funded by tax-deductible employer contributions, but team members are not allowed to contribute.

Retirement funds are highly regulated by the government through the Employee Retirement Income Security Act (ERISA) because of past negligence and abuse in the management of pension plans. Professional guidance from a broker is advised to determine which plan is best for the practice.

Retirement funds encourage team members to stay with the practice for the long term and reward team members for their dedication and hard work. The employer's match is tax deductible, making contributions a benefit for the practice.

Continuing Education: Continuing education (CE) should be available to all team members required to help the practice achieve strategic goals. Hospitals may determine a specific amount to be given to everyone on a yearly basis, allowing team members to attend CE that applies to the mission and vision of the practice. The set amount should include travel expenses, hotel, CE registration fees, and money to cover the cost of meals. If the practice would rather offer reimbursement for CE courses, then team members should submit all applicable CE expenses for payment. These receipts should be kept for year-end taxes.

Allowing a set dollar amount per team member can prevent overspending and holds team members accountable for their spending. They may choose CE on a local or state level, which ultimately saves money for the practice. CE benefits typically average between $2,000 and $3,000 per person (credentialed technician, associate DVM), for national or regional conferences, and include airfare, hotel, registration, and food (Well Managed Practices Benchmarks 2017).

VHMA PRACTICE DOMAIN TASK

Practice managers manage staff continuing education and licensure/certification.

Many local and state veterinary medical associations, along with manufacturers, hold CE events throughout the year, covering a variety of topics. Lunches or dinners are often offered at these free lectures, defraying some costs of attending. Technicians and veterinarians alike are normally invited to attend.

Holiday Pay: Practices may elect whether to pay team members for certain holidays. Holidays include New Year's Eve; New Year's Day; Martin Luther King, Jr., Day; Presidents Day; Easter; Memorial Day; Independence Day; Labor Day; Veterans Day; Thanksgiving; Christmas Eve; and Christmas Day. Some practices only observe the major holidays; others prefer to observe a day that is meaningful to the practice. Holiday pay is usually paid to a team member who would normally work those hours on days when the practice has chosen to close. Holiday pay is usually 8 hours of pay, and overtime is not paid when holiday pay has been accumulated.

Uniforms: If team members are required to wear scrubs, the practice should provide them or compensate individuals for their purchase. The benefit to the practice of providing scrubs is the ability to control the clothing appearance of team members. Team members should be held accountable for maintaining their uniforms in the best condition possible. Requiring all team members to wear the same color uniform on specific days adds to the professional appearance of the staff. Ask the team to pick the best colors and assign days to those colors. When having input, the team will comply much easier with the request. Many companies offer discounts when large orders are placed. Inquire with several companies to find the best price that fits the budget of the practice. Always replace scrubs that are looking worn, faded, or tattered as this reflects poorly on the practice. Build uniforms into the practice budget. Professional appearance is a long-term marketing strategy and must be maintained.

Membership Fees: Both veterinarians and credential technicians/nurses pay membership fees each year to state veterinary medical associations, national organizations, and specialty board memberships, just to name a few. Practices should analyze all potential dues and set a guideline to follow when choosing to cover such expenses.

Licenses: Licenses held by veterinarians and technicians are renewed each year or biannually with a fee. Practices may wish to cover this expense, including the state-controlled substance license, DEA license, state license, and any other license required to practice veterinary medicine.

The total cost of licensure fees and dues to organizations for one veterinarian averages $1,500 per year. Practices should remember that these fees could be considered a year-end tax write-off.

Employee Discounts: The practice has the discretion in determining team member discounts, and how much they should be. Many practices allow team members to purchase items at a reduced cost. Internal Revenue Service (IRS) guidelines must be taken into consideration when providing discounts to team members. Team member discounts on services greater than a 20% discount are reported as fringe benefits and must be reported as pay. Visit https://www.irs.gov/pub/irs-pdf/p15b.pdf every January for the most current update on fringe benefits. Practices not reporting fringe benefits risk paying back taxes and fines. In lieu of team member discounts, hospitals may wish to extend pet health insurance to team members and cover the premium associated with this benefit.

Code of Conduct: Team members are expected to maintain professionalism while on the premises. The code of conduct should define each area in which there are specific expectations of team members. Topics that should be addressed within a code of conduct (but not limited to) are appearance, confidentiality, quality of patient care, equipment care, and accountability for supplies and equipment.

Team member, client, and patient confidentiality is of utmost importance and must be addressed in the employee manual. Information must never be given out without team member or client consent.

VHMA PRACTICE DOMAIN TASK

Practice managers maintain confidential employee records.

If a pet is lost and an unknown person calls the practice indicating that they have found a pet, the practice should then call the client and pass on the information provided by the caller. Never give the client's name and phone number to an unknown person. The practice does not know whether the unknown person really has the pet, or the person has criminal intentions. The practice can be held liable for giving out confidential information if this scenario ever occurs.

Work Schedule Policy: All team members need to be aware of the work schedule policy. Veterinarians are expected to be available during set appointment hours, and vacation or personal time must be scheduled in advance to accommodate the request. All team members are expected to cover the shifts that have been assigned to them and must schedule vacation time in advance. Most practices will grant time off to team members if their shifts are covered. The practice must establish a policy, include it in the employee manual, and enforce it. Team members who do not follow policy must receive official discipline. See the section on termination procedures in this chapter for guidance on documenting and enforcing procedures.

Team members should be made aware of the issues that arise when the practice is short-staffed. Members must be held accountable for their shifts, and any absence (unless for an emergency or illness) is unacceptable. Team shortages contribute to increased stress levels, decreased team efficiency, and a decline in patient and client care. Shortages also produce individual resentment leading to decreased team morale.

VHMA PRACTICE DOMAIN TASK

Practice managers establish work schedules for staff.

Jury Duty: When team members are summoned for jury duty, they are obligated by law to attend. School, work, or any other excuse is not allowed. Team members should be encouraged to have their shifts covered before jury duty, and management should help with this coverage. Jury duty is a public service and should be served with pride.

Training Procedures: Training procedures should be clearly defined in the employee manual. New team members should be advised of the training schedule and when they are expected to master those skills (more information on developing a training program is provided later in this chapter). The manual should indicate whether there is a probationary period and the steps that follow the probation period (see section in this chapter, Probationary Period).

Employee manuals should also define how often performance evaluations will occur thereafter. It is recommended to provide (at minimum) yearly written evaluations for each team member, keeping copies in each team member's personnel file (covered later in this chapter). Coaching should occur daily in conjunction with yearly evaluations. Team members cannot be expected to improve without daily feedback and constructive criticism offered on an ongoing basis.

Noncompete Agreements: Some practices require veterinarians to sign a noncompete agreement (NCA) that protects the business, preventing an employee from working for another practice or opening their own practice within so many miles of the practice. NCAs are getting more difficult to enforce and detract from the practice's ability to attract veterinarians. While a high-producing doctor can take clients with the move, the likely financial impact is minimal. Legal costs to try and enforce an NCA may be higher and breed ill will in the culture of the practice. Practice managers and owners should consider eliminating NCAs and instead focus on creating a workplace environment with benefits that no doctor wants to leave.

Social Media Policy: Social media is a broad term for Facebook, Twitter, LinkedIn, Instagram, TikTok, blogs, or web pages. It has become a great way to communicate with clients, friends, and colleagues. However, it can also affect the practice negatively. Social media rules must be established, including identifying the social media manager and expectations of their role. The social media manager must review any information, pictures, or links before posting, and clients must authorize the use of patient photos before they can be used.

Team members must understand they are ambassadors for the practice, and responses to practice events on social media (even if just to friends) will be shared. Team members should be reminded to think twice before posting and should withhold comments they would not want their spouse, mother, or grandmother to read. They must be held accountable for what they post and reminded that the social media policy applies to not only those responsible for managing the practice's social media pages, but all team members employed. Consider the following statement to be a part of a social media policy:

Ultimately, you are solely responsible for what you post online. Before creating online content, consider the risks and benefits that are involved. Keep in mind that any of your conduct that adversely affects your job performance, the performance of fellow team members, clients, patients, and distributor/manufacturer representatives may result in disciplinary action up to and including termination. Inappropriate postings may include (but are not limited to) discriminatory remarks, harassment, threats of violence, or unprofessional comments.

The practice manager may also include the directive to refrain from using social media while on work time unless it is work-related and has been approved by management. Additionally, team members should not use the practice's email address to sign up for any social media networks, blogs, or tools for personal use.

Codes of conduct must include zero tolerance for harassment, the release of confidential information, or social media policy. Laws and regulations affecting social media change on a regular basis, and practice managers must remain vigilant when developing and maintaining policies. Visit the Society for Human Resource Management at https://www.shrm.org for the most up-to-date regulations and acceptable social media policies. Because social media laws change, remind team members the social media policy can be updated at any time.

Safety and Security Procedures: Team members should receive safety training during the first few days of employment; team safety should be of utmost importance. Chapter 15, Safety, covers the development and implementation of a safety program if one is not already in use. OSHA recognizes and enforces team member safety, and rules and regulations have been implemented that employers must enforce.

Security in and around the practice 24 hours a day is important. The outside premises should be well lit and secure for team members who are walking pets. Security cameras may be needed, depending on the location of the practice. The team member entrance door should always be locked, preventing the entry of clients or criminals. The door should only be locked from the outside to allow access out the door in the event of an emergency and quick escape from the building is needed.

The practice will on occasion, require that staff members have access to the facility after hours. Consequently, security becomes an individual matter. Each team member has the responsibility to see that the practice is secured if they are the last person to leave. Keys should be issued to team members at the discretion of the practice manager and returned at the end of employment or at the request of the practice manager or owner. The practice should install keypads, allowing codes to be engaged/disengaged accordingly.

Reporting Accidents: Any/all accidents should be reported to the owner and/or practice manager. Injuries can be serious and should not be hidden from management. When injuries occur, management should investigate and implement protocols to prevent the injury from reoccurring in another person. Recall the need for psychological safety (Chapter 2) in the workplace environment. People need to feel safe to report injuries without fear of management getting upset; leaders must demonstrate the behaviors to create a learning moment out of the safety incident.

Proper forms must be completed when an injury has occurred, and the practice manager is responsible for ensuring that the forms are forwarded to the proper authorities when warranted. Forms must be posted the following year for all team members to see, and annual reporting to OSHA is required, even when no injuries have been recorded for the year (see Chapter 15 for OSHA Forms 300, 301, and 301 A).

VHMA PRACTICE DOMAIN TASK

Practice managers document and report accidents and file appropriate reports.

Probationary Period: Many practices use a probationary period when hiring new team members. This trial period allows all parties to see if this is a good match for the practice. The probationary period should be clearly stated in the offer of employment letter and employee manual, including the length of the period. The practice's right to end employment without cause should also be stated.

If the new team member fails during the probationary period, the manual should indicate that the team member may be terminated. When the team member does succeed, the manual should indicate whether the team member will receive an evaluation and/or a raise after the probation period. On average, practices have a 30–60-day probationary period, with evaluations after 30 and 90 days, and raises may be provided after 90 days. Review state laws regarding lengths of probationary periods; states may require practices to pay unemployment if the length of time exceeded state requirements.

It is detrimental to maintain team members who do not fit into the practice. Poor work ethic, poor performance, and negative attitudes (usually demonstrated during the probationary period) are contagious and if team members with these habits are kept for long-term employment, they will negatively impact other team members.

Termination Procedures: Termination procedures are discussed in detail later in this chapter. Procedures should be discussed and clearly defined in the employee manual. Team members should be advised of the protocol and what to expect if a termination situation arises. Defined termination procedures also offer some protection to the practice if an unemployment claim or lawsuit ever arises.

JOB DESCRIPTIONS AND DUTIES

Now that the employee manual has been developed, job descriptions can be focused on. Job descriptions must be detailed and include the clear expectation of the role and how it ties to the overall strategic goals of the practice (Fig. 4.13). Team members cannot be held to expectations if the duty is not listed in the job description. The phrase "and any other task assigned by a supervisor" can be added to any job description. If the practice is large and has several departments, a description may include a statement such as "Every team member works for ABC Veterinary Hospital as a whole, not for a particular supervisor or department." It is clearly defined that each team member is to help anyone who needs help, not just those within their own department.

Examples of summarized job duties and descriptions in Fig. 4.16 are in no way complete. They can be added to or deleted. Each practice varies, and duties and descriptions should be developed for each hospital.

VHMA PRACTICE DOMAIN TASK

Practice managers create, review, and update job descriptions/manuals.

Both hard and soft skills must be included in job descriptions. Hard skills are competencies that are required for the position or could be learned through training. Examples of hard skills for veterinary technicians would include placing a catheter, giving vaccinations, or administrating tablets to a dog. Soft skills are competencies that are hard to teach and generally developed in individuals as they mature. Soft skills competencies include a strong work ethic, promptness, attentiveness, and leadership abilities. Both sets of skills are critical to evaluate when creating job descriptions and searching for the right candidate. Because hard skills can be trained and soft skills cannot, it is advantageous to hire a team member based on a strong set of soft skills. Each job description should address the following fundamentals:

A position title is the name of the role.

A summary highlights the responsibilities of the role.

Description of required skills and qualifications lists what degrees or skills are required for the role.

Duties and responsibilities include specialized and basic duties of the role. Essential skills such as lifting a 50-lb dog or providing client education, cannot be left out.

The wage range provides the minimum and maximum wages for the role. Some states require that salary information be provided within the job description itself, or when an ad is posted to recruit new talent. Review the practice's state law to ensure compliance.

Accountability states to whom this person or position will report.

Job descriptions and duties should be given to each applicant during the interview process. Applicants must fully understand the expectations of the role and how the rule contributes to the client and patient experience. This will allow the interviewer and candidate to compare skills and abilities and determine whether the applicant is a match for the position. Although providing job descriptions is not required by law in most states, they can certainly protect a practice against potential lawsuits, unemployment, and discrimination suits. Job descriptions add clarity and consistency for team members, helping each team member to know what duties and expectations are required for each role. Job descriptions must be tied to strategic goals with the core values, vision, and mission weaved in, along with clear performance expectations, then reviewed with team members during coaching and performance feedback sessions. Additionally, the descriptions and duties must be evaluated annually to check for any changes that may have occurred. Has the practice purchased new equipment? Have protocols changed? If yes, then job descriptions may need to be updated.

LEADERSHIP POINT

Take your job description to a trusted friend that is not familiar with veterinary medicine and ask them to review it. Once they have, ask them to tell you what would be expected of them if they applied for that role. If they cannot cover all the expectations you expect of a team member, rewrite the job description.

DEVELOPING TRAINING PROTOCOLS

The creation of a phased program for each role will ensure new team members are trained properly. Each practice is different, and development of these modules should be tailored to the specific practice. Tweaks and changes should be made to protocols to continue to produce the best quality of training. Training takes time and must be completed in phases, allowing each phase to be accomplished before moving on to the next phase (Figs. 4.14A and B).

VHMA PRACTICE DOMAIN TASK

Practice managers develop and manage personnel training and development programs.

An excellent protocol has different levels of training and allows team members reasonable amounts of time to master the skills within each phase. It is important that inexperienced team members understand why protocols are completed in such a manner, and that the protocols give examples of possible consequences of misinterpreted instructions. Skills should be detailed to ensure a complete understanding of each skill. For example, customer service has a variety of skills under its umbrella: answering the phone courteously, greeting clients as they enter the practice, and answering client questions.

Phase training should be tailored to each new team member depending on experience. Modules should contain detailed information with the expectation that team members learn the modules within a specific time frame.

New team members should be encouraged to read the team member procedures manual and the training modules. Once these are read, they can observe team members completing the skills, complete the skills themselves, and then be tested on the concept. Once a new team member has completed the first module with satisfaction, the second module can be started, with an estimated date of completion in mind.

Training should occur through multiple modalities, as adults learn by hearing, seeing, and touching. Reading training materials introduces the new team member to the concept, and the trainer must

SAMPLE OF SUMMARIZED JOB DESCRIPTIONS

KENNEL ASSISTANT

A kennel assistant will be expected to assist a veterinarian, veterinary technician, or assistant in the care of animals. This may include restraining, cleaning, and walking the patients. The kennel assistant will maintain the constant cleanliness of the kennels, cages, and ward area, including the care and feeding of all animals. Kennel assistants are expected to have knowledge of cleaning and disinfecting methods and use proper chemicals and equipment to complete the task safely and efficiently. The assistant should be able to patiently treat sick and debilitated patients as well as understand and carry out written and oral instructions. Kennel assistants must be able to lift and carry patients up to 40 lbs as needed and required by team members. If any problems arise, kennel assistants should report them to the practice manager immediately.

VETERINARY ASSISTANT

A veterinary assistant will be expected to assist the veterinarian and veterinary technician in the care of animals. This may include restraining, cleaning, and walking the patients; providing medical care assigned by the veterinarian; and providing communication to the client as specified by the veterinarian. The assistant will also perform laboratory analysis, take radiographs, and assist the receptionist with answering the phone and providing customer service as needed. An assistant is expected to always be pleasant, patient, courteous, and polite to clients and team members and contribute to keeping the office flowing in an organized, efficient manner. Assistants must have knowledge of vaccination protocols, pharmacology, nutrition, animal husbandry and care and must be able to lift and carry patients as heavy as 40 lbs as needed and required by team members. If any problems arise, assistants should report them to the practice manager immediately.

CREDENTIALED VETERINARY TECHNICIAN/NURSE

A credentialed veterinary technician/nurse is licensed in the state by the appropriate state licensing authority and will be expected to carry out duties as allowed by the state veterinary practice act, and under the supervision of a veterinarian. This role is also expected to assist the veterinarian in diagnosing, prescribing medications, and surgery. This may include restraining, cleaning, and walking the patients; providing medical care assigned by the veterinarian; and communicating with and educating the client. The technician/nurse will perform laboratory analysis, take radiographs, and assist the receptionist with answering the phone and providing customer service as needed. The technician/nurse may oversee the kennel and veterinary assistants and provide continuing education for these staff members. The veterinary technician/nurse is held to the highest standard of care and must ensure all patients receive the appropriate treatments and nutrition and be kept in a safe and clean environment. Veterinary technicians are expected to always be pleasant, patient, courteous, and polite to clients and team members and contribute to keeping the office flowing in an organized, efficient manner. Technicians must have knowledge of vaccination protocols, pharmacology, nutrition, and animal husbandry and care. Veterinary technicians must be able to lift and carry patients as heavy as 40 lbs as needed by team members. If any problems arise, veterinary technicians/nurses should report them to the practice manager immediately.

RECEPTIONIST

A receptionist is expected to provide the highest level of customer service and care. This is done by answering phones, scheduling appointments, answering client questions, creating/updating patient medical charts, checking clients in and out, and accepting payments. A receptionist will always maintain a professional appearance and behave in a professional manner, speak clearly and slowly for clients to understand, and relay reliable information to clients as directed by the veterinarian and/or veterinary technicians. If any problems arise, the receptionist should report them to the office manager immediately.

OFFICE MANAGER

An office manager is expected to provide the highest level of customer service and care. This is accomplished by answering phones, scheduling appointments, answering client questions, updating patient medical charts, checking clients in and out, and accepting payments. Office managers will always maintain a professional appearance and behave in a professional manner, speak clearly and slowly for clients to understand, and relay reliable information to clients as directed by the veterinarian and/ or veterinary technician. Managers are responsible for the training of receptionists and for overseeing all duties that are expected of them, accounts receivable, and any other activities as directed by the practice manager. The office manager is held to the highest standard and should ensure that all customers are satisfied and have received the value of service they have paid for. If any problems arise, office managers should report them to the practice manager immediately for guidance.

Fig. 4.13 Complete job descriptions set clear expectations for team members.

SAMPLE OF SUMMARIZED JOB DESCRIPTIONS (*continued*)

PRACTICE MANAGER

The practice manager oversees all roles in the veterinary practice and ensures that all team members receive proper training and adhere to Standard Operating Protocols, Standards of Care, charge capture, and providing a frictionless client experience. The practice manager oversees inventory management, team member scheduling, and maintenance of equipment. If problems arise, the practice manager should report them to the hospital administrator or owner for guidance.

VETERINARIAN

A veterinarian will see patients to diagnose and treat disease, perform surgery, and prescribe medications. A veterinarian must establish trust and rapport with the team, provide education to enhance the skills of the team, and will delegate duties associated with laboratory analysis, patient treatments and nursing, prescription filling, etc., to technicians/nurses and assistants, allowing more client/veterinarian interaction and education. Veterinarians are ultimately responsible for the care and treatment of patients and must advise clients of the best options available for their patients. Problems with training or with team members not completing their duties correctly should be discussed with the practice manager, hospital administrator, and owner of the practice.

HOSPITAL ADMINISTRATOR

A hospital administrator oversees the entire function of the veterinary hospital. The administrator is responsible for creating and maintaining budgets, finances, hospital protocols, and procedures. This position requires the use of accounting and financial tools, which must be used for the practice to be successful.

Fig. 4.13 Cont'd

verbally review the concepts to ensure the new team member hears and understands the skill that is being trained. The trainer must then demonstrate the skill, and then allow the new team member to try it. The trainer will need to provide coaching and words of encouragement as a team member tries to skill and builds confidence. Adults retain approximately 10% of what they see; however, this retention increases by 30% to 40% when they both hear and see. Adults retain 90% of training when they hear, see, and do.

CRITICAL COMPETENCY: RESOURCEFULNESS

The practice manager must have the ability to understand what it takes to complete the job by applying knowledge, skills, and expertise to perform tasks quickly and efficiently.

Basic training modules for kennel assistants should include kennel duties and tasks, including techniques, chemical usage, knowledge of diseases and their transmission, animal handling, restraint, exercise, and basic nutrition.

Veterinary assistants should be expected to know all the training materials for kennel assistants before proceeding to the next level. Surgery, laboratory, radiology, and pharmacology protocols can then follow. Credentialed veterinary technicians/nurses are expected to know all the modules, followed by all skills that are fully allowed by the state veterinary practice act.

Veterinarians also need a developed training protocol. New graduates should have a mentorship program built out (Chapter 6, Professional Development) allowing them to learn through coaching, observation, and seeing limited cases as they become familiar with SOPs, Standards of Care (SOC), and the functions that each section of the team carries out. Experienced veterinarians also need a protocol, and while mentorship would not be included in that plan, the remainder would.

It takes a team to train a team and using all team members to train new team members greatly improves efficiency. Ten people participating in training can offer more knowledge than if one person does all the training. However, one supervisor should oversee all training to ensure the team member can complete the procedures and techniques expected.

LEADERSHIP POINT

Take the time to collaborate with the team and develop very specific training vprograms for each role. Collaboration with the team will help them take accountability when training new team members, and a well-thought-out program develops a loyal team member who loves their job.

EMPLOYEE PROCEDURE MANUAL/STANDARD OPERATING PROTOCOLS (SOPS) AND STANDARDS OF CARE (SOC)

An employee procedure manual, known more commonly as SOPs, not only train new team members but also provide a guide to look up procedures as needed. SOPs take time to develop and must be updated frequently to provide consistency with all team members (Fig. 4.15).

Developing and Implementing Standard Operating Protocols

The practice should develop SOPs to include every procedure commonly used by the receptionist team, the medical team, and the kennel team. Team members can be asked to contribute by writing up all the

EXAMPLE OF PHASE TRAINING FOR KENNEL ASSISTANTS

KENNEL ASSISTANT MODULE ONE

- Policies and paperwork
- Team member personnel manual
- Team member procedures manual
- Team member expectations
- Professional ethics
- W -4, I-9, and benefits forms
- Time clock
- Dress code
- Cleaning
- Prevention of disease transmission through isolations and cleaning protocols
  - Keep all isolation cleaning items in isolation.
- Chemicals to clean with
- Chlorhexidine
- Rescue
- Chemicals to Not Clean with
  - Lysol
  - Ammonia
- Equipment
  - Scrub brushes
  - Mops and buckets
  - Brooms
  - Technique
  - Scrubbing
  - Contact time
  - Rinsing and drying
- Laundry
- Hot water
- Detergent and bleach
- Towels and blankets
  - Blanket safety: no holes or shredded blankets
- Proper Disposal of sharps and Biohazard Containers
- Proper disposal of bodies
  - Private burial
  - Mass or private cremation

KENNEL ASSISTANT MODULE TWO

- Nutrition
  - Knowledge of different types of food
  - Puppy, maintenance, and senior formulas; prescription formulas
  - Amount to feed each animal
  - Measure
  - NPO
  - PO
- Hospital sheets
  - Following treatments required
- Walking patients safely
  - Removing patients from cages/kennels safely
  - Slip leash
  - Three times daily, more if indicated
  - With IV fluids
  - With bandaging material, casts, or other
- Cats
  - Clay litter
  - Nonabsorbable litter
  - Paper litter

KENNEL ASSISTANT MODULE THREE

- Hospital maintenance
- Trash
- Sweeping/mopping
- Cleanliness
- Fans, display shelving
- Light fixtures
- Working light bulbs and ballasts
- Outside: weeds, animal waste, and front porch appearance

KENNEL ASSISTANT MODULE FOUR

- Restraint techniques
  - Dogs and cats
  - Psychological restraint
  - Lifting appropriately
  - Handling the fractious patient
  - Lateral recumbency
  - Sternal recumbency
  - Restraint for venipuncture (blood draw)
  - Jugular
  - Cephalic
  - Saphenous
  - Femoral
- Using precautions when necessary
  - Muzzles
  - Slip leash
  - Know when to hold tighter or use less restraint
  - Understand client concerns when restraining animals
- E-collars
- Normal vital signs
  - Temperature
  - Pulse
  - Respiratory rate
- Grooming
  - Combing and brushing
  - Ear cleaning
  - Nail trimming
  - Anal sac expression
- Bathing

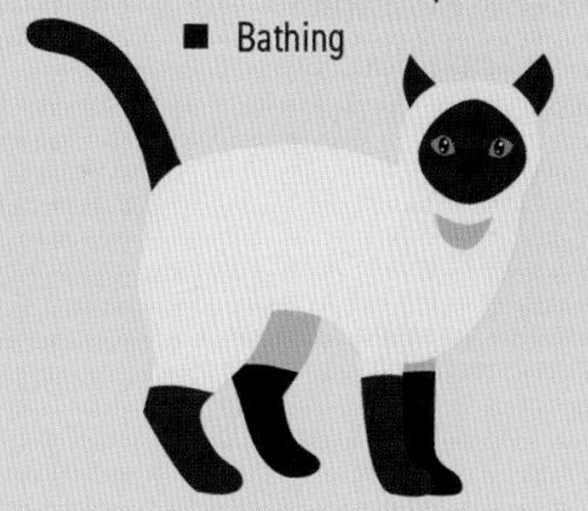

A

Fig. 4.14 Implement a phase training program for each role to prevent new employees from being overwhelmed.

procedures they perform daily. An outline can be created listing procedures by department or technique, which then can be developed into a table of contents. The SOP manual can then be organized in alphabetical order for easy and quick retrieval. Each SOP should be defined, outline steps needed to accomplish the procedure, and include "why" the procedure should be completed in that manner. This allows team members to completely understand and be able to explain procedures to clients when needed.

When team members participate in creating SOPs, they are more likely to help implement and make use of them. With the completion of each protocol, each team member should receive a copy, and a hard copy should be kept within the practice in a central location that is easy to find. Paperless practices can upload SOPs onto the practice server, allowing team members to access them from any computer in the clinic.

When new team members are hired, they should receive their own copy with training to occur over several weeks. Covering too much information too fast will overwhelm the new team member resulting in missed information. SOPs can also be used to develop phase training programs, and when team members question a protocol, they can reference the SOPs. In many cases, certain techniques are used so infrequently that their protocols are forgotten.

EXAMPLE OF PHASE TRAINING FOR VETERINARY ASSISTANTS

VETERINARY ASSISTANT MODULE ONE

- Kennel Assistant Modules One to Four

VETERINARY ASSISTANT MODULE TWO

- Interaction with clients and patients
- Treat animals as if they were your own.
- Ensure clients always feel comfortable
- Offer coffee or water to those that must wait extended periods of time.
- Listen to what clients say.
- Show you care.
- Offer to carry items and patients for clients.
- Always provide an answer. If you don't have the answer, find the correct answer as soon as possible.
- Cleaning between patients
- Prevention of disease transmission
  - Wash hands after each patient
  - Clean table and examination room between each patient
  - Clean instruments used between patients
- Animal care protocol
- Hospital sheets
- Proper food and proper feeding times for each patient
- Always provide fresh water unless otherwise indicated
- Always provide a clean blanket or towel unless otherwise indicated
- Prevention of nosocomial infections
- Patient monitoring
  - Observe patient for any bowel movement, urination, vomit, or abnormal condition. Indicate on hospital sheet and alert a veterinarian.
- Performing medicated baths
  - Be familiar with product and procedure for bathing.
- Medical records
  - Reading and understanding medical records
  - SOAP format
  - Writing a complete medical record
  - Abbreviations
  - Recording observations
  - TPR
  - Preparing room for veterinarian
  - Charge capture
- Cleanliness
- Stocking of inventory
- Sexing of animals
- Aging dogs and cats
- Mixing vaccines
- Filling syringes
- The Frictionless Client Experience
  - Greeting clients with a smile
  - Listening to what the client wants
  - Satisfying customer needs
  - Ensuring the customer perceives the value in the service they received
- Examination room SOPs, history taking, and client education
  - Common questions and concerns
  - Heartworm disease and products carries
  - Fleas and ticks; products carried
  - Nutritional needs and products carried
  - Shampoo (mediated and non-medicated) and conditioners carried and what each product treats
- Vaccination SOPs
- Laboratory analysis
  - Common tests and methods to complete
- Surgery SOPs (Exam Room)
  - Scheduling surgeries
  - Checking in patients
  - Routine procedures completed in the practice
  - Anesthetic consent forms
- Dental care SOPs (Exam Room)
  - Scheduling
  - Checking in patients
  - Routine procedures completed in the practice
  - Dental/anesthetic consent forms

B1

Fig. 4.14 Cont'd

Each time a vaccine protocol, laboratory procedure, or surgical prep technique changes, the SOP must be updated. Team members should receive a single sheet indicating the change, and team members should sign a form indicating they have received the update (like the employee manual protocol).

Changes can be hard for some team members to implement, especially when a routine with a procedure has been established. They may become resistant to the change, even though it has been formally established and they have signed the form indicating they are aware of the change. Some team members resist change because of their discomfort level with the change or new procedure. Training these team members with a different approach may improve compliance, including asking these team members why they may be resistant to the change. Review Chapter 2, Leadership, on change management.

LEADERSHIP POINT

Place an annual review of SOPs on the calendar 1 year from the date of implementation. Often, new equipment or procedures are implemented, and the updating of the SOP is forgotten about.

Standards of Care

Standards of care (SOCs) are guidelines and treatment protocols that have been established allowing the highest quality of medical care to be recommended for every patient. The veterinarian(s) develop the SOCs for the most common cases that a practice sees that includes diagnostic and treatment plans. When SOCs are established, every team member is on the same page in recommending the same treatment protocol

EXAMPLE OF PHASE TRAINING FOR VETERINARY ASSISTANTS (*continued*)

VETERINARY ASSISTANT MODULE THREE

- Surgical protocols for pre-op exams, pre-anesthetic, catheter placement, surgical prep, post op recovery and patient discharge
- Dental protocols for pre-op exams, pre-anesthetic, catheter placement, surgical prep, post op recovery and patient discharge
- Surgery logs
  - NPO (nothing by mouth)
- Preanesthetic and anesthetic drugs, dosage, side effects, when and how to administer
- Anesthetic planes
- Intubation
  - Selection of appropriate tube
  - Inflation of cuff
- Eye lubrication (how/why and product of choice
- IV fluids
  - Prepping site with aseptic technique
  - Catheters (18 g, 20 g, 22 g), length; how to choose appropriate size
  - Fluid Options (Normosol, NaCl, Plasmalyte, Dextrose)
- Surgical sterile fields
- Opening packs (instruments and gowns) and opening of
- Suture material (type, size of needle) and opening of
- Gowning the surgeon
- Monitoring the recovering patient
  - TPR
  - Removal of ET
- Release instructions (after care, medications, medical progress exams)
- Equipment
  - Surgical table (tilting, raising, and lowering of)
  - Monitors (Surgical monitor, Blood pressure machine, ECG)
  - Anesthetic machine
    - Proper use of, administration of gases, hose selection, bag selection
    - Refilling of anesthetic gas
    - Sofa lime (why it is used and how/when to change)
    - Maintenance of any scavenger system
    - Daily check for leaks
- Surgical instruments and packs
  - Names and uses of individual instruments
  - Proper cleaning and drying protocol
  - Cleaning protocol for wraps and gowns
  - Packing and wrapping packs
  - Autoclave protocol
- Maintenance of autoclave
  - Distilled water, gaskets, etc

VETERINARY ASSISTANT MODULE FOUR

- Radiograph procedures
  - Safety and equipment (thyroid collar, lead gloves, gowns, eye protection, dosimeter
  - Machine set up: patient and client name, view, etc
  - Anatomical positions
- Ultrasound procedures
- Endoscopy procedures
- Internal Laboratory Procedures
  - Common external parasites
    - Prepping for ear smear, skin scrape, cytology
  - Common internal parasites
  - Collecting fecal sample
    - Prepping and reading fecal
  - Urinalysis
    - Sample collection: free catch, cystocentesis, catheterization
    - Sample evaluation: microscopic, stick, specific gravity
    - Culture and Sensitivity
  - HCT/PCV Machine
  - Chemistry machine
  - CBC machine
  - Electrolyte machine
  - Microscope
    - Use, cleaning protocols, power levels, oil immersion
  - Cytology stains (when to stain and protocols for proper staining)
  - Refractometer (use, cleaning, and storage)
  - Centrifuge(s)
  - Tonometer (Use, calibration, and cleaning protocols)
  - Blood pressure machine (use, cuff size selection)
  - ECG machine (location of leads, how to use, storage of)
  - Blood tubes (types the practice has and when to use, proper filling protocols)
  - CBC/chemistry/electrolytes/blood gases
  - Urinalysis
  - Heartworm 4DX (heartworm, Ehrlichia canis, Lyme disease, and anaplasmosis)
  - FeLV/FIV/HWT
  - Parvo
  - Spec CPL
- External Laboratory Procedures
  - Laboratory forms
  - Common profiles and individual tests (Bile acids, Phenobarbital levels, ACTH stimulation, T-4, Total T-4, Equilibrium dialysis, Thyroid panels, etc)

B2

Fig. 4.14 Cont'd

EXAMPLE OF PHASE TRAINING FOR VETERINARY ASSISTANTS (*continued*)

VETERINARY ASSISTANT MODULE FIVE

- Patient discharge: instructions, medications, pet's personal items
- Pharmacology
- Handling controlled substances
- Amber bottle versus clear bottle
- Potential drug interactions of top 20% of medications used
- Normal dosing of each medication and labeling requirements
- Abbreviations
  - SID, BID, TID, QID, PRN, EOD
  - PO
  - IV, IM, SQ
  - AU/AD/AS
  - OU/OD/OS
- Providing instructions to the owner
- Administering medications to the patient: oral, aural, ocular, topical

VETERINARY ASSISTANT MODULE SIX

- Patient treatments
  - Injections: SQ, IM, IV
  - Oral
  - Topical
- Monitoring IV fluids and catheters
- Developing patient hospitalization sheets
- Developing patient release sheets and selecting client education documents

B3

Fig. 4.14 Cont'd

to clients. This enhances client compliance and communication. See Chapter 11 for more information on SOCs.

WAGE DEVELOPMENT AND MANAGEMENT

It is important for a manager to understand the entire payroll process. Becoming as organized as possible in its management will ensure a successful system. Payroll can be time-consuming and must be maintained by a motivated, trusted team member that must be held accountable for correct payroll procedures and ensuring that all tax payments are submitted on time. Many hospitals use an accountant, bookkeeper, or payroll that helps with payroll, the completion of tax forms, and the electronic submission of such forms. Either way, the payroll administrator must ensure the hours worked and wage rates are entered correctly.

Pay periods are defined as the length of time covered by each payroll period and generally cover weekly, biweekly, or semimonthly periods (Monday morning through Sunday night is an example). A practice can determine what pay period works best as well as days of the week to start and stop the period. Once pay periods have been determined and are set in motion, they cannot be changed.

Weekly pay periods generate 52 periods per year, paying team members weekly. The disadvantage of weekly pay periods is the administrative costs associated with processing payroll each week. Biweekly payroll decreases administrative costs by processing payroll every other week, producing 26 periods per year. Because there are not a balanced number of weeks in every month, there will be two months out of the year when payroll occurs three times within the month. This can make reports (for those two months) look incorrect because payroll percentages will be artificially high, lowering EBITDA. Semimonthly payroll eliminates this discrepancy in the analysis because payroll occurs evenly on the first and the fifteenth of each month and produces 24 pay periods per year.

Wage Determination

Determining wages for different levels of the team can be challenging. A balance must be made between achieving strategic goals and maintaining a knowledgeable and dedicated staff. Team members must be compensated for their skills while creating and maintaining an environment that is culturally strong.

When determining wages, the benefits package available must also be considered (team members should be reminded of benefits received during their total compensation review). The location of the practice within the United States also plays a factor in wage determination, as the cost of living in some areas is higher than in others. Practices in large cities, referral practices, and specialty centers will also have higher compensation rates than those in smaller cities and general practices.

VHMA PERFORMANCE DOMAIN TASK

Veterinary practice managers manage team member benefit programs.

To determine a pay scale (for new or established clinics), a chart can be developed to show minimum, average, and maximum rates for each position, as well as to determine any discrepancies a current practice may have in its pay scale system. It is critical to have consistent procedures for setting pay levels for each position.

List all the positions in the practice and the team members that fill those positions. Fill in the minimum and maximum pay wage for each position based on local wage demographics and the VHMA Compensation and Benefits, then add the current pay for team members. The chart will most likely reveal discrepancies when a pay scale has never been established. In general, wages have risen, but salaries of long-term team members have not, or raises were given for reasons other than performance-based. As previously stated, the location and type of practice are factors in pay scale, but a practice should at least be at or higher than the 75th percentile to recruit and retain excellent team members. Team members cannot be expected to complete highly skilled tasks and procedures for minimum wage. Higher-paid individuals will produce income for the practice while having team member engagement and greater accountability for their roles in the practice.

LEADERSHIP POINT

Developing levels within the practice allows team members to identify how they can grow within the practice while also being financially rewarded for such growth.

Different levels within roles can also be helpful. For example, the veterinary assistant role may have levels 1, 2, and 3. Level one is an entry-level role with limited skills and knowledge. Level 2 is average but not yet functioning at the highest level. Level 3 may be for an approved veterinary assistant, a veterinary assistant that has certifications, or an assistant that is attending veterinary technician school (or has yet to pass the VTNE and receive state credentialing).

Once levels are established, the minimum and maximum ranges established from VHMA, local demographics, and practice philosophy

SAMPLE TABLE OF CONTENTS FOR SOP MANUAL

- Animal bites
- Artificial insemination
- Bandages/splints/casts
    - Pressure bandages
    - Dry bandages
    - Wet-to-dry bandages (wound management)
    - Splints/casts
- Blood transfusions
    - Fresh frozen plasma
    - Whole blood
    - Equipment needed
- Catheters
    - Butterfly
    - Foley catheters
    - Intravenous catheters
    - Jugular catheters
    - Polypropylene catheters
    - Red rubber catheters
    - Tom cat catheters
- Common diseases
- Common emergencies
    - Cardiopulmonary resuscitation
    - Anaphylactic reaction
    - Blocked cat
    - Dyspneic animal
    - Dystocia
    - Gastric torsion
    - Seizures
    - Toxicities
- Dentals
    - Machine
    - Gum disease
    - Anatomy of the mouth
    - Determining age of cats and dogs
- Diets
    - Dogs, Cats
    - Ferrets, Rabbits
    - Reptiles, Snakes
    - Birds
    - Special diets (Hills, Waltham, Purina)
- Fluid therapy
    - Types
    - Additives
    - Catheter types and sizes
    - Catheter use and maintenance
    - Heparin bags and prep
    - Administration of fluids
    - Drip rate calculation
- Heartworm disease
    - Life cycle of the heartworm
    - Treatment
    - Prevention
- Instruments
    - Care and handling
    - Autoclaving
    - General pack
    - Cold sterilization
    - General cold pack
- Kennel care
    - Duties
    - Cleaning procedures
    - Blankets
- Laboratory equipment and procedures
    - Centrifuges
    - Microscopes
    - Hematology analyzer
    - Chemistry analyzer
    - Hemocytometer
    - Refractometer
    - Tonometer
- Diagnostic tests and laboratory work
    - Blood work abbreviations
    - Heartworm test
    - SNAP
    - Parvo
    - FELV
    - FELV/FIV/HWT
    - WBC
    - HCT or PCV
    - TP
    - UA
    - Fecal
    - DTM
    - Ear smear
    - Ear mite check
    - Skin scrape
    - Staining slides
    - Protocols for common blood work
    - ACTH stimulation
    - Bile acids
    - Phenobarbital
    - Thyroid
- Logs
    - Laboratory log
    - Surgery log
    - Controlled drug log
- Medications
    - Abbreviations
    - Weight conversions
    - Labels
    - Administration
- Pregnancy
    - Care of female
    - Care of puppies and kittens
    - Problems with pregnancy
    - Cesarean section
    - Gestation/reproductive maturity
- Radiology
    - Machine function
    - Server back up
    - Radiation safety
    - Aprons and care of
- Reproductive disorders
    - Cryptorchidism
    - Incontinence
    - Mastitis
    - Metritis
    - Prostate
    - Cystic hyperplasia
    - Prostate tumors
    - Pyometra
- Restraint (for examination and venipuncture)
    - Dog, cat
    - Ferret, rabbits
    - Reptiles
    - Birds
- Examination room
    - Room prep
    - Supplies
- Safety data sheets
    - Location
    - How to read
    - Safety plans and hazard communications (OSHA)
- Spaying/neutering pets
    - Age
    - Benefits
    - Risks associated with surgery
    - Postoperative care
- Surgery
    - NPO
    - Surgery prep
    - Biopsy prep
    - Anesthesia
        - Drugs
        - Endotracheal tubes
        - Monitoring
    - Anesthetic machines and maintenance
        - Isoflurane refill
    - Oxygen
    - Autoclave
        - Care and maintenance
    - Packs
        - Instrument packs
        - Cold pack
    - Gown and towel pack
    - Towel pack
    - Drapes
    - Needles and suture material
- Syringes
    - Varieties and gauges of needles
- Vaccines and protocols
- Dog, Cats, Ferrets

**ACTH stim, Adrenocorticotropic hormone stimulation; CPR, cardiopulmonary resuscitation; DTM, dermatophyte test medium; FELV, feline leukemia; FIV, feline immunodeficiency virus; HCT, hematocrit; NPO, nothing by mouth; PCV, packed cell volume; TP, total protein; UA, urinalysis; WBC, white blood cell count.*

Fig. 4.15 Standard Operating Protocols (SOPs) can help a practice stay aligned on both procedures and patient care.

can be equally split between the levels. This also helps team members grow in their roles. Levels should be established for credentialed veterinary technicians/nurses and receptionists as well.

> **CRITICAL COMPETENCY: CRITICAL AND STRATEGIC THINKING**
>
> Strategic thinking and planning are essential parts of financial forecasting and long-term plans for the growth of the practice. Managers must have the ability to identify questions, problems, and arguments relevant to these issues and to use logic and critical reasoning to identify the strengths and weaknesses of alternative solutions or approaches to problems.

Veterinarians

Hiring a veterinarian for a practice is very important. Not only should the person be able to fit into the practice, but they must be able to fit into the budget of the practice. To determine whether a practice can support another veterinarian, reports should be generated looking at the average number of clients seen on a yearly basis. To support a full-time–equivalent veterinarian, 800 to 1200 active clients are needed per year. Therefore, the practice needs to see at least an additional 800 clients per year to justify a new veterinarian.

Pro-sal (combination of production and salary), salary only, and production only are the three forms of compensation commonly used to pay veterinarians. If the practice commonly accepts after-hours emergencies, doctors may be paid additional money to compensate for their time. Under professional liability, veterinarians have a legal duty to accept emergencies or refer them to an emergency practice after hours.

While many veterinarians will have a minimal base salary when applying for a position, the practice must understand what they can pay, based on demographics, client spending, the standard of medicine, and client compliance. On average, a practice manager can take the assumed generated revenue that a new veterinarian will produce and divide it by 5. For example, if a veterinarian is expected to produce $700,000 in year one, $700,000 / 5 = $140,000. A base salary can be offered at $140k, with production as an incentive to achieve above and beyond. Another way to consider this equation is to take the veterinarians asking salary and multiply it by 5. If an applicant is asking $150,000 × 5, then the practice manager could assume the doctor will produce $750,000 in revenue. This equation is based on full-time equivalency (FTE) at 40 hours per week.

Practice managers and owners must be diligent about tracking production and sharing with doctors monthly. Those producing more than the goal should be rewarded, and those producing less need to be coached and mentored by the owner. Having conversations about revenue production should be positive, with the intent to "coach up." Seek to understand why production levels may be lower than anticipated. Consider:

Hours Worked: Is the doctor working 40 hours a week or less? Does the doctor cover shifts that historically have fewer visits?

Leveraging: Does the doctor feel they can effectively leverage duties to the staff so they can see the next patient?

Surgery: Does the doctor perform basic and advanced surgical procedures?

Service Mix: Does the doctor work up cases or make assumptions on diagnoses and send home medication? The goal of the practice is to have a service mix of 80% medical services and 20% inventory.

Invoicing: Are invoices coded consistently under the correct veterinarian?

All these factors impact the revenue production of each veterinarian. Create the winning team and ensure all areas are addressed.

It's the practice that pays production on any level; both inventory and procedures must be evaluated to determine the percentage of pay for each category. There are no set industry standards of what percent of each to pay, but a practice may consider:

- 20%–23% services, 10% inventory, with refills, diets, boarding, and grooming not included.
- 18%–20% flat production, regardless of what category.
- 20% service and 15% inventory, with refills, diets, boarding, and grooming not included.

DVM Salary-Based Pay: Salary-compensated veterinarians receive a set amount, regardless of the amount of revenue produced. Some practices prefer to pay veterinarians a set salary as opposed to any other form of payment because it seems to decrease the competition among veterinarians in the practice. It promotes a team environment in which all doctors and staff help each other accomplish all tasks, diagnoses, and treatments. Veterinarians are exempt from overtime under FLSA, but hours should be monitored to prevent burnout. Fig. 4.16 provides an example of salary pay.

Production: A production-only model compensates a veterinarian based on sales only. A production-only salary is easy to determine (Fig. 4.17).

Pro-Sal: The most common form of compensation is a pro-sal formula, also referred to as the *production reconciliation hybrid.* This allows veterinarians to receive a guaranteed base salary and a production bonus once a predetermined dollar amount has been reached. If this formula is chosen, the base salary must first be determined and is normally based on the veterinarian's experience. The practice must decide what percentage of the production will be paid as a bonus and whether the bonus is paid on a monthly or quarterly basis. When calculating the pro-sal rate, the salary is guaranteed, regardless of the production. The production total is then subtracted from the salary, and the veterinarian receives the remainder (Fig. 4.18).

The team member receives $100,000 in salary per year.

Payday occurs on the first and the fifteenth of each month:

$100,000 ÷ 24 = **$4,166.67 gross pay per pay period**

**Gross pay is the total amount earned before any taxes or other withholdings.*

Fig. 4.16 Example of salary compensation calculation.

A team member is paid 20% of production of all services and products.

- Payday occurs on the first and the fifteenth of each month.
- The payroll manager should pull a report of that specific team members production from the first to the fourteenth of the month. If the team member produced $35,000 during that period:

  $35,000 × 20% = **$7,000 gross pay**

- The second pay period report would run from the fifteenth to the thirtieth or thirty-first of the month. If the veterinarian produced $26,236 for that period, then:

  $26,236 × 20% = **$5,247.20 gross pay**

**Gross pay is the total amount earned before any taxes or other withholdings.*

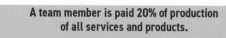

Fig. 4.17 Example of production-only compensation calculation.

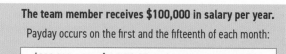

A veterinarian is paid $100,000 base salary per year with 20% production. Production is paid monthly for the previous month's production. Payday is on the first and the fifteenth of each month.

$100,000 ÷ 24 (24 pay periods per year) = **$4,166.67 per check**

- The veterinarian produced $53,000 for the previous month:

$53,000 x 20% = **$10,600**

$10,600 (production) - $4,166.67 (guaranteed salary) = **$6,433.33**

- The gross pay for the first of the month is **$6,433.33.**
- The gross pay for the fifteenth of the month is **$4,166.67.**

**Gross pay is the total amount earned before any taxes or other withholdings.*

Fig. 4.18 Example of pro-sal compensation calculation.

The advantage of percentage-based compensation is that it can motivate veterinarians to see more patients (by leveraging staff) and medically work up cases (SOC). It emphasizes the medical and business aspect of veterinary medicine and compensates veterinarians for their successful efforts and the skills involved in practicing high-quality medicine.

The disadvantage of paying on production is the overall team spirit may decrease, and it may foster competition among veterinarians. Some veterinarians will perform diagnostic procedures that may not be necessary to increase production numbers. This can lead to claims of price gouging from clients. Paying on production may encourage veterinarians to choose wealthy clients and big cases over yearly examinations, vaccines, and small procedures. It can also discourage veterinarians from participating in procedures that do not produce income, or that produce small amounts of income. For example, if the practice offers healthy shelter-pet checks for a reduced cost, production-only veterinarians may choose not to see them. In practices that have a positive culture, All the issues just discussed can be eliminated, producing a win-win situation for everyone involved.

The practice must determine which formula will work best for the practice. Some practices may find that competition is not a problem within the hospital, and that either a pro-sal or production-only formula yields the best results. Others may find the salary formula to be the easiest and least time-consuming formula to use. It is recommended to pay the same structure to all veterinarians to eliminate any negative emotions/competition, except for new graduates. Because many new graduates will need to experience some form of mentorship, they will be unable (and not have the confidence) to achieve production goals for the first year. New graduates may be offered a base salary for year one, then transition to a pro-sal formula thereafter.

Practices must be well staffed and trained for a pro-sal or production formula to work efficiently. Veterinarians must be able to effectively delegate duties, treatments, and diagnostics to technicians while they continue seeing patients. If they cannot delegate duties due to a lack of training, production goals will not be met.

Emergency Pay: If emergencies are accepted after hours, veterinarians may be paid salary plus emergency pay. Some practices pay the set emergency fee per animal seen; other practices may pay 30% to 50% of the examination cost, plus a percentage of the diagnostics performed before the office opens. Yet another option may be to pay 10% of the examination fee and 18% to 22% of the total client transaction.

Regular rate calculations:

- **Wanda is paid $18 per hour and works 34 hours per week.** Pay date is every other Monday; therefore, the work week is Monday, 12:00 a.m. through Sunday, 12:59 p.m.

34 hours per week x 2 = **68 hours per 2-week period**

68 hours x $18.00 = **$1224.00 gross pay**

**Gross pay is the total amount earned before any taxes or other withholdings.*

Overtime rate calculations:

- **This period, Ann has worked 44 hours during week one and 32-hours during week two.** She is paid $18 per hour; therefore overtime is paid at $27 per hour (1{1/2} times the regular rate).

WEEK 1:	40 hours x $18.00 = **$720.00**
	4 hours x $27.00 = **$108.00**
Week 2:	32 hours x $18.00 = **$576.00**

$720.00 + $108.00 + $576.00 = **$1,404.00 before taxes**

Fig. 4.19 Example of non-DVM payroll calculations.

Technicians, Assistants, Receptionists, and Kennel Assistants

Credential technicians/nurses, veterinary assistants, receptionists, and kennel assistants are compensated based on a combination of experience, demographics, and wage scales set by the practice period. Recall that nonveterinary roles are paid hourly and anything over 40 hours per week must be paid overtime pay. See Fig. 4.19 for non-DVM payroll calculation examples.

Groomers

Some groomers are paid on a production percentage, just as veterinarians may be paid, whereas others may be paid hourly. Independent groomers may simply be paid a fee for each animal that is groomed; others may rent the grooming space within the veterinary practice. Independent groomers must have their own tax identification numbers; therefore, taxes are not taken out of the groomers' paychecks. They are responsible for paying their own federal and state taxes. See the Independent Contractor section later in this chapter for more details.

Raise Determination

Team members should receive annual raises on a scheduled basis, but they should be based on performance, not seniority. The practice must establish a policy as to when raises will be considered for all team members. Yearly cost-of-living (COL) raises should be considered for those not receiving a raise based on performance and skill.

CRITICAL COMPETENCY: DECISION MAKING

The practice manager must be able to make good decisions based on critical thinking and problem solving as well as decisions that positively impact the practice. While many alternatives are available, the PM must be able to gather and effectively analyze relevant data and choose decisively.

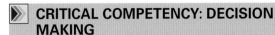

Develop a budget allocated to team member raises each year during the financial planning for the following year (Chapter 16, Finance, and Chapter 17, Strategic Planning). Use a percent of gross revenue to determine the total dollar amount; this can then be applied as needed for COL and performance. Don't forget about the veterinarians when budgeting. Those on salary-based pay should receive an increase; those on production receive an increase each time price increases go into effect.

If the practice's budget does not allow for team member raises, team members still need to be rewarded for excellent work and a one-time bonus should be considered. A bonus allows team members to know they are appreciated while impacting the bottom line less than raises. With that said, raises should not be overlooked because team members will seek employment at other practices offering higher pay.

Managing Payroll

QuickBooks is an excellent payroll software program. Frequent tax updates are provided, as well as tips for organizing payroll records. QuickBooks calculates the taxes withheld from the team member and those contributed by the employer, creates reports indicating where withheld funds should be allocated (retirement, health insurance, etc.), and creates pay stubs for each team member. If direct deposit is used, a link is available to complete the deposit. Payroll managers must take the time to enter the information initially, and QuickBooks does the rest.

CRITICAL COMPETENCY: PLANNING AND PRIORITIZING

Practice managers must be able to effectively manage time and workload to meet deadlines, thereby having the ability to organize work, set priorities, and establish plans to achieve goals.

Payroll Records: All states have different requirements regarding the length of time to keep team member payroll records, check with the state department of labor for current state regulations. All records should be kept in a locked cabinet for confidentiality purposes.

Team members should receive a payroll check stub with each paycheck (those with direct deposit should receive a stub on the day of payroll). Payroll stubs should indicate the team member's name, wage, and gross income (income before taxes and other withholdings), along with Social Security, Medicare, fringe benefits, contributions to an sIRA or 401(k) program, and/or any withholdings for insurance. Payroll stubs for full-time team members may also state the vacation and sick hours (PTO) available. A summary sheet for all team members should be kept on file for each payroll period.

Many practices and team members prefer to use direct deposit for payroll checks. The check is deposited directly into the team member's checking account on the date of payroll; the team member does not need to go to the bank to deposit the check.

Practices may contact their bank for direct deposit procedures. Normally, an authorization form is submitted from each team member to the practice's bank. The form includes the team member's name, address, current bank, and checking account number. The team member authorizing the direct deposit should also sign it. The bank may also request a voided check to ensure the correct routing number is entered when the initial deposit is set up. Paycheck amounts are usually due at the bank 2 to 3 business days before payday. This ensures that the funds will be transferred on payday.

Payroll Taxes: Several taxes are withheld from team members, and the employer is responsible for paying those as well as additional taxes. The practice bookkeeper, accountant, or team member responsible for payroll will determine this amount and must ensure that the taxes are paid on time. State revenue departments often penalize heavily for those that are late.

Social Security and Medicare: Taxes that are withheld from a team member's payroll check include income tax, Social Security, and Medicare. Social Security and Medicare fall under the Federal Insurance Contribution Act (FICA), wherein 6.2% of the gross pay is withheld for Social Security and 1.45% is withheld for Medicare. The employer is responsible for contributing the same amount to FICA. The total team member income taxes, as well as the team member and employer portions of FICA, are paid to the IRS through a federal tax deposit (FTD) system.

Federal Unemployment Tax Act: In addition to reporting FICA contributions on Form 941, employers are also responsible for taxes under FUTA, which are reported on Form 940. These taxes are paid solely by the employer and not withheld or deducted from the team member. FUTA collects $7000 (maximum) from the employer for each employee per year of employment. Some states may also have unemployment tax that is paid quarterly, and the amount of tax due depends on the schedule of payments.

Form W-4: Team members are required to fill out form W-4 (Fig. 4.20) once they are hired for employment. The form asks questions to determine how many deductions should be withheld from the payroll check, along with requiring the team member's Social Security number, address, and signature. This form should be kept in the team member's personnel file in a locked cabinet.

Form W-2: At the end of the year, when taxes are prepared, the accountant or bookkeeper will produce a W-2 form for each team member, summarizing their earnings for the year (Fig. 4.21). These forms include gross earnings, Social Security, Medicare, insurance, and retirement withholdings. These forms are due to team members no later than January 31 of each year (federal law). Don't forget to include the team member's total compensation statement as well (Fig. 4.12).

LEADERSHIP POINT

Create a well-organized payroll process to maximize efficiency and reduce processing errors.

Workers Compensation Insurance: As stated earlier, workers' compensation insurance protects the employer from injuries individuals might receive while on the job. Injuries include falls, animal bites, accidents, or exposure to harmful substances. Workers' compensation insurance is regulated by individual states, not the federal government; therefore, not all states require coverage. Depending on the state, a business may be able to contribute to a state fund, a private insurance fund, or a combination of both. Some states also allow practices to be self-insured. It is advisable to check with the state to ensure the practice complies.

If a team member is bitten, falls, or injures him- or herself in any way on the job site, workers' compensation insurance pays for physician visits, medications, and hospitalization that may be required. Insurance will also pay the team member's wages if more than 5 days of work are lost because of injury. Many practices do not require team members to visit a doctor when an accident has occurred because they are afraid that the cost of insurance will increase with each claim filed. However, if an injury worsens, and the team member does not seek medical attention, then the employer can be liable to pay for all medical costs. Workers' compensation may deny a claim if it is not filed within a specific number of days after the injury. To protect against future liabilities, all serious injuries including dog and cat bites, should at minimum, be examined by a physician.

When a team member is injured, a "first report of injury" form should be filled out. If medical attention is needed, the team member should be sent with the form provided by the company providing the insurance. The form should have the practice name, the policy number, and a place to input team member information. The form is then presented to the medical office, which files the claim.

Once the medical visit has been completed, the practice can submit the first report of injury and the insurance form to the insurance carrier. Workers' compensation should follow up with the rest of the

Form **W-4**

Department of the Treasury
Internal Revenue Service

Employee's Withholding Certificate

▶ Complete Form W-4 so that your employer can withhold the correct federal income tax from your pay.
▶ Give Form W-4 to your employer.
▶ Your withholding is subject to review by the IRS.

OMB No. 1545-0074

2022

Step 1: Enter Personal Information

(a) First name and middle initial | Last name | (b) Social security number

Address

City or town, state, and ZIP code

▶ **Does your name match the name on your social security card?** If not, to ensure you get credit for your earnings, contact SSA at 800-772-1213 or go to *www.ssa.gov.*

(c) ☐ **Single** or **Married filing separately**
☐ **Married filing jointly** or **Qualifying widow(er)**
☐ **Head of household** (Check only if you're unmarried and pay more than half the costs of keeping up a home for yourself and a qualifying individual.)

Complete Steps 2–4 ONLY if they apply to you; otherwise, skip to Step 5. See page 2 for more information on each step, who can claim exemption from withholding, when to use the estimator at *www.irs.gov/W4App*, and privacy.

Step 2: Multiple Jobs or Spouse Works

Complete this step if you (1) hold more than one job at a time, or (2) are married filing jointly and your spouse also works. The correct amount of withholding depends on income earned from all of these jobs.

Do **only one** of the following.

(a) Use the estimator at *www.irs.gov/W4App* for most accurate withholding for this step (and Steps 3–4); **or**

(b) Use the Multiple Jobs Worksheet on page 3 and enter the result in Step 4(c) below for roughly accurate withholding; **or**

(c) If there are only two jobs total, you may check this box. Do the same on Form W-4 for the other job. This option is accurate for jobs with similar pay; otherwise, more tax than necessary may be withheld . . . ▶ ☐

TIP: To be accurate, submit a 2022 Form W-4 for all other jobs. If you (or your spouse) have self-employment income, including as an independent contractor, use the estimator.

Complete Steps 3–4(b) on Form W-4 for only ONE of these jobs. Leave those steps blank for the other jobs. (Your withholding will be most accurate if you complete Steps 3–4(b) on the Form W-4 for the highest paying job.)

Step 3: Claim Dependents

If your total income will be $200,000 or less ($400,000 or less if married filing jointly):

Multiply the number of qualifying children under age 17 by $2,000 ▶ $

Multiply the number of other dependents by $500 . . . . ▶ $

Add the amounts above and enter the total here . . . . **3** $

Step 4 (optional): Other Adjustments

(a) Other income (not from jobs). If you want tax withheld for other income you expect this year that won't have withholding, enter the amount of other income here. This may include interest, dividends, and retirement income . . . . **4(a)** $

(b) Deductions. If you expect to claim deductions other than the standard deduction and want to reduce your withholding, use the Deductions Worksheet on page 3 and enter the result here . . . . **4(b)** $

(c) Extra withholding. Enter any additional tax you want withheld each **pay period** . . **4(c)** $

Step 5: Sign Here

Under penalties of perjury, I declare that this certificate, to the best of my knowledge and belief, is true, correct, and complete.

▶ **Employee's signature** (This form is not valid unless you sign it.) ▶ **Date**

Employers Only

Employer's name and address | First date of employment | Employer identification number (EIN)

For Privacy Act and Paperwork Reduction Act Notice, see page 3. Cat. No. 10220Q Form **W-4** (2022)

Fig. 4.20 Form W4.

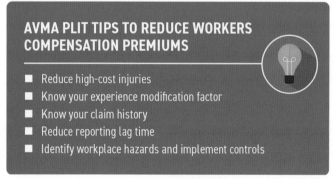

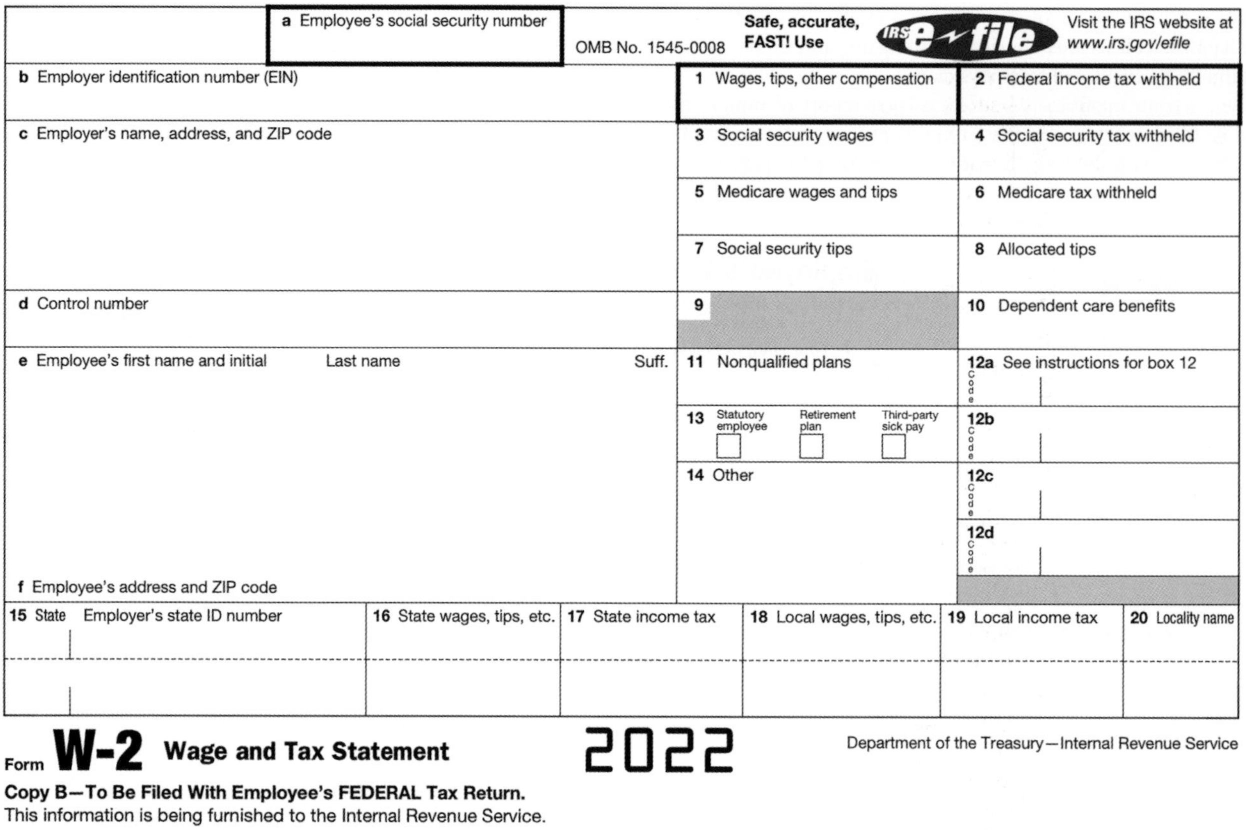
a Employee's social security number
OMB No. 1545-0008
Safe, accurate, FAST! Use IRS e-file
Visit the IRS website at www.irs.gov/efile
b Employer identification number (EIN)
1 Wages, tips, other compensation
2 Federal income tax withheld
c Employer's name, address, and ZIP code
3 Social security wages
4 Social security tax withheld
5 Medicare wages and tips
6 Medicare tax withheld
7 Social security tips
8 Allocated tips
d Control number
9
10 Dependent care benefits
e Employee's first name and initial Last name Suff.
11 Nonqualified plans
12a See instructions for box 12 Code
13 Statutory employee Retirement plan Third-party sick pay
12b Code
14 Other
12c Code
12d Code
f Employee's address and ZIP code
15 State Employer's state ID number
16 State wages, tips, etc.
17 State income tax
18 Local wages, tips, etc.
19 Local income tax
20 Locality name
Form W-2 Wage and Tax Statement 2022
Department of the Treasury—Internal Revenue Service
Copy B—To Be Filed With Employee's FEDERAL Tax Return.
This information is being furnished to the Internal Revenue Service.

Fig. 4.21 Form W2.

AVMA PLIT TIPS TO REDUCE WORKERS COMPENSATION PREMIUMS

- Reduce high-cost injuries
- Know your experience modification factor
- Know your claim history
- Reduce reporting lag time
- Identify workplace hazards and implement controls

Fig. 4.22 Workers' compensation premiums can vary based on the number of claims a practice has in a year.

documentation. If claims are not filed, the team member is responsible for the bill received from the medical office. This is also a good time to document the injury on OSHA 300 forms (Chapter 15, Safety) that must be posted the following year.

If the practice chooses not to carry workers' compensation insurance, the practice owner is exposed to liability. If a team member sustains an extensive injury on the job, the practice will be responsible for paying for the medical bills of the team member. Surgery can become costly, along with follow-up visits and physical therapy. Careful consideration should be taken if the practice chooses not to carry workers' compensation insurance. Fig. 4.22 provides tips from the American Veterinary Medical Association (AVMA) to save money on workers' compensation premiums.

BUILDING THE PERFECT TEAM

Now that the employee manual, job descriptions, training program, SOPs, SOCs, and wage ranges are complete, a plan can be created for building the perfect team. Part of this plan includes evaluating the current practice culture, values, mission, vision, and strategic goals of the practice (Chapters 2 and 17). Evaluate current team members. Does every team member support the goals? Are they positive, respectful to one another, and practice the values that have been established? If not, these team members must be coached up or coached out. Allowing toxicity to continue existing in the practice will kill any vision of the perfect team. Every team member, including leadership, must be held accountable for their behaviors and contributions; excuses for bad behavior cannot be tolerated. A culture of accountability may be new to the practice, and some team members may resist. That's OK. Allow them to spread their wings outside of the practice and explore other opportunities.

Perhaps the decision has been made to hire a new team member. But how does a practice manager know who to hire? What position will benefit the practice the most (veterinary assistant, credentialed veterinary technician/nurse, or veterinarian)? Having a plan in place will prevent a quick-to-hire mentality that practices often have. Practice managers must know who they want to hire and what qualifications and skills they are looking for. Having a plan prevents "emotional hiring" (hiring someone simply because you like them when they lack the skills or qualifications needed).

VHMA PERFORMANCE DOMAIN TASK

Veterinary practice managers recruit, interview, and hire new team members.

When and Who to Hire

Knowing which position to hire for can be difficult without a true evaluation of the hospital flow. Practice managers must be diligent about this decision, as it has a financial impact. Five key factors should be evaluated: veterinary/staff ratio, veterinary production, team members' production, hospital flow, efficiency, and staff payroll percentages.

Benchmarks show that the average number of full-time team members to one full-time equivalent veterinarian is 4.9, including kennel, assistants, credentialed technicians/nurses, and receptionists (WMPB, 2022). It is critical for veterinarians to have the ability to leverage duties to team members. If leveraging cannot occur (because of low staff numbers, skill of the team, or reduced efficiency) and veterinarians are doing the duties of technicians (versus only their duties of prescribing medications, diagnosing, and performing surgery) then it is time to hire a non-DVM role. Teams must be well staffed and efficient to generate income. Veterinary production numbers are also evaluated, but if the team is not leveraged, the veterinarian will produce less revenue. In the average general practice, the team's efforts will bring in approximately 50% of the income (passive income) and the veterinarian(s) will generate the remaining 50% (active income). If practices are not producing these numbers, staffing, leveraging, and training must be evaluated, and goals must be put into place to achieve maximal leveraging and efficiency.

Team member production is also critical. Perhaps a team is strong and assumes all the responsibilities it should, allowing the veterinarian to complete their duties diligently. However, if the team is overworked and understaffed, they may not be able to support the 50% passive income that every practice should strive for. In addition, overworked team members often neglect their work-life balance, which inevitably leads to burnout (Chapters 1 and 6).

Hospital flow and efficiency are just as critical to evaluate as the veterinary/staff ratio and veterinary/team member productions. The following questions should be asked:

- How many times does the phone ring before it is answered? Once answered, how long do clients have to wait on hold?
- How long does it take for a client to get an appointment? (Is the wait time 1 week, 2 weeks, etc.?)
- How long are clients waiting before they enter the examination room?
- How long are clients waiting before they are seen by the veterinarian?
- Are patient care standards being met?
- Are client service standards being met?

The ability to answer these questions can help determine what positions should be hired for. If there is a backlog of appointments, is it because the veterinarian is overbooked, or is the team too busy, therefore eliminating appointments? Can training and increased efficiency alleviate some of the backlog?

> **CRITICAL COMPETENCY: CREATIVITY**
>
> Practice managers must have the ability to creatively think through situations and embrace new and different ways to see opportunities by using imagination and collaboration, resulting in innovative solutions.

Most often, decreased efficiency is more of a problem than being short staffed. When team members are working harder instead of smarter, don't understand the goals of the practice, or have a toxic workplace, it can "feel" incredibly busy and unorganized.

What forms of technology can be implemented that can increase efficiency? For example, when clients make appointments online instead of calling the hospital, efficiency increases with the receptionist team (visit vetstoria.com for more details). When telehealth is an option, efficiency increases for receptionists, technicians, and doctors (Chapter 7, Telehealth; Chapter 8, PIMS; and Chapter 9, Medical Records).

Phones should ring no more than twice (Chapter 11, Client Experience), and chaos at the front desk can create a negative perception of the practice by clients. Can hiring a receptionist alleviate this issue? Can phones be moved to an area away from the reception desk to decrease chaos?

Patient care and customer service must be the number one priority of every practice. If either of these areas is compromised, an evaluation as to what, where, why, and how must ensue. Did the patient not receive treatments because the team is short staffed? Was the wrong treatment administered because of a lack of training? Did the customer not receive the service expected because the team was rushed?

Payroll percentages should always be monitored, along with overtime. Overtime will hurt the practice financially; however, it will also hurt the team member because long hours (and being underpaid) results in burnout. Team members experiencing burnout are less motivated, bring in less money, do not work well as a "team," and will likely leave the practice. Managers must not rely only on percentages; all the previous factors must be evaluated as well.

For comparison purposes, payroll percentages for non-DVM staff (including management) average 20%–22% (including taxes and benefits) of gross revenue (WMPB 2017) for general practice. Those with boarding facilities, urgent, emergency, or specialty care average higher. If a practice is a well-oiled machine that is incredibly efficient, the staff is leveraged appropriately and doctors can generate a high amount of revenue ($800 K+ per year), the payroll percentage will be lower, even when the team is well paid.

A team of highly motivated, positive team members with a strong work ethic can make a practice successful and take it to the next level; one team member who lacks motivation and enthusiasm can break the entire team. Practices need to hire for communication style (Chapter 11) and work ethic (soft skills) and train for the hard skill that is needed. One cannot hire for hard skills that are required and train for soft skills. Team members either have it or they don't. Don't hire a warm body just to fill a position; hire the right person that will help the practice achieve strategic goals.

> **VHMA PRACTICE DOMAIN TASK**
>
> Practice managers recruit, interview, and hire new team members.

Reviewing Resumes

Applicants share a resume for review when applying for a position within the hospital. Resumes should be short and to the point, with applicants clearly stating what they are looking for in a position. Do not make notes on resumes because they remain part of the personnel file if the applicant is hired. Notes should be made on a separate piece of paper. Also, remember that the threat involving claims of discrimination in the hiring process is real, so good defensive tactics must be practiced throughout the entire hiring process (treat all prospects the same; ask the same interview questions and check all references).

Using Social Media to Review Candidates: Employers looking to hire candidates must use caution; searching social media sites may reveal information about an individual's protected status under federal or state law. This information may include a person's age, race, political affiliation, national origin, or disabilities. At the time of publication, 28 states have laws that protect applicants from employers that may discriminate against them for engaging in lawful activities such as smoking (which may be revealed in social media photos). If an applicant feels that they did not get hired because of content on their social media page, they can bring a case of discrimination before the Department of Labor.

Interviewing: Asking the Right Questions

With the best team in mind, it is essential to ask the right questions when interviewing potential candidates (Fig. 4.23). Questions such as *"Tell me about yourself," "What do you know about our practice?"* and *"What is your single greatest achievement?"* stimulate discussion instead of eliciting a "yes" or "no" answer. *"Describe a typical day in your last job"* promotes discussion regarding work ethic. Questions should prompt the candidate to show their skill and potential. Open-ended questions allow the applicant to discuss the question asked. What, when, where, why, and how are excellent words to use when asking an open-ended question. Every applicant wants to relay an excellent work ethic and a great personality; the interviewer must be able to distinguish whether this is true. Closed-ended questions allow only a "yes" or "no" answer. One may also ask candidates if previous employers can be called; answers may provide a clue to the past employment history.

Questions should be heavily focused on skills that lead to the achievement of the practice's strategic goals, vision, mission, and core values. Develop questions around the practice's core values and ask candidates to define the value and provide an example of a past employee experience in which that value was exemplified or broken. At the end of the initial interview, the practice manager should be able to identify if the candidate is a right fit for the practice culture.

If a potential team member's original interview goes well, a working interview may be considered to help determine an individual's work ethic and skill. Many applicants may state they are qualified for the position, and a working interview will help determine whether certain skills are met. This also allows team members to weigh in and give their opinion of the potential hire. It is important to remind all team members what questions cannot be asked during this working interview.

Questions Not to Ask: The hiring process is highly regulated by federal and state laws, which exist for the protection of potential team members. Many questions cannot be asked in an interview, including any questions related to marriage, age, gender, religion, and military status. The interviewer cannot ask female applicants different questions than male applicants, nor if they have any children. See Fig. 4.23 for a list of questions that cannot be asked.

CRITICAL COMPETENCY: COMPLIANCE

Practice managers must be reliable, thorough, and conscientious in carrying out work assignments while having an appreciation for the importance of organizational rules and policies.

Reviewing Letters of Reference: It is important to follow up on any letter of reference. Some letters are written to ease a difficult termination; others may have been unwilling to express any reservations that were held at the time of the team member's resignation or termination. Therefore an outstanding letter of reference is not always a true reflection of the applicant's abilities. Phone calls are advised on all applicants; one candidate cannot be treated differently from another.

References: It is imperative to call all references listed. If a candidate has not provided a list of references with the resume and/or application, one should be asked for at the time of the interview. However, it can be difficult to obtain useful information when calling references or those that wrote letters of recommendation. Because of the increase in defamation lawsuits, past employers are reluctant to provide any information, either positive or negative. Information that is permissible

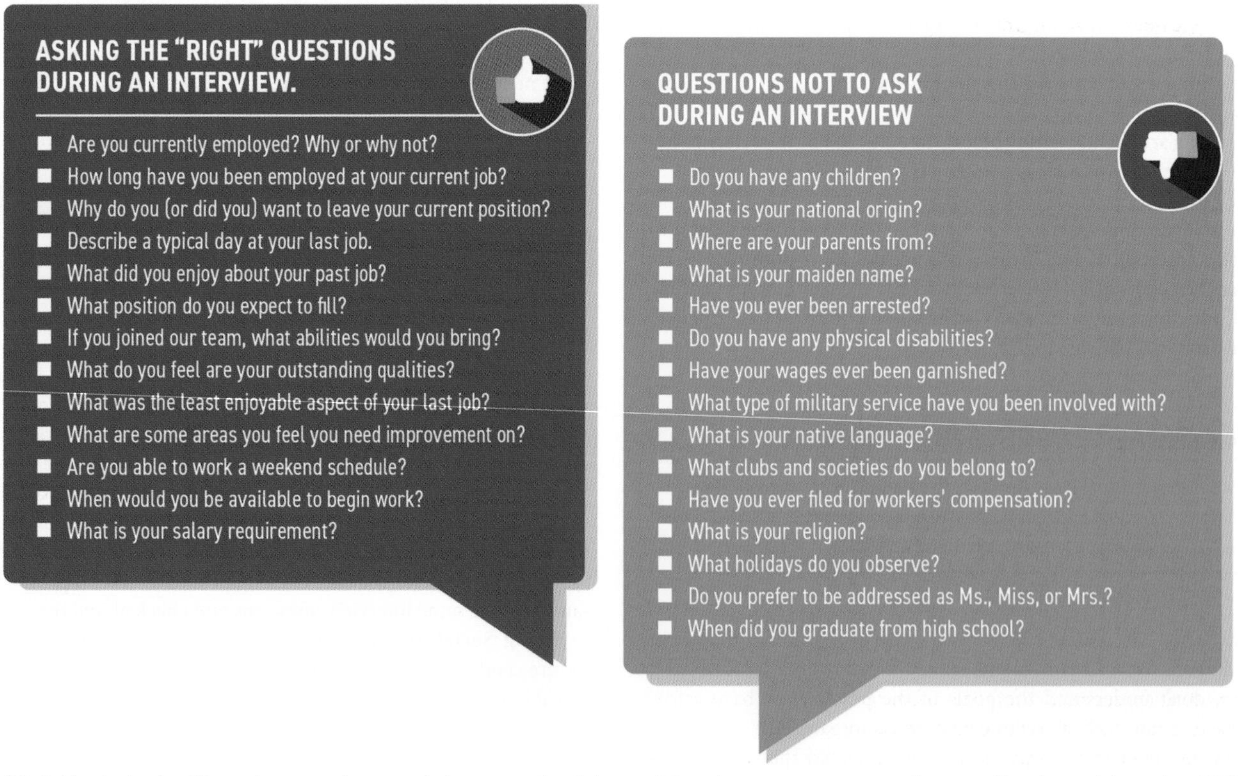
ASKING THE "RIGHT" QUESTIONS DURING AN INTERVIEW.
Are you currently employed? Why or why not?
How long have you been employed at your current job?
Why do you (or did you) want to leave your current position?
Describe a typical day at your last job.
What did you enjoy about your past job?
What position do you expect to fill?
If you joined our team, what abilities would you bring?
What do you feel are your outstanding qualities?
What was the least enjoyable aspect of your last job?
What are some areas you feel you need improvement on?
Are you able to work a weekend schedule?
When would you be available to begin work?
What is your salary requirement?
QUESTIONS NOT TO ASK DURING AN INTERVIEW
Do you have any children?
What is your national origin?
Where are your parents from?
What is your maiden name?
Have you ever been arrested?
Do you have any physical disabilities?
Have your wages ever been garnished?
What type of military service have you been involved with?
What is your native language?
What clubs and societies do you belong to?
Have you ever filed for workers' compensation?
What is your religion?
What holidays do you observe?
Do you prefer to be addressed as Ms., Miss, or Mrs.?
When did you graduate from high school?

Fig. 4.23 Asking behavioral interview questions can help source the right candidate; however, many questions are illegal to ask based on EEO.

must be factual and documented in written evidence. Questions that may be verified are dates of employment, attendance record, position, responsibilities, whether they would rehire the team member, and salary. Calling references can reveal any discrepancies with the applicant's resume and/or interview.

The most revealing question that provides useful information is whether or not the previous employer would rehire the employee. While they may not reveal the "why" behind their answer, the interpretation of the answer can be explored with the potential team member during a follow-up interview.

Negligent hiring is defined as hiring a candidate that the employer knew or should have known would be a risk to others in the workplace. Verifying references helps the practice manager reduce the risk of negligent hiring. It is also important to verify the candidates' credentials and ensure they are licensed to practice within the state.

Preemployment Screening

State regulations vary regarding prescreening tests. Most states require that an employment offer be made before the screening process can begin. The job offer may state something like "ABC Veterinary Hospital offers you a full-time position on the contingency that the background screen and drug test results are negative." Background checks are a matter of public record; managers should consider hiring a payroll firm to obtain the most complete, national background check. Local companies may only complete a local search; however, potential team members can have a history in any other state.

Independent/Contract Team Member Versus Employee

Some veterinarians and groomers prefer to be a contract employee instead of a permanent team member (for example, relief veterinarians or credentialed veterinary technicians/nurses). Independent/contract employees are responsible for their own taxes and are paid a straight fee; taxes are not withheld from their paychecks.

The IRS is strict regarding the classification of contract employment versus team member employment, and there are numerous variables in defining independent contractor status. It is always recommended to refer to IRS code and state regulations for current guidelines. A few defining points hold true in every case:

- A contractor does not solely rely on practice for income.
- The relationship cannot be permanent.
- The contractor services cannot be integral to the business but can contribute to profits.
- A contractor works at their own pace with minimal control by the practice, which may be defined by a working agreement.
- A contractor is not eligible for employer-provided benefits.
- A contractor retains a degree of control and independence and has the right to pursue other employment at will.
- Contractors are not required to follow instructions as to how to perform a task, duty, or job.

Although the independent contractor is their own boss, work does stay within the definitions of an oral or written contract and adheres to certain requirements. They usually are contracted to complete or deliver a set scope of work and are typically paid by the job, not the hour. Contractors are responsible for their own dues, licenses, and taxes.

An example of an independent contractor would be a specialist who comes into a practice, performs surgery, and leaves. These doctors do not develop a client/patient relationship, are paid for the job performed, and generally bring their own technician(s) to assist. An example of a relief veterinarian or credentialed veterinary technician/nurse is one that covers shifts for a short time, filling in for vacancies when full-time team members are on PTO.

Veterinarians who work as contract employees should have copies of all credentials, including state and controlled substance licenses and U.S. Department of Agriculture accreditation, on file. Verification of licenses should be checked with the state board of veterinary medicine; it is the practice's responsibility to ensure that proper documentation is verified. Additionally, practice managers should have independent contractors complete form W-9, providing their tax identification number. This tax identification number is then referenced on form 1099-MISC, which cites all money paid to the contractor during the fiscal year. Contractors are required to file 1099-MISC with their annual taxes (Fig. 4.24). The practices accounting firm that manages payroll and tax submissions should generate MISC 1099, which must be distributed by January 31st of each year.

THE FIRST DAY FOR A NEW HIRE

A new team member's first day can be intimidating, overwhelming, and daunting. The team member should be introduced to the rest of the staff, given a tour of the practice, and then taken to a quiet area to review practice policy and procedures. The new team member should fill out new hire forms, including Form W-4, state tax forms (if required), form I-9, forms for accepting or declining any team member benefit plans, and emergency contact information. Copies of any credentials should be made at this time. The team member should receive their own copy of the employee manual, review it verbally with a practice manager, and sign a document stating they have received, read, and understands the manual.

If a mentorship program has been established, the expectations of the program should also be discussed. And above all, take the time to reinforce the culture, vision, mission, and values of the practice.

> **CRITICAL COMPETENCY: LEADERSHIP**
>
> Practice managers must have the initiative to lead and take charge while simultaneously motivating and mobilizing others to achieve common goals.

The new team member should be given a copy of the practice's SOPs and SOCs and reassured that they are not expected to know all the information on the first day. The phase training program that the hospital has implemented should be explained, along with the expected dates of completion. The new team member should be allowed to observe the entire team for the rest of the day and encouraged to ask questions. Scheduling a team lunch away from the practice can be a great step toward initiating team building. Team members can ask questions and learn about each other out of the office. Overwhelming the new team member during the first week sets them up for failure, and it is ultimately a management issue. Team member loyalty builds the most in the first 60 days of employment. This period can make or break a great team member.

The success of a practice depends on the quality and quantity of training, and the adult learning theory must be applied (see developing training protocols earlier in this chapter). New team members with no or limited experience will take more time for the explanation and training of SOPs, while those with experience will take less. It is important to not skip steps or phases with those that have experience as SOPs and SOCs vary by practice. Provide the best experience possible for new team members by doing it right and building their long-term loyalty.

Don't stop with initial training. Continue the life-long development of team members, growing them to be thriving leaders in the practice

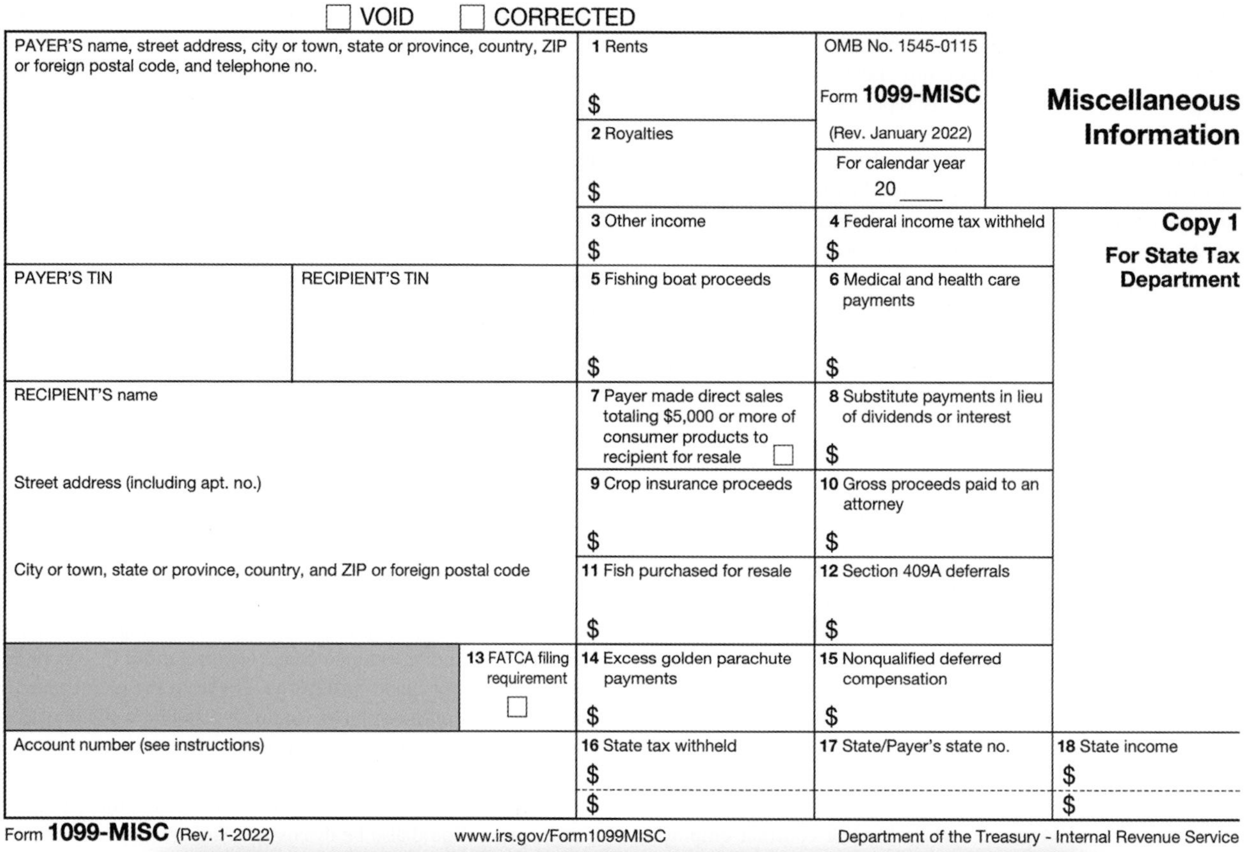

☐ VOID ☐ CORRECTED

PAYER'S name, street address, city or town, state or province, country, ZIP or foreign postal code, and telephone no.		1 Rents $	OMB No. 1545-0115 Form **1099-MISC** (Rev. January 2022)	**Miscellaneous Information**
		2 Royalties $	For calendar year 20____	
		3 Other income $	4 Federal income tax withheld $	**Copy 1** **For State Tax Department**
PAYER'S TIN	RECIPIENT'S TIN	5 Fishing boat proceeds $	6 Medical and health care payments $	
RECIPIENT'S name		7 Payer made direct sales totaling $5,000 or more of consumer products to recipient for resale ☐	8 Substitute payments in lieu of dividends or interest $	
Street address (including apt. no.)		9 Crop insurance proceeds $	10 Gross proceeds paid to an attorney $	
City or town, state or province, country, and ZIP or foreign postal code		11 Fish purchased for resale $	12 Section 409A deferrals $	
	13 FATCA filing requirement ☐	14 Excess golden parachute payments $	15 Nonqualified deferred compensation $	
Account number (see instructions)		16 State tax withheld $ $	17 State/Payer's state no.	18 State income $ $

Form **1099-MISC** (Rev. 1-2022) www.irs.gov/Form1099MISC Department of the Treasury - Internal Revenue Service

Fig. 4.24 Form 1099-MISC.

that strive daily to achieve the vision. Continuing education should be provided throughout the year, not just once a year outside of the practice. Ask team members to help build programs by asking them to teach what they learn at conferences (those who teach learn the topic more thoroughly than those who just listen to lecture).

Role playing is also an exceptional method of training that improves learning retention. Role playing can be uncomfortable for team members that lack confidence or are afraid of being judged by fellow employees. A psychologically safe space (Chapter 2, Leadership) must be created for any training environment, allowing everyone the freedom to ask questions and practice their roles before engaging with clients.

If a receptionist's or technician's job is to educate a client about heartworm disease, then team members should be able to recite the information to any other team member. Once they have mastered the ability to convey information to team members, they can better educate clients. When team members have confidence, they appear much more professional, communications become more effective, and compliance rates increase.

TEAM MEMBER RETENTION

Team member retention is both a leadership and human resource responsibility. Chapter 2, Leadership (What Do Team Members Need), covers leadership's role in retaining team members. But HR's responsibility in team member retention is to track turnover and identify specific causes of the turnover.

Currently, the average industry turnover rate (the number of employees that leave the practice within a 1-year period, either by means of termination or resignation) of credentialed veterinary technicians/nurses, assistants, and receptionists is approximately 25%. In other words, for every four team members hired, one leaves the practice. This impacts the practice's profitability and efficiency, and negatively impacts the client's bond to the practice. Long-term team members bring comfort and loyalty to clients by providing a frictionless client experience. High turnover breaks that bond. A practice goal of 13% or less should be set by leadership, and areas of improvement should be identified using a SWOT analysis and setting SMART goals (use templates in Chapter 12, Marketing).

Evaluate each area of the employee experience when examining current turnover trends in the practice:

Interviewing Process: Were the right behavioral questions asked to identify the team member's strengths and weaknesses?

Onboarding: What do team members experience during the first week of employment?

Training: What training protocols are in place, is Adult Learning Theory practiced, and do new team members feel they have been set up for success?

Continuous Development: Do team members receive continuous education throughout the year that leads to the achievement of practice goals?

Culture: What is the culture of the practice? Have recent anonymous team member surveys been obtained to identify potential issues?

Communication: How are team members communicated with, and do they feel that goals and initiatives are communicated clearly?

Psychological Safety: Do team members ALWAYS feel safe in the practice environment, creating a long-lasting bond with the practice?

Consider deploying surveys to both current team members (also known as stay surveys), as well as those that leave the practice to determine what needs to be improved to achieve the practice's desired turnover goal.

Team Member Surveys

To help evaluate current team member perception of the practice, periodic anonymous surveys should be deployed asking specific questions for areas of improvement. Anonymous surveys will yield honest results (whereas asking team members directly may result in false or misleading information if they are afraid to provide honest feedback). The key factor with team member surveys is doing something with the results. Team members need to know they were heard, that their opinion counts, and that leadership is implementing measures to correct the perception.

Surveys for those that left the practice may be harder to obtain the longer the time span between the departure of the employee and deployment of the survey. Employees that resigned will be more likely to complete the survey (anonymously) than those that were terminated; however, the practice leaders know why an employee was terminated and the questions above can help pinpoint areas of improvement to prevent the same issues from rising again with new team members.

Often, surveys identify issues that pertain to lack of communication, conflict resolution, training and development, psychological safety, goals, leadership, and poor culture. Platforms such as Survey Monkey can be used to deploy surveys by either email or text, making tabulation of results much easier.

The leadership team should also consider having yearly 360 evaluations completed by the team, evaluating their performance as leaders. While the anonymous team surveys mentioned above are similar, having a professional company deploy, evaluate, and provide follow-up coaching for leaders will help leaders grow professionally, ultimately improving the culture in ways that may not have been previously addressed. The 360 evaluations focus on competencies that embody emotional intelligence, conflict management, communication, and adaptability.

Succession Planning

Succession planning for team members is covered in Chapter 17, Strategic Planning, but it must be mentioned in this chapter as well. Succession planning is important to achieving practice goals while also empowering team members to grow to their maximum potential. Great team members that have an emotional investment in the practice should be developed to be future practice leaders, allowing leaders to grow leaders, and never leaving a gap when the practice loses a leader.

The succession of a team member does not happen overnight, and some team members are not the right fit for leadership roles. Succession planning requires the evaluation of team members for their current skills, and skills needed to achieve specific goals associated with specific leadership roles. Succession planning is different for everyone; therefore tailored, long-term plans must be developed.

Consider the role of an Inventory Manager. While this role is not a practice manager role, it is a critical role that oversees the success of the practice's second largest expense (and in some practices, the largest asset). It requires training, SOPs, coaching, and performance feedback. The same can be considered for a lead receptionist role, a lead veterinary technician role, and based on the size of the practice, perhaps a lead role for veterinary and kennel assistants.

Succession planning builds amazing teams that achieve goals together, never leaving a gap in a key role.

CRITICAL COMPETENCY: RELATIONSHIP BUILDING

Practice managers must develop and maintain constructive and cooperative working relationships to build trust and collaboration, resulting in the ability to settle disputes, resolve grievances and conflicts, and negotiate with others.

Performance Feedback/Performance Evaluations/ Performance Reviews

All team members want and deserve feedback on their performance. Additionally, team members want continuous feedback, not just once a year during an annual evaluation.

VHMA PRACTICE DOMAIN TASK

Practice managers provide regular feedback on employee performance.

This is also a great time to consider the definition of the term used (performance feedback/performance evaluations/performance reviews) and the perception it leaves for team members. "Evaluations and reviews" focus on past behaviors, leaving no interpretation or excitement for future growth and goals. Wouldn't it be healthier to address corrective behaviors in the moment through coaching, and focus on the future of the team member in an "individual strategic planning session"?

Before discussing individual strategic planning sessions, it is important to briefly identify the pitfalls associated with annual performance reviews and why they fail:

1. Everyone hates them. The practice manager hates prepping performance reviews as they need to recall events that occurred over the past year and find some positive points to provide accolades on. The team hates being evaluated on the past year's events and often won't participate in employee self-evaluations if asked to do so by management.
2. Because everyone hates them, it is easy to deprioritize them as other hot issues come up.
3. Performance reviews always focus on the past and often identify behaviors the team member never knew they demonstrated, and therefore does not know how to fix them.
4. Performance reviews leave team members feeling deflated, ultimately impacting team collaboration and efficiency.

To have the greatest impact on team members, coach behaviors that need to be addressed as soon as they happen. Help team members relate to the experience in the moment and the impact they had on others, clients and fellow employees alike. Coaching can be informal and be a side conversation. Practice managers can think of coaching employees to help them be the best of their ability. Chapter 2, Leadership, discusses coaching and when to document. This then allows practice managers to focus on the future with individual strategic planning sessions.

CRITICAL COMPETENCY: RESOURCEFULNESS

The practice manager must have the ability to understand what it takes to complete the job by applying knowledge, skills, and expertise to perform tasks quickly and efficiently.

Individual Strategic Planning Sessions

The term individual strategic planning sessions (ISPS) improves team member perception, supports succession planning and the overall practice strategic plan, empowers team members to contribute to the culture of the practice, achieve the vision, and decrease the employee turnover rate.

Practice managers and owners enjoy strategic planning much more than giving poor performance reviews, therefore, ISPSs are delivered on time, and team members are willing to complete their portion of the plan. ISPSs also give leaders the opportunity to follow up multiple times a year to make sure each team member is on track to achieve the goals set forth in the previous year.

To put ISPS in place, the practice manager and team member should discuss the strategic goals of the practice for the upcoming year. A SWOT analysis (of the team member) can then be completed together (Chapter 12, Marketing) to identify opportunities that not only grow the team member but also help the practice achieve its strategic goals. Leadership's role is then to find resources to help the team member achieve goals, behaviors, competencies, credentialing, or certifications identified in the SWOT analysis. Resources and goals should then be discussed with the team member using SMART goals (Chapter 12), ultimately putting the control in the hands of the team member to complete. One might argue to ask the team member to identify resources to achieve goals, however, the practice manager, owner, and potentially associate DVMs will have more knowledge of available resources (industry-wide) than a team member.

Use ISPSs as an opportunity to challenge the status quo. Performance feedback systems have failed team members for years. Take the opportunity to start coaching team members to greatness by energizing them, resulting in decreased mental exhaustion and burnout. Review Chapter 1 and remind yourself of the long-term challenges veterinary practices will have. Do everything in your power to build and keep great team members so that patients can continue to receive the care they deserve.

THEFT AND EMBEZZLEMENT

Team member theft and embezzlement are the leading causes of unexplained inventory reduction and cash flow. Excess inventory supplies available on the floor unfortunately invites team member theft. Team members may assume that taking one box of heartworm preventative is not going to hurt the practice, but if each team member took one box on a regular basis, the cost would be considerable. Unfortunately, theft typically does not stop with one box. Soon it becomes dog food or medication and, if the team member is not caught, can move to bigger, more expensive items. When team members purchase items, the practice manager should be responsible for entering charges for all team members. This can ensure correct charges for products and that all products are being charged for.

Team members can be crafty at embezzling cash. More than one person should be responsible for handling cash and balancing the cash drawer at the end of the night. Additionally, another person should be responsible for the deposits, and the practice manager must compare the completed deposit slip to the daily total.

If team member theft or embezzlement is suspected, the practice attorney should be contacted for further advice. Some practices may install cameras to try to catch team members in the act, as proof of theft will be required to file charges. Once the practice has proof, the team member can be terminated. See Chapter 16, Finance, for more information on theft and embezzlement.

TERMINATION

Termination procedures must be clearly stated in the employee manual and followed to protect the practice against unemployment claims, or worse, discrimination suits. Not following through with discipline decreases team member accountability (they know they can get away with bad behavior) and decreases team morale (other team members become upset because corrective action has not been taken). Further, if all team members are not treated the same regarding discipline procedures, the threat of discrimination is high. For example, if one team member is terminated for excessive tardiness and another is not, the terminated team member can claim discrimination. The threat of discrimination is real, and practice managers must take every action to prevent such accusations.

Termination is the final step after team members have been coached, a change has been asked for, and the team member has failed to comply. Termination must take place when a team member has been coached and written up for unsatisfactory performance of duties, behaviors that do not support the core values, excessive tardiness, or absenteeism.

VHMA PRACTICE DOMAIN TASK

Practice managers discipline and discharge employees.

If a team member has been coached but no change in behavior has been observed, an official written warning with a method to correct the behavior, mistake, accident, or violation must be given. The warning should be signed and dated by both the practice manager and the team member and filed in the personnel file (Fig. 4.25). Two or three written warnings are then allowed (the practice decides on the protocol), again each documented in the personnel file. The last warning must state that the next step is termination.

Dishonesty and unethical behavior, criminal activity within the hospital (stealing or embezzlement) or outside the hospital (drug use), and improper use of personal protective equipment (PPE) should be grounds for immediate termination (no warnings are needed). Immediate dismissal guidelines must also be stated in the employee manual.

The following guidelines should be used when the decision to terminate is final.

- Ensure that the team member was coached, all written warnings are documented, and that the team member understood the correction and signed each entry. No termination should be a surprise.
- Do not fire team members while upset, angry, or during an argument. When emotions are high, incorrect words, phrases, and actions can be said that may be inappropriate. Wait until the emotions subside and ensure that correct termination procedures are followed. This will help protect the practice against wrongful dismissal complaints.
- If the team member has insurance through the practice, the Consolidated Omnibus Budget Reconciliation Act (COBRA) requires continued coverage for a specified time. Be sure to initiate COBRA coverage through the practice healthcare provider.

Once a termination is reached, time and procedure are of the essence. Find a time in the practice when the potential to interact with other team members is least likely to happen. The practice manager should have a witness (owner or fellow leader) while having the conversation and will want to escort the employee out after retrieving the practice door key(s) or security card, signing termination papers, and helping them pack up any items they may have in the practice. Termination documents should indicate the reason for termination,

ABC Veterinary Hospital

Employee Warning Notice

Employee Information

Employee Name: Date:
Employee ID: Job Title:
Manager: Department:

Type of Warning

☐ First Warning ☐ Second Warning ☐ Final Warning

Type of Offense

☐ Tardiness/Leaving Early ☐ Absenteeism ☐ Violation of Company Policies
☐ Substandard Work ☐ Violation of Safety Rules ☐ Disrespectful to Customers/Coworkers
☐ Other: ______

Details

Description of Infraction:

Plan for Improvement:

Consequences of Further Infractions:

Acknowledgement of Receipt of Warning

By signing this form, you confirm that you understand the information in this warning. You also confirm that you and your manager have discussed the warning and a plan for improvement. Signing this form does not necessarily indicate that you agree with this warning.

Employee Signature: **Date**

Manager Signature: **Date**

Witness if Employee Declines to Sign: **Date**

Fig. 4.25 Example of a disciplinary form.

and the employee may or may not sign them; however, both the PM and the witness should. In addition, any passcodes should be removed from the security system or PIMS, and the practice manager should document the entire procedure immediately (before any facts are forgotten). All documentation and paperwork should be placed in the team member's file and locked in a file cabinet. It is imperative to remember that all information regarding the termination should be kept confidential and not shared with other team members.

If a team member resigns, the practice should ask for a letter of resignation, indicating the reason for leaving as the final date of employment. An exit interview should be completed before the last day of employment, providing the practice manager valuable information as to why the team member is resigning and suggestions for practice improvement.

Whether the team member resigns or is terminated, an employee separation report should be signed agreeing to the information that will be released when future employers are calling for a reference (Fig. 4.26).

ABC Veterinary Practice

Employment Separation Report

Employee Name:______________________________

Department/Position:______________________ Date of Separation:______________________

Starting rate of pay: ______________________ Leaving rate of pay: ______________________

Type: ______ Resignation (attach letter)
______ Mutual Agreement
______ Dismissal
______Other

Reason: ______ Absenteeism/Lateness
______ Health
______ Did not meet Standards
______ Changing Jobs/Career
______ Family reasons
______ Reduction in Force
______ Undisclosed
______ Other ______________

Employee Evaluation:

	Unsatisfactory		Fair	Satisfactory	Good
Excellent					
Attendance	☐	☐	☐	☐	☐
Cooperation	☐	☐	☐	☐	☐
Initiative	☐	☐	☐	☐	☐
Job Knowledge	☐	☐	☐	☐	☐
Client Service	☐	☐	☐	☐	☐
Quality of Work	☐	☐	☐	☐	☐

Employee Recommendation: Without reservation ☐ With some reservation ☐ Would not recommend ☐

Would this employee be considered for rehire?: Yes ☐ No ☐ Yes, with the following considerations: ☐

____

____

Manager / Team member comments:

____

____

____

____

____

____

____

____

My signature verifies my understanding of the reasons for employment separation. I also hereby acknowledge that the information on this form will be used to give references to any potential future employers contacting ABC Veterinary for a job reference.

Fig. 4.26 Example of a team member separation report.

LEADERSHIP ROLES IN HUMAN RESOURCES

There are many human resource-related tasks that seem unrelated to leadership. And while there are tasks, leadership is responsible for creating an environment where team members have emotional ownership in the practice, making the difficult part of HR easier. When team members are accountable for their actions, consistently exceeding expectations, and helping the practice to achieve goals, the "managing the people" part of HR is fun and rewarding. When poor culture, toxicity, and lack of accountability set in, HR is exhausting.

The leadership side of HR ties in closely with tasks related to specific topics that may/may not be required to be delivered by law. However, whether tasks (such as job descriptions, performance reviews, etc.) are required or not, setting clear expectations for employees and their safety clearly is needed to achieve practice goals. Implement all tasks/skills discussed in this chapter, along with Chapter 2 to create a strong culture that grows people and leaders to be the employer of choice.

PRACTICE MANAGER SURVIVAL CHECKLIST FOR HUMAN RESOURCES

- ☐ Determine workflow/staffing adjustments based on busy times.
- ☐ Manage overtime to prevent burnout of team members.
- ☐ Create and follow wage ranges as indicated by employee manual.
- ☐ Tie the mission, vision, and values into job descriptions, phase training programs, coaching sessions, and evaluations.
- ☐ Develop or annually update employee manual.
- ☐ Develop or annually update job descriptions.
- ☐ Develop or annually update and utilize phase training programs.
- ☐ Develop and embody exceptional team member onboarding plans.
- ☐ Develop or annually update and utilize a performance management system.
- ☐ Develop succession planning for team members.
- ☐ Develop termination procedures: the procedure, exit interview, and reference form.
- ☐ Develop a record-keeping system that includes team member files, performance reviews, and corrections.
- ☐ Monitor cost and compliance of team member benefits.
- ☐ Annually develop a year-end total compensation benefit statement for each team member.
- ☐ Maintain accurate paid time off records.
- ☐ Monitor team member discounts.
- ☐ Maintain I-9 forms for the required length of time.
- ☐ Update the W-2 form for each team member annually.
- ☐ Develop a records retention policy (review state and federal guidelines).
- ☐ Obtain legal counsel to review the employee manual and consult regarding human capital concerns.
- ☐ Post required posters and update as necessary.
- ☐ Post current DVM and credentialed technician licenses in public view (and monitor for expiration.
- ☐ Complete background checks implemented on all potential team members after a contingent job has been offered.
- ☐ Establish a drug-free workplace policy and utilize it as outlined in the employee manual.
- ☐ Develop a team member discount policy and follow it.
- ☐ Confirm the budget and strategic plan fit well together and that human resource policies support it.
- ☐ Create a policy for business credit card distribution to the staff.
- ☐ Evaluate whether staff compensation is comparable to other organizations of similar operating structures.
- ☐ Ensure leadership and management attend harassment prevention CE.

REVIEW QUESTIONS

1. Give two examples of questions that cannot be asked during an interview.
2. What is the FLSA?
3. What is USERRA?
4. What is OSHA?
5. What posters are required to be displayed in a practice?
6. Where should the required posters be displayed?
7. What is the benefit of developing an employee manual?
8. What payroll taxes are employers responsible for?
9. What is a contract team member?
10. Why should training be provided in phases?
11. When is a W2 form issued?
12. How many weeks does the FMLA cover a team member that wished to take unpaid leave?
    - **a.** 14 weeks
    - **b.** 6 weeks
    - **c.** 12 weeks
    - **d.** 8 weeks
13. Which act requires employers to pay minimum wage and overtime pay?
    - **a.** FMLA
    - **b.** EPPA
    - **c.** EEO
    - **d.** FLSA
14. What does NCA stand for?
    - **a.** National Contract-Team Members Association
    - **b.** Noncompete Agreement
    - **c.** No Contract Act
    - **d.** Nonimmigrant Control Act
15. Which of the following is a question you should not ask during an interview?
    - **a.** Why would you want to leave your current position?
    - **b.** What is your salary requirement?
    - **c.** What was the least enjoyable aspect of your last job?
    - **d.** When did you graduate from high school?

RECOMMENDED READING

Donnelly AL. *AAHA Guide to Creating an Employee Handbook*. 4th ed. AAHA Press; 2020.

Parker K. *A Practical Guide to Managing Employee Performance in the Veterinary Practice*. AAHA Press; 2017.

Hunt M. *Employment Law Guide*. 6th ed. Lawpack Publishing; 2003.

WTA Consultants. 2019 Well-Managed Practice® Benchmarks Study (WMPB) provides insights to the top veterinary practices in the country. WTA Veterinary Consultants. Published August 16, 2019. https://wellmp.com/2019-well-managed-practice-benchmarks-study-wmpb-provides-insights-to-the-top-veterinary-practices-in-the-country/

Wilson J. *Contracts, Management and Practice Management*. Priority Press; 2007.

US Department of Labor. Summary of the Major Laws of DOL. Accessed December 2022. https://www.dol.gov/general/aboutdol/majorlaws

5

Veterinary Ethics and Legal Issues

LEARNING OBJECTIVES

When you have completed this chapter, you should be able to:

- Differentiate ethics and law
- Define the branches of ethics
- Identify a veterinary practice act
- Differentiate criminal and civil law
- Describe informed consent
- Develop an informed consent form
- Clarify methods used to prevent malpractice and negligence
- Manage abandoned animals
- List the most common complaints in veterinary medicine

OUTLINE

KEY TERMS

Administrative Ethics
Civil Law
Code of Ethics
Consent
Contract Law
Criminal Law
DEA
FDA
Informed Consent
Law
Malpractice
Negligence
Normative Ethics
OSHA
Personal Ethics
Professional Ethics
Social Ethics
Standard of Care
Tort
Veterinary Ethics
Veterinary Practice Act
USDA APHIS

VHMA PERFORMANCE DOMAINS

Veterinary Hospital Managers Association (VHMA) Performance Domains

Performance domains applicable to ethics and legal issues include law and ethics, and organization of the practice. The practice manager understands and:

- Ensures compliance with appropriate regulatory agencies, including OSHA, DEA, FDA, state, and local agencies
- Monitors hospital violations and dangerous situations
- Documents and reports accidents and files appropriate reports
- Ethical requirements of veterinary practices, including the AVMA and CVPM Code of Ethics, and ensures that team members fulfill their ethical responsibilities
- Contract law as it pertains to associate DVMs, team members, and clients
- Ensures compliance with the legal and ethical guidelines surrounding confidentiality of clients, patients, and team members
- Acts as a liaison between the practice and professional services and agencies
- Maintains protocols for hospital procedures and risk management plans

Application of VHMA Performance Domains for Practice Managers

Integrating ethics and legal issues enhances the performance, knowledge, skills, and abilities of the practice manager by mitigating or eliminating risks that could put the practice, its clients, or its team members in jeopardy. The tasks related to legal and ethical standards require knowledge of state/provincial and federal laws, legal codes, government regulations, professional standards, and agency rules.

INTRODUCTION

Law and ethics in veterinary medicine have been integrated into most daily practices since the early 1970s. Ethics are woven into the culture of society and organizations have created standards that set behavioral expectations for their members. Regulatory agencies have been added in the US government to ensure workplace safety and well-being, patient safety, and the monitoring of controlled substances, just to name a few. These agencies also have an impact at the state and city level.

Three areas of ethics exist and affect team members on every level. Social, personal, and professional ethics are interrelated, yet they affect each person differently.

Social ethics are the consensus of principles adopted or accepted by society at large and codified into laws and regulations. Laws include those against murder, rape, and stealing, along with ordinances regarding pet ownership.

Personal ethics define what is right or wrong on an individual basis. This can include religious beliefs and values as they relate to relationships.

Professional ethics are developed specifically for a particular discipline, including rules, codes, and conduct for the profession to follow.

CODE OF ETHICS

Ethics is a branch of philosophy and a systematic, intellectual approach to the standards of behavior. A code of ethics consists of all the obligations that professionals must respect when carrying out their duties. It includes the core values of the profession and the behavior that should be adopted. It is a code of professional conduct.

The purpose of a professional code of ethics is to help members of a profession demonstrate high levels of behavior through moral consciousness and decision-making, and challenges veterinarians to determine right from wrong. Each organization within the profession also has a code of ethics for its members and is based on moral principles that reflect concern and care for the client and patient.

The American Veterinary Medical Association (AVMA) Principles of Veterinary Medical Ethics increasingly address moral and ethical issues related to animals and society. For example, Principle VIII states that a veterinarian shall recognize a responsibility to participate in activities contributing to the improvement of the community and the betterment of public health. Many states have incorporated the Principles of Veterinary Medical Ethics in their disciplinary rules, making them more than just voluntary (Fig. 5.1).

The Veterinary Hospital Managers Association (VHMA) holds a strong code of ethics for the profession, practice, and patient. Practice managers must protect the interest and integrity of the practice itself while also providing a proficient image for the profession (Fig. 5.2).

> **VHMA PERFORMANCE DOMAIN TASK**
>
> Practice managers understand the ethical requirements of veterinary medicine as outlined by the American Veterinary Medical Association and CVPM code of ethics and ensure that team members fulfill their ethical responsibilities.

AVMA PRINCIPLES OF VETERINARY MEDICAL ETHICS

Introduction

Veterinarians are members of a scholarly profession who have earned academic degrees from comprehensive universities or similar educational institutions. Veterinarians practice veterinary medicine in a variety of situations and circumstances. Exemplary professional conduct upholds the dignity of the veterinary profession. All veterinarians are expected to adhere to a progressive code of ethical conduct known as the Principles of Veterinary Medical Ethics (PVME). The PVME comprises the following Principles, the Supporting Annotations, and Useful Terms.

The AVMA Board of Directors is charged to advise on all questions relating to veterinary medical ethics and to review the Principles periodically to ensure that they remain current and appropriate.

The principles

1. A veterinarian shall be influenced only by the welfare of the patient, the needs of the client, the safety of the public, and the need to uphold the public trust vested in the veterinary profession and shall avoid conflicts of interest or the appearance thereof.
2. A veterinarian shall provide competent veterinary medical clinical care under the terms of a veterinarian-client-patient relationship (VCPR), with compassion and respect for animal welfare and human health.
3. A veterinarian shall uphold the standards of professionalism, be honest in all professional interactions, and report veterinarians who are deficient in character or competence to the appropriate entities.
4. A veterinarian shall respect the law and also recognize a responsibility to seek changes to laws and regulations which are contrary to the best interests of the patient and public health.
5. A veterinarian shall respect the rights of clients, colleagues, and other health professionals, and shall safeguard medical information within the confines of the law.
6. A veterinarian shall continue to study, apply, and advance scientific knowledge, maintain a commitment to veterinary medical education, make relevant information available to clients, colleagues, the public, and obtain consultation or referral when indicated.
7. A veterinarian shall, in the provision of appropriate patient care, except in emergencies, be free to choose whom to serve, with whom to associate, and the environment in which to provide veterinary medical care.
8. A veterinarian shall recognize a responsibility to participate in activities contributing to the improvement of the community and the betterment of public health.
9. A veterinarian should view, evaluate, and treat all persons in any professional activity or circumstance in which they may be involved, solely as individuals on the basis of their own personal abilities, qualifications, and other relevant characteristics.

Fig. 5.1 American Veterinary Medical Association. *AVMA Principles of Veterinary Medical Ethics.* (Courtesy of American Veterinary Medical Association, Schambaugh, IL.Last update by AVMA Board of Directors, 8/2019 and is under review as of August 2022.For principles with supporting annotations, please visit https://www.avma.org/resources-tools/avma-policies/principles-veterinary-medical-ethics-avma.)

VHMA CODE OF ETHICS

VHMA
Advancing Managers. Transforming Practices.
VETERINARY HOSPITAL MANAGERS ASSOCIATION

I pledge myself to: Comply with the principles and declarations of the Veterinary Hospital Managers Association, Inc.'s code of professional ethics. Maintain and promote the profession of veterinary practice management. I will assure my continued growth and development as a professional by utilizing, to the highest extent possible, the facilities offered to me for continuing the professional education and refinement of my management skills. Seek and maintain an equitable, honorable and co-operative association with fellow members of the Veterinary Hospital Managers Association, Inc. and with all others who may become a part of my business and professional life. Play a fundamental role in maintaining excellence and quality of care to our clients and their animals. Place honesty, integrity and industriousness above all else, and gainfully pursue my profession with diligent study and dedication so that service to my employer shall always be maintained at the highest possible level. Keep all information concerning the business or personal affairs of my employer confidential, except as may otherwise be required or compelled by applicable law or regulation. Protect the employer's funds and property under my control. Information gathered, maintained or produced within the veterinary practice is the property of the practice owner and will not be reproduced, shared or distributed outside the practice without consent of the owner.

Fig. 5.2 Veterinary Hospital Managers Association. *Code of Ethics.* (Courtesy VHMA.)

The National Association of Veterinary Technicians in America (NAVTA) code of ethics for veterinary technicians is a combination of professional ethics that focuses both on practicing medicine and protecting the profession (Fig. 5.3). NAVTA strives to provide excellent guidelines for its members as well as the public.

Veterinary Ethics

Four branches of veterinary ethics exist: descriptive, official, administrative, and normative. *Descriptive ethics* refers to the study of ethical views of veterinarians and veterinary professionals regarding their behavior and attitudes. This relates to what members of the profession think is right or wrong and does not involve making value judgments about what is moral or immoral in a professional's behavior. *Official ethics* involves the creation of official ethical standards adopted by an organization of professionals and imposed on their members. *Administrative ethics* involve actions by administrative government bodies that regulate the veterinary practice and activities in which veterinarians engage. Many veterinary organizations incorporate the AVMA's principles of ethics into their statutes or regulations. License revocation can result if any civil or criminal violation of these regulations occurs. *Normative ethics* refers to the search for correct principles of good and bad, right or wrong, and justice or injustice. The difference between ethics and law lies in enforcement; the government enforces laws, whereas the professional associations that develop ethics standards enforce them.

CRITICAL COMPETENCY: INTEGRITY

Practice managers must adhere to ethical principles and values, and be seen as honest, trustworthy, and sincere professionals (demonstrated through behaviors and words).

REGULATORY AGENCIES

The government agencies that have been developed over time have created laws that workplaces must abide by, and veterinary medicine is not exempt. Many traditional and rural practices were unfamiliar with laws that applied to them and have continued to do things as they have always done and therefore may be in violation of some laws. Fines for violations can be large, large enough to put a practice out of business. "I didn't know" is not a defense that will save even the best veterinary business.

The Occupational Safety and Health Administration (OSHA) ensures that every workplace is safe, regardless of the industry. All team members deserve to work in a business that places safety first. Employees have rights, as does the business, that must be abided by. Review Chapter 15, Safety in the Veterinary Practice, for requirements, reporting, and training that must be completed by every practice, every year. Some states have more stringent requirements for safety; become familiar with state and local laws to ensure the practice complies.

The Drug Enforcement Administration (DEA) oversees the controlled substances ordered, administered, or prescribed for patients. Chapter 14, Controlled Substances, outlines requirements that the DEA established for every practitioner that either brings controlled substances into the facility for administration or prescribes them to patients under their care. Heavy fines are in place for those that are not in compliance with record keeping and reporting. In addition to DEA, some states have a more stringent controlled substance reporting policy and may have some drugs labeled as controlled substances when the DEA has not yet listed them as such.

The Food and Drug Administration (FDA) regulates food, drugs, medical devices, radiation-emitting products, tobacco, cosmetics, vaccines, and biologics, and is charged with protecting human and animal health. Most of the products used in the practice are FDA-approved, with the expectation of diets and nutraceuticals.

The United States Department of Agriculture (USDA) Animal and Plant Health Inspection Service (APHIS) regulates the accreditation of veterinarians and the ability to issue health certificates to patients that will be traveling across state and international boundaries.

EMPLOYMENT LAW

The employment laws that apply to every business are covered in Chapter 4, Human Resources. However, this chapter would incomplete if there was not a call out for this very important area. Many employers with less than 20 employees are unfamiliar with the laws that apply to them; some feel they are too small for employment laws to affect them. The exact opposite is true; while some laws only legally apply based on the number of employees that work for the business, it does not mean that every employer should not strive for excellence and meet compliance regardless. Review Chapter 4 for details on the Fair Labor Standards Act, Civil Rights Act of 1964, Family and Medical Leave, Workers' Compensation, Federal Unemployment Tax Act, Employment Retirement Income Security Act, COBRA, HIPPA, Mental Health Parity Act, Employee Polygraph Protection Act, Uniformed Services Employment and Reemployment Act, and the Affordable Care Act. Also, take note that some laws require current posters to be posted in a highly visible area of the practice for team members to see. These posters are available free of charge from the state department of labor office.

VHMA PERFORMANCE DOMAIN TASK

Understand and ensure compliance with employment/labor law.

NAVTA CODE OF ETHICS

Each member of the veterinary technology profession has the obligation to uphold the trust invested in the profession by adhering to the profession's code of ethics. No code can provide the answer to every ethical question faced by members of the profession. They shall continue to bear their responsibility for reasoned and conscientious interpretation and application of the basic ethical principles embodied in the Code to individual cases.

A veterinary technician shall uphold the laws/regulations of his/her state or province that apply to the technician's responsibilities as a member of the veterinary medical health care team.

Preamble

The Code of Ethics is based on the supposition that the honor and dignity of the professional of veterinary technology lies in the just and reasonable code of ethics. Veterinary technology includes the promotion and maintenance of good health in animals, the care of diseased and injured animals, and the control of diseases transmissible from animals to man. The purpose of the Code of Ethics is to provide guidance to the veterinary technician for carrying out professional responsibilities so as to meet the ethical obligations of the profession.

Code of Ethics

- Veterinary technicians shall aid society and animals through providing excellent care and services for animals.
- Veterinary technicians shall prevent and relieve the suffering of animals.
- Veterinary technicians shall promote public health by assisting with the control of zoonotic diseases and informing the public about these diseases.
- Veterinary technicians shall assume accountability for individual professional actions and judgments.
- Veterinary technicians shall protect confidential information provided by clients.
- Veterinary technicians shall safeguard the public and the professional against individuals deficient in professional competence or ethics.
- Veterinary technicians shall assist with efforts to ensure conditions of employment consistent with the excellent care for animals.
- Veterinary technicians shall remain competent in veterinary technology through commitment to life-long learning.
- Veterinary technicians shall collaborate with members of the veterinary medical profession in efforts to ensure quality health care services for all animals.

Ideals

In addition to adhering to the standards listed in the Code of Ethics, veterinary technicians may also strive to attain a number of ideals. Some of these are:

- Veterinary technicians shall strive to participate in defining, upholding, and improving standards of professional practice, legislation, and education.
- Veterinary technicians shall strive to contribute to the profession's body of knowledge.
- Veterinary technicians shall strive to understand and support the attachment between a person and his/her companion animal.between a person and his/her companion animal. e competent veterinary medical clinical care under the terms of a veterinarian-client-patient relationship (VCPR), with compassion and respect for animal welfare and human health.

Fig. 5.3 National Association of Veterinary Technicians in America. *Code of Ethics.* (Courtesy NAVTA.)

LEGAL ISSUES

Laws are bodies of rules developed and enforced by government to regulate people's conduct. Veterinarians are faced with legal obligations daily. Many laws stem from society's moral and ethical concerns for life, death, and how people conduct themselves. The Veterinary Practice Act of each state defines the requirements necessary to practice veterinary medicine within that state. Veterinary standards of care are developed from both the practice act and statutory law. Principles of ethics also govern veterinary medicine and are implemented for the protection of the profession and society itself.

Each practice should have reliable legal counsel licensed in their jurisdiction who is knowledgeable about contracts and business relationships. Ideally, counsel would understand veterinary practice standards, but not required. In addition, each practice should have at least one team member who is thoroughly familiar with the state practice act and regulations (preferably all veterinarians, credentialed technicians, and the practice manager) (Fig. 5.4).

Veterinary Practice Act

The Veterinary Practice Act emphasizes that the right to practice veterinary medicine is a privilege granted by state law and is thus subject to regulation to protect and promote public health, safety, and welfare. This statute is enacted as an exercise of the powers of the state by ensuring the delivery of competent veterinary medical care. Individuals who practice veterinary medicine are expected to possess the personal and professional qualifications specified in this act. AVMA has created a model practice act that most states follow when developing their state veterinary practice acts.

Veterinary practice acts are umbrella laws that govern the practice of veterinary medicine and changes cannot be made easily. Changes must be submitted to the House and Senate, approved by both parties, and then ultimately signed into law by a governor. State associations and veterinary medical boards may circulate proposed changes among members of the veterinary and veterinary technician communities, soliciting opinions and changes that members may recommend. Once the board and associations agree, a lobbyist can be hired to find state senators and representatives to support the bill and introduce it into the legislative process. Throughout this process, amendments and updates will occur various times before the final product is approved by both chambers; it is only then that the bill is presented to a governor for acceptance. A governor can then accept or deny the bill but cannot make changes.

LEADERSHIP POINT

Review the State Veterinary Practice Act to ensure the practice leverages credentialed veterinary technicians/nurses appropriately and to the fullest extent allowed.

Practice acts are then regulated and enforced by the state board of veterinary medicine (BVM), which oversees veterinarians. In most states, the BVM also oversees credentialed veterinary technicians; however, this can vary as few states are self-regulated. The BVM is

SUMMARY OF AVMA MODEL VETERINARY PRACTICE ACT UPDATED JANUARY 2021

Preamble
Section 1 Title
Section 2 Definitions
Section 3 Board of Veterinary Medicine
Section 4 License Requirement
Section 5 Veterinarian-Client-Patient Relationship Requirement
Section 6 Exemptions
Section 7 Veterinary Technicians and Technologists
Section 8 Status of Persons Previously Licensed
Section 9 Application for License: Qualifications
Section 10 Examinations
Section 11 License by Endorsement
Section 12 Temporary Permit
Section 13 License Renewal
Section 14 Discipline of Licensees
Section 15 Impaired Veterinarian or Credentialed Veterinary Technician
Section 16 Hearing Procedure
Section 17 Appeal
Section 18 Reinstatement
Section 19 Veterinarian-Client Confidentiality
Section 20 Immunity from Liability
Section 21 Cruelty to Animals—Immunity for Reporting
Section 22 Abandoned Animals
Section 23 Enforcement
Section 24 Severability
Section 25 Effective Date

Fig. 5.4 American Veterinary Medical Association Model Veterinary Practice Act. Updated January 2021. (Courtesy of American Veterinary Medical Association, Schambaugh, IL.Visit https://www.avma.org/sites/default/files/2021-01/model-veterinary-practice-act.pdf for full explanation of each section.)

responsible for testing and licensure, collection of renewal fees, and the evaluation of complaints presented by the public. With adequate evidence of wrongdoing, boards can revoke any professional veterinary license. The most common complaints are listed later in this chapter.

States may adopt administrative regulations or rules to implement statutory practice acts, which are enforceable by law and should be reviewed for compliance as carefully as the practice acts.

CRITICAL COMPETENCY: ORAL COMMUNICATION AND COMPREHENSION

The practice manager must have the ability to express thoughts verbally in a clear and understandable manner, and the ability to actively listen and attend to what others are saying.

Definitions of Law

A law generally consists of established rules, statutes, and administrative agency rules that can be enforced to establish limits of conduct for governments and individuals in society. Laws are divided into two categories: civil and criminal.

Civil law relates to the duties between individuals and society. A contract dispute between a veterinarian and an employee is an example of a civil law case.

Criminal law prosecutes crimes committed against the public. Most criminal laws focus on acts that injure people or pets or offend public morality. Violation of civil law generally results in fines paid to the opposing party, whereas violation of criminal law results in jail time and/or fines.

Civil law can be further broken down into tort and contract law.

Tort law involves a civil offense to an opposing party in which harm has occurred and permits people to sue for relief of an injury that occurred because of damages inflicted on their bodies, to their families, or to their property. Furthermore, tort law can be determined as intentional or unintentional and must be proven to the court. An *intentional tort* is defined as an intentional action that has taken place in which harm has occurred to another member of society. Examples of intentional torts include assault and battery, defamation of character, invasion of privacy, immoral conduct, and fraud. An example of an unintentional tort claim would be the failure to practice the standard of care. If a veterinarian did not practice the standard of care that has been developed by veterinary professionals and an animal suffered injury because of neglect, the veterinarian could be guilty of an unintentional tort of negligence. Torts are generally resolved with a civil trial and a monetary settlement.

Contract law deals with duties established by individuals because of contractual agreements. This area of law was developed to ensure that promises made by people would be fulfilled; if they are not fulfilled, a breach of duty is established.

VHMA PERFORMANCE DOMAIN TASK

Understand and ensure compliance with contract law as it pertains to associate veterinarians, staff, and clients.

A crime is an unlawful activity against a member of the public and is prosecuted by a public official, normally the district attorney or the attorney general's office. A crime is further classified as a misdemeanor or a felony. A misdemeanor charge is less serious than a felony and usually results in less jail time.

Negligence is the performance of an act that a reasonable person under the same circumstances would not perform. Malpractice can be considered a form of negligence and is considered intentional or unintentional. Overall, malpractice can refer to any unprofessional, illegal, or immoral conduct. Malpractice is the dereliction of duty, resulting in injury to the patient. Fig. 5.5 lists the most common errors in veterinary practice that can result in malpractice claims.

Consent

Consent is the voluntary acceptance or agreement to what is planned or is done (for a patient) by another person. Informed consent is when a veterinary practice has given information to a client regarding the proposed treatment, allowing the client to make an informed decision regarding whether to proceed with a treatment for their pet. Courts have established several elements that must be fully addressed to have complete informed consent.

- The consent must be given freely, and the treatment and diagnosis must be given in understandable terms.
- The risks, benefits, and prognosis of the defined procedure must be stated, as well as the prognosis if no treatment is elected.
- The practice must provide a statement of alternative treatments or procedures along with the risks, benefits, and costs of each.
- The client must be given the right to ask questions and have them answered.

ACTS OF MALPRACTICE

- Incorrect drug administration
- Incorrect strength of drug administration
- Failure to clean animals that have defecated and/or urinated on themselves
- Abandonment
- Leaving foreign objects in a patient after surgery
- Failure to exercise good judgment
- Failure to communicate
- Loss or damage to patients' personal property
- Disease transmission
- A patient attacking another while in the veterinary practice
- Use of defective equipment or medication

Fig. 5.5 Malpractice is the dereliction of duty that results in injury to a patient.

Fig. 5.6 is an example of an informed consent form; the pet owner and technician sign each section together after the risks and benefits have been discussed and understood by the owner.

If informed consent is challenged in a court of law and these conditions have not been met, the court may conclude that the client did not consent to the procedure and the veterinarian may be held liable. Documentation of the discussion must be in the record; if a record does not indicate that risks were discussed, the court can assume the discussion did not occur. A signed consent form does not indicate that informed consent occurred because many people sign consent forms without reading them. Therefore, a verbal discussion must also occur. Practices should never rely on clients who state "Do what is best" because this is not informed consent; they have not been provided the education on the risks and benefits of the procedure. The average client does not possess the skill or knowledge to make informed decisions without all the available information.

Information should be given to clients in a manner that they can understand. Each client should be evaluated for the level of education, skill, and knowledge that he or she possesses with which to comprehend

ABC Veterinary Clinic
Surgery, Anesthesia, and Treatment Consent Form

Client Name ______________________ Patient Name ______________________
Date ________ Procedure ______________________________ Male/Female

Your pet has been scheduled for a procedure requiring sedation or anesthesia. By signing this form, you authorize ABC Veterinary Clinic and its agents to administer tranquilizers, anesthetics, and analgesics that are deemed appropriate. Please be aware that all drugs have a potential for adverse side effects in any particular animal. The chances of such occurrence are extremely low; however, death can result in any anesthetized patient.

Owner initials ________ Tech initials ________

In an effort to ensure your pet's safety and to anticipate any problems before they occur, we advise pre-anesthetic bloodwork and electrocardiogram prior to anesthesia. Bloodwork will determine the kidney and liver functions, which participate in the metabolism of anesthesia. An electrocardiogram can detect abnormal arrhythmias, heart rate, and conductivity.

I accept/decline bloodwork I accept/decline an electrocardiogram

Owner initials ________ Tech initials ________

IV fluids are advised for all patients undergoing anesthesia. IV fluids help maintain blood pressure of the patient while offering support for the kidneys to metabolize the medications. Pets may take longer to recover without IV fluids.

I accept/decline IV fluids

Owner initials ________ Tech initials ________

Heartworm tests are recommended for dogs over 6 months of age. Heartworm disease can cause anesthetic complications. We advise FeLV/FIV testing for cats. FeLV or FIV infection can delay healing of any surgical site.

I accept/decline heartworm test I accept/decline FeLV/FIV test

Owner initials ________ Tech initials ________

Vaccinations are important for disease prevention in your pet. We advise that pets be current on vaccines. Rabies vaccination is required by law; every pet must receive a rabies vaccine.

Vaccines due (booster?): DHPP FVRCP FeLV Rabies

Owner Initials ________ Tech Initials ________

Fig. 5.6 Example of an informed consent form.

Did pet eat this morning?	Yes	No
Has pet had any allergies or vaccine reactions in the past?	Yes	No
Are we declawing the pet?	Yes	No
Are we removing dewclaws?	Yes	No
Does the pet have 2 testicles?	Yes	No
If the pet is pregnant, can we continue with surgery?	Yes	No
Does the pet have an umbilical hernia?	Yes	No
May we repair?	Yes	No
Does the pet have retained teeth?	Yes	No
May we remove?	Yes	No
Does the pet need an Elizabethan collar?	Yes	No
Dental: OK to extract teeth?	Yes	No
OK to take dental radiographs if indicated?	Yes	No
OK to apply Doxirobe gel if indicated?	Yes	No
Is pet currently on antibiotics?	Yes	No
When was last dose? ________		
How many pills are left? ________		
Growth Removal: Histopath?	Yes	No
Location of growths: ________		

You may contact me **today** at: ________

Alternative contact phone number: ________

I understand that anesthesia is a risk and authorize the above procedures. I understand that I will be contacted first if any changes in the discussed protocol occur.

Client signature ________ Date ________

Fig. 5.6 cont'd

LEADERSHIP POINT

Hospitals must have a policy in place that ensures every client consent form is verbally reviewed with, and understood, by the client.

the information. If judgment is deemed to be impaired (by minor age, mental illness, intoxication, etc.) or whether their understanding of the information is questionable, acceptance of consent should be made with extreme caution.

The best consent form available is one that is tailored to the specific patient and the procedure being recommended. If anesthesia is advised to complete a procedure, the consent form should clearly indicate a risk of death. A signature should be placed next to this statement for both the client and the reviewing team member. All risks, benefits, and prognoses should be listed as such and initialed by both individuals. This will help the court determine whether each topic was fully addressed and whether the client was fully informed before signing the form.

Emergency Care

Veterinary practices often face a dilemma when a Good Samaritan brings in a pet that has been hit by a car. Can the practice treat this emergency? Who is the owner? Can the owner be contacted? Is the Good Samaritan responsible for the bill? The first thought that most practices experience is that there is no consent to treat the animal. However, if the owners are found, they may hold the practice liable for not performing lifesaving techniques.

According to the AVMA Code of Ethics, veterinarians have an ethical responsibility to provide essential services for animals when necessary to save life or relieve suffering. Such emergency care may be limited to euthanasia to relieve suffering, or to stabilize the patient for transport to another source of animal care.

The *law of unjust enrichment* allows protection for the practice if critical factors are met. If there is value to the pet, the courts may allow a recovery of cost; the more valuable the pet appears, the greater the chance of recovery. Value can be based on either economic or emotional attachment with respect to the human-animal bond. The severity of the injuries must be proven. Photographs documenting injuries and supportive treatment will help ensure the client and the court that unnecessary procedures were not completed. Attempts to reach the owner must be documented in the record with the name of the person trying to make contact, phone numbers, time of the calls, as well as the number of attempts made. Once the patient is stable, only supportive care should be rendered. Plating a fracture would not be considered supportive care for a trauma patient unless it was a lifesaving technique.

Historically, the only way for a practice to recover the costs associated with emergency care has been to take the client to court (if the owner was identified). This has led to many practices refusing to treat animals without owners (which then leads to an ethical dilemma: does the practice treat the pet or let it suffer?). There is no law that states that practices must treat. In fact, by law, the duty to treat is only initiated once a valid client-patient relationship has been established. Once a valid client-patient relationship has been established, a practice must continue the treatment until the animal recovers, the veterinarian has completed all the treatments agreed upon, the patient dies, or the client terminates the client-patient relationship.

Treatment can be declined by the practice because of the client's inability to pay; however, once treatment has begun, it is extremely difficult to terminate treatment if the result would be neglect or harm to the animal. If treatment by the veterinarian must be terminated for any reason, including nonpayment of services, the veterinarian should make a good faith effort to find a veterinarian that will continue the treatment.

VHMA PERFORMANCE DOMAIN TASK

Understand and ensure compliance with the legal and ethical guidelines surrounding confidentiality of staff, clients, and patients.

Veterinary practices are ethically obligated to provide emergency services to their clients after hours (as stated in the AVMA Code of Ethics); if they do not provide services themselves, they must refer their clients to a location that accepts emergencies after hours.

Recently, several states have adopted laws that allow a veterinarian (and in some cases, any person who boards or treats an animal under contract with the owner) to place a lien on the animal and detain it until payment is made. There are some states that allow officers of the peace to take an animal into possession after he or she determines that the animal is being treated cruelly, is being neglected, or is abandoned. The officer may then place a lien on the animal for the costs associated with caring for the animal and detain the animal until the debt is paid.

Although many states differ in their enforcement of the lien laws, the general rule is that if the debt is not paid within 10 to 20 days of giving proper notice to the owner, the veterinarian or caregiver may sell the animal, or, in some cases, euthanize the animal or turn it over to a humane society. In most states, a lien attaches once the debt becomes due; however, in a couple of states, a veterinarian or caregiver must perfect the lien by filing a financial statement with the secretary of state's office. Only a handful of states require that the lien be enforced through a legal process.

The general rule in most states is that once the veterinarian or caregiver sells the animal, they may use the proceeds to pay the debt due as well as any costs associated with putting the animal up for sale.

Malpractice

Lawsuits against veterinarians and veterinary technicians are almost always based on neglect versus breach of contract, defamation, or breach of warranty. *Negligence* is defined as performing an act that a person of ordinary prudence would not have done under similar circumstances (or failure to perform an act that a person of ordinary prudence would have done). If a veterinarian or technician is sued for negligence, four basic elements must be proven in a court of law. The first is the establishment of a valid client-patient relationship. This is rarely an issue because most client-patient relationships were established when the patient was presented to the practice by the pet owner. Second, breach of duty must be proven. *Breach of duty* is the failure of the veterinarian or technician to act in accordance with the standard of care. This breach can occur by either performing an act that should not have been performed or not performing an act that should have been performed. Third, *proximate cause* must be established. Proximate cause is the connection between the negligent act of the veterinarian and/or technician and the harm to the patient caused by the act. Fourth, damages or harm incurred by the patient because of the negligent act must be displayed.

The *standard of care* can be defined as the duty to exercise the care and diligence that is ordinarily exercised by a reasonably competent veterinarian under normal circumstances. With the availability of specialists in many metropolitan and suburban areas around the United States, the standard of care may be held to the specialist level. This means that veterinarians should refer or recommend referrals to a specialty center when a case is complex and requires the intervention of a specialist. Veterinarians may be held liable if they do not make the recommendation and/or do not document the referral recommendation in the record. If the client declines the referral, the declined treatment should be clearly documented.

To help avoid a malpractice lawsuit against a veterinarian or practice, several topics should be addressed with team members. Medical records must be complete and include every detail of the case. "If it is not in the record, it did not happen" is a common standard considered by the court of law. Every treatment and recommendation must be clearly documented along with any refusals the client has made. Clients must be informed when making decisions, and proof of informed consent must be included in the record.

Most veterinarians purchase liability insurance through AVMA, which is supported by Professional Liability Insurance Trust (PLIT). This insurance provides coverage for veterinarians, veterinary technicians, and support staff that are engaged in activities involved in the practice. Each veterinarian in the practice must carry his or her own liability insurance.

Abandoned Animals

Animals may be left at practices unclaimed, especially puppies with parvovirus or other incurable or expensive ailments. Practices must make repeated attempts to contact the owner and document these attempts. After repeated attempts to contact the owner, a certified letter should be sent to the owner indicating the confirmation of abandonment of the pet. Because a valid client-patient relationship was developed when the owner dropped off the pet, the practice is responsible for providing treatment that will prevent harm or neglect to the patient. The practice is not required to perform lifesaving techniques; however, the pet cannot receive injury by withholding treatment. Local and state laws should be reviewed indicating the length of time the practice is required to hold the pet to confirm abandonment. A second certified letter might be required by some municipalities. If there is no response from the owner within the stated time, the pet can be considered abandoned, and the practice can make the pet available for adoption or euthanize it, whichever provides the best outcome for the practice.

IMPENDING LAWS

Ownership Versus Guardian Issues

State and local laws have been amended in several cities/states so that animals may no longer be considered property, but rather as animals cared for by guardians. This can affect the veterinarian-client relationship in many ways. In human cases, a guardian is usually given the authority or designation to care for a person who is a minor, incapacitated, or disabled. A *guardian ad litem* is a person appointed to protect the interests of a minor or legally incompetent person in a lawsuit or, in this case, an animal.

> **LEADERSHIP POINT**
>
> Monitor your state veterinary medical association website to stay informed of pending pet ownership/guardian changes.

Change in the status of owner to guardian can present many issues. Who will determine what is best for the animal: the guardian or the veterinarian? Could the veterinarian be sued for wrongful death on behalf of the pet? Other questions will certainly be raised by this designation of guardianship, as well as concerns about animal abuse or neglect by veterinarians. If a veterinarian does not immediately provide pain relief for an animal or send home postoperative pain medication, the practice may be held liable for neglect. Visit the AVMA website (https://www.avma.org/advocacy/state-and-local-advocacy/state-local-ownership-vs-guardianship-issues) frequently to check for updates.

> **CRITICAL COMPETENCY: COMPLIANCE**
>
> Practice managers must be reliable, thorough, and conscientious in carrying out work assignments while having an appreciation for the importance of organizational rules and policies.

Compounding Medications

Compounding is defined as any manipulation of an FDA (Food and Drug Administration)-approved drug (beyond that stipulated on the product's label) to provide individualized medication for a specific patient with special needs not met by FDA-approved drug products. Manipulation includes mixing, diluting, concentrating, flavoring, or changing a drug's dosage form to accommodate a specific patient's needs.

Compounded preparations can provide effective therapies for treating painful or life-threatening medical conditions in patients and provide much-needed therapeutic flexibility for veterinarians, especially considering the wide range of species and breeds treated in the veterinary practice. However, if done incorrectly or inappropriately, the use of compounded preparations can lead to prolonged treatment needs, adverse events (including treatment failure), liability, or even enforcement action by federal or state authorities.

Ideally, compounding should be implemented to meet the medical needs of a specific patient. State regulations vary regarding the use of compounding medications for office use and the dispensing or reselling of compounded medications. At the time of publication, Fig. 5.7 shows states that have compounding regulations in place. Visit https://www.avma.org/advocacy/state-local-issues/administration-and-dispensing-compounded-veterinary-drugs for current updates.

To ensure US Pharmacopeia (USP) standards have been met by a compounding pharmacy, the Pharmacy Compounding Accreditation Board (PCAB) offers accreditation to compounding pharmacies that meet high quality and practice standards. Visit www.pcab.org for a listing of accredited compounding pharmacies.

> **VHMA PERFORMANCE DOMAIN TASK**
>
> Understand and ensure compliance with state and local agencies.

Extra-Label Drug Use in Patients

Before Congress passed the Animal Medicinal Drug Use Clarification Act (AMDUCA) in 1994, federal law did not permit extra-label drug use in animals. The AMDUCA provisions amended the FD&C Act to allow veterinarians to prescribe approved human and animal drugs for extra-label uses in animals under specified conditions:

- A valid veterinarian-client-patient relationship must exist.
- General conditions for extra-label drug use must be met, including an animal's health being threatened or where the animal may suffer or die without treatment. In addition, one of the following general

State laws and regulations that allow veterinary offices to administer compounded products and dispense the products to clients but may be subject to conditions or limitations in some cases:	State laws and regulations that allow veterinary offices to administer compounded products but do not specifically address or the law is not clear regarding dispensing products compounded by a pharmacy:	State laws and regulations that allow veterinary offices to administer compounded products but specifically prohibit them from dispensing or reselling products compounded by a pharmacy:	States that prohibit compounding for office use:	Compounding is not addressed in state laws or regulations
Arizona Arkansas California Colorado Delaware Florida Georgia Illinois Iowa Maine Maryland Massachusetts Michigan Minnesota Mississippi Missouri Nebraska New Mexico Ohio Tennessee Texas Virginia	Idaho Montana Nevada New Hampshire New Jersey Oregon South Carolina	Alabama Alaska Connecticut Kansas Kentucky Louisiana North Carolina North Dakota Oklahoma Rhode Island Utah Vermont Washington West Virginia Wyoming	Ney York Rhode Island	Hawaii Indiana Pennsylvania South Dakota Wisconsin

Fig. 5.7 Compounding regulations by state.

conditions must be met before a veterinarian can legally prescribe an approved human or animal drug for extra-label use:

- No animal drug is approved for the intended use.
- An animal drug is approved for the intended use, but the approved drug does not contain the active ingredient needed for treatment.
- An animal drug is approved for the intended use, but the approved drug is not in the required dosage form (for example, a liquid form is needed, but the approved drug is only available in a tablet form).
- An animal drug is approved for the intended use, but the approved drug is not in the required concentration (for example, 5 mg is needed, but the approved drug is only available in 50 mg).

CRITICAL COMPETENCY: ADAPTABILITY

Practice managers must be open to change and flexible work methods and can adapt behavior to changing conditions or the latest information.

Fairness to Pet Owners Act

For years, some members of Congress have pushed for new federal regulations implementing prescription mandates. This legislation would force veterinarians to provide written copies of all prescriptions they issue for companion animals, even if the client does not want a written copy or if the medication is only available through a veterinarian.

In 2019, Congress introduced prescription mandate legislation called the "Fairness to Pet Owners Act." The AVMA opposed (and continues to oppose) this legislation because it will require veterinarians to spend more time on paperwork instead of what's most important: caring for patients. Many veterinary practices are small businesses with limited administrative resources; therefore, the extra regulatory burden will affect the number of patients that can be seen and will increase pet care costs for clients.

The AVMA's Principles of Veterinary Medical Ethics (PVME) advises veterinarians to provide written prescriptions when asked, and most states have similar laws or policies. For further information on this issue, visit https://www.avma.org/advocacy/avma-opposes-prescription-mandate-legislation.

LEADERSHIP POINT

Give clients the opportunity to purchase medications online through the practice's reputable online pharmacy platform.

Clients wishing to obtain a prescription for their pets' medications should be advised to ask the practice for a prescription prior to requesting the medication from the online pharmacy. Practices can choose to write a prescription or call the internet pharmacy direct to authorize the prescription. It is the veterinarian's responsibility when filling a prescription (whether in-house or through another pharmacy) to explain the risks and benefits of the medications, including potential side effects, and recommend a pharmacy that is accredited with the National Association of Boards of Pharmacy (NABP). The NABP ensures that the pharmacy is licensed and that veterinary standards are met, along with other program requirements (www.nabp.net).

MEDICAL RECORDS

The laws concerning the legal ownership of records vary from state to state; however, in general, medical records are owned by the practice, not the pet owner. The owner can request a copy of the medical record at any time, and in fact, most clients request copies of records when they are changing veterinary hospitals.

Clients should sign a medical record release for medical records to be copied and released to someone other than the client. This includes faxing or emailing records to other hospitals, boarding facilities, or new pet owners. The only time medical records should be released without consent is if the patient has a reportable disease that must be reported to the state or U.S. Department of Agriculture.

Keep in mind that all medical records are legal documents. Therefore, they must always be complete and legible. Medical records are generated to ensure consistent and accurate care as well as protect the veterinarian in the event of a malpractice suit. Inaccurate, incomplete, and illegible medical records could be interpreted as professional incompetence with substandard care. If evaluated by a court of law, the following stance may be upheld: "If it was not written down, it did not occur."

LEADERSHIP POINT

Allow every client full access to their medical records through the practice's pet portal or practice app.

If mistakes are made in a paper medical record, a single line should be drawn through the mistake, initialed, and corrected. Correction fluid or blackouts are not permitted because this could be interpreted as an alteration of records, rendering them inadmissible in a court of law. Electronic medical records should be set up correctly so that when a copy of the EMR is printed for the referring veterinarian, a complete understanding of the case can be obtained (see Chapter 9 for more information on medical records).

VHMA PERFORMANCE DOMAIN TASK

Maintain an appropriate medical records system that complies with legal standards.

THE MOST COMMON COMPLAINTS TO THE BOARD OF VETERINARY MEDICINE

A complaint is a formal action noting dissatisfaction with the services of a licensed veterinarian or credentialed veterinary technician. A complaint is filed with the state veterinary medical board, which then sends a letter to the veterinarian and/or technician. An investigator is assigned to the case and completes all needed interviews and record reviews. The complaint is then evaluated by a review committee and submitted to the full veterinary board for consideration. The board either acts against the veterinarian or technician or can dismiss or settle the case without a hearing (continuing education and fines may be imposed). If the complaint is found to be severe, a Notice of Contemplated Action is sent requesting a hearing. The result of the hearing may impose continuing education, fines, license suspension, or revocation. All decisions can be appealed.

VHMA PERFORMANCE DOMAIN TASK

Maintains protocols for hospital procedures and risk management plans.

Unsatisfied Experience

Patient owners tend to file complaints because of dissatisfaction resulting from experiences at the practice and usually rise because of customer service or communication that did not fulfill their expectations. Clients may be upset when they did not fully understand the procedure their pet would be undergoing, the potential risks associated with it, or the potential outcomes (refer to section on informed consent). For example, a cast or splint may have been too tight, resulting in cast or bandaging sores, or a pet chewed off a cast and removed their sutures or staples (when the veterinary team had not instructed the owner how to keep the pet from chewing).

Clients may be unhappy with the results of a surgery or treatment. Many fractures do not heal properly, and the client believes the veterinarian is responsible. The team must recommend the best procedure available to repair fractures, regardless of whether the practice provides that procedure. When applicable, the patient should be referred to a practice that provides the best outcome. If the client declines the referral and opts for the lesser treatment, it must be noted in the record. The recommendation should also be written on a release sheet that the owner signs when the patient is discharged; this provides proof that the owner was made aware of the recommendation.

Team members treating clients disrespectfully can cause loss of clients for the practice and can also result in formal complaints being made. Disrespect may include being rude to a client, not listening to client wishes, gossiping about another client, or not returning client calls for any reason.

Lack of Communication

Poor communication is the top board complaint. Communication is integral to most aspects of veterinary practice, from the receptionist to the veterinarian and every team member must place client communication as a key priority. Chapter 11 states clients must hear a recommendation three times to fully accept the importance of such a recommendation. The same can be said for informed consent; it is the practice's responsibility to ensure clear communication has been delivered to the client.

Occasionally, credentialed veterinary technicians relay too much information and overstep their professional boundaries as they cannot diagnose disease; only veterinarians are permitted to do so. In the process of providing information to the client before the veterinarian has seen the case, the technician may give incorrect or invalid information, and the variability in the information provided by both the veterinarian and veterinary technician can confuse the client (resulting in a complaint).

When patients are discharged from the hospital, a signed copy of the information provided to the client must remain with the record; this covers the practice if the client states they did not receive the information. When a patient is discharged, the team member must ensure that the client fully understands home care instructions.

Occasionally, when a patient incurs severe trauma, the team is dedicated to caring for the patient's immediate needs. The cost, aftercare, and prognosis of the pet are often the last items communicated to the owner resulting in clients becoming upset about the expense of saving a pet. They feel that if they had known the prognosis and the amount of aftercare required, they may have chosen to euthanize the pet instead. The entire treatment process, from immediate care to prolonged aftercare, must be communicated to the owner and documented in the record to prevent this complaint. Consider how one might apply the above to a diabetic ketoacidosis case.

Many times, clients are dissatisfied with an invoice after a procedure. Written estimates must always be provided to owners, and a copy of the estimate must remain in the medical record for future reference. If the estimate should change in any way, the client must be notified immediately. If the owner did not approve services, a formal complaint may be filed.

Unexpected Death

The unexpected death of a patient is an unfortunate situation and the source of a common complaint. If a client brings a pet to the practice for treatment, regardless of the use of anesthesia, the owner must sign a treatment authorization form. As stated earlier, informed consent must be discussed with the owner, listing the risks and benefits of treatments or procedures. The client must be fully informed that death may result from numerous unexpected situations. A seemingly simple blood draw on an unhealthy cat can induce a sudden, unexpected death. It is imperative that risks be discussed with the owner.

Conduct, Record Keeping, Premises, and Pharmaceutical Issues

Conduct, record keeping, premises, and pharmaceutical citations are four common violations given in veterinary medicine. Conduct is defined as veterinarians shall exercise the same degree of care, skill, and diligence in treating patients as are ordinarily used in the same or similar circumstances by reasonably prudent members of the veterinary medical profession in good standing. A veterinarian shall not use or participate in any form of representation, advertising or solicitation containing false, deceptive, or misleading statements or claims.

Record keeping is a difficult challenge for many practices; however, records must be fully completed to prevent a violation (see Chapter 9).

The most common premise violation is that a surgery room must be a separate room from all other rooms, reserved for aseptic surgical procedures requiring aseptic preparation. Only items used for surgical procedures may be kept in the surgical room (dental machines cannot be stored in the surgical room as they are not part of an aseptic procedure).

Common pharmacy violations include veterinarians not honoring a client's request to dispense or provide a written prescription for a drug that has been determined by the veterinarian to be appropriate for the patient.

Many other complaints arise in veterinary medicine for malpractice and negligence; however, the examples previously listed are the most common and can be easily prevented by the veterinary healthcare team through exceptional customer service and clear communication.

LEADERSHIP'S ROLE IN VETERINARY ETHICS AND LEGAL ISSUES

A primary responsibility of the practice manager and owner is to manage become familiar and stay current with employment law, and legal issues/ethics that impact the veterinary practice. Impending laws covered in this chapter may have a significant impact on the way veterinary medicine is practiced, as well as the administrative burden that may result. Last must not least, owners and managers must ensure that SOPs and SOCs are created and followed, client service is expectational, and that all team members embody the importance of client communication to prevent (or mitigate at minimum) the risk of board complaints and lawsuits.

PRACTICE MANAGERS SURVIVAL CHECKLIST FOR VETERINARY ETHICS AND LEGAL ISSUES

- ☐ Develop a hospital policy regarding the shredding of documents (client, employee, or business).
- ☐ Develop liability releases for volunteers, interns, and students.
- ☐ Follow AVMA for current updates regarding the Fairness to Pet Owners Act and compounding regulations.
- ☐ Develop medical record standards, including SOAP (subjective, objective, assessment, and plan) format, abbreviations, data entry, and required password protection.
- ☐ Develop standard protocols to handle client communication, conflict, and complaints.
- ☐ Ensure practice protocols meet state requirements daily, not just when inspected.

REVIEW QUESTIONS

1. Define civil law.
2. Define contract law.
3. Define negligence.
4. Define malpractice.
5. Why are ethics important to the veterinary profession?
6. Why is informed consent imperative?
7. Why would a consent form be upheld in court?
8. What branch of law does animal abuse fall under?
9. What is PLIT? Whom does it cover?
10. Why is medical record legibility and completeness important?
11. Which association created the Principles of Veterinary Medical Ethics?
    a. AVMA
    b. NAVTA
    c. VHMA
    d. PLIT
12. What does the acronym VCPR stand for?
    a. Veterinary-client public records
    b. Veterinarian-client-patient relationship
    c. Veterinary cardiac pulmonary resuscitation
    d. Veterinary conduct and professional responsibilities
13. Which of the following is considered a branch of veterinary ethics?
    a. Normative
    b. Descriptive
    c. Administrative
    d. Official
    e. All of the above
14. What are the two categories of law?
    a. Civil and federal
    b. Criminal and common
    c. Criminal and civil
    d. Federal and criminal
15. What is the correct definition of an *intentional tort?*
    a. An intentional action that has taken place in which harm has occurred to another member of society
    b. Crimes committed against the public as a whole
    c. A civil offense to an opposing party in which harm has occurred
    d. An injury occurring to a member of society as a result of negligence

RECOMMENDED READING

Wilson JF. *Laws and ethics for the veterinary profession*. Priority Press; 1990.

Wilson JF, et al. *Contracts, benefits, and practice management for the veterinary profession*. Priority Press; 2009.

Wilson JF. *Legal consents for veterinary practices*. 4th ed. Priority Press; 2006.

6

Professional Development

LEARNING OBJECTIVES

When you have completed this chapter, you should be able to:

- Identify the importance of professional development
- Differentiate between compassion fatigue and burnout
- Understand what causes compassion fatigue and burnout
- Know how to manage compassion fatigue and burnout
- Identify and achieve becoming positively unbalanced
- Measure the success of resolving burnout/compassion fatigue
- Understand how to be proactive regarding suicide
- Approach someone you are concerned about
- Discuss career fields that are available
- Explain how to develop an effective resume
- List methods used to prepare for an interview
- List questions to ask a potential employer
- Discuss how to follow up after an interview
- Differentiate offers of employment
- Discuss retirement savings

OUTLINE

KEY TERMS

Awareness
Burnout
Compassion Fatigue
Personal Skills
Resume
Substance Abuse
Suicide
Transferable Skills

INTRODUCTION

Professional development applies to all employees. It is a leader's responsibility (practice manager/owner/department leader) to develop the team. In a 2016 survey on practice culture, the American Animal Hospital Association (AAHA) found that supporting career development for all employees was rated as one of the top attributes of a positive workplace culture.[1] Positive workplace environments can help improve employee retention, client satisfaction, and overall profitability. There are many ways that veterinary practices can support the professional development of all employees, regardless of their role.

While veterinarians normally receive dollars and days off to use specifically for professional development, credentialed technicians don't always. In the 2016 NAVTA demographic survey, 70% of technician respondents reported receiving a CE stipend, but only 50% received time off to pursue their CE training as part of their benefits package.[2] Many practices want to be the employer of choice, and professional development opportunities must be provided for all. See Chapters 2

(Leadership) and 4 (Human Resources) for more benefits of CE allotment for the team.

VHMA PERFORMANCE DOMAIN TASK

Manage personnel training and development programs.

Professional development should be looked at in a variety of ways. One may wish to self-develop to better themselves, better the practice, or better the industry. Some may wish to pursue all. Lifelong education refills the soul and drives passion. The success of each individual may vary, as one may feel success as being paid well with an important title, while others view success as being happy and enjoying what they are doing in their professional life.

When the practice is providing monetary benefit for professional development, it is important that the practice tie professional development into the strategic plan. CE may focus on developing a new profit center such as rehabilitation or exotics. The new skills learned by the veterinarians, the practice manager (pricing strategy and marketing techniques), and the credentialed technicians are essential for the success of the new profit center. In a practice with a great culture, this will also drive personal satisfaction, resulting in increased employee retention.

There are also professional development opportunities that may not directly tie to the success of the practice; however, the practice indirectly benefits from such benefits. Veterinarians, practice managers, and credentialed veterinary technicians are encouraged to get involved in organized medicine (national and state associations and organizations) by volunteering time, skills, or intellect, and by running for board positions in various organizations, or contributing to community growth and service opportunities (Fig. 6.1). Many of these organizations provide leadership training and aid in skills development associated with communication, professionalism, speaking, and writing.

LEADERSHIP POINT

Continuing education should be a practice benefit provided for the entire team resulting in each team member having the ability to achieve the highest level of Maslow's Hierarchy.

Community growth and service opportunities may be related or unrelated to the profession (such as Habitat for Humanity, Shelters for Domestic Violence, or homeless shelters). Opportunities related to veterinary services may include volunteering for Veterinarians without Borders (http://vetswithoutbordersus.org) or Rural Area Veterinary Service (http://www.ruralareavet.org).[3]

It is also critical to maintain a network of friends, mentors, and advisors (outside of the practice) who will always challenge the status quo, lend an ear, or be a guide through the various levels of career development. Leaders need mentorship from those who have been in the industry for several years, have served in different positions, and bring energy and enthusiasm outside of the walls of the practice. Mentors and advisors may serve in areas outside of veterinary medicine and bring skills to the conversation that create excitement, and help you develop transferrable skills that can be used in many walks of life.

Professional development starts with a self-assessment. What competencies would you (or your team member) like to gain? When attending continuing education, who motivates you? What did they do that was so inspiring? Was it the skill or the way it was delivered? Subjects may be diverse: conflict management, change management, building self-confidence, leadership influence, professional speaking skills, or veterinary-specific skills related to case management.

With professional development comes self-perceived barriers. Often, leaders and team members are afraid of reaching out and asking for help or advice. It is also common for people to be afraid of taking on

EXAMPLES OF ORGANIZATIONS THAT VETERINARY TEAM MEMBERS CAN GET INVOLVED WITH TO FURTHER THEIR PROFESSIONAL DEVELOPMENT

Organization	Potential Opportunities for
American Veterinary Medical Association (AVMA)	Veterinarians, Credentialed Technicians,
American Animal Hospital Association (AAHA)	Veterinarians, Practice Managers, Credentialed Technicians, Veterinary Assistants
National Association of Veterinary Technicians in America (NAVTA)	Credentialed Technicians, Veterinary Assistants
Veterinary Hospital Managers Association (VHMA)	Practice Managers
State Veterinary Medical Association	Veterinarians
State Veterinary Technician Association	Credentialed Technicians, Veterinary Assistants
Veterinary Association specific to interest such as Emergency and Critical Care, Rehabilitation, Internal Medicine, Shelter Medicine	Veterinarians, Practice Managers, Credentialed Technicians, Veterinary Assistants
Publications such as *Today's Veterinary Nurse, The NATVA Journal, DVM 360, Todays Veterinary Business, JAVMA*	Veterinarians, Practice Managers, Credentialed Technicians, Veterinary Assistants
National and Regional Conferences such as Western Veterinary Conference (WVC), VMX, Southwest Veterinary Symposia, IVECCS, Fetch, AVMA, Connexity by AAHA	Veterinarians, Practice Managers, Credentialed Technicians, Veterinary Assistants

Fig. 6.1 Volunteering in organized veterinary medicine is an excellent way to build leadership and professional development skills.

new challenges, skills, or stretching boundaries. Barriers are likely due to a lack of self-confidence or not having a mentor to help push limits. Getting outside of the comfort zone is the best way to learn! Having a mentor or a network of trusted colleagues who will challenge the status quo (the way you have always done things) encourages outside-the-box thinking while also providing motivation.

CRITICAL COMPETENCY: ADAPTABILITY

Practice managers must be open to change and flexible work methods and can adapt behavior to changing conditions or new information.

As a leader in your practice, evaluate how you can help others grow and move past their barriers. This form of "coaching" also helps develop your skills and find your next "why" in the professional development journey.

MENTORING PROGRAMS

Another area of professional development includes being an effective mentor and/or developing a mentoring program that positively impacts those being mentored. Mentor programs are especially important for new graduates, veterinarians, and credentialed technicians alike. One of the top reasons veterinarians leave their first job is the lack of or a negative mentorship program.[4,5]

The heart of mentorship is the development of a relationship that is built on mutual respect and trust between mentor and mentee. In establishing the relationship, both parties must set clear expectations and goals for each other and the outcomes they want to achieve. Ultimately, when done well, the relationship is mutually beneficial to both mentor and mentee, supporting personal and professional development for all involved.

Areas that should be focused on when developing mentor skills include influential leadership, trust, communication, emotional intelligence, psychological safety, compassion, and empathy (see Chapter 2). These are all soft skills; it matters "how" the content is delivered that will have the most positive impact on the mentee.

Developing a Mentorship Program

Developing a mentorship program that has a positive influence on the mentee starts with a plan: What is the end goal for the program? For example, if the mentor program is for a new team member, the program should be specific to the role the team member plays within the practice, yet always be tied to the goals (vision, mission, and core values; Chapter 2).

CRITICAL COMPETENCY: LEADERSHIP

Practice managers must have the initiative to lead and take charge while simultaneously motivating and mobilizing others to achieve common goals.

The components of any mentorship program must include:

- **Emotional Well-Being:** Team members need to have healthy techniques for dealing with stress, be able to maintain an appropriate work-life balance, and be able to manage debt that often contributes to increased stress.
- **The WHY:** For team members to succeed, they need to understand how what they do impacts the practice and the goals established.
- **ADL:** All training needs to encompass the Adult Learning Theory (see Chapter 4, Human Resources). Adults must read it, hear it, see it demonstrated, then do it themselves with positive coaching.
- **Transparency and Clarity:** Always be honest and provide feedback in the moment as much as possible. Often, people don't recall that they showed an undesirable behavior when called on it later.
- **Timelines:** Create timelines for the mentees to learn each skill, followed by when the new employee is expected to master said skill.
- **Scheduled Check-Ins:** Mentors should establish check-in points with mentees and ask questions like "How do you feel about XX skill? What would you rate your confidence level of this skill on a scale of 1 to 5?" While this is more on the side of soft skills, it is critical to show empathy and compassion and have confidence in the mentee.
- **Always ensure physiological safety** (Chapter 2).
- **Coaching**. Treat every opportunity as a coaching moment; "coach up" mentees to be the best they can be.
- **Mistakes happen!** Coaching allows for mistakes; allow them to happen and make it safe for them to happen. People learn from mistakes and will make mistakes as they learn new skills; that's OK! Have double checks in place so that the mistake does not impact the customer/patient in some way.
- **Develop a team-driven support network**. The more team support the mentees receive, the quicker they develop, resulting in a robust program.

The length and intensity of the program depend on the team member being mentored. New graduates will need to be mentored in both clinical and surgical skills for several months. Credentialed veterinary technicians/nurses (depending on previous skills) will also need to be in these areas for several months. Veterinary assistants and receptionists should have phased training programs (Chapter 4) as well as a mentorship program that results in team member loyalty to the practice.

SELF-MARKETING

There are many professional development opportunities for veterinary team members in the practices, but you or other team members may be ready to spread your wings and try something new. That is when it is time to create a personal marketing plan, develop a resume, and prepare for interviews!

When career changes are needed, it can be overwhelming to start the process of looking for new employment. Self-confidence may falter, and suddenly the skills that once seemed so strong may now seem useless. It is common to feel this way, but it is easy to turn that mindset around. The skills that one has acquired over the years are essential for survival. Skills such as interpersonal and verbal communication, critical thinking, writing, and leadership are all valuable resources for any employer. In addition to these essential skills, self-discipline, excellent morals, outstanding ethics, and creativity are skills that should be reflected on to help rebuild confidence. Consider the value of the following soft skills to help build confidence when developing a self-marketing plan.

LEADERSHIP POINT

Bragging about oneself can be extremely uncomfortable for some. Practice bragging about yourself with a trusted colleague or friend that will help you attain a position at your desired employer.

"Team players" excel quicker than those who choose to work as "individuals." This does not mean that people must depend on a team to succeed, but it shows that they have been successful in adjusting to a team environment as well as sharing and empowering responsibilities effectively.

Positive attitudes are contagious, and those with positive attitudes excel faster than those with toxic negativity. People prefer to be around happy, energetic, and enthusiastic individuals as they tend to be creative problem solvers and contribute to a team environment.

A strong work ethic is an excellent attribute to possess. A team member with a strong work ethic strives for the best and excels at finding tasks to complete. These tasks are then completed quickly and efficiently with excellent and consistent results. A strong work ethic cannot be taught; it is a trait that one either possesses or does not. Team members exhibiting a strong work ethic should be selected for higher-level positions, more responsibility, and, ultimately, promotions.

Education is the key to professional development. College courses enhance current skills, develop new skills, and teach independence. Continuing education is required of credentialed veterinary technicians, veterinarians, and certified veterinary practice managers to help maintain the skills obtained, while also learning new techniques. Science, medicine, and laws continually change, and it is imperative to stay current with the latest information, up-and-coming trends, and updated treatment protocols. Further, education stimulates innovative thinking, critical thinking, and problem solving.

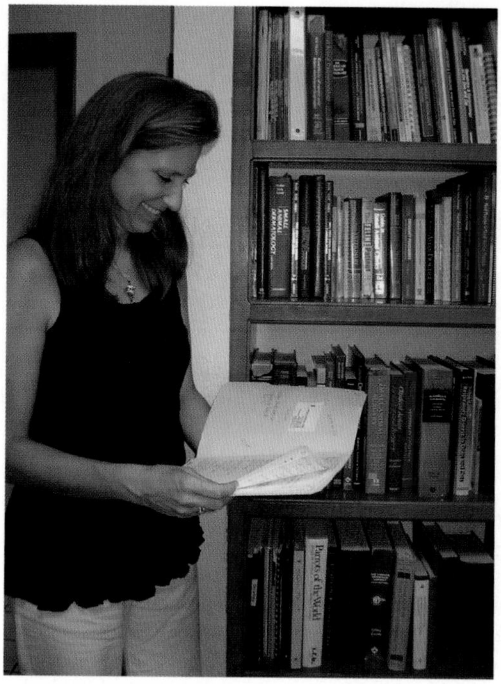

Fig. 6.2 A professional appearance is a marketing tool that projects quality.

CRITICAL COMPETENCY: RESILIENCE

Practice managers must have the ability to cope effectively with pressure and setbacks. Additionally, PMs must be able to handle crisis situations effectively and remain undeterred by obstacles or failure.

Marketing Skills

All the previously mentioned skills help individuals market themselves while they look for employment. Team environments look for positively motivated individuals to join their staff. Self-confidence and a positive personality must be demonstrated through action words in a resume, securing an interview for the applicant.

Marketing oneself starts with personal interactions within a profession or within the industry being considered. Individuals must present themselves professionally and confidently while they explore employment opportunities (Fig. 6.2). Many benign conversations lead to interviews for a successful networker. Maintaining contact with associates, sales representatives, vendors, and colleagues in all areas within the profession pays off with employment opportunities.

Team members must have personal goals as well as employment goals. It is important to not forget oneself and work-life balance when looking for new employment opportunities. Dedicated and hardworking team members must actively take vacation and personal time off (PTO) on a regular basis.

DEVELOPING A PROFESSIONAL RESUME

Frequently, the first impression an applicant makes on a potential employer is by the quality of the resume submitted. Care must be taken to develop a professional resume conveying positive attributes and a strong work ethic. Hiring managers are looking for team members who "fit" their culture. Therefore, resumes are used to not only highlight where and when you worked but why you would be a fit in this new role.

A resume is a marketing tool tailored to the specific job in which the applicant is interested. The goal of a resume is to be granted an interview. As a rule, resumes should be concise and limited to one or two pages in length, and abbreviations and acronyms should be avoided. Formatting matters when presenting concise information that attracts the reader. The font must be easy to read; consider soft fonts like Arial, Calibri, or Century Gothic. The font should not be smaller than 10.5 point or larger than 12-point size, and margins should remain at 1 inch on all sides.

When creating or updating a resume, consider the following questions:

- What is the potential employer looking for?
- What qualifications is the employer looking for?
- What attributes are needed?

These qualifications and attributes should be emphasized in the resume.

All resumes should have contact information listed first, at the top of the first page. This includes the applicant's name, address, telephone number, and email address. An objective statement follows, which is a brief description of the position that is being applied for and how the applicant's unique skills can contribute to the position. Education may be cited next or listed last, listing schools by full name and address. Education should be arranged in reverse chronologic order, listing the most current first. Degrees should be listed, along with any majors, minors, or certifications (Fig. 6.3). When an applicant has just completed school, education is usually listed first. If the applicant has been in the profession for several years, education is often listed last.

LEADERSHIP POINT

Consider having a professional resume writer review and update your resume.

The order of experience and skills can vary in presentation on a resume. No one order is correct; the goal is simply to market the applicant in the best possible manner. Reverse chronologic order lists employment history starting with the most current position held. Skills-based resumes may be used when changing careers; education and work history are minimized, whereas the skills used to accomplish tasks are embellished. This may be of benefit when trying to match the target

GUIDELINES TO BUILDING AN EFFECTIVE RESUME

- Avoid lengthy job descriptions or descriptions of nontransferable job duties.
- Be consistent. Use the same format throughout the resume.
- Use headings that allow the reader to find needed information quickly.
- Construct a resume using action verbs, adjectives, and key words that describe skills.
- Describe accomplishments quantitatively where appropriate; emphasize qualities and experience.
- Leave off unrelated personal information (age, weight, height) and photographs.
- Only make statements that can be backed up with examples or proof.
- Avoid using the word "I".
- Only include salary information (from previous work experience) if requested.
- Limit the number of graphics and length. One page should be sufficient unless extensive professional experience is included.
- Ensure the resume typed, single sided, and free of spelling, grammatical, and typographical errors.
- For printing, select resume paper that is light in color and has a plain background; print using a laser jet or very clear inkjet printer.
- Save resume document as a PDF prior to submitting via email or company portals.

Fig. 6.3 Organized and professional resumes attract potential employers.

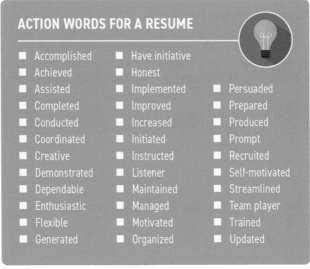

ACTION WORDS FOR A RESUME

- Accomplished
- Achieved
- Assisted
- Completed
- Conducted
- Coordinated
- Creative
- Demonstrated
- Dependable
- Enthusiastic
- Flexible
- Generated
- Have initiative
- Honest
- Implemented
- Improved
- Increased
- Initiated
- Instructed
- Listener
- Maintained
- Managed
- Motivated
- Organized
- Persuaded
- Prepared
- Produced
- Prompt
- Recruited
- Self-motivated
- Streamlined
- Team player
- Trained
- Updated

Fig. 6.4 Use action words in resumes to attract attention to demonstrated behaviors and achievements.

skills to the position available. Mixed resumes offer a combination of both chronologic and skills-based resumes, focusing on individual skills.

Employment history includes the name and location of the employer, employment dates, and a summary highlighting responsibilities and accomplishments using action words (Fig. 6.4).

Volunteer experiences are listed after employment history, especially if volunteering was a large part of a previous employment period. Previous volunteer experience may also be vital to the skills targeted for the open position. Just as for employment history, the name and location of the organization should be listed along with volunteer dates in chronological order. A brief description of duties should be included as well.

Membership organizations should be listed after volunteer experiences, especially if a leadership position has been held. A brief description of roles, responsibilities, and highlights should be documented.

Reference lists are no longer necessary. Instead, add an annotation at the end of the resume that "resources are available upon request." Then make sure that sheet (saved as a PDF) is readily available when asked.

If several jobs have been held with some relating to career goals and some not, rather than using a reverse chronological order, use the heading "related experience" as a section header that highlights all career-related jobs (that are applicable to the position in which is being applied for). Other jobs can then be listed under the heading "supportive experience" where descriptions of those experiences can be highlighted.

A trusted friend or professional should meticulously proofread the resume. The writer is bound to make typographical errors that will be overlooked or not caught by spellcheck; a fresh set of eyes will pick up the errors before the target reader does (who will then form a negative perception regarding the professionalism of the applicant). A good friend will also scrutinize the information and offer tips for improvement. If a good friend is not available for review, a local college is sure to have excellent resources and staff available for such tasks.

LEADERSHIP POINT

Write a cover letter when submitting a resume that highlights your skills and why you would be a good fit for the role. This is a great place to highlight soft skills (leadership, values, work ethic) that may get lost in the bullet points of a resume.

Many companies prefer accepting resumes online either by submission through a company portal or by email. It is important to know that applications can change the configuration of resumes that are created in a Word document. Therefore, always save the resume as a PDF file, allowing it to be viewed exactly as it was created.

PREPARING FOR AN INTERVIEW

Depending on the type of company and position, wearing business casual attire or a suit may be appropriate. For example, when interviewing for a role as a manufacturing representative, a suit may be more appropriate, whereas business casual apparel would be appropriate for a veterinary healthcare team member. Hair should be well groomed and professional looking. Appearances make a critical impression that can last forever; it is imperative to dress appropriately. If there is any question, always dress a step above what might be expected.

Preparing for an interview is like completing homework for a college course; one must present homework in a professional and logical manner (Fig. 6.5). Preparing for an interview allows for a professional, calm, and personal interview. Preparation includes rehearsing frequent questions that will be asked, as well as knowing about the practice/company and services provided (Fig. 6.6).

Applicants should expect to answer questions about previous employment, gaps in employment history, or frequent changes in jobs. Skills, aptitudes, and responsibilities should be thought about when prepping for the interview.

Common Interview Questions

"What are your long-term goals?" A potential employer wants to know what the goals of the applicant will be. Where would this potential employee like to be in 1 year, 5 years, or 10 years? Will they benefit the company in the long term? On a personal level, the applicant must determine goals, understand that goals can change, and be willing to accept challenges that come along the way.

"How are you going to achieve your goals?" Additional schooling, employment opportunities, or volunteering experiences may help achieve goals and dreams. A particular job may provide an opportunity to fulfill a dream or goal the applicant has; if so, it is important to take the right steps to obtain that goal.

"What are your strengths and weaknesses?" It is advantageous to determine one's strengths and weaknesses. This question will likely be asked in an interview, and the potential employer will appreciate a well-thought-out answer. In many cases, a veterinary team member's greatest weakness is the inability to say no. They take on too many projects, become overwhelmed, and perhaps do not complete any of them on time or above the expected level. A great asset may be leadership and influence. A great team member that builds relationships and achieves goals has a superpower that is highly desirable. A great employee may talk a lot, but clients love team members who are social, listen, and reply with valuable knowledge.

"What type of benefits or salary are you looking for?" Benefits and salary are generally decisive factors when determining employment, so full thought and consideration should be given to this topic before an interview. The topic may or may not evolve during the interview process; it will, however, evolve by the time an offer of employment is made. Veterinarians, veterinary technicians, and practice managers can refer to the Veterinary Hospital Medical Association, American Animal Hospital Association, or Well Managed Practice Benchmarks for standards of pay in the region in which they reside or will potentially reside. Other considerations are benefits that are available to team members. Many times, benefits packages far outweigh salary, and consideration must be given to both. See Chapter 4 for benefits that are usually offered and Fig. 6.6 for more common interview questions.

Applicants should learn about the business to which they are applying. Mission statements, values, and services offered can often be gained

INTERVIEW GUIDELINES

- Ask questions.
- Safe the salary discussion for last. Learn about the job first and share why your knowledge and skills can fill that role.
- Show enthusiasm, dress professionally, and make eye contact.
- Do not talk excessively or appear too aggressive; use proper grammar.
- Do not chew gum.

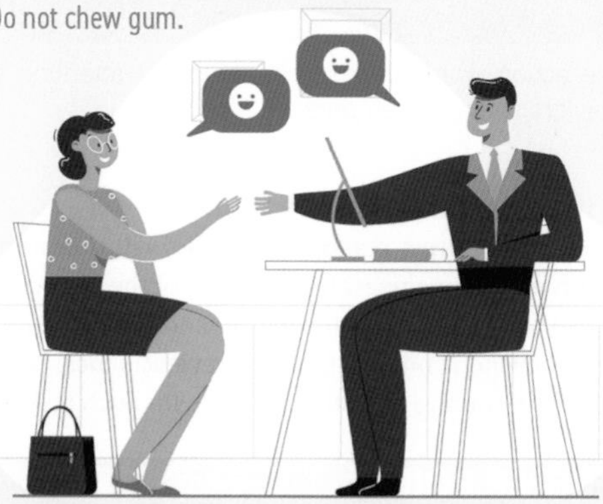

Fig. 6.5 Interviews are a two-way street; candidates should ask the potential employer questions to help identify if this is the "right fit."

COMMON INTERVIEW QUESTIONS

- Are you currently employed?
- Describe yourself.
- How did you learn about this profession?
- What are your goals? Five years from now? Ten years from now?
- What can you bring to our team?
- What formal education have you received?
- What is your ideal job?
- What is your strongest asset?
- What is your weakest asset?
- What responsibilities have you enjoyed the least at your previous jobs, and why?
- What responsibilities have you enjoyed the most at your previous jobs, and why?
- What salary do you expect?
- Why are you interested in this company?
- Why do you feel you are qualified for this position?
- Why do you wish to change jobs?
- Why should our company hire you?

QUESTIONS TO ASK POTENTIAL EMPLOYERS

- Tell me about your open-door policy regarding communications, problem solving, and personnel issues?
- Share with me how you value your team members.
- How many team members are employed?
- What are short-term goals for this practice/company?
- What are the long-term goals of this practice/company?
- What benefits are generally offered with this position?
- What do you feel is the biggest strength of this practice/company?
- What is the staff turnover rate?
- What do you feel is the weakest attribute of this company

Fig. 6.6 Being prepared with questions that a potential employee may be asked, or that can be asked of a potential employer demonstrates confidence and improves the flow of the interview.

from company websites. If the applicant knows any current employees of the company, questions may be asked in advance about company policies, benefits, opportunities, and incentives. Social media posts are also a great way to see how the company interacts with clients and consumers. You want to know that the employer will be a good fit for you, as much as the hiring manager wants to know you will be a good fit for them.

LEADERSHIP POINT

Do your homework before any interview. Know about the company you are applying for a position with, practice your interview in the mirror (what does your body language say?), and practice your answers to the most common interview questions.

Interviews should be a two-way street, in which the applicant prepares relevant questions for the potential employer (Fig. 6.6). There is no need to waste the applicant and employer's time if their values and goals do not match. A small notebook can be taken to the interview to remind the applicant of questions and to make notes from the interview. If the interview is successful, the next step might be asking to meet the staff, interviewing with the direct position manager, or observing the practice for a day (if applicable). Evaluating the working environment can be extremely helpful for the applicant to know if "this is the right fit."

Always arrive early for an interview. Latecomers are automatically assessed a penalty. Lateness may indicate a work pattern of the employee and shows a lack of respect for the time of the employer. If you can't make the interview, always let the hiring manager know. The veterinary community is small and word travels fast! Be pleasant with everyone in the veterinary practice; you are being evaluated by the entire team as to whether you will be a great fit.

Ask to mingle with the team after the initial interview. Observe the team member's interactions with one another; are they pleasant and respectful, and do they communicate well? Ask why they like working there, and what their favorite attribute of the practice is.

There are a few common mistakes individuals may make when interviewing. Being prepared is the key.

Not fully answering an interview question. It's OK to not know an answer, but don't simply leave it at that. Part of interviewing well is showing the ability to think on demand. A great response starts with *"that is a great question that I do not know the answer to, however…"* then share the thought process and how one would find out the information or resolve the situation.

Failing to share what you bring to the hospital. A good interviewer will ask how the applicant will contribute to their team. Be prepared to share passions, skills, and knowledge that have been acquired through past work experiences. If the question was not asked during the interview, bring up those passions and skills before the conversation closes.

Trying to be someone you're not. Be genuine, professional, and courteous throughout the interview. But if the interview reveals this is not the "right fit," say that. It is better to wait for the right job, because "faking it till you make it" is not a long-term strategy.

Follow-Up After an Interview

A follow-up letter or thank-you note should always be sent 1 or 2 days after the interview, reiterating the interest in the position. A letter should thank the interviewer for their time and once again highlight the qualifications of the candidate and how the applicant's assets will benefit the company. After the interview process, if the applicant chooses not to pursue an employment opportunity, a letter should be written again, thanking the interviewer for their time and stating that you have decided to pursue other options. This not only saves the employer time and money, but you may wish to seek employment with this company in the future if the chosen opportunity did not work out.

RECEIVING EMPLOYMENT OFFERS

Not every job offer received may be the "right one." Take time when evaluating potential opportunities. What feels right? After all, a career is not just about money. Consider the following tips when evaluating offers:

- Know your value. Research hourly/salary rates in the area.
- There's more to pay than salary. Consider PTO, health insurance, work-life balance, pet care benefits, CE allotment, tuition reimbursement, or retirement contributions.
- Will you have a commute? How much time will it take (coming and leaving work) and what the cost of gas (and time) be?
- Will you need to move? If yes, what is the change in the cost of living?
- Will you have an opportunity to learn and grow in this role?

It is advisable to receive any offers in writing, including the agreed-upon salary, the raise and evaluation structure, and any benefits that are offered at the time of employment. Some employees may be put on a trial period that prevents benefits from immediately being offered; the rules of the trial period should also be clearly stated in the offer.

If more than one offer has been received, all offers should be considered before making a final decision. Potential employers should be told that several offers exist for employment and that a response will be available in a stated time. Be careful not to extend this time too far out, because potential employers may hire someone else. Individuals must consider their goals: *"What kind of employer do I want?" "What kind of work environment do I want?" "What is my goal for hours and salary?"* Once most expectations have been met, a decision can be made.

RETIREMENT

Retirement should not be ignored while developing one's career. Whether an individual is entering the veterinary profession or developing a new career, retirement is important to consider. Previous generations have had Social Security to rely on. Although it does not produce a wealthy income, it at least provided money for food and shelter. Future generations may not have Social Security to depend on, so long-term strategies must be implemented.

If companies do not offer a retirement fund as a benefit, it is up to the individual to start one for him- or herself. A financial planning professional can help determine what type of account would be best. It is best to find an advisor who is willing to educate and spend time finding the correct investments for each client. Coworkers, friends, and professionals in the community may be able to offer recommendations.

It takes discipline to save money now and will be well worth it later. Many practices or companies allow funds to be deducted directly from a payroll check and deposited into a savings or retirement account, in some cases before taxes. This is helpful for enforcing a savings plan for those who lack the discipline to do so.

EMPLOYMENT OPPORTUNITIES BY ROLE

There are many opportunities in the field of veterinary medicine, both in practice and in industry, regardless of role. General and specialty practices offer very rewarding careers, with general practice seeing a variety of animals, diseases, and treatments. Specialty and referral practices specialize in specific areas such as internal medicine, surgery, dermatology, dentistry, or emergency and critical care.

Research and development can add challenges and rewards to any career by developing new products, foods, or treatments for a variety of species and diseases. In the past, medical research has had negative connotations because the media often assumes that research involves harming animals. This is not always true and exceptional research facilities offer many employment opportunities.

Veterinary manufacturers and distribution companies are always seeking qualified practice managers, credentialed and experienced technicians, and veterinarians. Some companies require a bachelor's degree for employment; it may be imperative to finish a bachelor's program if a career change is contemplated. Completing a bachelor's degree can lead to additional opportunities in management and leadership and increases in pay wages.

Teaching may also be an option for practice managers, credentialed technicians, or veterinarians. Both online programs and campus programs employ experience-based instructors to continue growing and supporting veterinary medicine.

Practice Managers

There are diverse employment opportunities available for experienced practice managers. Business skills are essential to every business, regardless of industry, just as culture and leadership are. Consider the following areas:

- A larger practice, perhaps one that has larger growth potential or a specialty practice
- Manufacturing or distribution companies
- A company that analyses vet data
- Consulting (which usually leads to writing articles and lecturing to fellow constituents)
- Teaching for a veterinary practice management program

A PM may also wish to further their credentialing by obtaining their Certification in Veterinary Practice Management (CVPM) through VHMA, a certification in Human Resources, Compassion Fatigue, or DISC/Myers Briggs personality profiles.

Practice managers can locate employment opportunities on websites at VHMA, AVMA, AAHA, NAVC, Indeed, and state veterinary medical/practice management association job boards, through word of mouth from distributor or manufacture reps, on the careers page of corporations, and at regional and national conference job boards.

Credentialed Veterinary Technicians

Management of a general or specialty practice takes time, patience, and leadership, and can be extremely rewarding. Technicians who have exceeded expectations in practice are often promoted to practice managers. Although the technician portion may have been easy to master, running an entire business is a whole new ballgame. Management skills can be acquired by attending online courses and national conferences that focus on management (as well as learning from peers) and will help even inexperienced businesspersons succeed.

Excellent technicians are often excellent educators. They have experience teaching clients as well as other team members about veterinary medicine. Those who enjoy educating others can find very rewarding careers in teaching. There is nothing more gratifying than seeing a student progress and become a distinguished individual in the veterinary profession, and those with outstanding teachers often become outstanding teachers themselves (Fig. 6.7).

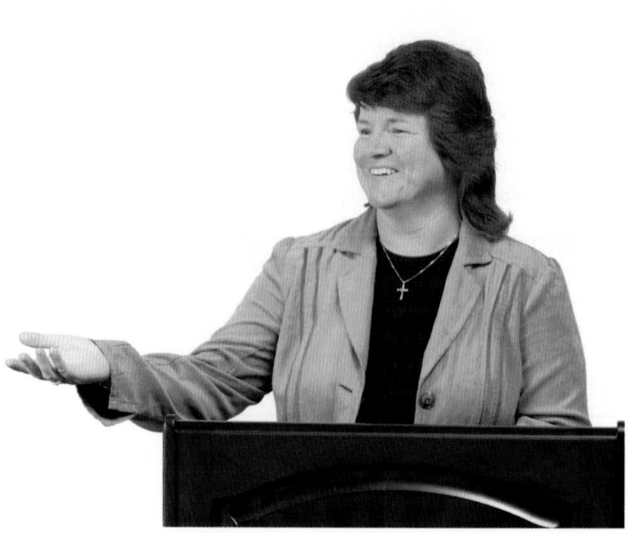

Fig. 6.7 Many veterinary professionals choose teaching as a second career. (Courtesy Kara Burns.)

Other areas of employment to consider:

- A larger practice, perhaps one that has larger growth potential, or a specialty practice
- Manufacturing or distribution companies
- Providing relief work throughout the region
- Research
- Telehealth companies

A credentialed technician may also wish to further their credentialing by obtaining their Veterinary Technician Specialist (VTS) in specific areas of interest through NAVTA (Chapter 3): Compassion Fatigue, Fear Free, rehabilitation, or pain management.

Credentialed technicians can locate employment opportunities on websites at AVMA, AAHA, NAVC, Indeed, veterinary technology programs, and state veterinary technician association job boards, through word of mouth from distributor or manufacture reps, on the careers page of corporations, and at regional and national conference job boards.

Veterinarians

DVMs have many opportunities to further their career, both in and out of practice. While in practice, veterinarians may want to choose a specialty with the American Board of Veterinary Practitioners (ABVP) and/or work in a specialty practice to refine their skills/passions.

Other areas of employment to consider:

- Manufacturing or distribution companies
- Providing relief work throughout the region
- Research
- Telehealth companies
- USDA
- Teaching in veterinary technology programs
- Speaking/writing

Professional development is up to the individual to peruse growth. Mentors can advocate for individuals, but the "want" must come from within. That "want" is usually driven by a life-long passion to continue learning. This prevents individuals from plateauing in their careers or burning themselves out of the profession. Identify boredom early. Professional development is fueled by looking for challenges that stimulate thought and passion and by "challenging the way things have always been done."

People will limit their development with perceived barriers that then turn into excuses. Both barriers and excuses can be overcome with passion, drive, and aspiring to love your career (not just a job).

EMOTIONAL WELL-BEING

Emotional well-being is a concept that must be embraced and demonstrated by leadership, as well as developing a sense of emotional wellbeing of all employees. Maslow's Hierarchy (Chapter 2, Leadership) states that team members must feel safe in physiological safety (food, shelter, and sleep), working conditions, and psychological safety before they can advance further in their careers in the practice. Compassion fatigue, burnout, and suicide must all be addressed to assure team members are in a healthy state of well-being.

CRITICAL COMPETENCY: ORAL COMMUNICATION AND COMPREHENSION

The practice manager must have the ability to express thoughts verbally in a clear and understandable manner, and the ability to actively listen and attend to what others are saying.

Compassion fatigue and *burnout* are likely the most common terms used in veterinary medicine to describe how team members are feeling, but it must be questioned if they are being used in the correct manner. If not identified and managed appropriately, compassion fatigue can lead to burnout, but the two are very different. The first step is understanding the differences by defining each term, and second, the causes of each must be explained. Third, symptoms must be understood along with knowing how to treat them. Think of it like diagnosing a condition. If you don't address all factors, then the treatment will not be successful.

In combination with personal stressors (consider the stress COVID had on team members), unmanaged compassion fatigue and burnout can exacerbate the chances of suicidal ideation. Suicide is an uncomfortable term to talk about, and often one that is whispered when it needs to be spoken. However, the veterinary industry cannot afford to whisper any longer about something that needs to be yelled.

As with any change management process in a practice, it starts with the leaders. If the leaders are involved in educating and recognizing symptoms, then their team will understand the importance and recognize symptoms as well. "It's not a problem in my/our practice" is a detrimental mindset to have. Veterinary medicine is notoriously a reactive industry. It cannot afford to be reactive regarding compassion fatigue, burnout, and suicide. It's not a problem in the practice, until it is. And then it is too late.

COMPASSION FATIGUE AND BURNOUT

Compassion fatigue (CF) is defined as the cost of caring and has an immediate impact on team members through listening to clients and helping them through their fears, pain, and suffering as they care for their pets. Two things must be present for someone to experience CF: the ability to have and show empathy, and a caregiving relationship.

A differentiating factor between burnout (BO) and compassion fatigue is that CF can only occur in a caretaking role, while BO occurs in every industry. Empathy is the ability to put oneself in another's shoes and feel what the other may feel. Depending on life experiences, the level of empathy can change from situation to situation. For instance, think of an elderly client who comes to the practice to euthanize their senior pet. They share stories about adopting the pet with their significant other who recently passed away. This pet may be a last reminder of that person. The listener then begins to experience empathy for this client. Some professionals find themselves experiencing higher levels of empathy when certain breeds are present that remind them of their own pets (current or past).

Discussing what CF *is* is just as important as discussing what it is *not*. CF gets confused with BO, and although they have similar symptoms, they are very different.

- Compassion fatigue has a shorter onset and can occur from just one incident. Burnout occurs slowly, over time.
- Because of the longer onset, burnout takes longer to resolve and sometimes cannot be resolved until the employee leaves the place of employment. CF can often be resolved by taking some time away from the caretaking role (i.e., vacation).
- Burnout can be defined as an overall decrease in job satisfaction.
- CF is not the absence of compassion; it is the fatigue felt because of the immense compassion veterinary professionals provide daily.

Why CF Is Important

The impact CF has on both personal and professional elements is profound. Many publications speak to CF being contagious, and this is apparent when one considers the impact CF can have on people in their personal life. The impact of being a caregiver does not end after a work shift. Emotional stress spans the personal decisions that are made outside of work, causing professionals to distance themselves from friends, family events, and significant others. Emotional stress can cause a rift in the most important part of managing CF, which is having a connection to others. Connection is the "C" in the "ABCs" of anticipating and managing CF. This topic, along with a 75-year Harvard study, will be discussed further in the Managing section.

Within the practice, CF has a cyclical impact on staff, patients, and clients. Although it is not always a causal relationship, Fig. 6.8 shows the impact when staff experience CF and do not manage it effectively. When left unmanaged, CF ultimately impacts patients (medical errors) and client satisfaction.

Adverse and sentinel events occur most frequently in practices/departments that have unmanaged CF and BO. A decrease in communication and team member happiness impacts clients, causing them to seek alternative care for their pets. In summary, CF impacts every aspect of the business. It can be the ultimate reason why staff leave the practice. Team members may move to other practices because they are running away from the effects of CF but are unaware of what to call it. They soon realize that what they were running away from is being experienced again in the new practice, resulting in them ultimately leaving the profession.

Causes of Compassion Fatigue

In the book *Compassion Fatigue in the Animal Care Community*, Charles Figley shares a study that was conducted by the American Society for the Prevention of Cruelty to Animals (ASPCA) that surveyed thousands of veterinary professionals asking what the top stressors were in practice. Veterinarians' responses included difficult or noncompliant clients, not having enough time with clients, and discussing or disputing fees with clients. Veterinary support staff agreed the number one stressor is difficult or noncompliant clients, followed by difficult team members and not having enough time to complete duties and client relations.

It is important to note that the above stressors are part of the daily situations that all veterinary professionals experience. These stressors

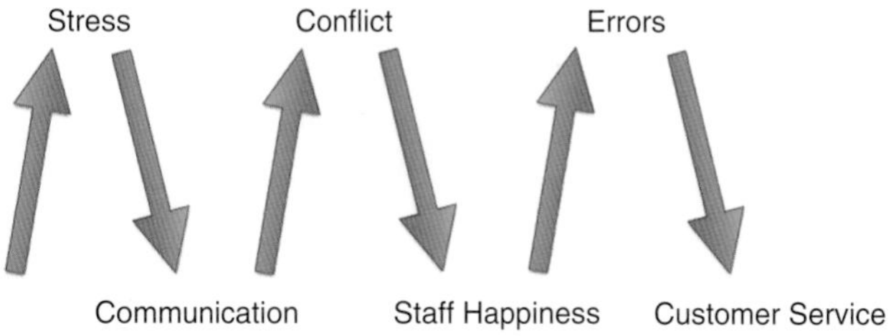

Fig. 6.8 Compassion fatigue has a cyclical impact on staff, patients, and clients.

aren't likely to go away, which emphasizes the importance of providing all staff members with the necessary tools to "anticipate and manage" their stress.

Although these stressors are not always the direct cause of CF, they increase a team member's susceptibility. As stress increases, the ability to think through the cause of stress and manage it significantly decreases. Other common stressors include:

- Overall demands of the job
- Lack of clarity about responsibilities
- Management/ownership pressures
- Lack of work-life balance

Many of these stressors can be reduced with a good leadership team that creates a culture of support, clear communication regarding the goals of the practice and of each team member, and monitoring of the work-life balance of team members (Chapter 2, Leadership).

Symptoms

CF manifests very similarly to BO. In both situations, individuals can experience symptoms in one or more of the following categories: cognitive, emotional, behavioral, spiritual, interpersonal, or physical. Understanding these categories and being aware of the symptoms caused by CF or BO is part of the "A" in the ABCs, Awareness.

It is important to note, some of these symptoms can also be a part of someone's general personality, thus "normal" for that person. For instance, someone could be a naturally forgetful person. This does not mean that they are necessarily experiencing CF/BO (Fig. 6.9) However, if there is a sudden onset or change in these symptoms, leadership should consider a coaching conversation with that team member.

Anticipating and Managing Compassion Fatigue and Burnout

Because CF and BO may be unavoidable, the best approach is to anticipate and manage the symptoms. The goal is to practice the ABCs to the point that one can predict and manage the impact that the stressors will have on them. The ABCs are designed to empower the veterinary professional to take charge of their own job satisfaction. The "A" represents awareness, the starting point of any change process. The "B" represents work-life balance, and arguably the most important is "C," which stands for connection.

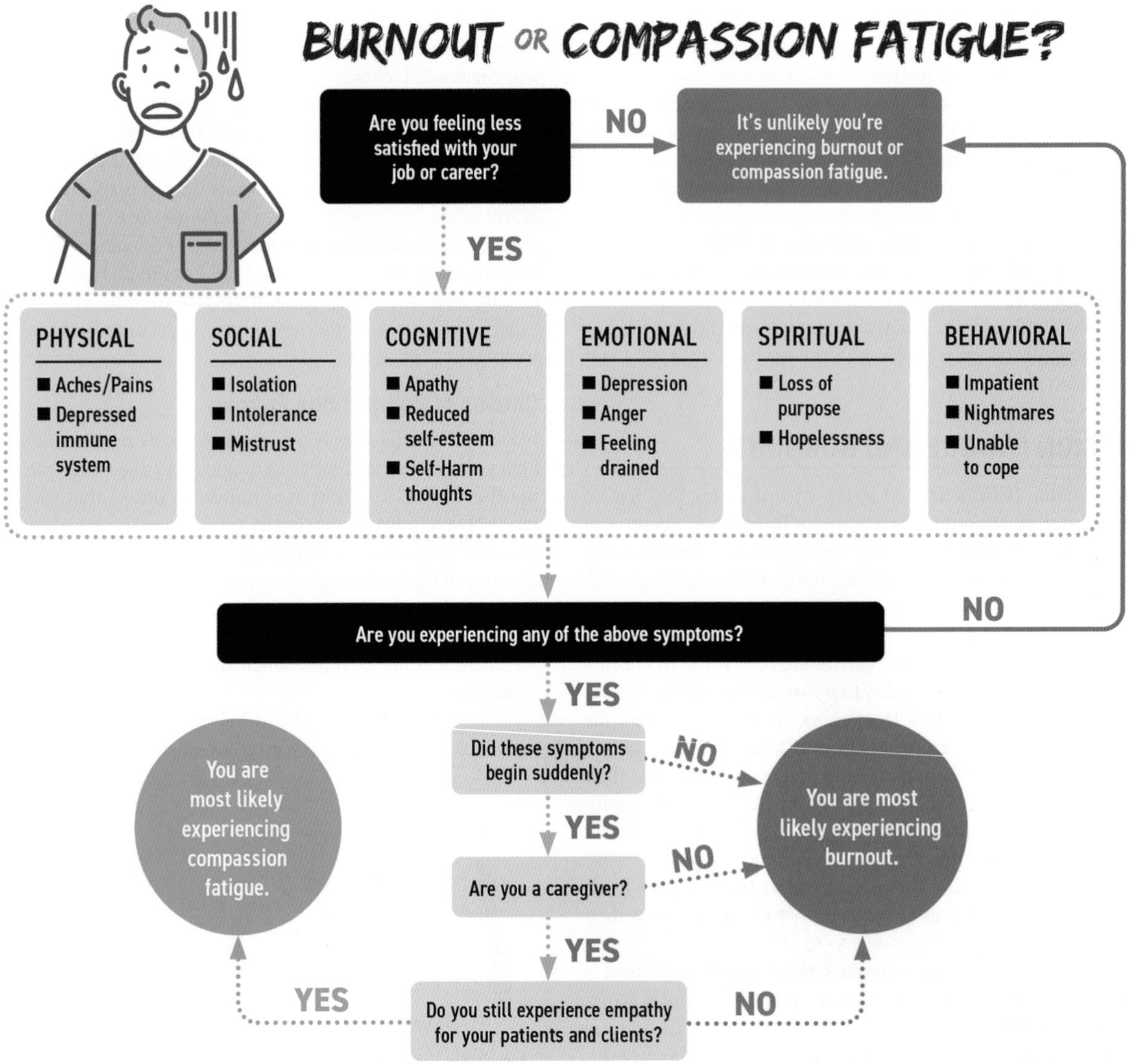

Fig. 6.9 The ABCs of Avoiding Compassion Fatigue.

Awareness

Practicing awareness is the first step after understanding what needs to change, and that awareness increases in steps. The first step is looking back at past events that caused CF/BO that may have been caused by interactions with certain clients, patients, breeds, or life stages. After reflecting on the past, the second step is to look at current situations that could, or are currently, causing symptoms. Practicing step two will ultimately allow transition to step three, increased awareness so that the effects of CF/BO can be predicted. The following questions can be asked to start the process:

- "What are my CF triggers?"
- "How does my BO manifest itself?"
- "Have my feelings changed about my career choice?"

Successfully achieving improved awareness comes together with increasing personal ownership, emotional intelligence, and control of the response.

There are events that occur in everyday life that are beyond one's control. How one responds dictates the outcome. Therefore, if the outcome is not desirable, one can change their response to result in an improved outcome.

Emotional intelligence is one's awareness of their emotions, communication, and impact on others. Someone who can stop a conversation, address a nonverbal response from another person, and prevent the conversation from turning into a conflict is practicing an elevated level of awareness and emotional intelligence (Chapter 2).

Balance

Work-life balance is an elusive goal for many veterinary professionals. One of the biggest pitfalls is feeling pressured to establish an equilibrium between the two. A second pitfall is assuming that the definition is the same for everyone. There are many factors that play into someone's definition of work-life balance: personal demands (children, family, etc.), extracurricular activities, professional demands, personal expectations, and generational differences. The current generations present in the workplace have different definitions of what work-life balance means to them. This highlights the need to not look at a standard definition of work-life balance, but rather to meet the needs of each individual team member (Fig. 6.10).

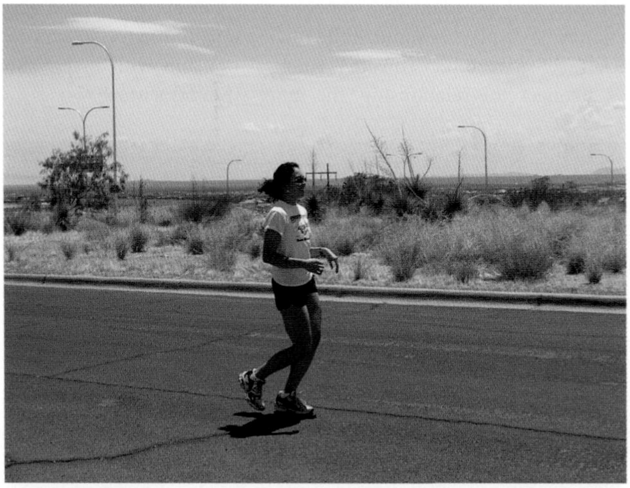

Fig. 6.10 Exercise can alleviate stress and create equilibrium in the work-life balance.

Setting Boundaries

The essence of setting boundaries is individual. What does work-life balance mean to each team member? Will work always be heavier than life? If so, how does one increase the quality of time spent experiencing life? Set goals, practice emotional intelligence, set boundaries, and respect the definition of others to manage CF and BO.

Setting boundaries can be uncomfortable but an essential step for all veterinary professionals. Consider the following questions when setting boundaries:

- "Have you put unrealistic expectations on yourself?"
- "What boundaries can be drawn (even if it's just once a month) that will improve job satisfaction?"
- "Will the boundaries affect your ability to complete job responsibilities?" If you are not sure, you should discuss it with your supervisor before setting it.
- "What impact will this boundary have on others?"

Measuring Compassion Fatigue and Burnout

The most popular quantitative assessment that has been normalized in many caretaking industries is the Professional Quality of Life (ProQOL5). This assessment measures the following:

- Compassion satisfaction: The pleasure derived from the ability to do work well. The higher the compassion satisfaction, the lower the compassion fatigue.
- Burnout: Feelings of hopelessness and difficulties in dealing with work or in doing the job effectively.

A newer assessment is the Veterinary Employee Wellness Assessment, created by Brandon Hess, CVPM, CCFP, with the guidance of a PsyD-level clinician. This assessment is tailored to the veterinary industry but has not been normalized to the extent of the ProQOL. It quantifies both burnout and compassion fatigue and can be found at https://www.vetsupport.com/compassion-fatigue/. The ability to quantify the CF/BO is a great way to measure change over time. Consider assessments a diagnostic tool, much like bloodwork. By having an idea of where one started, one can measure progress.

Connectivity

Harvard's Grant and Glueck[6] study highlights the importance of connection to others. During this 75-year study, Harvard studied two groups of individuals: one from a low-income area of Boston, and another of Harvard graduates from upper-income backgrounds. Annually, the study researched the happiness of each participant and what correlation could be drawn to that level of happiness, physical and mental health, and the success of their personal lives. The study found that participants that lived the longest with the most fulfilling lives were not those with the most money or successful careers, but rather those with the strongest (quality, not quantity) relationships.

Professional relationships are driven by practice culture, and the value that the leadership team puts on developing them. The following factors influence both practice culture and team member connection:

- Leadership's mindset, emotional intelligence, and vulnerability
- Trust among the staff
- Communication and conflict resolution
- Team meetings: how often they occur and how effective they are
- Practice accountability: the goal is not only for accountability to be driven by the leadership team but also for the team to hold each other accountable
- Level of understanding regarding each other's personality and communication style

LEADERSHIP POINT

Practice managers should have a strong enough relationship with team members to identify abnormal behaviors, have confidence to approach the subject tenderly, and listen to the team member's responses (verbally and nonverbally).

When someone is experiencing high levels of CF and/or burnout, people tend to disengage with each other and stay in their comfort zone at home. Getting out and connecting with others is a way to manage CF and BO. Encourage team members to connect with others by organizing team activities, sending them to local/regional/national conferences, having cross-departmental meetings, and/or encouraging them to have an accountability partner. The idea of an accountability partner is that there is someone within the practice (ideally) who they trust and who will hold them accountable when needed. An accountability partner might be able to say, "Matt, I can tell you are a little off today, is everything OK?" or "Matt, you're being a little bit abrasive today, is everything OK?" Matt's accountability partner would be coming from a good place, and Matt would know this. They would be responsible for bringing things to one another's attention that otherwise may not be addressed.

Suicide Awareness

This is not a topic that the veterinary industry can afford to be reactive about any longer. Proactive steps must be taken to educate team members. By making education a priority and putting tools in place, practices can have a positive impact on the suicide rate in the industry.

Suicide rates in veterinary medicine are one of the highest in any caretaking industry (Fig. 6.11). However, 80% to 90% of people who seek treatment for depression are treated successfully.[7]

There are unique stressors within veterinary medicine that do not occur within other industries that contribute to the high rate. Debt-to-income ratios, euthanasia, ethical dilemmas, lack of work-life balance, compassion fatigue, perfectionism, and easy access to drugs are a few stressors that contribute to the high rate.

Although some of these stressors occur in other healthcare industries, euthanasia and the level of ethical dilemmas are unique. Compound these with personal stressors and the stigma that accompanies seeking help, and an understanding of "why" begins to emerge. Two predicting factors of suicide are mental disorders and substance abuse, both at staggering rates in the veterinary industry (Fig. 6.12).

Resources

To help the team overcome the stigma of asking for help, ensure resources are available that don't have to be "asked for." A one-page PDF can be posted in the break room and restroom with local and national suicide hotlines, veterinary-specific hotlines, and numbers for the Employee Assistance Program (EAP). EAPs are a cost-effective benefit to provide team members with resources that work through personal problems and/or work-related issues that may impact their job performance, health, and mental and emotional well-being. Some practices may already have EPAs placed through company-provided health insurance plans, disability insurance carriers, or payroll companies.

When there is concern over an individual who is feared of contemplating suicide, there are some common misconceptions:

- "Offering support or concern will increase the chance of a suicide attempt." Many people considering suicide are needing/hoping for others to show concern for them. If you are seeing warning signs, it may be someone reaching out for help. Offering concern does not increase the chance of suicide.
- "There are always warning signs." This is not the case. If someone wants to hide suicidal thoughts or plans, they will. Through interviews with those who have lost a loved one to suicide, many said they firmly believe there were no warning signs. Often, the only time signs become present is in hindsight, post suicide.
- "Suicide is a selfish decision." The Canadian Mental Health Association defines the suicidal state of mind as "constricted, filled with a sense of self-hatred, rejection and hopelessness." Most people considering suicide feel as if they are a burden on their friends and family.

Warning Signs

Every suicide attempt is unique. There are, however, some consistent signs that could be a precursor to suicidal ideations. The following is a list of behaviors that the National Suicide Prevention Lifeline suggests being aware of:

- Increased, or sudden, substance use/abuse
- Controlled substances missing on shift
- Talking about wanting to die or kill oneself
- Asking about ways to kill oneself or searching for resources to do so
- Talking about feeling trapped, in unbearable pain, or being a burden to others
- Behaving recklessly
- Sudden attendance and/or performance issues or changes in behavior and/or emotions (mood swings)

Approaching Difficult Conversations

Perhaps you have identified someone that you are concerned about that may be displaying some of the suicide warning signs. To approach such a sensitive topic, consider your relationship with that person. The stronger the relationship, the more straightforward you can be

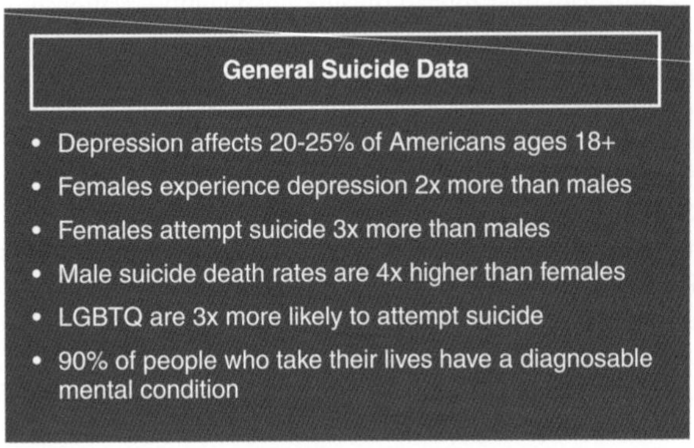
General Suicide Data
• Depression affects 20-25% of Americans ages 18+
• Females experience depression 2x more than males
• Females attempt suicide 3x more than males
• Male suicide death rates are 4x higher than females
• LGBTQ are 3x more likely to attempt suicide
• 90% of people who take their lives have a diagnosable mental condition

Fig. 6.11 Suicide levels are high in veterinary medicine. (Courtesy Brandon Hess, CVPM, CCFP.)

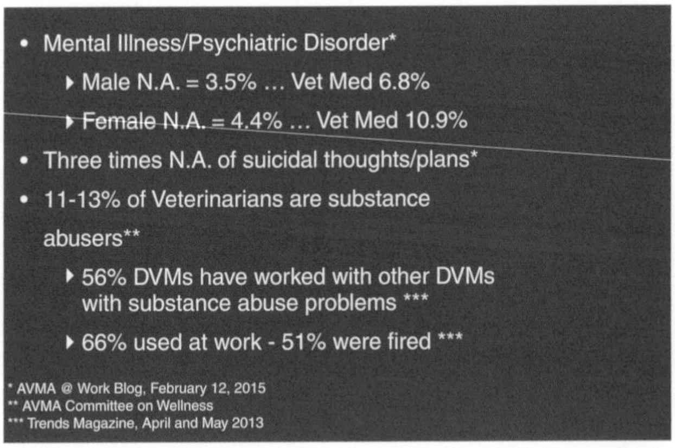
• Mental Illness/Psychiatric Disorder*
▸ Male N.A. = 3.5% ... Vet Med 6.8%
▸ Female N.A. = 4.4% ... Vet Med 10.9%
• Three times N.A. of suicidal thoughts/plans*
• 11-13% of Veterinarians are substance abusers**
▸ 56% DVMs have worked with other DVMs with substance abuse problems ***
▸ 66% used at work - 51% were fired ***
* AVMA @ Work Blog, February 12, 2015
** AVMA Committee on Wellness
*** Trends Magazine, April and May 2013

Fig. 6.12 Mental health disorders and substance abuse are predicting factors of suicide. (Courtesy Brandon Hess, CVPM, CCFP.)

ASK	"I've noticed you have been a little off lately, is everything ok?" Don't accept "yup" as an answer if you know something is wrong.
LISTEN	Do not compare things you are going, or have gone, through to what they are. They need a listening ear, not a competing voice.
EMPATHY	Regardless of their reasons, try to understand. By being judgmental you will only create a barrier between you and them.
REASSURE	Tell them they are important, and loved. Reassure them that you are there to support them. NOTE: This does not mean you have to be the solution!
SUPPORT	As noted above, you do not have to be the solution, and in fact should not be. Let them know that you would like to help them find professional support.
FOLLOW-THROUGH	Check in on them. If you say you will call, or meet with them, make sure to do it!

Fig. 6.13 Steps used to approach someone you may have a concern about.

If you are concerned about someone or know someone who is concerned about the well-being of another, please share the following resources with them:

- National Suicide Hotline: 1-800-273-8255
- National Crisis Text Hotline: Text 741741 anywhere in the United States

with your wording and questions. Fig. 6.13 demonstrates the steps of approaching someone you are concerned about.

Suicide is not a comfortable subject to talk about, but by being proactive through education, practices can have a positive impact on the suicide rates in veterinary medicine. Should a suicide affect your practice, reach out to a counselor to help support the team and yourself.

LEADERSHIP'S ROLE IN PROFESSIONAL DEVELOPMENT

A primary responsibility of the practice manager and owner in professional development is to coach and grow team members to be the best they can be, develop a sense of purpose and pride in the veterinary practice, and empower them to take emotional ownership of the veterinary hospital. Professional development is a lifelong process and stimulates enthusiasm when a plan is created. Additionally, leadership must ensure the emotional well-being of team members is a top priority in the practice. While exceptional practice culture, empowerment, and sense of purpose (Chapter 2) decrease compassion fatigue and burnout, leaders must stay astute for behavioral changes in team members that may indicate something more severe is occurring. Great leaders care and have courageous conversations with team members to grow and positively challenge them, while also caring about their personal well-being.

The author would like to recognize Brandon Hess, CVPM for his contribution to the above content.

PRACTICE MANAGER SURVIVAL CHECKLIST FOR PROFESSIONAL DEVELOPMENT

- ☐ Develop mentor programs for all positions.
- ☐ Hep team members find challenging opportunities. Coach others to greatness, even if they take their talents elsewhere. They will be back!
- ☐ Develop a resume and update it biannually.
- ☐ Continuously seek education to improve self and prevent burnout.
- ☐ Always represent professionally; hidden opportunities are always lurking.
- ☐ Post a suicide helpline PDF as a resource for team members.
- ☐ Develop practice education that embodies compassion fatigue, burnout, emotional balance, and recognition of suicide warning signs.

REVIEW QUESTIONS

1. What is the difference between CF and burnout?
2. What causes CF and burnout?
3. Which has a rapid onset? CF or burnout?
4. Why should one prepare for an interview?
5. When would one use a skills-based resume?
6. Why should one ask potential employers questions?
7. How should one dress for an interview?
8. Why is professional development important to maintain?
9. What is the purpose of a follow-up letter?
10. Prepare a chronologic resume.
11. What is the "A" in the ABCs of care?
    a. Acknowledgement
    b. Acceptance
    c. Awareness
    d. Avoidance

12. In the ASCPA stress study, which was NOT a stressor listed commonly by veterinarians?
    a. Difficult or noncompliant clients
    b. Difficult staff members
    c. Not enough time
    d. Discussing/disputing fees
13. Marketing oneself starts with:
    a. Cover letters
    b. Resumes
    c. Benign conversations
    d. Interviews
14. Cover letters are:
    a. Required
    b. Recommended
    c. Not needed
15. A successful interview encompasses all of the following except:
    a. Interviewing the potential employer
    b. Interviewing the potential candidate
    c. Answering questions with confidence
    d. Arriving to the interview late

REFERENCES

1. Fukami C., et al. Understanding the impact of organizational culture in veterinary practice [white paper]. Accessed August 2022. https://specialtyvets.com/wp-content/uploads/2017/05/Jensen-AAHA-Paper-Org-Culture-reference-info.pdf
2. National Association of Veterinary Technicians in America. NAVTA 2016 Demographic Survey Results. Accessed April 2019. https://navta.site-ym.com/page/Demographic_Survey?
3. Zunz A. Clinic Champion: Windu Wojdak. Today's Veterinary Nurse. Summer 2022. Accessed August 2022. https://todaysveterinarynurse.com/personal-professional-development/clinic-champion-windi-wojdak/.
4. Gates MC, et al. Experiences of recent veterinary graduates in their first employment position and their preferences for new graduate support programs. *NZ Vet J*. 2020;68(4):214–224. Accessed October 202. https://doi.org/10.1080/00480169.2020.1740112.
5. Jelinski MD, et al. Factors associated with veterinarians' career path choices in the early postgraduate period. *Can Vet J*. 2009;50(9):943–948.
6. Mineo L. Good genes are nice, but joy is better. *The Harvard Gazette*. April 22, 2017. https://news.harvard.edu/gazette/story/2017/04/over-nearly-80-years-harvard-study-has-been-showing-how-to-live-a-healthy-and-happy-life/. Accessed October 2022.
7. Figley C. *Compassion fatigue: Coping with secondary traumatic stress disorder in those who treat the traumatized*. Brunner/Mazel; 1995:1.

RECOMMENDED READING

Veterinary Mental Health and Wellbeing and How to Improve Them. Accessed August 2022. https://merck-animal-health-usa.com/wp-content/uploads/sites/54/2022/02/2021-PSV-Veterinary-Wellbeing-Presentation_V2.pdf.

Figley CR, Roop RG. *Compassion Fatigue in the Animal-Care Community*. Humane Society Press; 2006.

Becker C. Resumes: Putting Your Best Foot Forward. *Today's Veterinary Nurse*. November 15, 2021. Winter 2022. Accessed November 2022.https://todaysveterinarynurse.com/personal-professional-development/veterinary-nurse-technician-resumes/

Becker C. Preparing for an Interview. *Today's Veterinary Nurse*. March 11, 2022. Spring 2022. Accessed August 2022. https://todaysveterinarynurse.com/personal-professional-development/veterinary-nurse-technician-interviewing/.

7

Telemedicine

LEARNING OBJECTIVES

When you have completed this chapter, you should be able to:

- Compare and contrast telehealth, telemedicine, teletriage, and teleconsult
- Identify key components of a telehealth strategy
- Fairly evaluate platform providers
- Develop an exceptional client experience with telehealth
- Integrate work-life balance for team members with the use of telehealth

OUTLINE

KEY TERMS

AVMA Model Practice Act
Barrier to Patient Care
Remote Patient Monitoring
Teleconsult
Telehealth
Telemedicine
Teletriage
Veterinary client-patient relationship
Veterinary Practice Act

INTRODUCTION

Forms of telehealth have been around for years through the means of providing advice or tentative diagnoses over the phone. Most of these calls are with current clients of the practice that have a veterinary client-patient relationship established; however new clients also call with questions and may/may not schedule an appointment with the practice based on the experience they had with the veterinary practice.

The pandemic of 2020–2022 highlighted the need for the use of more formal telehealth programs; however, the topic was met with resistance by regulators and traditional veterinarians. As practices tried to navigate local, state, and federal restrictions, curbside service became the norm. Because curbside took more time than traditional (in-person) appointments, clients adopted pets at rates higher than previously seen, and clients were home with their pets 24 hours a day (to observe abnormalities), clients began experiencing a barrier to receiving pet healthcare. Meanwhile, practice teams were burning out and experiencing their own COVID hurdles in their personal lives (Chapter 1). The impact of the pandemic will have a long-lasting effect on clients (due to poor client experiences) and team members (decreased well-being resulting in labor shortage).

What can be learned from these challenging years? The implementation and use of technology to meet the needs of clients and team members alike must be integrated into the practice immediately. This will increase efficiency, allowing team members to work smarter (not harder) to continue serving the patients and clients that bring a sense of purpose to each team member. While communication technologies have been discussed in various chapters (Chapters 8 [PIMS], 9 [Medical Records], 10 [Appointments], and 11 [Client Experience]), this chapter will focus solely on understanding and integrating Telehealth into the practice setting.

DEFINITIONS

Veterinary telehealth is the use of telecommunication and digital technologies to deliver and enhance veterinary services, including veterinary health information, medical care, and veterinary and client education.[1] Technologies used to deliver telehealth may include e-mail, text messaging, video conferencing, and the use of remote patient monitoring devices. Providing telehealth outside of the brick-and-mortar building requires electronic medical records (EMR), allowing all forms of communication to be documented immediately after the services are provided. Some telehealth platforms will integrate information immediately into the medical record as well. Other requirements and recommendations needed to implement telehealth are discussed throughout this chapter.

LEADERSHIP POINT

Telehealth should not be thought of as a separate discipline within the profession, but rather another tool that the practice should provide to meet client needs (and increase team efficiency).

Telemedicine can be defined as the communication between a veterinary team and a client that has established a veterinary-client-patient relationship (VCPR). State veterinary practice acts (VPAs) vary regarding the specific definition and requirements of a VCPR (some do allow a VCPR to be established electronically), therefore it is important that each practice know what their state VPA says and implement protocols appropriately.

Teleconsulting is established when the veterinarian (that has a VCPR) consults with a veterinary specialist regarding a specific case. By definition, the specialist does not have a VCPR with the client and would not be able to initiate a teleconsult directly with the client. However, if the referring DVM, specialist, and client are on a telemedicine video conference together, the criteria would be met for the specialist to provide recommendations of care.

Teletriage is often already delivered by team members that answer the phone and schedule appointments for the patient to be seen. Teletriage and teleadvice are often given by the veterinary healthcare team, with careful navigation to not provide a diagnosis or prognosis, but rather schedule an appointment to be seen (for those without a VCPR) or to create a telehealth appointment with a DVM. Teletriage can be taken a step further in which the veterinary healthcare team can suggest an immediate appointment, a referral to an urgent care facility (if the practice is overbooked with urgent cases, or the call comes in after hours), or a referral to an emergency center.

All teleservices provide patient and client-centered care that engages the entire team. Many considerations must be thought through, planned, and implemented to ensure the client experience is one that will have clients raving about the exceptional service.

VETERINARY TELEHEALTH CONSIDERATIONS AND APPLICATIONS

First and foremost, telehealth, telemedicine, teletriage, and teleadvice have been offered in human healthcare for years. The structure of these programs includes a fee; the result is a decrease in barriers to patient care. These applications are also already occurring in the veterinary practice; however, it is a free service that has no structure and does not use advanced communication techniques.

Consider your ability to leave work to see your physician; we often put off medical and wellness visits for ourselves because it is difficult to schedule the time to leave the practice. By utilizing telehealth services that are available, you would not have to leave work to see your primary care physician, or to be referred to a specialist that may be in another city or state, within the same week of your inquiry. This is more convenient for you and decreases the barrier to receiving self-care. That is what our clients want as well, and they are willing to pay for the service to receive immediate answers regarding their concerns.

Consider revenue centers that can be expanded and delivered by the veterinary healthcare team (not necessarily a DVM) that do not take up an exam room. Behavioral observations, recommendations, and training; nutritional consultations to recommend a specific diet, calorie consumption, or obesity scoring; hospice coaching for clients that need reassurance they are making the right decisions and address concerns for their companion; post-vaccine observations and education about puppy/kitten behavior, boosters, and dental care; and postop surgery video calls to check on the patient and answer questions are only a few examples. Team members can provide client and patient-specific training for topics such as the administration of SQ fluids, insulin, ophthalmic ointment, wound care, and bandaging.

Consider how telehealth decreases the barrier to patient care when the practice has no appointments available, for clients who drive excessive distances, or those with a disability making it difficult to bring their pet in. Telehealth and telemedicine make it easy to do business with your practice.

Telehealth platforms can also enhance the care of hospitalized patients by allowing pet parents to have a live update of their pet's status and be able to see and talk to their pet. Services like this set your practice apart from competitors in the area.

Today's clients want and expect 24/7 access to care. While the practice may be closed in the evenings and on weekends, providing comfort via telehealth allows the practice's veterinary team members to recommend coming into the practice the next day, or visiting a recommended urgent care facility or emergency center, based on presenting conditions. When clients can talk to someone they trust, their perception of client service, compassion, and empathy increases 10-fold.

In addition to implementing telemedicine, DVMs may find remote patient monitoring systems (RPM) useful to aid in a diagnosis. RPMs are newer in the veterinary market and are a useful diagnostic tool that provides live parameters such as patient heart rate and temperature and can provide continuous monitoring of glucose concentrations in diabetic patients. This technology will further develop in the near future to provide more diagnostic parameters.

WHERE TO START

Understanding the VCPR: The first step in implementing a formal telehealth program is to become familiar with your state's definition of the VCPR. The AVMA Model Veterinary Practice Act has been used in many states and defines the veterinarian-client-patient relationship as the basis for veterinary care. To establish such a relationship, the following conditions must be satisfied:

1. The licensed veterinarian has assumed responsibility for making medical judgments regarding the health of the patient(s) and the need for medical therapy and has instructed the client on a course of therapy appropriate to the circumstance.
2. There is sufficient knowledge of the patient(s) by the veterinarian to initiate at least a general or preliminary diagnosis of the medical condition(s) of the patient(s).
3. The client has agreed to follow the licensed veterinarian's recommendations.
4. The licensed veterinarian is readily available for follow-up evaluation or has arranged for:
   a. Emergency or urgent care coverage, or
   b. Continuing care and treatment have been designated by the veterinarian with a prior relationship to a licensed veterinarian who has access to the patient's medical records and/or can provide reasonable and appropriate medical care.
5. The veterinarian provides oversight of treatment.
6. Such a relationship can exist only when the veterinarian has performed a timely physical examination of the patient(s) or is personally acquainted with the keeping and care of the patient(s) by virtue of medically appropriate and timely visits to the operation where the patient(s) is(are) kept, or both.
7. Patient records are maintained.

Both the licensed veterinarian and the client have the right to establish or decline a veterinarian-client-patient relationship within the guidelines set forth in the AVMA Principles of Veterinary Medical Ethics.

When conducting telemedicine consults across state lines, it is advisable and may be required for the veterinarian to be licensed both in the state where they are located and the state where the patient(s) is located. Should issues arise, being licensed in both states ensures the veterinarian is legally authorized to practice. Just like an appropriately established VCPR, licensure in both states protects veterinarians, patients, and clients.[1]

Integrating a Seamless Service: The second step to take before implementing a telehealth program is to not only evaluate potential service providers (covered in the next paragraph) but also how telehealth can be an integrated service that is delivered by the practice in addition to (not just a substitute) in-person visits. Brick-and-mortar and telehealth should be seamlessly integrated to deliver high-quality patient care. For that to work together seamlessly, consider the following points:

Space: What space is available in the practice to provide a quiet, professional, uninterrupted telehealth experience? If telehealth will be provided off-site, consider what that DVM or team member will need (equipment, technology, internet bandwidth, professional background, etc.) to exceed the client's expectations of this service.

Technology: What technology will be needed to deliver telehealth professionally, what are the expenses of that technology, and who will install, maintain, and troubleshoot that technology to ensure it is easy for the team to deliver a high-level experience?

Scheduling: How will the practice integrate telehealth appointments into the current appointment schedule?

Team Member Support: Will the team members' work schedules need to change to adapt to the additional telehealth appointments? Will new team members need to be added to support the service?

Approach to Diagnostic Workups: How will doctors approach diagnostic workups? What tests will be recommended and what will the process be (within the flow of the veterinary practice) to accommodate the diagnostics needed? Will the practice provide any type of concierge service to obtain samples from the patient's home environment (eliminating the need for the client to visit the practice)?

PIMS Integration: Can the chosen platform easily integrate with the medical records and appointment calendar of the current PIMS?

Medical Record Entry: How will medical records be completed (who enters what information and where)?

Medications: How will medications be filled and in what time frame? Will some medications be filled in the practice whereas others can be scripted to the practice's online pharmacy and be sent directly to the client? If medications are filled in-house, is the client expected to pick up the medications or will the practice provide delivery?

Practice Flow: How will the team coordinate the care of the patient? If a patient needs additional care, diagnostics, medications, or a medical progress exam once the initial consult is completed, who handles that to ensure no element is dropped? Does the practice consider the role of a telehealth patient coordinator?

Team Training: How will the team be trained? What role does what? Who will lead the telehealth service and ensure the client's expectations are being met?

Client Awareness: How will the clients be made aware of the new service, and how will the team provide clear expectations of what the service delivers?

The Client Experience: What does the client experience look like? Put your client hat on—what would you expect from a service that would have you asking for this service again?

Client Consent: How will the doctors and/or the team obtain client consent to perform diagnostics through this service? Will estimates and treatment plans be developed and emailed or sent via text to clients for signature? If yes, what digital platform can be used to increase the efficiency of this process?

Pricing: How will the practice price the service? Per individual consult, by length of consult, as a bundle package? See the section on pricing for more considerations.

Invoicing: How will clients be invoiced for this service? Will they be expected to pay prior to the consult, or after? How will that money be collected?

Marketing: How will the service be marketed to existing clients? Text messages, emails, blogs, social media, website, practice app, practice portal, and/or in-clinic signage?

Success: What defines success for the program? Number of consults per day? Client satisfaction? Team satisfaction and work-life balance? Profitability?

Backup Plans: Technology can fail. Collaborate and determine what failures could occur and create back plans (loss of power, internet, client inability to access the platform, etc.).

Liability Insurance: Check with your insurance provider to ensure claims associated with telehealth are covered.

With the above considerations, consider what the practice workflow would look like (Fig. 7.1).

Provider Evaluation: Now that the ideal service has been determined by the team, the next step is to evaluate technology and service providers that can help the practice achieve its goal. Be sure to evaluate multiple providers and choose a provider that can not only help the practice easily achieve the goal through its capabilities but is easy to work with. A more expensive service that provides outstanding support supersedes a cheaper platform that negatively impacts the client's experience and leaves the team feeling frustrated. Questions that the practice will want to ask include:

- What are the full capabilities and costs of the platform?
- What technology is required for both the practice and the clients?
- What equipment is the practice required to have to run the platform effectively?
- What internet speed/bandwidth is required for both download and upload activity? Is that bandwidth available in the demographic the practice supports?
- Can the platform allow the practice to host more than one consult at the same time (in different rooms)?
- How much support is provided by the company during and post-integration?
- How often are updates completed, and how are they deployed to the practice?
- What is the cost of the platform for the practice (fixed monthly fee or per consult)?
- What team training is provided? Does training cover troubleshooting equipment and technology?
- Are any marketing services provided to help promote the service to clients?
- Do service providers protect client information (i.e., not sell to or use client information for any other purpose?
- Does the service integrate with the practices' PIMS?
- Does the platform accept client payments on behalf of the practice?
- Do the capabilities of the service include text/email/video conferencing?
- Can the platform send and receive images?
- Can clients and team members access via computer, tablet, iPad, and smartphone?

Pricing Considerations: Pricing new services appropriately can be difficult. Many times, practice owners call a colleague that is already providing the service and price in a similar fashion. But every hospital is different, and what covers expenses in one practice may not cover expenses in another. Be sure to estimate all costs of the service before implementation to ensure that a pricing structure is not outside of what the local demographic can pay and should not be higher than the cost of an in-person visit.

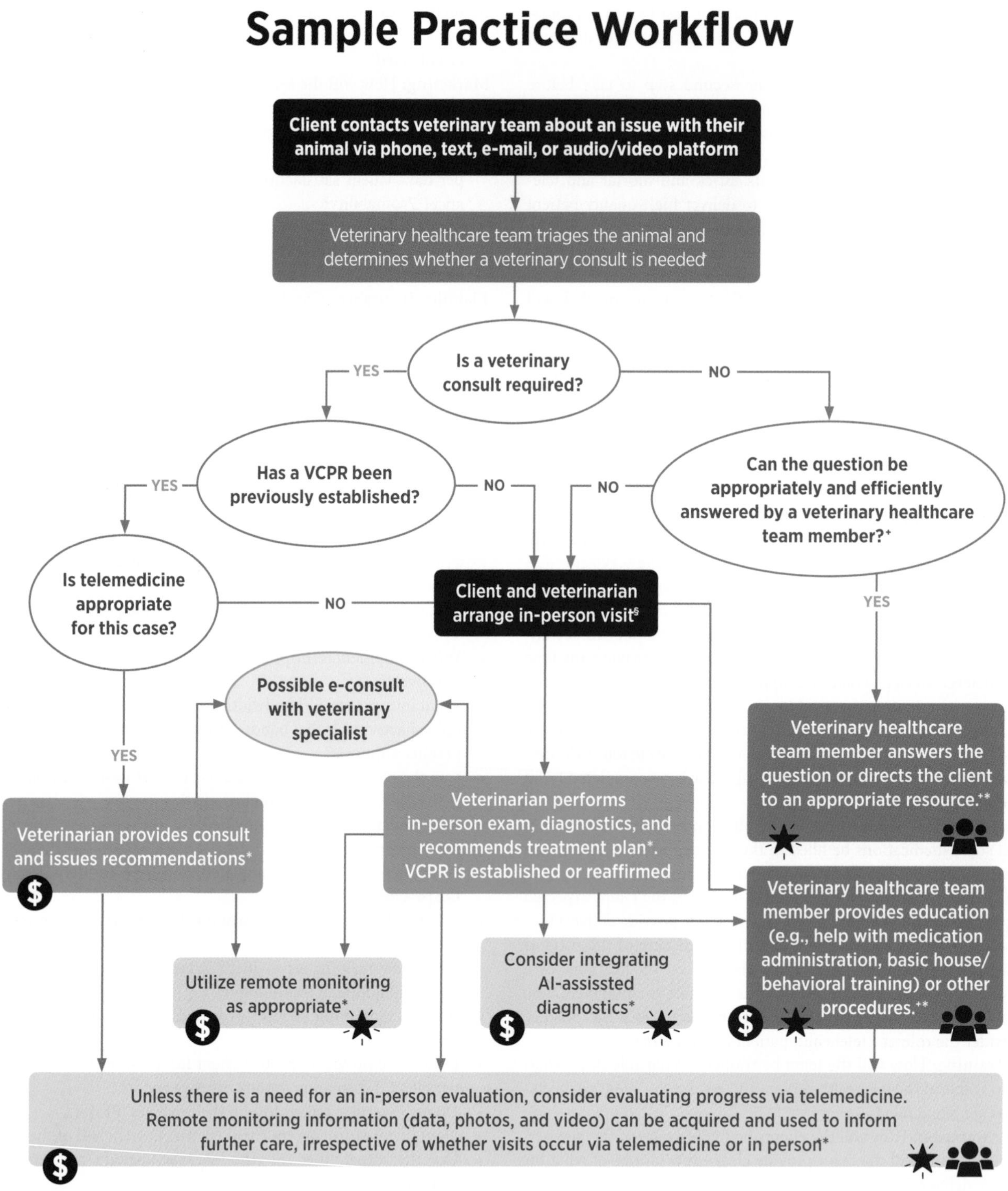
Sample Practice Workflow
Client contacts veterinary team about an issue with their animal via phone, text, e-mail, or audio/video platform
Veterinary healthcare team triages the animal and determines whether a veterinary consult is needed*
Is a veterinary consult required?
YES
NO
Has a VCPR been previously established?
Can the question be appropriately and efficiently answered by a veterinary healthcare team member?+
Is telemedicine appropriate for this case?
Client and veterinarian arrange in-person visit§
Possible e-consult with veterinary specialist
Veterinary healthcare team member answers the question or directs the client to an appropriate resource.+*
Veterinarian provides consult and issues recommendations*
Veterinarian performs in-person exam, diagnostics, and recommends treatment plan*. VCPR is established or reaffirmed
Veterinary healthcare team member provides education (e.g., help with medication administration, basic house/behavioral training) or other procedures.+*
Utilize remote monitoring as appropriate*
Consider integrating AI-assissted diagnostics*
Unless there is a need for an in-person evaluation, consider evaluating progress via telemedicine. Remote monitoring information (data, photos, and video) can be acquired and used to inform further care, irrespective of whether visits occur via telemedicine or in person*

* All interactions should be captured in the medical record

\+ Any assessment or procedures performed by a member of the veterinary healthcare team must be within the team member's scope of practice.

§ Pertains to situations where a VCPR must be established via an in-person examination

$ Potential telehealth income ★ Increases efficiency Better utilize veterinary healthcare team

Fig. 7.1 The Flow of Telehealth in the Veterinary Practice. (Courtesy AVMA.)

- What are all costs associated with delivering telehealth? Consider the service provider fee, equipment, credit card merchant fees, etc.
- How many team members will be required to deliver telehealth and how much time will each appointment take from start to finish?
- How many minutes will be allotted for telehealth appointments and is this different than in-person appointments?
- Can the practice run multiple telehealth visits at once (i.e., a technician is obtaining patient history and subjective information in one video room while the DVM finishes another consult in a different room)? The key to this consideration is efficiency. Running two rooms at the same time increases patient volume, therefore decreasing staff costs associated with the service.
- Once you know this information, use the pricing strategy covered in Chapter 16 to determine break-even costs associated with delivering the service. Once the break-even price point is known, consider the next three bullet points as options.
- If a telehealth consult leads to an in-person visit, do you bundle the fees together?
- Do you charge by consult with a maximum DVM time (one-time visit or after hours)?
- Would bundled pricing with a practice visit be considered (consider behavior counseling, nutrition modification, hospice care, etc.)?
- After the service is established, a practice may want to consider a simple subscription fee with unlimited visits.

There is no one thing that fits every practice. Do what is right for the business (cover expenses and ensure profitability), the team (work-life balance), and the client and patient experience.

TEAM TRAINING

While one of the considerations/questions above asked what training is provided for the team by the service provider, it is also up to the practice to implement a successful training program for every member of the team. Team members must understand *why* this service is so critical to patient care, correlate the "why" with the practice values, mission, and vision, and understand how their role plays a significant part in achieving the goal. Practice managers must consider team member concerns, allow collaboration, and bridge the gaps that are identified while collaborating with the leaders of each team (receptionist, assistant/credentialed technician, and the doctor team).

It is common to experience resistance when implementing an innovative technology such as telehealth. Review Chapter 2 to identify reasons for team resistance, successfully address and influence change management, and encourage the staff to challenge the status quo to meet client expectations.

When the telehealth program is near completion, facilitate role playing with the team to ensure every team member is confident when talking about the program and making recommendations to clients. If even one person lacks confidence, does not believe in the service, or consistently points out the challenges/hurdles in a negative manner, the team morale will decrease, and the manager will have a difficult time launching the program successfully.

THE CLIENT EXPERIENCE

It was stated above to step into the client's shoes and define what the client experience should feel like. Collaborate with the team when identifying topics/hurdles that need to be addressed; each role brings a different perspective to ensuring the client experience is exceeded.

One area that is often missed during the collaboration is how to successfully set the expectations of the service for the client. For many, this is the first time they are using a service like this, therefore the team must be patient and kind. Many clients may be technology challenged; prepare for that hurdle and make it a fun experience for them.

- Explain to clients how telehealth/telemedicine flows, including technology, the scope of services, scheduling, and payment expectations.
- Add time at the beginning of the telemedicine appointment to ensure the client can connect to the platform and has both audio and visual tools working. This should be delivered by a nonveterinarian, allowing the DVM to maximize their time when the appointment begins. This also keeps the telehealth appointments running on time. As clients return for the service, the added time on the front of the appointment can be reduced as they become more familiar and confident with the platform. Communicate with clients as to why additional time is needed on the front end. Set clear expectations and provide assurance that a team member will guide them through that process.
- Expect technical failure to happen; communicate the backup plan for clients before a failure occurs (i.e., have the client's phone number handy to call, etc.).
- With each consult provided, clients should know what the next steps are, which veterinary team member will coordinate them, and when they will occur.
- Inform clients that for the best experience, they should be in a quiet, well-lit, distraction-free area for their appointment (avoid backlighting so the veterinarian can easily see the patient). Additionally, using a camera that is moveable and can zoom in on the area of interest (i.e., smartphone) allows the medical team to best see the presenting problem.
- For client expectations to be exceeded, the practice must deliver a professional experience. Ensure consults delivered by the team are in a room that is distraction-free and uninterrupted. Lighting should be adequate with the camera at eye level. The team member should be centered in the middle of the screen, and the backdrop must be professional in appearance. Ensure bandwidth, resolution, and internet speed are adequate to prevent glitches. The viewing screen should be large enough to see the patient well and monitor behavior, the environment, incisions, skin conditions, etc. If using a portable device, ensure it is connected to a screen that provides clarity for the team member (without having to get incredibly close to the screen).
- If a portable device is used (tablet, iPad, Laptop), place it on a solid surface (not the knees) so the device does not wobble while the team member is typing.

Keep in mind that, for the long-term success of any telehealth service, the client experience must be the same or better than what they receive in practice to keep them returning.

KEY PERFORMANCE INDICATORS TO MONITOR

As with any revenue center provided in the practice, the practice manager must measure and monitor results. This allows the practice to determine if the revenue center is successful through profitability, team member, and client expectations. Review Chapter 16, Finance, for details on revenue center management. When creating SMART goals (Chapter 12, Marketing) to implement the telehealth service, be sure to establish KPIs that will be measured. When KPIs are not being met, the practice can adjust to ensure the future success of the program. Consider (at a minimum):

- Anonymous client experience surveys
- Anonymous team member surveys
- Usage reports
- Average client transactions
- Compliance rates
- Team efficiency

Maintain a spreadsheet of monthly KPIs and share them with the team. Collaborate monthly and determine what is working/not working and pivot as needed.

BEFORE THE LAUNCH

Once the entire program is set up, complete several trial runs with team members who are offsite. Check links, picture quality, sound, lighting, and background image, and listen for an echo in the audio. Send and receive photos, radiographs, lab results, videos, or documents that may be needed in a real case. Use this as a training opportunity to identify hurdles that need to be overcome to avoid a poor client experience.

SUMMARY

Telehealth is here to stay, and practices must consider how it may become a natural part of patient care delivery. Telehealth increases practice efficiency while embodying a work-life balance for the team. At the same time, patients receive the care they need because it does reduce the barrier to care. When work-life balance is present within the team and their purpose is fulfilled (Chapter 2), employee retention increases. Additionally, a successful telehealth program allows the practice to employ remote team members who can seamlessly communicate with the practice team and the PIMS.

In the future, remote areas that have no current veterinary care may be able to use the telehealth model, allowing credentialed veterinary technicians to travel to the remote area to observe and gather data, lab work, etc., while the DVM is on video. This is known as telesupervision (as defined by the AVMA). While this is an innovative service that would further decrease the barrier to patient care and utilize the credentialed veterinary technician to the highest degree, the regulatory process has yet to catch up. Currently, the term supervised, or indirect supervision as stated in the VPA, would need to be modified or clarified to serve this category.

REVIEW QUESTIONS

1. Define Telehealth.
2. Define Telemedicine.
3. When a VCPR is absent, what form of telehealth is delivered to the client?
4. How does your state's VPA define Telehealth?
5. Identify 5 KPIs that should be monitored.

REFERENCES

1. Implementing connected care. AVMA guidelines for the use of telehealth in the veterinary practice. AVMA.org. Accessed January 2023. https://www.avma.org/sites/default/files/2021-01/AVMA-Veterinary-Telehealth-Guidelines.pdf

8

Practice Integrated Management Software

LEARNING OBJECTIVES

When you have completed this chapter, you should be able to:

- Identify the difference between PMS and PIMS
- Describe how each function of a practice integration management system cross-functions with another
- Identify third-party vendors that can increase efficiency
- Describe why setting up a practice integration management system correctly is important
- Compare and contrast the benefits of a cloud-based or local-based server

OUTLINE

KEY TERMS

Bundled treatment plans
Cloud-based server
Diagnoses codes
Gap analysis
Practice integration management software
Pet portals
Templates
Third-party integrations
Whiteboards

INTRODUCTION

Practice Management Software has been referred to by two different acronyms in the past: PMS, Practice Management Software; and PIMS, Practice Information Management System. However, based on the evolution of the software, a more current term would be PIMS, Practice *Integration* Management System. The software has evolved from a simple invoice and pricing database to a complex, cross-functional space that increases efficiency in every aspect of the veterinary practice.

PIMS: THE INTEGRATION SOFTWARE

The PIMS ties together medical records; medical, boarding, and grooming appointment scheduler; reminders; invoices; credit card processing; imaging and lab requisitions and results; inventory management; and reporting that impacts financials, controlled substances, and time clocks. It also enables the practice to utilize third-party applications to help the practice continue to grow, maintain efficiency, and provide a frictionless client experience.

The problem? Change management. It can be difficult to move from antiquated software that has not improved cross-functional abilities, thereby allowing the practice to continue functioning at suboptimal levels. The veterinary industry can be complacent; this has prevented software companies from updating the successful software that was developed many years ago. Some PMS (and simply that, a practice management system) have built additional modules over time to meet the needs of progressive practices. But when the modules don't cross-function and support one another efficiently, the team works harder, not smarter.

Imagine, a PIMS that follows the flow of the practice. A PIMS that is intuitive and easy to use and has a similar appearance to common systems used on many platforms today. A PIMS that is built with a strong base so while entries are being made in one area, it is autopopulating

VHMA PERFORMANCE DOMAINS

Veterinary Hospital Managers Association (VHMA) Performance Domains

Performance domains applicable to practice integrative management software include marketing and client relations, organization of the practice, and financial management. The practice manager:

- Coordinates and plans client service programs, client education, and communication processes, and monitors client retention and satisfaction.
- Is responsible for maintenance of medical record systems, inventory controls, and implementing technology systems.
- Analyzes financial reports, maintains financial accounting, and monitors financial trends.

Application of VHMA Performance Domains for Practice Managers

Integrating an efficient and effective practice integrative management software improves the performance, knowledge, skills, and abilities of the practice manager to enhance client service communication, medical records, inventory processes, and the implementation of technology to improve client satisfaction and retention

another area. A PIMS reduces missed charges on the invoice because the invoice is being built as medical records are being completed. *No more imagination is needed; the possibility is here!*

CRITICAL COMPETENCY: ADAPTABILITY

Practice managers must be open to change and flexible work methods and can adapt behavior to changing conditions or new information.

In today's fast-paced practice that is short-staffed and has excess client demand, practice managers must take into consideration every opportunity to increase the efficiency of the team, helping them work smarter, not harder. With the rise in costs, a practice cannot afford to lose revenue through missed charges, and the cost of team burnout is intangible. One might add up the cost of the turnover of the team member and the cost to train a new team member, but one cannot estimate the impact that burnout has on clients, the mental health of the team, and the long-term damage to this industry that continues to lose team members in droves.

Specific functions of PIMS are listed below with a high-level summary of how each area must cross-function to create optimal efficiency. Additionally, third-party applications (or features already built in) that can further enhance efficiency are covered (Fig. 8.1).

Medical Records

Main Points of Function: Medical records are required by state veterinary practice acts and serve as documentation for any services provided to owners (as well as all communication). Medical records must include the presenting complaint, assessment, plan, diagnosis, and prognosis. To support the diagnosis, all supporting laboratory results and imaging must be included (along with interpretations of the results). Medical records should be seen as documentation that proves what recommendations have been made, accepted, or declined by the owner, and delivered by the practice, should a board investigation or lawsuit entail. See Chapter 9, Medical Records, for a complete discussion. For accurate reporting and reducing the potential risk associated with medical record alteration, medical records should have a lockout period. If a correction or change needs to occur, an addendum can be added, but the previous record should not be altered.

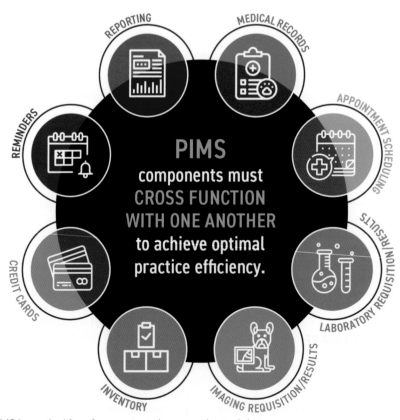

Fig. 8.1 A cross-functional PIMS is required for a fast pace veterinary practice to thrive.

Cross Functions With:

Treatment Plans: When medical recommendations are made for a patient, a treatment plan needs to be developed to provide an estimate of the cost of services. Recommendations should be made in the medical record which autopopulates a treatment plan. Technicians then review the treatment plan with clients, acknowledge what has been accepted or declined, and document it all in the medical record, finalizing the treatment plan (this should also autopopulate).

Consent Forms: When a client is given a recommendation for a service for their pet, the consent form must be signed. When the recommendation is generated in the treatment plan, a client consent form should autopopulate with the pet's name, date, recommendation(s), and a place for the client to electronically sign.

Treatment Whiteboard: When treatment plans are created and accepted for patients staying in the hospital, the treatment whiteboard should autopopulate, providing the patient's name, doctor, lead technician/nurse, and what treatments the patient should receive and when. When the treatments are completed by the technician/nurse, the procedure or medication autopopulates the invoice (Fig. 8.2).

Invoicing: When medical records are being completed and a treatment plan has been accepted by a client, the treatment plan should then autopopulate the invoice.

Reminders: When services have been completed for a patient that requires a reminder (annual or biannual exams, vaccines, bloodwork monitoring medications or long-term diseases, parasiticide prevention, etc.) reminders should be automatically generated.

Client Education Documents: When medical records are completed and a diagnosis has been made, supporting client education materials should be made available to print, email to a client directly, and/or be visible in the patients' pet portal.

Diagnostic Requisitions and Results: When a treatment plan has been created and a client accepts, appropriate lab requestion forms should be generated with the correct labwork request and all patient data. This also allows the results to autopopulate when they are ready (either outside reference labs or in-house lab equipment).

Recommendations and Compliance Reports: When services or medications are recommended in a medical record, they should be tagged, allowing compliance reports to be generated indicating what percent of clients have accepted specific recommendations, which doctors have the highest compliance rates, etc.

Financial Reports and Key Performance Indicators (KPIs): All entries made, and transactions linked to medical records produce *correct* financials. If medical records are incomplete and charges are missed, compliance reports, financial reports, and KPIs will be inaccurate.

The medical record lockout period impacts the medical record itself, invoicing, recommendations and compliance reports, and financial reporting. If there is no lockout period set, any transaction can be altered at any time, increasing the risk of embezzlement and the inability to reconcile appropriately.

Third-Party Functionality:

Pet Health Insurance: Increase efficiency by granting a preferred partner access to the medical records and invoicing. Reports can be generated for the provider, allowing quicker turnaround time for client reimbursement or practice payment. This improves the efficiency of the team and enhances the frictionless client experience.

Pet Portals or Practice App: To best serve client expectations, more than just reminders need to be present in portals or apps. Give clients the opportunity to print or share their pets' medical records with ER or specialty/referral practices, or print spay, neuter, and rabies certificates. All reminders should be made available, including diagnostic bloodwork, medication refills, vaccines, and physical exams in the pet portal or practice app.

Two-Way Text Messaging: Ensure that clients can send a text to the practice and the practice can respond. This allows reminders to be sent automatically via text, helps the practice respond to appointment requests efficiently, and the practice can send photos and updates to clients while their pet is hospitalized or undergoing a procedure.

Companies That Facilitate Wellness Plans: Access to medical records allows the company to track what has/has not been completed as a part of the plan, which impacts accurate client invoicing at the time of checkout.

Telehealth: Integrating telehealth applications seamlessly allows the team to efficiently enter the medical record notes, create recommendations, prescriptions, and appointments, and invoice the client if appropriate.

Appointment Scheduling: The ability for clients to schedule appointments online via the practice website, pet portal, practice app, or social media. Grant the application access to the PIMs so that appointments are booked directly into the appointment calendar, reducing call volume by nearly 60%.[1]

Appointment Scheduling

Main Points of Function: The appointment scheduling function serves many roles, including hosting boarding reservations, grooming,

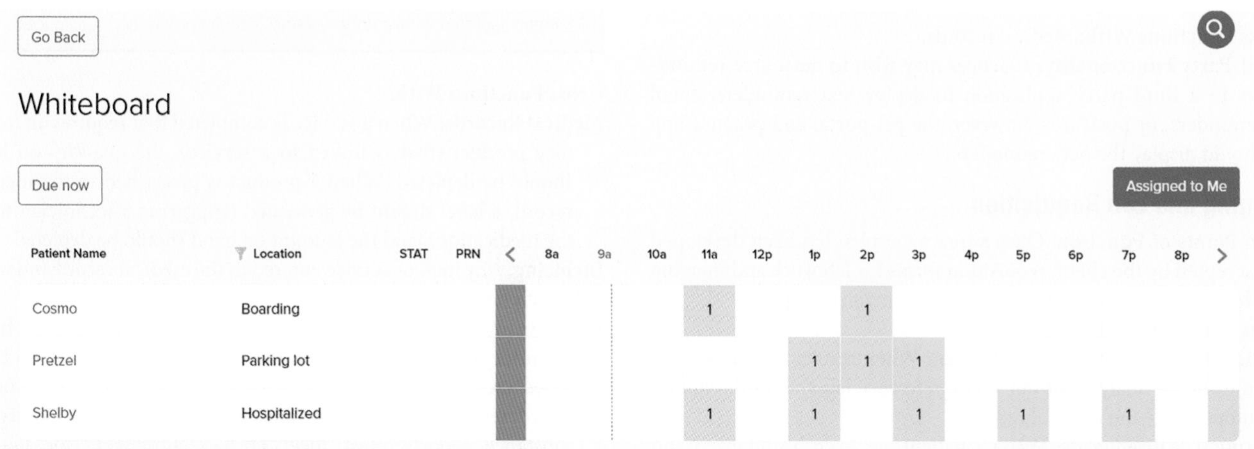

Fig. 8.2 Image of the whiteboard functionality in Shepherd Practice Management Software. (Courtesy Shepherd Practice Management Software.)

and bathing appointments, as well as the standard medical-based appointments for the doctors, technicians, surgery, and dentals. The appointment function aids in the control of the practice flow; scheduling appropriately can decrease the chaos and help develop a work-life balance with the team. See Chapter 10, Appointment Management, for specific details.

Cross Functions With:

Inpatient and Outpatient Whiteboards: This feature allows appointments that are checked in to be viewed on an outpatient whiteboard (wellness and medical exams), or an inpatient whiteboard (surgeries, dentals, or hospitalized patients), increasing efficiency, and directing doctors and technicians "where to go next." Reporting can also be tied to this feature, helping the practice manager determine how long each step of the outpatient process took, and identify steps to increase efficiency where needed.

Invoicing: Once the patient is checked in, the invoicing process is initiated.

Reporting: Practice managers must be able to track no-show rates and implement strategies to decrease them.

Third-Party Functionality:

Vetstoria: The ability for clients to schedule appointments online via the practice website, pet portal, practice app, or social media. Grant the application access to the PIMs allowing appointments to be booked directly into the appointment calendar, reducing call volume by nearly 60%.[1]

Pet Portals, Practice App: Allow clients to view and secure appointment times.

Telehealth: If the practice utilizes a third-party platform for Telehealth, appointments should be integrated to allow clients to book appointments through the website, social media platforms, pet portals, or the practice app.

Reminders

Main Points of Function: Reminders are a critical function of any PIMs system. But they can only remind for services that have been set up correctly. In addition, cell phone numbers, email addresses, and client mailing addresses must be correct to deploy reminders (text, email, postcard). Clients should receive reminders for annual or biannual physical examinations, vaccines, annual or biannual lab work, chronic medication refills and lab work, dental prophylaxis, and parasiticide prevention at a minimum. See Chapter 12, Marketing, for more specific details.

> **VHMA PERFORMANCE DOMAIN TASK:**
>
> Develop and maintain a client reminder system.

Cross Functions With: Medical records.

Third-Party Functionality: Practices may wish to outsource reminders to a third-party application to deploy text reminders, email reminders, or postcards; however, the pet portal and practice app should display the pet's reminders.

Imaging and Lab Requisition

Main Points of Function: Once a treatment plan has been developed and accepted by the client, requisition forms for lab work and imaging should be autogenerated, then populate the invoice (Fig. 8.3).

Cross Functions With:

Medical Records and Treatment Plan: When results are ready from an in-house analyzer or out-house reference lab, the results should autopopulate the medical record.

Treatment Whiteboards: When a patient has been hospitalized and lab work or images are completed, they should autopopulate the invoice.

Third-Party Functionality: Reference laboratory and in-house analyzers.

Invoicing and Credit Card Processing

Main Points of Function: Once a client moves to the check-out process, it should be fast, efficient, and easy. Clients are either overwhelmed, mentally checked out, irritated that the wait has been so long, or (hopefully) happy with all services. Accurate and efficient invoicing and credit card integration are essential to ending the frictionless client experience on a positive note. The invoice should be ready for the client when they check out, whether that is in the exam room or at the front desk. On average, practices lose 5%–10% of annual revenue through missed charges that never get added to the invoice; invoices should be built off all previous points discussed, allowing a quick review by the lead technician upon checkout. In addition, credit cards should be integrated with PIMs to reduce manual entry errors and increase efficiency.

Cross Functions With:

Medical Records and Treatment Plan and Treatment Whiteboard: When medical records are completed and the treatment plan has been executed, the treatment plan should then autopopulate the invoice.

Wellness Plans: If clients are enrolled in a plan, the invoicing feature must be integrated to ensure accurate invoicing based on the clients' package.

Third-Party Functionality

Debit/Credit Card Integration (VISA/MC/AMEX/CareCredit): Should be a click feature within the PIMS that automatically prompts the swipe of the card, autopopulating the amount to be charged. Manually entering the amount of the charge (in either the PIMS or the credit card machine) increases the risk of human error.

Wellness Plans: Must be integrated with invoicing to ensure clients are charged correctly for services rendered based on what the client has used or not used in the plan.

Telehealth: If the practice utilizes a third-party platform for Telehealth, invoicing should be integrated to autocapture charges for the service.

Inventory

Main Points of Function: Maintain accurate inventory counts; report low quantities and alert to reorder; maintain accurate pricing of inventory products by tablet/capsule or bottle, and by mL or bottle; add dispensing fees, injection fees, and minimum prescription fees; be linked to service items and automatically reduce count number when either a service or product is invoiced.

> **VHMA PERFORMANCE DOMAIN TASK:**
>
> Maintain appropriate inventory systems, including controlled substances.

Cross Functions With:

Medical Records: When a service is completed that requires an inventory product (that is linked to a service), the quantity on hand should be depleted. When a product is prescribed in the medical record, a label should be generated (triggering a technician to fill the medication), and the amount on hand should be depleted.

Invoicing: Any item or service entered in the medical record and treatment plan should auto-invoice.

Reports: Inventory reports determine an accurate quantity on hand, the price paid for the product, the value of the inventory on hand based on the price paid, the client price, how often the product is ordered, and who the product was ordered from. Controlled substance reports must meet DEA requirements for logging (Chapter 14, Controlled Substances) and be available for random audits if requested.

LAB USE ONLY

ZOETIS
REFERENCE
LABORATORIES

ORDER MANIFEST

CLINIC INFO

Clinic ID : 900
ZZZTest Hospital 1
123 Main Street - Suite B (Hosp)
Chula Vista, CA 91913
P : (212) 555-1212

PATIENT INFO

Family : Hinds
Pet : Meeka
Age : 7 years
Sex : Female Spayed
Species : Canine
Breed : German Shepherd

ORDER INFO

Order Date : 09/24/2022
Spec Date : 09/24/2022
Doctor : TEST Bertot

Requisition Number : 997796

TESTS ORDERED

#	CODE	TEST NAME	SOURCE
1	CBCC	Comprehensive CBC, Canine/Feline	-

For cases where this information is important:

Please provide a brief clinical history for this case: ______________________

What anatomic location has been sampled in this case? ______________________

What is your clinical differential diagnosis? ______________________

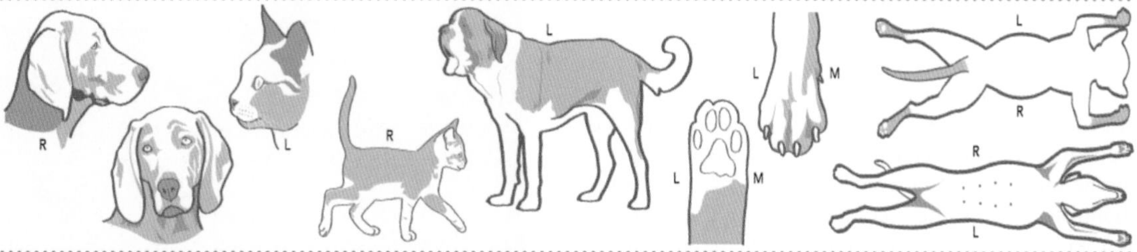

Fig. 8.3 Image of an autopopulated lab requisition form from Shepherd Practice Management Software. (Courtesy Shepherd Practice Management Software.)

Third-Party Functionality: Distributors and manufacturers can automatically import invoices into the PIMS when an order is shipped, or an automated medication dispensing machine (i.e., Cubex) can place orders when reorder points are achieved.

Reporting

Main Points of Function: PIMS should be able to print a variety of detailed reports allowing the Practice manager and owner to analyze the business. Reports should be easily generated with specific timeframes.

VHMA PERFORMANCE DOMAIN TASK:

Practice managers must analyze practice financials and client retention processes.

Cross Functions With:

Medical Records: Entries must be made in medical records to be able to track and report services (surgical, procedures, lab, etc.) and products recommended, completed, and sold.

Invoicing: Reports can be generated that include the Average Doctor Transaction (ADT), the Average Client Transaction (ACT), the Average Revenue Per Patient (ARPP), the number of transactions, the number of patients seen, etc. More report suggestions are found in Chapter 16, Finance.

Compliance: Compliance reports track what was recommended and what was accepted.

Reminders: Reminder reports allow the practice manager to track when clients responded to a reminder (several reminders for the same service should be set up and cleared when the service is invoiced) for a service or product.

Inventory: Reports should include the amount of product that has been ordered, the current amount on hand, the amount sold and clients who purchased the product, which doctor prescribed the product, etc.

Third-Party Functionality: QuickBooks or any accounting software.

SETTING UP AN EFFECTIVE PIMS

To achieve the most efficient PIMS, the "base" must be set up correctly. Consider the base as the bottom of the pyramid. Efficiency begins when the base has been set up to support all functions of the PIMS. This area cannot be skipped or even completed 50%; the result will be an inefficient and frustrated team, 5%–10% of lost revenue per year for missed charges, and a poor client experience that will leave clients searching for another veterinary provider. Templates, diagnosis codes, problem lists, bundled treatment plans by diagnosis, client education documents, and inventory must be set up correctly. Use the software to its fullest potential to be as efficient as possible (Fig. 8.4).

Templates: Templates can be set up for any routine standardized procedure to maximize the team's efficiency. Review areas of the practice that are routine and identify how templates may increase efficiency in that area. Templates can also be useful for ensuring that required data is gathered and not skipped. For example, when completing a *medical progress* exam, obtaining vitals should still be required. If the data is not obtained, the user should not be able to move to the next task. Physical exams (wellness, illness, and medical progress exams) templates will prompt for vitals, the assessment of each body part, and the SOAP portion of the medical record (Chapter 9, Medical Records). A surgical template is applicable for routine ovariohysterectomies, castrations, TPLOs, etc. Anesthesia templates can be created based on current protocols. Fig. 8.5 provides examples of templates to consider.

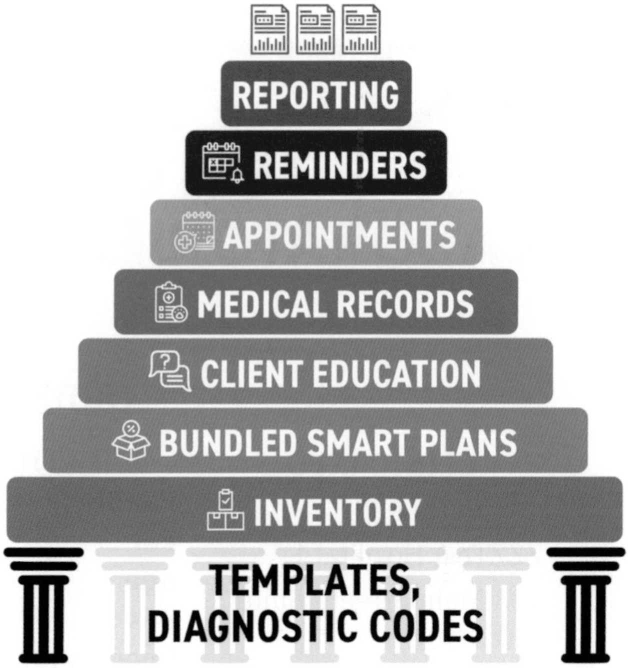

Fig. 8.4 Implementing PIMS without building the base will result in a frustrated team and poor client experiences.

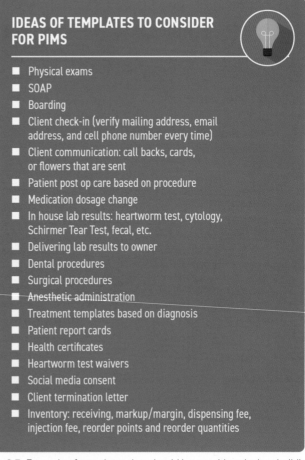

IDEAS OF TEMPLATES TO CONSIDER FOR PIMS

- Physical exams
- SOAP
- Boarding
- Client check-in (verify mailing address, email address, and cell phone number every time)
- Client communication: call backs, cards, or flowers that are sent
- Patient post op care based on procedure
- Medication dosage change
- In house lab results: heartworm test, cytology, Schirmer Tear Test, fecal, etc.
- Delivering lab results to owner
- Dental procedures
- Surgical procedures
- Anesthetic administration
- Treatment templates based on diagnosis
- Patient report cards
- Health certificates
- Heartworm test waivers
- Social media consent
- Client termination letter
- Inventory: receiving, markup/margin, dispensing fee, injection fee, reorder points and reorder quantities

Fig. 8.5 Example of templates that should be considered when building an effective and efficient PIMS base.

Diagnosis Codes: Diagnosis codes can be used to increase the efficiency of the team when a diagnosis has been made (patients often have more than one diagnosis). These diagnosis codes should be linked to bundled treatment plans (aka estimates) and client education literature. Consider the most common diagnoses the practice sees: abscesses, aural hematomas, lacerations, periodontal disease grade 3, pancreatitis, and parvovirus. These codes must be developed to create effective bundled treatment plans and improve efficiencies.

Bundled Treatment Plans by Diagnosis: These smart plans list considerations a patient would receive when they have been diagnosed with a specific condition. It is much easier to remove treatments, medications, or lab tests than to remember to get them all on the plan. Recall that every client should be offered the best medicine and bundled treatment plans should follow SOPs/SOCs developed by the practice. Consider the example above, an aural hematoma. Based on the age of the pet and if a heartworm test is current or not, the team member creating the treatment plan would need to remember to add a heartworm test. Because it is not directly related to the procedure, it can be easily forgotten. If the test was positive, it may change the treatment plan to treat the diagnosis; if the pet is current on a test and on heartworm preventative, the test can simply be removed from the treatment plan. This allows for the best medicine for every case. Recall from the earlier discussion that once the treatment plan is executed and marked complete on the whiteboard, the items should automatically roll to the invoice. Setting up bundled codes saves the team a significant matter of time, allows the best medicine to be recommended to clients, and prevents missed charges.

Client Education Literature: Clients need to have a full understanding of what their pet has been diagnosed with. On average, clients only retain about 30% of the information presented in the exam room (Chapter 11, Client Leadership). Automatically linking diagnosis codes to literature allows the information to be emailed or printed and reviewed with the client, increasing understanding, and therefore impacting compliance. It is also important to link inventory products (prescriptions and OTC if available) that are sold to client education literature that lists potential drug interactions and side effects. Linking literature to the diagnosis codes and inventory increases the efficiency of the team member, while also documenting in the medical record that the client received the literature.

VHMA PERFORMANCE DOMAIN TASK:

Practice managers must develop and manage client education protocols and processes.

THIRD-PARTY INTEGRATIONS

There are many third-party integrations that should be considered when purchasing or upgrading a PIMS. Some PIMS don't play friendly with third-party integrations, but they significantly increase the efficiency of the team. Another important consideration (which is PIMS-specific) is if the third-party application can write back to the PIMS. As an example, the practice partners with an online pharmacy to fill prescriptions for clients. The practice must either write the script for the client or, the client requests the product through the online pharmacy and the practice authorizes filing the product. Regardless of either choice, the medical record must document the prescription (name of the product, strength, dose, label instructions, and DVM authorization). What if the online pharmacy integrated with the medical record and added that information automatically to the medical record? That is the power of efficiency and accuracy, and why more third-party integrations are important to consider. Fig. 8.6 provides applications that integrate with PIMS at the time of publication. However, a new technology comes to the market every year. Keep an open ear and eye for technology that can continue impacting efficiency in the practice.

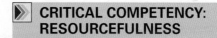

POTENTIAL THIRD-PARTY PIMS INTEGRATIONS FOR MAXIMAL EFFICIENCY

- Care Credit or other financing options
- Pet health insurance
- Wellness plans
- Pet portals
- Practice specific app
- Two-way texting and email to enhance communications with clients
- Vetstoria: giving the clients the opportunity to make appointments online
- AVA; the artificial intelligence receptionist that can handle overflow and prescription refills
- Internal messaging to help keep the team aligned
- Quick Books: import practice revenue centers from PIMS for accurate P&L statements and balance sheets
- Time clocks for team members to clock in, and import to Quick Books for payroll
- Telehealth
- Voice dictation for medical records

Fig. 8.6 Example of third-party integrations that should be considered when building an effective and efficient PIMS.

CRITICAL COMPETENCY: RESOURCEFULNESS

The practice manager must have the ability to understand what it takes to complete the job by applying knowledge, skills, and expertise to perform tasks quickly and efficiently.

Another type of integration that is important to clients is pet portals or practice apps. Historically in veterinary medicine, practice owners have been afraid to share all the client's data for many fears that are not real.

- "Clients might share their records with another veterinarian for a second opinion." Practices copy records when clients leave regardless.
- "Clients will research on the internet and try to self-diagnose." They do anyway.
- "A client might sue the practice." Perhaps if they have reason to, and they still will (but that is why we practice standard of care, all the time).

Defining the term "data" is important, but more important is the outcome of the transparency when data is shared. Data that the practice should share includes vaccine administration and certificates, reminders, lab results, radiographs, and, for full transparency, the medical record. Consider a client that needs to take their pet to the emergency room over the weekend or at night when the practice is closed. Being able to share medical records with the ER doctor saves time and money and allows more precise patient treatments. When clients have access to their medical records, they (records) must be completed by the doctor at the completion of each visit.

Clients should have the ability to text the practice to provide updates for their pet, make an appointment, and refill medications. Take the burden off the reception team and allow clients to interact through a practice portal or app versus calling the practice. In addition, direct messages can be sent to clients through integrated options when the practice is closed for holidays, bad weather, etc.

When clients have full transparency and easy access to their medical records, they feel empowered and a part of their pet's healthcare, resulting in trust and compliance, therefore strengthening the client-practice bond and leading to long-term client retention.[2]

CHOOSING THE IDEAL PIMS

The ideal PIMS is different for each practice. Finding the one that meets the practice needs can be overwhelming. Start with a gap analysis of the current state and future state of the PIMS (consider 10 years from now). What slows efficiency today with the existing PIMS? What does the practice wish the PIMS could do easier, faster, and more efficiently? Moving to Electronic Medical Records (EMR) from paper records or changing an existing PIMS due to gaps may be perceived as a scary change, and the concept can be rejected when a comfort zone is established with the current system. When completing a gap analysis (see Chapter 12 for an example), every position within the practice should be represented to establish software needs. Receptionists have important client check-in/check-out features that the technician team does not, and technicians have whiteboard needs that the receptionist may not. Managers would need to have the ability to easily generate reports, while veterinarians may be most concerned with the ability to dictate medical records (Fig. 8.7).

CRITICAL COMPETENCY: DECISION MAKING

The practice manager must be able to make good decisions based on critical thinking and problem solving, and their decisions must positively impact the practice. While many alternatives are available, the PM must be able to gather and effectively analyze relevant data and choose decisively.

VHMA CRITICAL COMPETENCY

Analytical Skills

The practice manager must have the ability to grasp complex information, analyze information and use logic to address problems accurately, quickly, and efficiently.

Appoint an in-house IT person who can support the integration/upgrade and understands internet bandwidth and the impact it has on PIMS efficiency, printers, and how they are connected to labels, client

FACTORS TO CONSIDER WHEN CHOOSING A PRACTICE INTEGRATED MANAGEMENT SYSTEM

SOFTWARE CONSIDERATIONS

- Evaluate which software will meet the current and future needs of the practice.
- Does the software integrate with third-party applications (for example: to calculate drugs and alert for potential interactions with other previously prescribed medications for the patient)? Consider that apps are released every year. Can the PIMS integrate with new technology, or only integrate apps developed by that specific PIMS company.
- Can the software be tested in a 'sandbox environment'? A demo shows all the bells and whistles but doesn't let you play in the sandbox and to see if it is the 'right' software.
- Does the existing PIMS have an electronic medical records version?
- What training options are provided? Does a consultant train onsite or just virtually?
- What is the PIMS process to convert data if changing software providers?
- Does a seat license need to be purchased per user or per workstation?
- Does the software support a whiteboard set up allowing treatments to be auto invoiced when completed?
- Reporting: can files be exported in Excel and PDF for analyses?

CONNECTIVITY CONSIDERATIONS

- What is the bandwidth of internet that serves the practice?
- What cabling exists in the practice, and will it need to be upgraded to support the fastest bandwidth possible?
- Will more electrical outlets need to be added to support additional workstations?

EFFICIENCY CONSIDERATIONS

- Where should workstations be placed for optimal efficiency?
  - Check in and out for CSR
  - Phone room
  - Exam rooms
  - Lab area
  - Pharmacy
  - Multi in treatment area
  - DVM office
  - Tech office
  - Boarding kennels
- Consider how the practice will scan existing medical records and upload PDFs into the new EMR.
- Determine what templates, diagnostic codes, and treatment bundle codes should be created.

HARDWARE CONSIDERATIONS

- Review hardware requirements that the PIMS needs on each workstation to always work efficiently.
- Consider tablets or iPads, allowing electronic consent forms to be reviewed and signed with the owner.
- Is a digital camera needed to take pictures of patients?
- How will old radiographs be scanned and imported into medical records?
- Calculate an estimate of all costs, including hardware and software acquisition.

Fig. 8.7 Choosing the right PIMS to meet practice needs can be difficult when all factors have not been considered.

education literature, or electronic client consent forms. PIMS have glitches; having a team member onsite that understands the technology portion of the PIMS reduces the stress load on leadership and the team.

Cloud Base or Local Server for PIMS Backup

Cloud base is defined as all data being stored "in the cloud" versus on a server that stays at the practice. Practice leaders traditionally have been fearful of placing data in a cloud-based system, but with the help of a knowledgeable IT expert that has experience with encrypting files, the cloud is safer than a local server. I.T. Guru is a veterinary-specific company that specializes in IT infrastructure, security monitoring, business continuity, and cloud-based migration services, all while having a broad knowledge of most PIMS in the veterinary industry. An IT professional is only expensive when you don't have one, experience the loss of data, or worse yet, a cyberattack in which all client data is stolen and held for ransom.

Cloud base systems allow a continuous backup to occur, never losing data. This is the best and safest method to secure data when one considers potential theft, fire, or damage from natural disasters. If a local server is chosen to store data on, computers should be backed up ideally every hour, daily at a minimum. In addition, backups must be tested to ensure the backup is in fact occurring, and that data can be restored when a server crashes. Servers should be stored appropriately on a rack in a cool room, not on a floor that has the potential to flood and collects hair and dust (Fig. 8.8).

Another advantage of a cloud-based PIMS is the auto updates that occur when new solutions are implemented. If there is a configuration error, a software engineer can remote into the PIMS and immediately correct the issue. Cloud-based PIMS tend to be a bit more innovative and are always looking for ways to improve security, functionality, and efficiency. In fact, cloud-based PIMS take pride in continuously monitoring threats and are responsible for security management.

Practices that choose a local-based server normally have higher hardware costs associated with maintenance and replacement of equipment, as well as the initial upfront purchase of the software (or upgrade from a paper version). Cloud-based PIMS have lower costs associated with equipment maintenance, have fewer requirements, and usually pay on a per-month basis for a subscription to the platform.

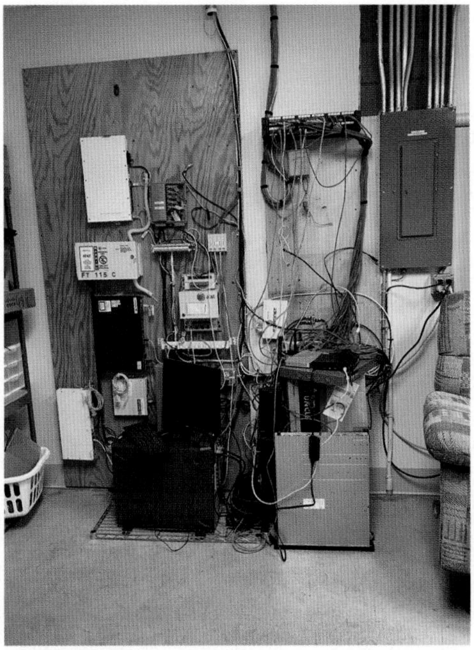

Fig. 8.8 PIMS equipment must be stored properly to reduce the risk of data loss.

There is always a concern about losing electrical power and the inability to utilize any PIMS. While battery backups may work for local workstations, the practice would still likely not have internet. Therefore, a secondary plan for cloud-based PIMS is to be able to access from any personal mobile device, allowing records to still be accessed.

Preparing the Team for Change

The greatest obstacle to any PIMS conversion is the team. There will be bumps in the road that must be addressed; learning new processes always slows efficiency and causes temporary frustration. Identify team members who may be most resistant to change and create a plan to work closely with them. Chapter 2 discusses the causes of change resistance and offers methods to keep the team forward focused. When a substantial change of this nature is to take place, introduce the concept to the team early, get them involved in the gap analysis, and get them excited. Reassure that training and support will be built in, resulting in reduced errors and misfiles and increased efficiency, in addition to the gaps that were identified in the initial analysis. Complete a change planning form (Fig. 2.24) to effectively prepare.

> **VHMA CRITICAL COMPETENCY**
>
> **Critical and Strategic Thinking**
>
> Strategic thinking and planning are essential to financial forecasting, marketing plans, and long-term plans for growth of the practice. Managers must have the ability to identify questions, problems, and arguments relevant to these issues and to use logic and critical reasoning to identify the strengths and weaknesses of alternative solutions or approaches to problems.

Common Barriers

A small percentage of team members will always experience barriers to change. That is a normal process. A great leader storms through barriers and carries the team to success. Some of the largest barriers experienced with moving to a new PIMS (or upgrading) are the fear of technology, being unable to efficiently type, and not having paper charts in front of them when visiting with clients.

Address fears head-on. Acknowledge that change is scary, but with training, the support of a strong team, and the ease of use of the chosen software, technology will help the practice achieve goals identified by the gap analysis.

Older-generation team members are afraid of not being able to type efficiently and "feel" it will slow the process. Typing with efficiency takes practice, as does everything. However, dictation software and/or the use of veterinary assistants/technicians can help any doctor that is worried about decreased efficiency. Ensure the chosen software has dictation as an embedded feature, or that a third-party application can be integrated. In addition, having a support team member entering the exam findings (in PIMS) as the doctor verbalizes them to the client brings efficiency to a new level. When clients "hear it and see it," their understanding and compliance dramatically increase (Chapter 12).

Removing paper charts from doctors is stressful and understandable. This is a change of years of habit. Remind the doctors that the information is still present in the medical record, and is simply getting used to the new location. Address the emotional component that a doctor may feel like they look incompetent in front of a client while they adjust to the computer format reviewing the history. Remind them that it takes time to get comfortable with a new process and help the veterinarian look great in front of the client by assigning a support team member to the doctor(s) to ease any fear, concern, or frustration.

CRITICAL COMPETENCY: LEADERSHIP

Practice managers must have the initiative to lead and take charge while simultaneously motivating and mobilizing others to achieve common goals.

Security of PIMS

A practice integrative management system is the heart of the practice, and it must be secure. Every team member must be set up with security levels to ensure that records are not changed, payments are not deleted, and the price of services and inventory cannot be altered. Consider the roles of each individual and what they should have access to. A receptionist, veterinary assistant, veterinary technician, and doctor who does not have management responsibility should not be able to access reports, change the appointment calendar setup, or delete line items or closed invoices. A lead receptionist may have access to the appointment calendar setup, accounts receivable functions and reports, and end-of-day/month reports. A lead technician may have access to a whiteboard and inventory functions. The practice manager and owner should have access to all and be the only individuals that can change security settings for any other team members.

IMPLEMENTATION OF NEW OR UPGRADED PIMS

Creating an implementation plan is critical to the success of software changes. Build in time to build the base right. The more work put into the program at the beginning yields greater success in the end. It can take 6 months to a year to pick a system and implement it; the more prepared the practice is to accept change, the easier the process. Be sure to choose the right PIMS for the practice; the one that impacts team efficiency and the client experience the most.

CRITICAL COMPETENCY: PLANNING AND PRIORITIZING

Practice managers must be able to effectively manage time and workload to meet deadlines, thereby having the ability to organize work, set priorities, and establish plans to achieve goals.

Most software vendors provide a consultant to aid in the process of converting the practice data and helping the practice manager/owner set up the new system. Questionnaires may need to be completed by the practice manager, helping the consultant create a guide to success. In addition, consider the value of having the consultant/trainer onsite with the practice team during the first few days of implementation. They have the experience, answers, and a support team that can remote in when needed and can make suggestions to help ease the stress throughout the first few days. This will be an added charge but may be completely worth it, depending on the comfort level of the team with virtual learning.

Successful implementations are strategically planned, have team buy-in, and are well-executed. Celebrate each day of implementation week. Each day is a win as the team learns processes. Acknowledge the stress and hard work of every team member and give thanks. PIMS integrations is a team sport! Fig. 8.9 provides implementation guidelines.

LEADERSHIP'S ROLE IN PIMS

The Practice Integrative Management Software is the heart of the practice that drives efficiency, customer service, exceptional medicine, and patient care. But it must be set up right, and all elements of the system must be used to maximal capacity. There are many third-party integrations that can be added (depending on the PIMS) that will further enhance efficiency and help the team work smarter, thereby decreasing burnout, client complaints, and missed patient treatments. The practice manager and owner must set time aside to look for opportunities for improvement (which may include a change in software) for the long-term health of the practice. Once maximal capacity is identified in all areas, reevaluate on a yearly basis to see if software upgrades and/or new technology can be implemented to further drive efficiency and enhance the frictionless client experience (Chapter 11).

PRACTICE MANAGER'S SURVIVAL CHECKLIST FOR PIMS

- ☐ Ensure PIMS is secured against medical record alteration.
- ☐ Set security access levels in the PIMS, preventing changes to pricing, appointment schedule template, invoice deletion, client list, etc.
- ☐ Create a protocol for database backup (including dental and general radiographs and laboratory results).
- ☐ Research available technology that will integrate with existing PIMS to enhance efficiency.
- ☐ Build templates, diagnostic codes, and bundled plans.
- ☐ Attach client education literature to templates, diagnostic codes, and inventory items that are prescribed.

STAGES OF PIMS IMPLEMENTATION

PLANNING STAGE (ONCE A PIMS HAS BEEN CHOSEN)

- Set goals up front. Pick a go live date and work backward from that date. Consider a slower season to go live.
- Determine how paper records will be converted to EMR, which clients will be converted (active vs inactive), and the equipment needed to efficiently scan (consider renting verses purchasing). If deciding not to scan inactive clients, review record retention laws for remaining paper charts.
- Determine how radiographs (both dental and skeletal) will be stored.
- If an onsite sever is chosen for data storage, determine the process for hourly backups, and a contingency plan should the server crash.
- Outline protection protocols to mitigate the risk of hacking.
- Identify where workstations will be placed for maximal team efficiency.
- Build in time for building the 'base' and establishing set protocols for templates, diagnostic codes, bundled treatment plans, and client education literature.
- Develop a plan to move the team to electronic whiteboard use.
- Determine the timeline and process to convert and test data to ensure conversion accuracy.
- Determine the fears/barriers of the staff and develop change management plans to overcome.
- Establish security levels and a sensible entry lock out time.

MONTH 1

Develop an implementation team: a project leader that is responsible for implementation, a superuser, and a transition team (one receptionist, technician, and veterinarian).

Have the implementation teamwork through the following areas:

- Planning the ideal practice workflow. Assess current workflow and determine what the ideal workflow is (gap analysis) when:
  - Making appointments
  - Checking in/checking out clients
  - Credit Card integration
  - Reminder integration (or outsource)
  - The exam room flow:
  - Medical record entry
    - Development of treatment plans
    - Determine templates, diagnostic codes, treatment bundle codes, and client literature that needs to be set up
  - The treatment room flow:
    - Whiteboard
    - Treatment/patient data/observation entries into medical record.

MONTH 2

- Set up templates, diagnostic codes, treatment bundle codes, and client literature.
- Tie services, diagnostic codes, treatment codes to reminders, call backs.

MONTH 3

- Data integration should begin if not sooner. Test data in a "sandbox" with updates templates, diagnostic codes, treatment bundle codes, client literature and assumed workflow.
- Be open to adjustments!

MONTH 4

- Begin to train the team in the sandbox.
- Start transitioning paper records to electronic (scan and import)—ask the vendor for support/suggestions to make this efficient.

GO LIVE TIPS:

- Plan on making tweaks the day of.
- Extend appointment times for the week, add additional team members for support, block some appointments to "catch up" if needed.
- Have 2 assistants in exam rooms; one to hold the patient, 1 to capture medical record notes.
- Let clients know you are bringing in a new system through social media and posted signs, ask for their patience as the practice strives to bring greater efficiency and service for them.
- Have food. Have fun. Celebrate each day. It's a win with a new system!

Fig. 8.9 Strategically plan for a PIMS integration to yield the best outcome for the team, clients, and patient experiences.

REVIEW QUESTIONS

1. Describe how critical competency resourcefulness applies to the evaluation and management of a PIMS.
2. How does critical competency adaptability apply to the implementation of new technologies?
3. How does the PIMS play a role in practice efficiency?
4. Why is it important to implement the online feature that allows clients to make their own appointments?
5. Explain why it is important for credit card terminals to be integrated with the PIMS.

REFERENCES

1. Brice M. Testimonial on Vetstoria website. Accessed August 2022. https://www.vetstoria.com/
2. Jones L. Top 5 Perks of Having a Pet Portal Directly in your Practice Management Software. July 13, 2022. Shepherd Veterinary Practice Management Software. Accessed August 2022. https://www.shepherd.vet

9

Medical Records Management

LEARNING OBJECTIVES

When you have completed this chapter, you should be able to:

- Identify components of a medical record
- Discuss the importance of obtaining an accurate patient history
- Define each component of SOAP
- Identify common abbreviations
- Explain how to purge medical records
- Identify when a medical records release is needed
- List the most common medical record violations and explain methods to mitigate each violation
- Discuss the advantages of EMRs
- Define leadership's role in medical records management

OUTLINE

KEY TERMS

Client discharge instructions
Diagnosis
EMRs
Medical Records
Medical Records Release Form
Primary Complaint
Prognosis
Record Retention
SOAP

INTRODUCTION

Medical records are the most important documents in veterinary medicine, and medical record management is one of the most important management tasks. A medical record is a permanent written account of the professional interaction and services rendered in a valid patient-client relationship. Medical records serve several purposes in medicine, most importantly providing an accurate historical account for the veterinary health care team and owner, enabling any veterinary team member to review the patient history, assess current needs, and document recommendations for future needs. Medical records provide team members with a means of communication, alert them to a patient's special needs, serve as documentation for referrals and as evidence in a court of law, and are an asset to the veterinary practice. Records must always be complete, legible, and easily accessible.

Most practices started with paper medical records and have transitioned to electronic medical records (EMR) over the years. Inactive records (clients that have not been seen for 12 months or more and likely paper records that were never converted to EMR) must be kept for a certain length of time (covered later in this chapter) and can be purged after a set period. The most important thing to remember is that all communication with the owner must be documented in the medical record, either verbally or in any written material. A medical record and all the supporting documents can become evidence in a civil suit, malpractice suit, or board investigation. The old saying *"if it was not documented, it did not happen"* is true and serves as the only evidence that the practice has in its defense.

During the COVID pandemic, more than 23 million households adopted a pet. At the same time, owners became accustomed to technology such as zoom and FaceTime to maintain connectivity with colleagues and family. Immediate adaption to technology and the expectation to have immediate access to data became the norm.[1]

With staff shortages, increased demand for services, and expectations from clients, veterinary practices must continue finding ways to increase efficiency and make it easy for clients to do business with

VHMA PERFORMANCE DOMAINS

Veterinary Hospital Managers Association (VHMA) Performance Domains

Performance domains applicable to medical records include law and ethics, and organization of the practice. Practice managers must:

- Understand and ensure compliance with appropriate regulatory agencies, including local, state, and federal authorities.
- Ensure compliance with legal and ethical guidelines surrounding the confidentiality of clients, patients, and team members.
- Maintain an appropriate medical records system that complies with legal standards and establishes policies for the use of technology in the practice.

Application of VHMA Performance Domains for Practice Managers

Ensuring that medical records are compliant with regulatory agencies mitigates the risk of potential board complaints, fines, and lawsuits while enhancing the performance, knowledge, skills, and abilities of the practice manager. Tasks in this domain require a working knowledge of medical terminology and requirements for medical procedures (radiology, safety, anesthesia, biohazards).

the practice. EMRs can integrate with third-party applications and is essential to remaining competitive, meeting client demands, and developing work-life balance for the team. While paper practices can still share data with the most current software version, what can be shared is minimal, likely creating a friction full client experience.

Examples of third-party applications include pet portals, a practice-specific app, two-way texting, reminder services, and an online pay portal (see Chapter 8, PIMS).

CRITICAL COMPETENCY: RESOURCEFULNESS

The practice manager must have the ability to understand what it takes to complete the job by applying knowledge, skills, and expertise to perform tasks quickly and efficiently.

COMPONENTS OF A MEDICAL RECORD

Each medical record must have the same information, regardless of the type of pet, client, or veterinary software used. The organization of the medical record depends on practice preference; however, most hospitals use a reverse chronological order system, with the most recent records being visible first. The following list is required of all medical record entries, regardless of paper or EMR.

VHMA PERFORMANCE DOMAIN TASK

Maintain an appropriate medical records system that complies with legal standards.

Client/Patient Information Sheet: It is critical that the owner complete the client information with as much detail as possible online, through their portal, the practice app, or upon arrival. Additionally, client information must be verified at each visit to ensure the cell phone number and email address are still current.

Previous Medical History: If a patient has been seen by another veterinarian and received prior medical treatment, the patient's history should be entered. The medical record from the previous practice can be stored as a PDF and a synopsis can be recorded in the first exam and the master problem list.

Vaccination History: Each patient should have some type of vaccine history unless it is a young puppy or kitten. Dates and types of vaccines administered should be entered. Once the patient has established a history with the practice, the vaccine history will be updated automatically. It is important to document where vaccines have been administered to the pet's body for future reference.

The Primary Complaint: This will accurately summarize the client's complaint and the history of the presenting problem. The complaint is provided by the owner and is the reason for their visit. They may also provide a history of the presenting complaint which should also be documented.

LEADERSHIP POINT

When veterinarians examine a patient, they may find more issues than just the primary complaint. While some of those issues may be more critical, always ensure the primary complaint is addressed or the client will feel that their concern was not "heard."

Physical Examination (PE): The results of the pet's PE must be documented for each visit. If the animal is hospitalized, the patient must receive progress examinations daily. These too must be documented in the record. Temperature (T); weight (WT); respiratory rate (RR); heart rate (HR); pain (P); body condition score (BCS); mucous membrane color (mm); capillary refill time (crt); eyes/ears/nose/throat (E/E/N/T); auscultation of the chest (H/L); palpation of the abdomen (Abd); examination of the lymph nodes (LN); musculoskeletal system (MS); and urogenital (Uro) must be documented. Many team members abbreviate terms, descriptions, and abnormalities. Please see the appendixes for common abbreviations used in veterinary medicine. If a PE is omitted from the medical record, or a particular body system has been omitted, it is assumed that the examination did not occur. Templates should be used to help ensure that body systems are not missed during an exam.

Diagnosis and/or Possible Diagnosis: Diagnosis is the identification of a disease by analysis and examination. The patient may have one or several diseases and all must be documented.

Laboratory Reports: All laboratory results (normal and abnormal), including radiographs, ultrasounds, and electrocardiograms, must be documented. If a consult was completed by a specialty veterinarian, that also must be documented in the record (date, method of consult, results, and any follow-up communications). See the section on the SOAP format in this chapter for more details on laboratory interpretations.

Treatment: Any treatment recommendations and/or medications must be documented in the medical record. See the section on the SOAP format for more details on notating medications.

Prognosis: A prognosis is the prediction of the outcome of the disease. The prognosis must be communicated to the client and documented in the record. The prognosis may help the client decide what medical route to take when treating a pet. The prognosis will likely change with treatment, laboratory results, and surgery. When it does change, the record must be updated.

Surgical report: Any surgical procedure must be described in detail (including anesthesia used and duration of, size of the intubation tube, type and size of suture material, patient monitoring, and the initials of all technicians and veterinarians working the case, just to list a few). Include complications that might be expected postoperatively.

Treatment Plans (Estimates) and Consent Forms: Each client must give consent for treatment. If a treatment protocol has been recommended, it should be documented in the medical record and clients should receive an estimate. Both the consent to treat form and the client estimate should be signed. If a client declines any of the recommended treatments, that must also be entered into the medical record.

VHMA PERFORMANCE DOMAIN TASK

Ensure a full understanding of contract law as it pertains to treatment plans and consent forms.

A master problem list is an extremely beneficial summary of the patient's medical history and is autogenerated by EMRs but is a manual process that should be created for paper practices. A master problem list should include the patient's name, gender, species, breed, age, diet, allergies (including any environmental, food or to medications, vaccines, or anesthetics), current medications, and any vaccinations the pet has received. Although the master problem list is not required to complete the medical record, it increases the team's efficiency when refilling medications and determining vaccines for which the patient may be due. Fig. 3.27 (Chapter 3) provides an example of a master problem list.

Obtaining an Accurate History

An accurate history is one of the most important aspects of the medical record. All the information the owner has presented must be summarized in the objective section of the medical record. This allows the doctor to easily review the presenting facts and may help diagnose the case more rapidly and accurately. Often clients will chat with team members and give valuable information that the client did not realize was pertinent. For example, a client may indicate that they were recently on vacation in Florida (and how great it was), but Fluffy is presenting with diarrhea.

- Did the pet go on vacation with the owners?
- Was the pet exposed to a new environment?
- Was the pet fed a new diet? Did the pet drink water from the ocean?
- Did Fluffy eat bird droppings on the beach?
- Were any special treats given?
- If the pet did not go on the trip, who stayed home with Fluffy?
- Did a house sitter stay with Fluffy? Or did Fluffy go to a boarding kennel?

These are all important questions that should be asked during a conversation about a client's recent vacation (Fig. 9.1).

SOAP Records

A standard SOAP format (**S**ubjective, **O**bjective, **A**ssessment, and **P**lan) is followed for medical records in the veterinary profession.

Subjective information is the most important element for the reception staff, veterinary technicians, and assistants. Subjective details include the reason for the office visit, the history, and observations made by the client. The opinions and perceptions of the client represent the most subjective information.

LIST OF QUESTIONS TO ASK WHEN OBTAINING PATIENT HISTORY

NUTRIENT INTAKE
- Is the pet eating normally?
- What is the pet fed?
- When was the last meal?
- How much did the pet eat?
- How often does the pet eat?
- What treats are offered? How often?

DRINKING
- Is the pet drinking the same amount of water as usual?
- How often?
- How much? Or how often is the water bowl filled?

VOMITING
- How often is the pet vomiting?
- What color is the vomit?
- What does the vomit consist of?
- Has the pet eaten any toys, blankets, or towels?

BOWEL MOVEMENTS
- Is the pet defecating normally?
- What does the stool look like (color and consistency)?
- How often is the pet defecating?
- Any straining to defecate?
- If the patient has abnormal bowel movements, when did the abnormal signs start?

URINATION
- How often does the pet urinate?
- Is the pet urinating the same amount as always?
- Is the urine a clear, steady stream?
- Any straining to urinate?
- If the patient is having abnormal urination, when did the abnormal signs start?

COUGHING
- Does the pet cough or gag?
- If so, how often?
- When did the coughing start?
- How often does the pet cough?
- How long does the episode last?

SNEEZING
- When did the pet begin sneezing?
- Does the pet have any discharge from the eyes and nose with the sneezing?
- If yes, what color is the discharge?

WALKING
- Is the pet walking normally?
- If not, when did the abnormal signs begin?
- Is the pet limping or not bearing weight on an extremity?
- If yes, which one?
- Did the owner see any trauma happen to the pet?

GROWTH(S)
- What is the location of the growth?
- How long has the growth been present?
- Has any previous diagnostic work been completed before?
- Has it increased in size? How much?
- Has the growth changed color? How much?

MISCELLANEOUS
- Swelling: Where is the location of the swelling?
- Swelling: When was the swelling noticed?
- Discharge from the eyes: When was the discharge first noticed?
- Discharge from the eyes: What color is it? Is the pet squinting the eye(s)?
- Is pet scratching? If yes, how often and where?
- Have any parasites been seen?
- Have you noticed fowl breath or trouble eating?

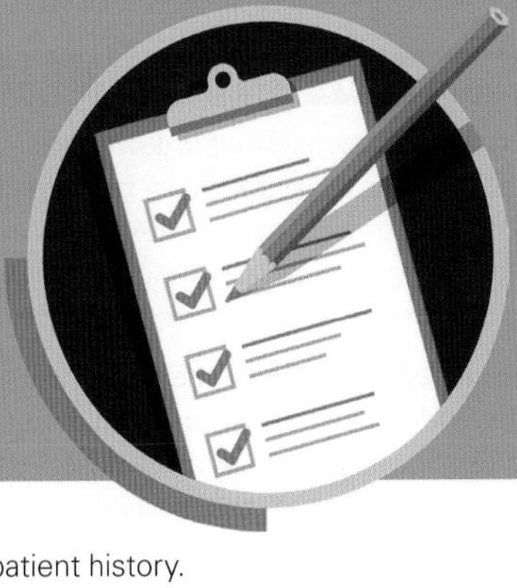

Fig. 9.1 Both open- and closed-ended questions should be used when obtaining a complete patient history.

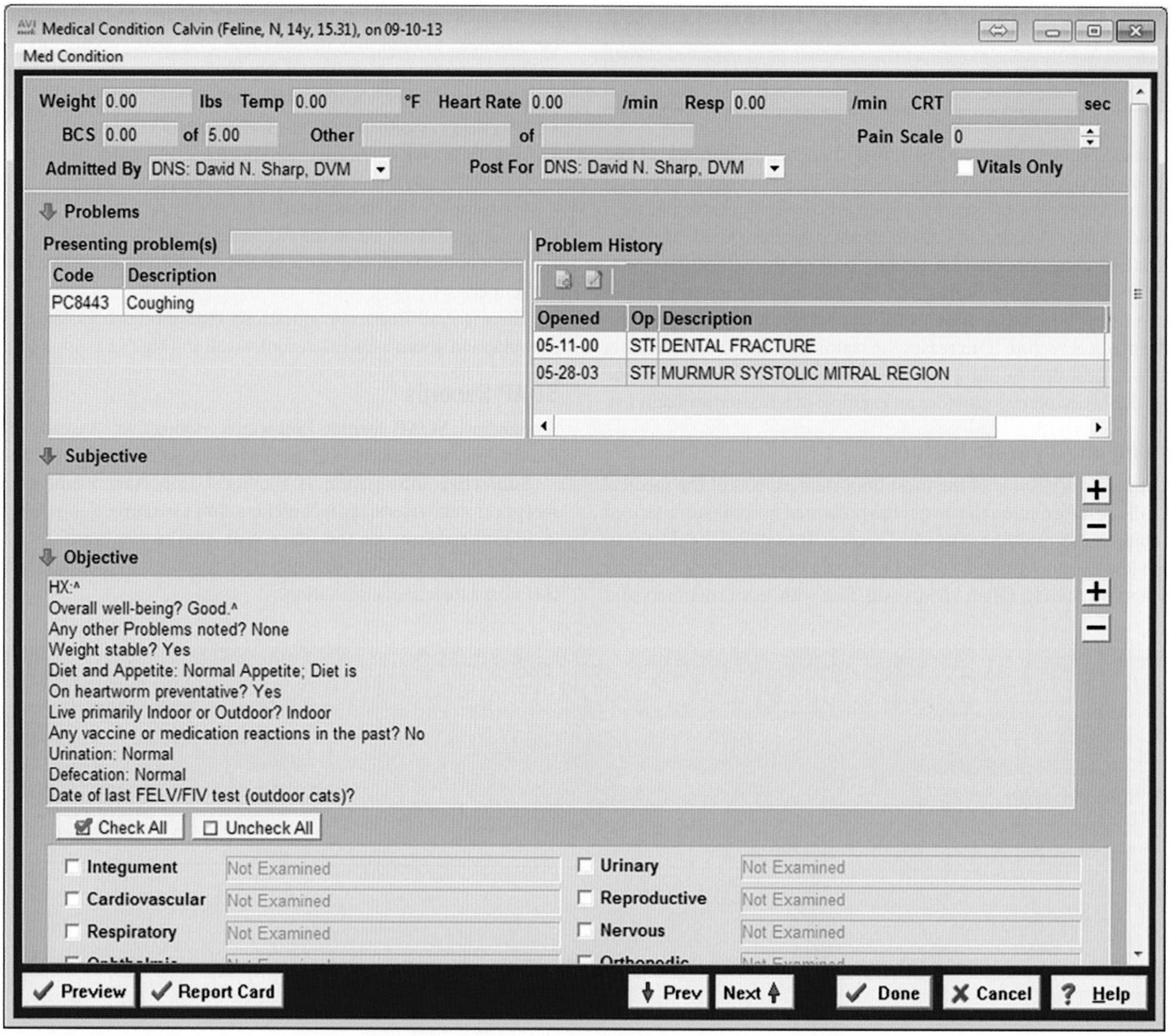

Fig. 9.2 Example of AVImark's medical record, SOAP format. (Courtesy AVImark, LLC, Piedmont, Mo.)

Objective information is gathered directly from the patient during the physical examination and the vitals. Objective information is factual information (Fig. 9.2).

The **Assessment** includes any conclusions reached from the subjective and objective sections and includes a definitive diagnosis. If there are multiple, or tentative diagnoses, they should all be documented, along with a list of "rule-ins" (R/I) or "rule-outs" (R/O). R/I can be classified as any disease the patient could possibly have as well as diagnostic work that must be completed to rule out specific diseases.

LEADERSHIP POINT

By leveraging experienced team members to deliver treatment plans to clients, veterinarians can see the next patient. When treatment plans are accepted by with client, the team member can then execute the plan and update the veterinarian when they have finished with the current patient.

A **Plan** is developed according to the assessment and includes treatment, surgery, intended diagnostics, and all communication with the owner. This can also be a list of options that will be presented to the client.

A prepared treatment plan with all costs should be given to the client. Full transparency of price and client education should be delivered by an experienced team member (not a doctor) and documented in the record. Once a client agrees to the specific recommendations, treatment can begin.

Progress notes will then follow in which the veterinarian must interpret the results, not just document them. Abnormal laboratory work values must be acknowledged in the medical record. Interpretation is defined as analyzing the results and explaining why abnormalities may be present. The list of rule-ins (R/Is) and rule-outs (R/Os) can be completed +/- the recommendation of further diagnostic workup. If previous lab work is used for comparison, that should also be documented in the progress notes. At this time, a prognosis of the case should be stated along with updated communications to the owner. A prognosis can be labeled as poor, guarded, fair, or excellent.

Patients must have a daily physical exam (PE) during hospitalization and receive medications as recommended by the doctor. Results of the PEs, an updated prognosis, medications administered (drug, dose, route of administration, who administered, and what time), urination, bowel movements, and/or vomiting must be documented in the progress notes. Hospitalization sheets can be used to help keep track of patient status while they are hospitalized for paper records, while whiteboards are used with EMRs. When a patient is hospitalized and a treatment plan/estimate is created in an EMR, it can be loaded into the whiteboard. Once treatments are completed, observations are made, or medications are administered, the notes should autopopulate the medical record and charges should be sent to the invoice.

Diligent team members can often catch common errors and omissions in a medical record before the record is locked (EMR) or filed (paper). Some of the most common errors include missing lab work interpretation, progress notes while the patient is hospitalized, preoperative physical examinations, administered anesthetic drugs, and/or initials of the author(s) documented in the record. The use of templates in EMRs can reduce potential errors.

Medication names, doses, and route given must be accurately written in the medical records. For example, "0.2 mL cefazolin IV" is an incorrect notation. This description does not indicate how many milligrams were given. The entry should read, "0.2 mL cefazolin (100 mg/mL), IV," or it may read "20 mg cefazolin, IV." Many drugs come in different strengths; it is important to identify and document the correct strength of medication. The same drug may also be administered using different routes (some drugs will have a different dose depending on the route administered); it is therefore important to document by which route the medication was administered (Fig. 9.3).

If fluids are administered to patients, records must clearly indicate the name of the fluid(s), the amount the pet is receiving, and the route given (IV or subcutaneously). If a pet is simply receiving Plasmalyte under the skin, the attending veterinarian or technician should indicate the number of milliliters administered. However, if a patient is receiving a drip intravenously, the rate must be indicated. "Plasmalyte, 66 mL/kg/24 hours = 100 mL/hr IV" is an acceptable entry.

When medications are dispensed, the same principles apply. The name of the drug must be recorded, along with the strength, route of administration, frequency, and duration of treatment. If a team member has administered the medication in the examination room, it must be documented in the medical record as well. Team members should always initial labels on prescriptions they have filled and indicate in the medical record that they filled the request.

Radiographs

Patient radiographs are an integral part of the medical record. Digital radiographs are auto-labeled with the veterinary hospital name and address, client's last name, patient's name, date, and view. In EMR practices, the views can be requested via the PIMS, therefore allowing the images to autopopulate the medical record. A paper practice with digital radiography will have views stored in a PACs- or cloud-based system that must be accessed to view. To attach old films to a new PIMS, a picture of the radiograph can be taken and uploaded into the medical record.

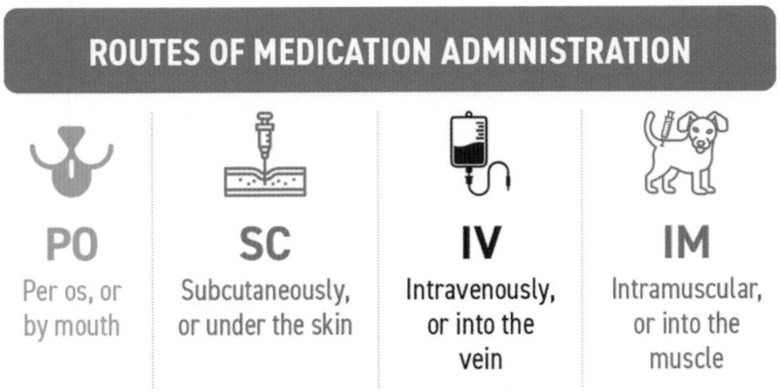

ROUTES OF MEDICATION ADMINISTRATION
PO
Per os, or by mouth
SC
Subcutaneously, or under the skin
IV
Intravenously, or into the vein
IM
Intramuscular, or into the muscle

Fig. 9.3 All team members, including receptionists should be familiar with common abbreviations used in medical records.

> **CRITICAL COMPETENCY: CRITICAL AND STRATEGIC THINKING**
>
> Strategic thinking and planning are essential to financial forecasting, marketing plans, and long-term plans for growth of the practice. Managers must have the ability to identify questions, problems, and arguments relevant to these issues and to use logic and critical reasoning to identify the strengths and weaknesses of alternative solutions or approaches to problems.

Client Discharge Instructions

Client discharge instructions are very important (Fig. 9.4), as clients will only remember 30% of the information provided while they were in the practice. EMR practices can autogenerate client instructions based on diagnosis codes or treatment plans, with an electronic copy saved in the medical record. In paper practices, team members should print out or email materials to the owner. These instructions and materials must be reviewed verbally with the client before discharging the patient. It is also a good idea to keep a copy of the materials given to the owner in the record, or at least make a note of the materials provided. It may also be beneficial to have the owners sign an acknowledgment of the materials received.

COMMON ABBREVIATIONS

Standard abbreviations are standard operating procedures (SOP) in veterinary practices and literature, increasing the efficiency of the team. Memorizing and using abbreviations are strongly recommended for every team member; examples of abbreviations are in the appendixes of this book. Consider the following example and the impact abbreviations have on efficiency:

- IV Normosol fluids maintenance rate; NPO ×12 hrs: sx in a.m.: 12 mg cefazolin IV pre/post sx; increase fluids to sx rate; 3 mg buprenorphine SQ pre/post op.
- This can be interpreted as meaning that the patient will be receiving IV fluids with Normosol at the maintenance rate of 66 mL/kg/24 hours. The pet will receive nothing by mouth (NPO) for 12 hours before surgery (sx) and will have a surgical procedure in the morning. The patient will receive 12 milligrams (mg) of cefazolin IV both before and after surgery. The patient will also receive 3 mg of buprenorphine before and after surgery.

> **LEADERSHIP POINT**
>
> The use of correct, industry-relevant abbreviations dramatically improves practice efficiency.

MEDICAL RECORDS RELEASE FORM

Medical records are confidential and can only be released with owner consent. Clients should be required to sign a records release form that must be kept in the medical record. This includes releasing records to any other veterinary hospital, specialty clinic, boarding or grooming facilities, or transferring records to a new owner of the pet. A practice can be held liable for the release of records without the owner's written consent. It is important for the entire team to understand the Privacy Act and that no records may be released without a client's authorization. The Privacy Act of 1974 states in part:

No agency shall disclose any record, which is contained in a system of records by any means of communication to any person, or to another agency, except pursuant to a written request by, or with the

ABC Veterinary Clinic 555-555-5555
Dr. Roe, Dr. Morton, Dr. Larsen
Post-anesthesia Release Sheet

Please provide clean, dry bedding and a quiet place for your pet to recuperate. Please notify the hospital with any concerns.

DIET:
( ) Wait a few hours after arriving home to offer your pet water. Please give only a small amount. If no vomiting occurs, you may offer more water about an hour later. You may feed a small amount (1/4 normal amount) if water stays down.
( ) You may continue to feed your pet normally.
( ) Special diet instructions ____________________

ACTIVITY:
( ) Restrict exercise for 1 day. NO RUNNING, JUMPING, CLIMBING OR BATHING.
( ) Restrict exercise for 7 days. NO RUNNING, JUMPING, CLIMBING OR BATHING.
( ) Other ____________________

OTHER:
( ) Please use paper strips or pinto beans in place of litter for 7 days.
( ) Please booster vaccines in 3-4 weeks.
( ) Your pet's metabolism may permanently decrease after surgery. You may need to decrease the amount of food you feed to prevent obesity.

INCISION:
( ) Watch for swelling, redness, or drainage. Prevent scratching, rubbing, and licking of the incision. Please ask for an E-collar if you think your pet will lick the site.
( ) Ice incision for 5 minutes, 3 to 4 times daily for the first 72 hours.

MEDICATION:
( ) Give pain medication ____________________
( ) Give antibiotics ____________________
( ) Give other medication ____________________
____
( ) Start medication ____________________

FOLLOW-UP VISITS:
( ) Recheck in ________ days.
( ) There is no need to return for suture removal; the skin was closed with absorbable suture or tissue adhesive.
( ) Not necessary unless you feel there is a problem.

Comments:

Doctor ____________ Tech ____________ Client ____________ Date ____________

Fig. 9.4 Example of discharge instructions.

prior written consent of, the individual to whom the record pertains (US Department of Justice).

A client is entitled to a copy of their record. The original record is the property of the hospital, along with any diagnostic images and laboratory results; however, a client may request copies at any time. When a client is referred to a specialist, a copy of the record should be emailed, along with relevant images that have been taken.

All records must be kept confidential. Medical records cannot be discussed with other clients; the privacy of both the client and the pet must be respected.

If a client has access to their pet's portal and the practice allows all aspects of the medical record to be shared, then the client can share their pet's medical record. Pet portals give the ability to share vaccine status, medical history, lab and imaging results, medications, etc. When clients share their records with boarding facilities, groomers, or specialists, it saves the practice time by not having to prepare records to be sent. See further discussion on Pet Portals and third-party applications in Chapter 8, PIMS.

MOST COMMON MEDICAL RECORD VIOLATIONS

Euthanasia Without Consent: This seems like an unusual scenario, but it is not uncommon. How can pets be euthanized without consent? Surprisingly, some practices do not obtain a signature on a euthanasia consent form before performing the procedure. Case in point in this unfortunate example: A wife typically brings a pet to the hospital for care and her name is on the medical record. On this occasion, the husband brings in the pet and provides a legitimate reason for euthanasia, and the practice euthanized the pet at his request. Several weeks pass and the wife sues the hospital for negligence stating she did not authorize the procedure. The wife won the case because she did not consent to euthanasia, no consent form was signed, and her name (not his name) was listed on the medical record. The outcome of this lawsuit makes it clear that practices must always have complete medical records (both owners' names if applicable) and must include a consent to euthanize form signed by an authorized owner of the pet that is listed on the medical record.

The "Routine" Definition: The medical record states: "Routine castration or routine ovariohysterectomy was performed." What does routine mean? What may be routine in one hospital may not be routine in another. Procedures must always be documented in detail and thoroughly describe what treatment was completed. This can be averted with EMR templates.

LEADERSHIP POINT

Create templates that describe routine processes and procedures to improve medical record standards and efficiency, and mitigate the risk of a medical records violation.

Missing Physical Exam: If PE is not written in the record, it is assumed it was not completed, at all. This can be averted with EMR templates.

Client Refusals: Any time a client declines a service, procedure, or product, it must be indicated in the medical record. If the refusal is not documented in the medical record, a court of law will assume the service, procedure, or product was not offered as the practice cannot prove it was offered. This can be averted with EMR templates.

Legibility: Illegible records are a serious issue and contribute to errors made by the veterinary team that could injure a patient. Unreadable records may also contribute to a court ruling against a practice for lack of clear documentation, which can be averted with EMR.

These violations can be avoided with EMR templates, or stringent protocols regarding records completion in paper practices. Many violations occur due to lack of training, loss of focus, and poor time management. Practice managers must ensure every team member is trained on the proper procedures of medical record completion and implement time management strategies to aid in thorough completion.

HERD HEALTH RECORDS

It is impossible for large-animal veterinarians to have individual records for each food animal they examine. Herd health records refer to the practice of recording information for an entire herd, including medications and vaccinations on one record. Individual records may be kept if surgical procedures or special treatments are completed on one animal.

PURGING MEDICAL RECORDS

The length of time a practice must keep an inactive medical record varies from state to state. An inactive medical record is defined as a client who has not been seen by that practice for a year or more. Most states require medical records to be retained for at least 3 years, but some states have 7-year requirements (Fig. 9.5). Because some vaccine protocols have changed to administration every 3 years, some clients only return when vaccines are due. It is therefore more cost-effective for veterinary practices maintaining paper records to keep inactive files in a storage room on the premises where records can be easily accessed for the minimum number of years required by state law.

Most practices have limited space, and by purging and moving inactive records to another area of the practice, space can be freed up for current records. By reducing the number of active records, the possibility of loss from misfiling, misspelling, and misplacement, is reduced. Long-term storage can be arranged at an offsite storage facility until state law allows purging. Purged records must be shredded so that confidential information is not accessible and includes all laboratory work results, client informational sheets, or any authorization/release sheets that were signed by the client.

ELECTRONIC MEDICAL RECORDS

Practices that wish to improve team efficiency, morale, work-life balance, and client satisfaction have no choice but to upgrade to EMR. Paper and paper light practices are less efficient, have higher expenses, and have a significantly higher number of missed charges. Industry standards estimate that veterinary practices miss 5%–10% of annual revenue due to missed charges. For every $1 million in revenue,

Medical Record Retention by State

Length of time from last visit (including deceased animals)	State
3 years	AL, AZ, AR, CA, CO, DE, DC, FL, GA, ID, IN, KS, MD, MI, MN, MT, NE, NY, NC, ND, OH, OK, OR, PA, SC, TN, VA, WA, WV, WI, WY
4 years	MA, NV, NM
5 years	AK, IL, IA, KY, LA, MO, NH, NJ, RI, TX, UT
7 years	CT, VT

Patient medical records include laboratory reports, radiographs, rabies tag data, and health certificates.

Fig. 9.5 The length of time a practice must maintain medical records for patients varies by state.

$50,000-$100,000 is lost annually due to poor charge capture.[2] Allowing an EMR to autopopulate charges based on treatment plans and medical record entries significantly increases efficiency while recapturing lost revenue.

CRITICAL COMPETENCY DECISION MAKING

The practice manager must be able to make good decisions based on critical thinking and problem solving and their decisions must positively impact the practice. While many alternatives are available, the PM must be able to gather and effectively analyze relevant data and choose decisively.

In addition to charge capture, an EMR that is set up correctly can:

- Integrate with outside labs to order tests then auto-sync results when they are ready
- Auto-sync radiographs
- Create automatic discharge instructions and auto-generate client handouts when a diagnoses or treatment code is entered
- Allow reminders to be set for refills of medications, vaccines, or bloodwork
- Track inventory by subtracting medications and supplies based on medical record entry, set reorder points and reorder quantities
- Run and download reports to analyze business data

Some EMRs are excellent at providing medical record lockout periods; these lockout periods prevent medical record alteration after 24 hours (addendums can always be added with the date of the entry). Others do not have a lockout period, allowing records to be altered days or even months later (impacting financial reports). This disadvantage must be considered when choosing software for the practice.

Advantages of EMRs

The greatest advantage of EMRs is that they can be accessed from any computer. The most efficient practices have many workstations throughout the practice, allowing any team member immediate access. Having to wait for a workstation to become available brings efficiency to a grinding halt. Multiple workstations must be in the reception area, the phone room, the lab and pharmacy area, the treatment area, and one in each exam room, surgery, radiology, and kennel area (at minimum). Some practices also have tablets that team members can carry around; however, one must put down the tablet to carry a patient, also decreasing the efficiency as they must go back to retrieve the device (Fig. 9.6).

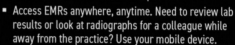

REASONS PRACTICES SHOULD CONSIDER MIGRATING TO ELECTRONIC MEDICAL RECORDS

- Increased efficiency
- No more searching for lost files; decreased stress on the team and allows them to spend more face time with clients and patients
- Access EMRs anywhere, anytime. Need to review lab results or look at radiographs for a colleague while away from the practice? Use your mobile device.
- Records are completed within the patient visit; spend more face-to-face time with clients, and no more after hours spent completing medical records
- Improved patient care and documentation with the use of templates
- Improved client service with the integration of patient portals and third-party applications (clients expect digital access to their pet's information)
- Improved charge capture with cross functioning templates that create estimates that when approved become treatment plans; when treatments are completed, they are invoiced; when diseases and conditions are diagnosed, client education materials are autogenerated
- Improved accuracy eliminating misinterpretation from illegible handwriting
- Autopopulating daily treatments, vitals, and patient observations
- Upload photos of lesions, tumors, lacerations, etc. into EMR to watch progression of treatment plan
- Electronically read and signed consent forms that can be emailed to clients
- Use of a template-based approach decreases the chance of missed steps in treatment protocols by aligning the medical standards of the veterinary team improving both team and client communications
- Space once used for paper medical records can be converted to a new profit center or improved workspace to for the team
- Improved staff morale, practice image, and marketing efforts

Fig. 9.6 Electronic medical records increase the efficiency of the team, allowing them to focus on delivering a frictionless client experience.

VHMA PERFORMANCE DOMAIN TASK

Established policies for the use of technology in veterinary practice.

LEADERSHIP'S ROLE IN MEDICAL RECORDS

A primary responsibility of the practice manager and owner is to manage medical record protocols. The paper practice manager should ensure records are being maintained thoroughly and consistently and completed daily. The EMR practice manager must ensure templates are being followed and team members are not taking shortcuts during data entry points. If managers note that medical records are not completed at the time of the patient visit, inefficiencies must be identified and changes implemented. Incomplete medical records at the time of invoicing and collecting payment from a client are leading causes of missed charges.

Practice managers should audit medical records on a regular basis to ensure accurate documentation is being entered, abbreviations are used correctly, records are completed, and all charges are captured. Improved PIMS options can eliminate many missed charges and improve team efficiency. See Chapter 8 for more details.

PRACTICE MANAGER'S SURVIVAL CHECKLIST FOR MEDICAL RECORDS

- ☐ Ensure PIMS is secured against medical record alteration.
- ☐ Create a protocol for the database backup.
- ☐ Develop protocols to protect client data and set PIMS security features that support the protection.
- ☐ Educate team members and have them sign a statement of confidentiality indicating they understand and will not release or share client, patient, or team member information outside of the practice.
- ☐ Confirm that common abbreviations are being used correctly.

- ☐ Create a medical records audit policy.
- ☐ Ensure that all medical records are completed in SOAP format that includes rule-ins/rule-outs, prognosis, and diagnosis.
- ☐ Ensure team members are documenting all recommendations in the medical records.
- ☐ Ensure that declined services by clients are documented in the medical record.
- ☐ Create a protocol for how often paper medical records are purged.
- ☐ Create a policy for shredding paper documents with client names on them.
- ☐ Ensure team members have limited access to software capabilities, depending on their position.
- ☐ Require clients to sign a record release before medical records are released to anyone other than themselves.

REVIEW QUESTIONS

1. Why is legibility so important in medical records?
2. Why should medical record auditing be a critical function of practice managers?
3. What is the earliest that records can be shredded?
4. Why is history taking critical for a medical record?
5. What is a SOAP progress note? Give an example of each acronym.
6. What items are mandatory in a medical record? Why?
7. Why are discharge sheets vital?
8. Does a client record belong to the client? Why or why not?
9. Who owns the radiographs of a pet?
10. What is EMR and what is the benefit of using EMRs?
11. Abbreviations are only used in medical records.
    a. True
    b. False
12. Medical records:
    a. Can be released to any person asking for a copy
    b. Must be released to the owner only
    c. Must have an owner's consent to be released to any person asking for a copy
    d. b and c
13. The objective portion of the SOAP format includes:
    a. Chief complaint of the client
    b. Observations of team members upon check-in
    c. Physical examination
    d. Diagnosis
14. Purging medical records:
    a. Increases lost records
    b. Is required by law
    c. Allows inactive records to be shredded
    d. Moves inactive medical records to another storage area
15. The advantage of EMRs is:
    a. Access from any computer
    b. Improved patient care
    c. Third-party application integration
    d. All of the above

REFERENCES

1. Barnes C. Letting your Practice Management Software for the Work for You. July 2022. Shepherd Veterinary Practice Management Software. Accessed August 2022. https://www.shepherd.vet
2. Jones L. Top 5 Perks of Having a Pet portal Directly in your Practice Management Software. July 2022. Shepherd Veterinary Practice Management Software. Accessed August 2022. https://www.shepherd.vet

RECOMMENDED READING

Guenther J. 10 rules for record keeping. DVM 360. Published March 1, 2004. Accessed October 2022. https://www.dvm360.com/view/10-key-rules-record-keeping

SECTION II

Veterinary Operations

10

Appointment Management

LEARNING OBJECTIVES

When you have completed this chapter, you should be able to:

- List factors that impact appointment scheduling
- Effectively make appointments
- Discuss the importance of reminding clients of upcoming appointments
- List methods used to increase the production and efficiency of the team by managing appointments
- List methods used to manage clients who walk into the practice with minor emergencies

OUTLINE

KEY TERMS

Appointments
Calendar template
Forward booking
Medical progress exams
Patient drop-off
Reminders
Treatment Plan
Urgent care

VHMA PERFORMANCE DOMAINS

Veterinary Hospital Managers Association (VHMA) Performance Domains

The performance domain applicable to Appointment Management is organization of the practice. The practice manager:

- Coordinates and plans client service programs, client education, and communication processes, and monitors client retention and satisfaction.
- Is responsible for implementing technology systems.

Application of VHMA Performance Domains for Practice Managers

When practice managers use technology to enhance the appointment and manage integrations well, it allows them to pivot in the moment and adapt to changing needs. Well-managed systems improve client satisfaction and retention while bringing improved work-life balance and reduced stress to the veterinary team, to improve team morale, culture, and employee retention.

INTRODUCTION

Effectively managing an appointment scheduling system is a critical task in the veterinary practice. Appointments control the flow of clients and the chaos that sets in each day by offsetting critical cases and wellness examinations. It also allows for improved staff scheduling; by having more team members during heavily scheduled appointment times, a frictionless client experience can be delivered.

Practices must also be innovative and determine how best to best work in urgent care cases. These are cases that normally cannot wait to be seen; however, trying to work them into an overbooked schedule impacts the ability of the team to function optimally, eventually leading to team burnout.

Schedule templates are normally built out by the practice manager and owner. However, these often need to be modified over time. Economic challenges, staffing shortages, and veterinary shortages pose scheduling challenges in the practice which practice managers must quickly adapt to decrease the impact on the business.

Receptionists must be fully trained on the practice's appointment scheduling program, gaining a full understanding of what appointments are scheduled for specific lengths of time, why those lengths of time are important, and how such appointments affect the entire team (for example, a limping pet may require radiographs and a longer appointment time with additional technician staff to obtain the radiographs).

CRITICAL COMPETENCY: RESOURCEFULNESS

The practice manager must have the ability to understand what it takes to complete the job by applying knowledge, skills, and expertise to perform tasks quickly and efficiently.

BALANCING APPOINTMENTS, WALK-INS, AND URGENT CARE

Scheduled appointments are essential to controlling the flow of the practice. Team members know what to expect from the day's schedule, which clients are coming, and for what type of exam. Team members can prepare medical records for appointments, morning huddles can allow the team to review the cases that are scheduled and make a "game plan." In a perfect world, only scheduled appointments show up and the day goes as planned. But that world does not exist in veterinary medicine. Pets don't get sick on a schedule; in fact, illness happens at the most inconvenient times. Practice team members must accept the fact that walk-ins and urgent care cases will arrive daily. It should be the culture of the practice to figure out "how to" accept patients with a positive, can-do attitude. The pandemic of 2020–2022 sent many practices in a downward spiral, trying to accommodate all clients and patients, leaving no time for the self-care of team members. Fortunately, patient visits returned to normal, pre-pandemic levels in late 2022, allowing for more balanced daily routines. The practices that are innovative with scheduling and have a great team culture that is supported by values are those that are thriving the best.

CRITICAL COMPETENCIES: ADAPTABILITY

Practice managers must be open to change and flexible work methods and can adapt behavior to changing conditions or new information.

LEADERSHIP POINT

Practices with innovative scheduling are built on strong values, culture, exceptional leadership, team collaboration, leveraging, efficiency, and built-in work-life balance for the team.

When clients call the practice to have their pet seen, it is important that the team member hears the concern and offers potential solutions versus telling a client that no appointments are available. A client may call and indicate they need to get their pet in as soon as possible because the patient is shaking its head/ears. If there are no open appointments that day, the team member member may offer the following options:

"It sounds like Fluffy really needs to be seen, so here is what we can do.

- *We can take her as a walk-in after 3:00 p.m. today if that works for you, but we do have scheduled appointments so there will be a short wait time to be seen.*
- *We could also schedule her for tomorrow; we have an appointment at 9:30 a.m.*
- *You can also drop Fluffy off with us this morning and we'll check her as soon as we can, between appointments without keeping you waiting."*

This offers multiple solutions to the client; accommodating client requests is part of offering exceptional service.

Tricks to Balance Appointments, Walks-Ins, and Urgent Care

Alter Wellness With Illness Appointments: When receptionists can alter an easy case with a difficult case, it allows the team to have 1–2 minutes to "catch up" both mentally and physically. Having critical cases back-to-back can be exhausting and can set the team behind when trying to complete diagnostics requested by the doctor. If clients will leave pets for diagnostics, it allows a bit more time for the team to complete those tasks. Wellness exams bring pet kisses and happy clients, both helping the team to mentally recharge.

Offset Appointment Times: To reduce the chaos at the front desk for check-in, stagger the appointment times for each doctor. Fig. 10.1 demonstrates Dr. A's first appointments starting at 8:00 a.m., Dr. B starting at 8:10 a.m., and Dr. C starting at 8:20 a.m.

Leave Appointments Open for the "Day Of": This will help accommodate walk-in clients that need veterinary care. Pre-pandemic, practices could estimate how many walk-ins they would have in a day and leave that number of appointments open. The pandemic changed the number of walk-ins greatly, as practices could not keep up with demand. However, since visits have reverted to more normal quantities, this can be reinstituted. The risk is walk-ins not coming and having open appointments. If this happens, receptionists should call clients that have set appointments for later in the day or week and see if they can fill those slots.

Add an Urgent Care Column: Adding an urgent care column is a newer concept. Walk-ins used to be considered the "urgent care" of veterinary medicine, but some walk-ins are for vaccines, wellness, and simple diarrhea cases. Urgent care cases are dog fights, lacerations, proptosed eye, etc. The most important reason for an urgent care column is for the mental wellness of the team. When a team is put together that only handles urgent care for the day, they are mentally prepared for crazy, challenging cases, and receptionists know they can get those cases in without having to ask the team for permission. By having a team that is mentally prepared for the challenge, burnout is much lower. It is still critical to allow this team to see scheduled appointments on some days to get the balance of knowing what is scheduled, frequent kisses, and happy clients. There is always a possibility that urgent care slots will not always fill up; if that is the case, this team can see nonurgent walk-ins, appointments, and drop-offs, alleviating the burden on the appointment team.

Navigating Emergencies: If an emergency arrives that sets the team back (e.g., the patient needs to go to surgery), the reception team may need to proactively call clients scheduled for the day and explain that an emergency has caused appointments to fall behind. Team members can politely reschedule appointments for later in the day or for another day if that works better for the client's schedule. Yearly examinations should always be asked first to reschedule; those appointments should have lower priority over a client who has a sick pet.

Drop-Off: Offer to drop off pets that cannot wait for an extended period to help balance the schedule and keep the team running on time. Drop-off patients can be worked in as time permits, starting with the doctor's exam (who can then empower the team members to carry out diagnostics and client communications), allowing the doctor to continue seeing exam rooms and ensuring the appointments run on time. See the next section for more details.

Create a Credentialed Technician/Nurse Column: Having a credentialed technician/nurse column for appointments allows the doctors to see more appointments that require a diagnosis. Technicians can

Appt Time	Dr. A	Dr. B	Dr. C	Urgent Care
8:00	**Angela Jones** Cassidy-K9, Yearly Exam	Block	Block	HOLD FOR DAY OF
8:10		**Sabrina Patterson** Sheba- Fe, Ear Inf	Block	
8:20	**Nikki Ewing** Sundance-Hamster Vomiting		**Kimberly Olsen** Lily-K9 OVH	
8:30				
8:40		**Julie Denmartin** Oscar, K9, Ortho Exam		HOLD FOR DAY OF
8:50	Block		**Vicki Edwards** Fluffy-K9 OVH	
9:00	**Sue Bacal** King-Av, Wing Trim			
9:10		Block		
9:20		**Brenda Rosales** Geo-K9 Yealy Exam	**Matt Peirson** Kane-K9 Neuter (Mastiff)	HOLD FOR DAY OF
9:30	**Denzel Britton** Joy-K-9 PU/PD			
9:40		**Valarie Goodwill (NC)** Sasha-K9, Consult		
9:50			**Lance Baldwin** Sushi-K9 Dental Grade 1	
10:00	**Jenny Taylor (NC)** Stich-K9 New Puppy			HOLD FOR DAY OF
10:10				
10:20		**Clint Short** Gus-K9, Sr Exam		
10:30	HOLD FOR DAY OF			
10:40			**Laura Blevins** Tootsie - K9, Hip Rads	HOLD FOR DAY OF
10:50		Block		
11:00		**Rita Morales** Lady-Fe, Yearly Exam	**Kendra Basinger** Mimi-Fe OVH	
11:10	**Debbie Miller** Gauge-K9 Yealy Exam			
11:20		HOLD FOR DAY OF	**Candiss Hartraft** Bullie-K9 Growth Rem	Block
11:30	Block			HOLD FOR DAY OF
11:40	**Linda Block** Jackie-K9, Eye Drainage			
11:50				
12:00				

Procedure ■ Dental ■ Surgery ■ Wellness Exam ■ Illness Exam ■ Extended Illness Exam ■ Release hold on day of appt

Fig. 10.1 Staggered appointment blocks keep multiple clients from walking in at the same time.

see appointments for nail trims, anal gland expression, suture removal, vaccine boosters, and some medical progress exams; if the technician has questions, they can grab a doctor to look at the patient.

> **LEADERSHIP POINT**
>
> The maximal leveraging of credentialed veterinary technicians/nurses allows improved appointment management by allowing the veterinarians the opportunity to see other cases that need to be diagnosed, while the credentialed technician/nurse completes appointments where a doctor is not immediately needed.

Clients that choose to walk in must be advised up front that there are scheduled appointments that will be seen first, and the team will work them in as they can. A receptionist should never promise how long the wait will be, as that time may change with the arrival of critical patients.

There is an inherent risk of saying "no" to walk-ins and urgent care clients. Clients are quick to voice their displeasure with a practice for not seeing their baby on social media. A comment like *"I have been a client here for 20 years and they don't have time to see my dog that is going to die"* is reputation damage that can be hard to overcome. But team balance is also critical. That is why team collaboration is critical; where/how can the team become more efficient so that they do not have to say no and still maintain a work-life balance? The balancing act is critical and can be achieved with team collaboration, great culture, and amazing leadership.

ACCOMMODATING PATIENT DROP-OFFS

Drop-off patients can be more efficient for the team and prevent the client from having to wait, resulting in happy teams and happy clients. The key is for the veterinary technician/nurse to gather a detailed history and chief complaint from the owner. The doctor can then examine the pet and the technician/nurse can call the owner with an update and a treatment plan. The technician/nurse must be able to convey the "why" behind the treatments to get buy-in from the client.

Once the treatment plan is approved by the client, the technician can move forward with diagnostics or procedures recommended by the doctor as time permits. Once the diagnostics are complete and the doctor reviews the results, a diagnosis and a final treatment plan can be developed. The technician/nurse can prepare discharge instructions and the doctor can call the client between appointments (the technician/nurse MUST ensure the doctor calls within a reasonable time). Once the client arrives to pick up the pet, the technician can review the discharge instructions and medications, and schedule a medical progress exam.

LEADERSHIP POINT

An efficient medical team that multitasks well can manage multiple drop-offs in a short time, create treatment plans for each, and well-leveraged team members can review with the client, obtain approval, and execute the plan.

Multiple drop-off patients can be managed by one technician and doctor throughout the day, allowing the doctor to see multiple cases at the same time and in between appointments. This accommodates the client's needs and provides the patient care that the pets deserve. To improve efficiency, one efficient technician/nurse may be assigned to drop-off cases. If cases are not dropped off, that technician can float with appointments, help with treatments, or call clients to check on pets that were dropped off the previous day.

The credentialed technician working in this capacity must be organized, efficient, and extremely knowledgeable in medical diagnostics and treatments. The doctor handling this volume must be able to multitask with multiple cases, be organized, and trust the credentialed technician they are working with. An effective PIMS (Chapter 8) with EMR (Chapter 9) is critical to the efficiency of this team.

THE IMPORTANCE OF MANAGING WAIT TIMES

It is critical to monitor client wait times. Clients easily become frustrated with prolonged wait times, especially when there is no communication from the team. The result is decreased compliance. Studies indicate that clients regard on-time performance to be a more important factor than the practice fee structure. Clients that are irritated are less likely to accept recommendations and will only choose "what they feel is important." They are also less likely to return for medical progress exams or wellness/preventive care. Team members must keep clients informed why wait times are prolonged and provide value through client education and personal conversation (Chapter 11).

VHMA PRACTICE DOMAIN TASK

The practice manager must establish work schedules for staff (that accommodate the heavier client appointment times).

The most common reasons practices run behind schedule is due to a mismanaged schedule, a higher-than-normal volume of critical cases, inefficiency, and veterinarians and team members "chit-chatting" in the exam room. It is a common misconception that meeting the needs of one client in the examination room is the primary factor in providing good customer service. The multiple clients who are waiting for appointments must also receive exceptional customer service; perfecting the balance between the two is critical. Handling wait times appropriately will keep even the most irritable clients returning to the practice for future services.

CRITICAL COMPETENCY: CRITICAL AND STRATEGIC THINKING

Strategic thinking and planning are essential parts of long-term plans for the growth of the practice. Managers must have the ability to identify questions, problems, and arguments relevant to appointment management and use logic and critical reasoning to identify the strengths and weaknesses of alternative solutions or approaches to problems.

SCHEDULING FOR A FRICTIONLESS CLIENT EXPERIENCE

When creating or updating an appointment template that the practice will follow for client appointments, several factors should be considered.

Client needs: Consider the demographic of the clients served by the practice. An older retired demographic may be available all day and would not prefer evening appointments. The working class would need appointments that are late afternoon or evening. And working parents may need more availability on the weekends. To exceed client service expectations, the practice should have appointments most available to serve the largest demographic. In an ideal world, staffing would not be an issue, and a practice could be open seven days a week to meet the needs of all clients. Since staffing is a dilemma in veterinary medicine, meeting the need of the largest demographic the practice serves is a priority. Another option is to schedule appointments through the common lunch period. Team members can rotate lunch hours so that everyone still gets a break, or team members that work half days can alleviate those that leave once the morning shift has wrapped up. If the afternoon shift handles the appointments, the morning team can finish up their tasks, treatments, and client check-ins.

Appointment length: On average, veterinary appointments last 20 minutes, with some practices extending to 30- or 40-minute appointments. The length of time depends on the goals of the practice. Higher volume reduces the cost per minute of doing business (Chapter 16, Finance). If the practice has a set revenue and profitability goal for examinations the year, that goal should be broken out per day, which then sets appointment length expectations (X number of appointments must be seen, with an average transaction of X dollars to achieve the revenue and profitability goal for exams the year). Twenty-minute appointments will result in an average of 24 appointments per day per DVM (8-hour appointment day), 30-minute appointments will average 16 appointments per day per DVM, and 40-minute appointments will average 12 appointments per day per DVM. The ability to keep shorter appointments on time highly depends on an educated, well-trained team that is leveraged, trusted, and efficient.

LEADERSHIP POINT

Appointment availability must meet the needs of the largest demographic whom the practice serves. This may include evening and weekend hours.

Scheduling for Efficiency: Doctors should be able to delegate tasks to well-trained team members while the doctor continues seeing appointments. If diagnostic work has been advised for a patient in an exam room, the patient should be turned over to the veterinary technician/nurse who can complete the tests the veterinarian has advised. Once results are available, the doctor can review the results and a treatment plan created. The doctor should continue to the next appointment, keeping the schedule running on time (no need to wait on results for one patient before moving to the next). Technicians/nurses can also keep appointments running on schedule by asking the client to wait in a consultation room while in-house laboratory work is being performed. This allows the examination room to be freed up for the next appointment and prevents a delay for waiting clients.

Patient medical record reviews should occur before the client arrives at the practice. Receptionists should be auditing the medical record to help the medical team be more efficient (Fig. 10.2) by looking for items that may be overdue, such as vaccines, heartworm tests, bloodwork to monitor long-term conditions and medications, or refills of parasiticide prevention or chronic medications. The receptionists can then address lapses in care with the client upon check-in and make notes for the medical team as well. This starts the efficiency

ABC VETERINARY CLINIC- PATIENT AUDIT

Client ______________________

Pet ______________________

Age ____________ Date ____________

PUPPY/FIRST VACCINATION SERIES:

DHLPP Yes/No Booster? Yes/No
Bordetella Yes/No Booster? Yes/No
Rabies Yes/No
Is the pet exposed to Rattlesnakes? Yes/No
Dewormer? Yes/No
Puppy Kit? Yes/No
Fecal Yes/No Advised? Yes/No
Heartworm Preventative Yes/No
☐ 1 month ☐ 6 month ☐ 12 month
Flea/Tick Preventative Yes/No
☐ 1 month ☐ 6 month ☐ 12 month
Microchip Yes/No

YEARLY EXAM/REGULAR EXAM

DHLPP Yes/No Due Date ____________
Rabies Yes/No Due Date ____________
Bordetella Yes/No Due Date ____________
Rattlesnake Yes/No Due Date ____________
Urinalysis Yes/No Advised: Yes/No
Heartworm/E-Canis/Anaplasmosis/Lyme Test Yes/No
Heartworm Preventative Yes/No
☐ 1 month ☐ 6 month ☐ 12 month
Flea/Tick Preventative Yes/No
☐ 1 month ☐ 6 month ☐ 12 month
Microchip Yes/No

SENIOR WELLNESS: CANINE

DHLPP Yes/No Due Date ____________
Rabies Yes/No Due Date ____________
Bordetella Yes/No Due Date ____________
Rattlesnake Yes/No Due Date ____________
Heartworm/E-Canis/Anaplasmosis/Lyme Test Yes/No
Heartworm Preventative Yes/No
☐ 6 month ☐ 12 month
Flea/Tick Preventative Yes/No
☐ 6 month ☐ 12 month
General Health Profile/EKG Yes/No Advised: Yes/No
Urinalysis Yes/No Advised: Yes/No

Client ______________________

Pet ______________________

Age ____________ Date ____________

KITTEN/FIRST VACCINATION SERIES:

FVRCP Yes/No Booster? Yes/No
FeLV Yes/No Booster? Yes/No
Rabies Yes/No
Dewormer? Yes/No
FeLV/FIV/HWT Yes/No
Kitten Kit Yes/No
Fecal Yes/No Advised? Yes/No
Heartworm Prevention Yes/No

YEARLY EXAM/REGULAR EXAM

FVRCP Yes/No Due Date ____________
FeLV Yes/No Due Date ____________
Rabies Yes/No Due Date ____________
Felv/FIV/HWT Yes/No Advised? Yes/No
Urinalysis Yes/No Advised? Yes/No
Heartworm Preventative Yes/No

SENIOR WELLNESS: FELINE

FVRCP Yes/No Due Date ____________
FeLV Yes/No Due Date ____________
Rabies Yes/No Due Date ____________
Felv/FIV/HWT Yes/No Advised? Yes/No
Urinalysis/T-4 Yes/No Advised? Yes/No

Fig. 10.2 Patient audits help team members identify services or products the pet may need while visiting the hospital.

and education process, resulting in better patient care and a frictionless client experience.

Exam Room Efficiency: In most practices, a veterinary assistant or credentialed veterinary technician/nurse brings the client into the exam room and obtains a history with the vitals. Once completed, they get the doctor, and the history is reviewed again. To increase efficiency, the tech should bring the client into the exam room where the doctor is waiting, allowing the client to tell the story one time. This can save about 7 minutes of time (making 20-minute appointments a reality).

Medical Record Efficiency: Medical record charting can slow the doctor significantly when efficiency measures have not been put in place. Electronic medical records should have templates, diagnostic codes, and bundled treatment plans built out (Chapter 8, PIMS), allowing the doctor to move through record entry quickly. In addition, having a scribe in the room while the doctor verbalizes the exam to the client allows the scribe to capture the medical notes, allowing the client to become "a part" of the exam. Verbalized exams add value to the client experience as the doctor "teaches" what they are looking for. This also yields greater compliance when recommendations are made. The scribe enters the notes in a template and creates a treatment plan or prescription label(s) while the doctor verbalizes the plan to the client. Once the exam is complete, the medical record is 90% complete, and the doctor can take a few moments to finish the remaining 10%. The more integrated the PIMS is, the more efficient the team will be to accommodate 20-minute appointments. In this example, the scribe should be a team member who is extremely familiar with the doctor's exam process, types well, navigates the PIMS quickly, and possess strong medical knowledge.

LEADERSHIP POINT

Allow scribes to increase the efficiency of the medical team. This creates balance for doctors not having to stay late (after their shift) to complete medical records.

Designing the Calendar Template

The template is the outline of the appointment calendar and should be established before implementing a new system and should be updated as needed (i.e., to accommodate the pandemic). Updating the template after appointments have been created can cause issues; to be prepared, capture all appointment entries before updating the template, and reenter appointments if necessary.

Several factors impact appointment scheduling that must be considered when building or updating the template. The hours of appointment availability should be set first, including weekends. Be sure to block off lunches (if the staff does not rotate shifts), team meetings, and holiday closures. Permanent flextime (that allows the team to catch up) should also be blocked so that team members cannot accidentally remove or book an appointment in that slot. Generally, a practice manager or owner creates the template and is the only one who has access to modify it.

CRITICAL COMPETENCY: DECISION MAKING

The practice manager must be able to make good decisions based on critical thinking and problem solving that will positively impact the practice. While many alternatives are available, the PM must be able to gather and effectively analyze relevant data and choose decisively.

Practice managers should manually block off doctors' schedules when they intend to take PTO or CE. This will prevent overbooking, and for clients that ask for a specific doctor, appointments can be made with another doctor during that time. Ideally, the other doctors in the practice will help pick up some appointment times, or a relief doctor can be found far enough in advance to cover shifts while the vacationing doctor is away.

The next step is to determine the length of the appointments. The previous section covered methods to increase the efficiency of the team, allowing 20-minute appointments to be achieved successfully. Another factor to consider is that some doctors may need more time than others. New graduates will need longer appointment times as they learn to navigate their new careers. New doctors to the practice may need temporarily longer appointment times as they adjust to the new practice. Relief doctors may be incredibly efficient and rely heavily on the team and can utilize the current set schedule. Lastly, the type of appointment will impact the length of the appointment. Wellness exams may take 20 minutes while orthopedic exams may take 40 to 50 minutes. Medical Progress and Technician Exams may take 10 minutes. One must consider how to integrate the various lengths of time into a set template.

A 10-minute flex system is an option that will accommodate the above factors. This will allow team members that schedule appointments based on the doctor, and to analyze the client's needs and estimate the length of time needed for an appointment. Several 10-minute blocks can be lumped together to create the perfect appointment time. Fig. 10.1 has different appointment types scheduled, each with various times based on client and patient needs. Team members who schedule appointments must be knowledgeable about diseases, procedures, and client needs to schedule effectively.

To determine how many minutes should be allotted to each appointment type, the practice manager should be in alignment with the medical team and come to an agreement about the average length of time for average exams and procedures. An example of procedures can be found in Fig. 10.3. Providing general guidelines can help the reception team schedule more efficiently.

Types of Appointments

Surgery: The number of surgeries scheduled each day depends on the efficiency, skill, and leveraging of the team, the length of time it takes the veterinarian to complete a procedure, and the amount of time available to complete the procedures. One veterinarian may be faster at a particular procedure and able to complete more procedures per day than another. Larger practices may have two surgical tables and are thus accommodating a larger number of surgical patients per day (Fig. 10.4).

Dental Procedures: Practices may have either one or two dental tables and prophy units available, increasing the number of dental procedures a practice can accommodate in one day. Several credentialed technicians/nurses can complete dental prophy's concurrently while nonsterile procedures are performed on another table, while sterile procedures are completed in the surgical suite. The length of time allotted for dentals should depend on the severity of the disease.

Nonsterile Procedures: Abscess debridement, anal sac expression or flush, ear flushes, and patients that need to be sedated for radiographs all take time away from the treatment team (Fig. 10.5). Time should be allotted to complete these procedures if possible, helping prevent the team from running behind on appointments. An excessive number of unscheduled, nonsterile procedures can place increased stress on the team and the practice schedule.

Client Education: Client education must be provided by a credentialed veterinary technician/nurse or a skilled assistant, and having time scheduled prevents the client from having to wait when they are ready to take their pet home. A pet may have been diagnosed with

TYPE OF APPOINTMENT	APPROX. TIME REQUIRED
EXAMS	
New Client- Healthy Exam	30 minutes
Booster Exam	10 minutes
Yearly Exam	20 minutes
Senior Exam	30 minutes
Orthopedic Exam	30 minutes
Avian/Exotic Exam	30 minutes
New Client Illness Exam	40 minutes
Exisitng Client Illness Exam	30 minutes
Medical Progress Exam	10 minutes
NONSTERILE PROCEDURES	
Radiographs w/ Anesth	20 minutes
Ear Flush w/ Anesth	20 minutes
Anal Gland Flush w/Anesth	20 minutes
Sedate/Nail Trim	10 minutes
Abcess	20 minutes
Dental Grade 1	50 minutes
Dental Grade 2	70 minutes
Dental Grade 3	90 minutes
Client Education	10 minutes
STERILE PROCEDURES	
K9 Neuter	20 minutes
K9 OVH	30 minutes
Fe Neuter	10 minutes
Fe OVH	20 minutes
Growth Removal (ask DVM)	30 minutes

Fig. 10.3 A list of the most common appointments and surgical procedures when listed by length of time, help decrease scheduling errors.

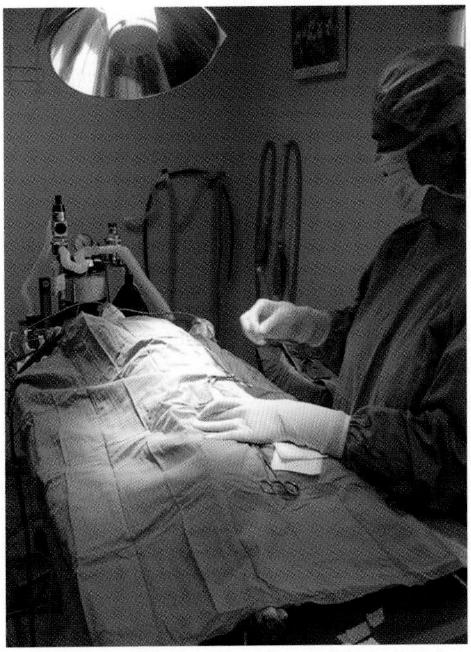

Fig. 10.4 Surgical procedures require longer appointment times.

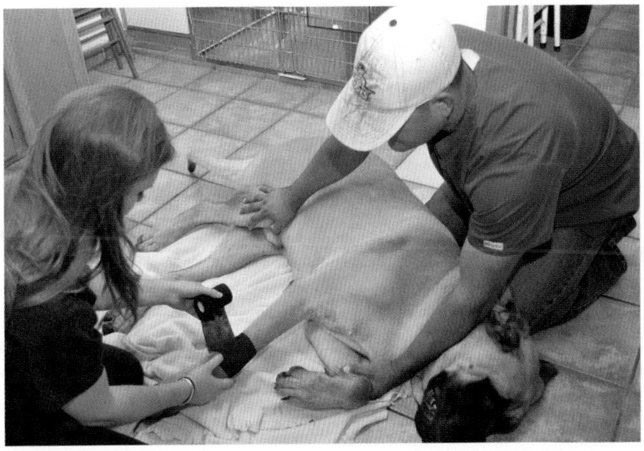

Fig. 10.5 Building additional time into the schedule for nonsterile procedures keeps the practice from running behind.

a chronic disease or had a major surgery while in the hospital, and the client will need to receive client literature regarding the patient's disease and treatment. Scheduling client education can significantly increase client compliance and understanding while establishing a lasting client-practice bond.

Another option to provide education to clients when the number of exam rooms is limited is to use telehealth platforms. The client can be briefed upon discharge, and those that require extensive education (diabetes, pancreatitis, etc.) can be scheduled for a video conference call to provide further detail and answer client questions.

SPECIAL CLIENT CONSIDERATIONS

Certain clients will always take longer than others simply because they like to talk, share stories, and ask multiple questions. Team members should be able to identify these clients right away and add extra time for their appointments. These clients are likely in the top 10% of the practice's producing clients because they have a strong bond and trust with the practice. By accommodating these clients during the scheduling process, team members can prevent appointments from running behind. The top 20% of clients usually contribute to 80% of the practice revenue. Accommodating these clients makes great business sense!

Habitually Late Clients: There will always be clients who are late. Practices may post a sign indicating that any client who is more than 15 minutes late will be considered a walk-in; they can either be rescheduled or treated as a walk-in and seen as time permits. To enforce this policy, practice appointments must also be on time or clients will become irate. If clients are asked to respect the doctor's time by being on time, then practices must respect the client's time as well.

Once a client has been rescheduled due to tardiness, it is unlikely they will be late for the following appointment. Clients can also be politely addressed regarding their constant tardiness when the appointment is made. *"Mr. Collins, the nature of Spot's appointment requires the full time allotted for your appointment. Please remember your appointment is set for Tuesday, June 5, at 3 p.m."* This kindly lets the client know that the practice has recognized the tardiness in the past and will be expecting him to arrive on time.

If a client calls ahead and lets the team know they will be late, the receptionist should check the schedule to make sure the client can still be accommodated without delaying the rest of the appointments. If it will be a tight squeeze, ask the client if the appointment can be rescheduled.

No-Show Appointments: All practices have clients who do not show up for appointments. Emergencies occur, clients forget, or a pet may disappear for a few hours (cats especially!). Being proactive can alleviate some of the no-show appointments. Team members should confirm the appointment with clients the day before through a text message that has a link to click that confirms the appointment. If the client doesn't respond, the receptionist should call the client. Providing simple reminders can easily offset no-show rates. Always ask clients how they prefer to receive reminders for appointments and services.

When a client does not show up, a team member should always call and attempt to reschedule the appointment. It should be noted in the record that the client did not show up for the appointment and that a team member attempted to reschedule the appointment. Documenting the no-show can help defend the veterinary practice should something tragic happen to the pet because of an injury or disease process; the practice can demonstrate the client never showed up for a scheduled appointment.

Specific clients may be frequent no-shows and should be documented in the record as well. Honest and kind communication is critical with these clients; nicely advised them that they have missed a few appointments and will need to come as a walk-in or be able to drop off the pet that will be seen as time permits. PIMS allows for client alerts to be entered, informing team members when they access the account to make the appointment.

Clients Who Arrive on the Wrong Day: On occasion, clients arrive for appointments on the wrong day. If the practice schedule permits, team members should work the client in if possible since they have taken the time to bring in their pet. However, if the schedule doesn't allow for seeing them at that time, the client should be asked if they will drop the pet off, or if their original appointment time works. If neither option works, the appointment can be rescheduled. Sincere apologies should be given to the client regarding the misunderstanding and inconvenience, no matter whose fault (team member or client), keeping in mind they may have taken time off work or driven some distance for the appointment. Remember, excellent customer service is the goal, and being able to satisfy a client is very important.

FORWARD BOOKING

Forward booking an appointment is defined as scheduling the patient's next appointment before they leave the practice. Forward booking should be in place for medical progress examinations, booster vaccines, laboratory follow-up visits, dentals, surgeries, and annual preventive vaccine/healthcare examinations. Forward booking ensures patients receive the highest quality of care, on schedule. When appointments are scheduled in advance, owners are more likely to keep the appointments, supporting increased compliance, stronger client relationships, and better patient care.

Forward booking is common practice in dental practices, hair salons, chiropractors, etc., yielding improved compliance rates. Clients get busy; by the time they remember to make the appointment, the pet is overdue, and the practice is likely booked for several weeks. Forward booking secures those appointments.

LEADERSHIP POINT

Forward booking is a team sport and starts with the veterinarian setting expectations that the next appointment will be set before they leave the practice.

Forward booking is a team sport. It starts with a conversation in the exam room with the doctor and veterinary technician. If the pet has been seen for a wellness exam, the doctor would wrap up the exam by saying *"Fluffy looks amazing this year! Unless she has any issues that pop up, we will see you next year! Brenda will get that appointment scheduled for you before you leave, ensuring Fluffy has a spot on the appointment calendar. And no worries Mrs. Smith, if you need to change that appointment as it gets closer, just give us a call."* If the technician, Brenda, is checking Mrs. Smith out in the exam room, she can schedule that appointment on the same day and time the following year. If Brenda will be taking Mrs. Smith to the reception desk, Brenda will ask the receptionist to schedule that annual exam. The receptionist then needs to complete that task first (before checking the client out). Steps in this order ensure the appointment is listed on the client receipt and catches the client before they mentally check out (many clients mentally check out once they have paid the bill).

Correct reminder setup is critical in forward booking. A reminder should be sent to the client one month in advance, indicating that if that time does not work, to call the practice and reschedule. A second reminder should be sent one week before, and a third reminder two days before. It is important to identify how clients want to receive reminders; typical options include postcards, email, or text. Many clients prefer email and text over postcards, but assumptions should not be made regarding client preference. Obviously, reminders one week out and 2 days out need to be in a digital format. It is therefore critical to ensure the email and cell phone numbers on file are correct.

APPOINTMENT ENTRY

The PIMS appointment calendar has far more features than just scheduling appointments. When a team member fills an appointment slot with an existing client, the software can show alerts reminding the team of overdue vaccinations or lab tests, previous no-show appointments, or poor credit status. When the client account is accessed, all pets owned by that client will be available, allowing the reception team to either schedule an appointment for multiple patients owned by the same client or to remind the owner of overdue services for any of the pets.

If a client chooses to cancel or change an appointment, the receptionist can cut and paste, keeping all pertinent client information together. The receptionist will not have to reenter client and appointment information.

Integrated PIMS appointment calendars can enhance the experience of a client by allowing them to make their own appointments through the website, the pet portal, or the practice app.

Specific information, including the client's first and last name, is needed to enter appointments. As stated above, existing client data will prepopulate, while new clients will need to have the data entered with the name of the patient, sex, breed, etc. Both existing clients and new clients will need to have a reason for the appointment as well as a verified cell phone number where the client can be reached. This information allows the veterinary team to prepare for the appointment; team members know when and which client will be arriving, what procedure to expect, and what equipment or laboratory work may be required. This increases the overall efficiency of the team.

____

has an appointment

on

☐ MON ☐ TUES ☐ WED. ☐ THURS. ☐ FRI. ☐ SAT.

______________________________ AT __________ A.M. / P.M.

If unable to keep appointment, kindly give 24 hrs. notice.

Fig. 10.6 Appointment cards remind clients of their scheduled appointment times and decrease no-shows.

Once the appointment information has been completely entered, the team member should read the appointment back to the client, ensuring no miscommunication has occurred. *"Mr. Lockridge, we have Rosie scheduled for her yearly examination on Monday, January 21, at 9 a.m. with Dr. Bresiger. Is there anything else I can help you with until we see you on the twenty-first?"* This is an excellent way to confirm the appointment (the date has now been repeated twice; once while making the appointment and the other while reviewing), and an opportunity to ask further questions has been offered.

Some clients still prefer receiving appointment cards for their upcoming appointment, while others will add to the calendar on their cellphones. Appointment cards contain the name of the practice as well as the address, phone number, email, and website on the front, and an open slot for the appointment on the back. The date, day, and time of the appointment should be written in along with the patient's name (Fig. 10.6). It is a good idea to include the office policy regarding no-show appointments on the back of the card. This reminds clients that the veterinary practice's time is valuable.

If a surgical procedure has been scheduled, preoperative instructions for the pet should be given to the owner with their appointment reminder. These patients are generally held off food and water before surgery, are dropped off at a specific time, and may be picked up at a specific time. Clients should be given these instructions both verbally and in writing (to take home for review) (Fig. 10.7).

APPOINTMENT PREPARATION

Managing the schedule, making new client appointments, forward booking future appointments, and providing reminders are all important steps in managing appointments. Efficiently preparing for each patient appointment is the next step. A medical records audit should be completed for every patient, every time. For example, a patient may be seen for an ear infection but may also be overdue for a heartworm test or parasite prevention medication. Clients would prefer to visit the practice once for all services needed (especially when visiting for anything other than the yearly examination), instead of receiving a reminder one month later for services still needed.

The medical team should also be prepared for the client and pet by reviewing the medical record and medical record audit, identifying the reason for the visit, and having all expected diagnostic tools in the exam room. This prevents the team from leaving and returning, saving several minutes of time thus increasing efficiency.

APPOINTMENT REMINDERS

Appointment reminders are critical when implementing forward booking into the schedule, but so are reminders for other services. Review Chapter 12 for additional appointment reminder tips. Don't forget to identify how the client wants to receive reminders: postcards, email, text messages, or app notifications.

Other services that require reminders are surgery, dentals, boarding, etc. If a surgical procedure or laboratory work has been scheduled, reminders are the perfect way to reiterate specific appointment instructions. Clients who don't follow (or remember) these instructions fall into the same category as missed appointments; a canceled surgical procedure equals lost revenue and the opportunity to have scheduled another patient needing treatment.

VHMA PERFORMANCE DOMAIN TASK

Practice managers develop and manage reminder systems.

PIMS, pet portals, and the practice app should be interactive and have the added benefit of allowing clients to confirm appointments from the reminders sent. When a client confirms an appointment via text, email, or app, the receptionist no longer needs to make a reminder phone call. However, if a client has not confirmed an appointment, then the reception team should make reminder phone calls. Missed appointments represent gaps in the schedule when other patients could have been seen, lost income, and missed patient care opportunities.

LEADERSHIP POINT

Ask clients what their preferred method is to receive reminders. Postcards are costly and time-consuming and should be reserved for those that wish to continue receiving them.

TRAINING NEW EMPLOYEES TO USE THE APPOINTMENT CALENDAR

Once team members have experience scheduling appointments, making appointments becomes an easy, efficient task. However, learning the art of scheduling appointments causes anxiety for new team members. A training program should be implemented to ease this stress and decrease the chance of mistakes. The appointment calendar as a template helps guide appropriate times for appointments, but conditions that require extra time need to be fully understood. A list of conditions, diseases, and treatments with the preferred length should be made available for trainees. A list like the one shown in Fig. 10.3 can be created to assist new employees.

A list of clients who require extra time should also be made available to new employees if alerts have not already been added to these clients' accounts.

LEADERSHIP'S ROLE IN APPOINTMENT MANAGEMENT

Practice managers and owners must ensure the appointment templates are created to best serve the veterinary practice, as well as the client demographic in which it serves. Managing and revising the appointment schedule to adapt to changing needs is required; however, those that can make changes and block times must be reserved for a select few. It is common for doctors (and occasionally team members) to block the schedule at the end of the day without the knowledge of the leadership team.

Thorough training on the appointment system should be provided to all new employees (built into a phase training program), and daily team huddles to review the schedule should be implemented at the beginning of each shift (to engage the team and increase efficiency).

ABC Veterinary Clinic

Pre-operative Instructions for Healthy Dogs and Cats:

- No food after 6 pm
- No water after 10 pm

If your pet is over 7 years of age, please remove water first thing in the morning.

Please drop off your pet between 8 and 9 am

Please allow 10-15 minutes for a technician to ask you questions regarding your pet's health.

Your pet may be ready at 3 pm; please call before arrival to be sure your pet is ready.

- Pre-anesthetic blood work is available for each pet. Blood work is recommended the day of surgery to minimize the risk of anesthesia.
- Postoperative pain medication is available for each pet. Please inform us if you do not want pain medication for your pet.
- Blood work and pain medication are available for an additional cost and are highly recommended.

What can I expect after surgery?

- Your pet may be groggy from the anesthesia. Each pet may react differently to the medication. Each pet's health is evaluated before anesthesia administration.
- Provide your pet with a clean, quiet bed for recovery.
- Restrict exercise for 7 days.
- Check the incision daily. Do not allow your pet to lick the incision. If it is red and irritated, please return for a recheck.

Please call our clinic with any questions or concerns.
We are here to provide your pet with the best possible care.
123 Inspiration Lane
Anytown, MI
555-555-5555
Please give 24 hour advance notice of cancellations.

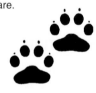

Fig. 10.7 Preoperative instructions should be sent home with clients, providing them with all the details needed before their pet's procedure.

Appropriate setup and use of the appointment system in the PIMS, integrating third-party applications to increase efficiency and enhance the client experience, and forward booking appointments will help control the chaos that can occur daily in the practice, and must be planned and well-executed by the leadership team.

PRACTICE MANAGERS SURVIVAL CHECKLIST FOR PIMS

- ☐ Ensure the practice's core values, mission, and vision, and are tied into training of the appointment system, enabling all team members to accommodate client needs, based on the values of the practice by providing a high standard of care and exceptional customer service.
- ☐ Ensure client expectations are always met when scheduling appointments, solidifying the brand of the practice.
- ☐ Ensure the facility's appearance is clean, welcoming, and modern for clients.
- ☐ Develop internal team training programs for the reception team to ensure client and patient needs are met with every interaction.
- ☐ Ensure the website is well-developed, answering client queries when possible and enticing them to call when not.
- ☐ Update the website yearly and evaluate often for changes to services offered, team members, or recommendations.
- ☐ Ensure the online store is marketed by team members.
- ☐ Develop a practice app and/or portal to allow appointments to be made (in addition to online booking for new clients) to further meet and exceed client expectations.
- ☐ Measure appointment compliance through appointment reminders, tracking no-shows or cancellations, and the average number of reminders sent to increase compliance.

REVIEW QUESTIONS

1. How can urgent care appointments reduce the burnout of team members?
2. How can a receptionist proactively prevent appointments from running behind when an emergency arrives?
3. What are the benefits of clients dropping off patients?
4. What factors impact efficiency in the exam room?
5. Why should an appointment be established for client education?
6. Explain how to handle clients who are always late for their appointments.
7. What factors affect appointment scheduling?
8. Specific clients always take longer for appointments. Why give those specific clients more time than other clients?
9. Why should walk-in clients be seen?
10. What information is vital when scheduling appointments?
11. The goals of an appointment system include which of the following?
    - **a.** Maximize productivity
    - **b.** Reduce stress on team members
    - **c.** Control traffic within the veterinary hospital
    - **d.** All the above
    - **e.** None of the above
12. The longer a client waits to be seen for an appointment, the more likely:
    - **a.** Compliance will increase
    - **b.** Compliance will decrease
    - **c.** Compliance will not change with appointment wait times
13. To help reduce client overload at the front desk, appointments should be:
    - **a.** Set every 10 minutes
    - **b.** Staggered
    - **c.** None of the above
14. Appointments should be set for:
    - **a.** Client education
    - **b.** Surgery/dental procedures
    - **c.** Technicians
    - **d.** All the above
    - **e.** None of the above
15. Appointment lengths may vary for all the following except:
    - **a.** Specific client
    - **b.** Appointment type
    - **c.** Veterinarian
    - **d.** Patient
    - **e.** All the above

11

The Client Experience

LEARNING OBJECTIVES

When you have completed this chapter, you should be able to:

- Define a frictionless client experience
- Describe the importance of written client materials
- Describe the importance of professional verbal skills
- List methods used to communicate in a positive, professional manner
- Identify methods used to educate clients with a variety of techniques
- Describe the importance of providing estimates for clients
- Define client needs
- Clarify barriers that prevent effective client communication and list methods that can improve verbal image
- Develop effective phone techniques
- Describe how to control telephone conversations with clients
- Identify techniques for handling multiple phone lines
- Identify techniques used to turn phone "shoppers" into appointments
- Define the liability associated with giving medical advice over the phone
- Describe methods used to greet clients effectively
- Effectively discuss invoices with clients

OUTLINE

KEY TERMS

Body language
Client communication
Client compliance
Client retention
Client survey
Estimates/treatment plans
Fear Free®
Forward booking
Frictionless client experience
Human-animal bond

Nonverbal skills
Paraverbal skills
Recalls
Reminders
Standard of care
Standard operating protocol
Verbal skills

VHMA PERFORMANCE DOMAINS

Veterinary Hospital Managers Association (VHMA) Performance Domains

Performance domains applicable to the client experience include law and ethics, marketing and client relations, and financial management. The practice manager:

- Understands local and state regulations
- Ensures compliance with contract law
- Ensures compliance with client, patient, and staff confidentiality
- Monitors client retention
- Handles client complaints
- Obtains and reports feedback on client service
- Responds to client questions
- Manages client education
- Establishes and enforces credit client policies

Application of VHMA Performance Domains for Practice Managers

Ensuring that a frictionless client experience is delivered to every client every time takes the integration of advanced technology, team member education, and a culture built on values and goals. Practice managers that build the base to "make it simple for a client to do business" will have improved key performance indicators, a team with improved work-life balance, and decreased team member turnover.

Veterinary Hospital Managers Association Critical Competency Knowledge Requirements

The tasks related to client services and education requires knowledge of the principles and processes for providing customer and personal services, including customer needs assessment and methods for evaluating customer satisfaction.

INTRODUCTION

The Client Experience is an important concept to both appreciate and develop. The experience clients have every time they interact with the practice is what drives the best medicine, the best compliance, and the best marketing. Clients that trust a veterinary practice accept recommendations made by the veterinary healthcare team, and when they have trust, they become loyal. And loyal clients brag to their friends about how great their experience was at your practice. Word-of-mouth referrals are more powerful than any external marketing that the practice can do. Best of all, their pet gets the best care, and that is why every team member entered the veterinary profession.

What does the ideal client experience look like? It is simply exceeding client expectations. Think of a time that you experienced phenomenal service outside of the veterinary industry. Perhaps it was at a restaurant, a hotel, or a business. Why was it phenomenal? The team member providing the service likely communicated well (professional, well spoken, was able to address all questions, was genuine, not rushed, listened to your needs, and was honest with expected outcomes), was prepared to take care of you (organized, knew what you needed before you asked, and efficient), and made it easy to do business. The veterinary practice can also exceed client expectations. It is a team effort, and every team member must understand how they contribute to this experience (Fig. 11.1).

But it all starts with leadership and culture. Leaders must implement training for the team, instill the culture and values into every team meeting, build processes and tools to help the team be successful, and hold those accountable for not delivering on the values, vision, and mission of the practice, all of which support the exceptional client experience.

Also important is the concept of client leadership. Team members lead clients to make the right decision for their pets, and clients expect team members to guide them through difficult decisions. Each team member leads clients every day, whether that is on the phone, in person, or virtually (telehealth, text, pet portals, or a practice app). Changing this simple terminology to client leadership changes the mindset of how teams relate to clients. Leading clients opens the door to unlimited relationship building, resulting in greater client retention, compliance, and loyalty.

Studies prove that consumers will pay more for exceptional service. They value businesses that go above and beyond for them and will remain loyal to these providers even when prices are higher than competitors. Every team member contributes to the client experience; most clients do not have any healthcare experience, so they cannot rate the medicine of the practice, but they can certainly rate (and rave about) the service.

CREATING A "WOW!" SERVICE EXPERIENCE

Practices never get a second chance to make a first impression. In fact, if you get a second chance, it can take over 3 years to overcome a negative perception that was formed. On average, one person tells 13 other people about a bad experience they had with service. If a practice has one client that experienced poor service each day, 260 people could hear about the bad service at your practice per month, equating to 3120 people per year! Now add social media into this equation. How fast does word travel through social media outlets? Creating a "WOW!" experience has never been more important.

First impressions are made by the tone of voice of team members, appearances, actions, smiles, and word choice, all of which will be described throughout this chapter. And clients know when customer service is good or bad. Fortunately, and unfortunately, when customer service is exceptional, clients feel the quality of medicine is great. When customer service is poor, clients feel the level of medicine is subpar.

To further support the "WOW!" factor, teams should be prepared for each client visit. Prep every medical record before the client arrives (compliance check, consent forms, verify client phone number, and email address), allowing team members to have a tailored, individual approach for every client every time they visit the hospital.

It is time to stop thinking about transactions and focus on creating interactions that build strong client relationships and memorable experiences, not just mediocre experiences. (Fig. 11.2). If service is only mediocre, the client-practice bond won't be established and clients will eventually change hospitals looking for better service and for team members they connect and bond with. Team members must strive to

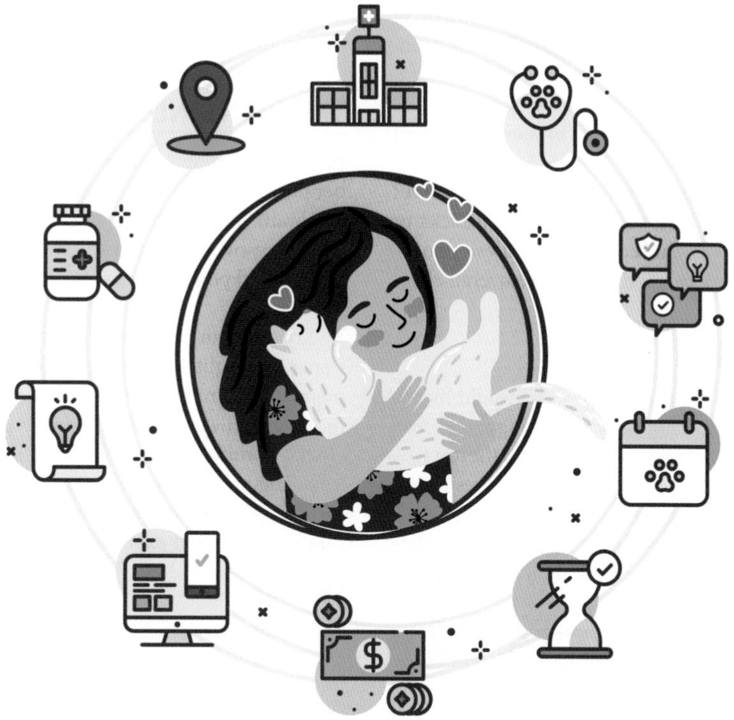

Fig. 11.1 A frictionless client experience must be delivered by the team, bringing value to clients, and improving compliance rates. That experience is driven through the implementation and use of technology that makes it easy for the client to do business with the practice.

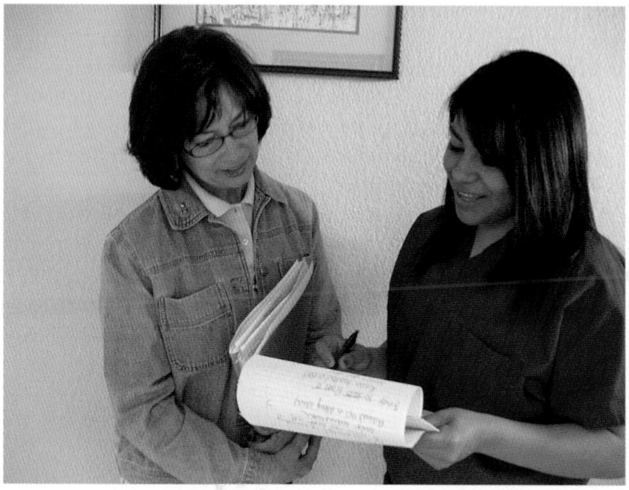

Fig. 11.2 Building relationships with clients includes providing client education in a manner that clients understand and relate to.

create long-lasting bonds with clients that will drive loyalty, as clients are no longer loyal to a particular doctor, but rather to the brand that has been established by the team. Brands are developed when bonds are created, and when consistent service is delivered every time the client calls or enters the practice.

LEADERSHIP POINT

During the team meeting, ask team members to think of a business that has provided exceptional service for them. Have them define the service that was provided, what made it great, and how it made them feel. Capture all ideas and present them to the team to see how your practice might be able to implement the memorable experience they had.

Review the areas of communication that occur with each client. This includes the initial telephone conversation, checking clients in and out, and the examination room experience. Every aspect of the client's visit is built around communication (verbal, paraverbal, and nonverbal). What does it sound like when clients call the practice? The receptionist must be warm, friendly, inviting, and conversational. The first impression starts here; ensure clients feel valued and not like just a number in the deli line at the local grocery store. Work to continue that conversation when the client arrives at the practice. Do not make the client repeat the entire reason for making the appointment. Instead, add great notes in the PIMS, and ask questions that acknowledge the client's concern. Take the time to "teach and lead" clients in the examination room, not "sell" to clients.

Offer the best standards of care (SOC) to every client, every time. Veterinary team members are guilty of prejudging client finances and making recommendations based on that assumption. This not only provides a poor client experience, but the patient (the one we are advocates for) suffers the most. When SOCs are not offered every time, the loyalty to the brand that is consistently striven for gets broken. SOCs are covered later in this chapter.

Client Perception

Client perception impacts the client experience (both in good and bad ways). Perception is defined as the ability to see, hear, or become aware of something through the senses. If a client perceives a lack of confidence in a team member, a poor culture of the practice, a disagreement between team members, or distrust that a veterinarian may have in a team member, the overall trust in the practice is questioned.

Place yourself in your client's shoes for at least 5 minutes every day. Start by walking through the front door. "What does it smell like?" If your answer is "like a veterinary practice" then you have a mission for the day. It is not OK for a practice to smell like a veterinary practice; those odors include urine, feces, and anal glands. Clean smells give clients a positive perception of the practice.

Next, ask, "What does it sound like when I sit in the lobby or in an examination room for 5 minutes?" Do you hear gossip from team members? Do you hear animals waking from anesthesia? Keep in mind the perspective of a client. How would they perceive these sounds? What can be done to make sounds have a positive influence on client perception?

While sitting in the lobby or examination room, what do you see? Look at baseboards, picture frames, fans, vents, and behind racks or tables. Any negative perception the client receives from these visuals, sounds, or smells impacts the client's perception, and the overall client experience.

What Do Clients Really Want?

It is helpful to know what the practice clients expect or would like to see, allowing the team to implement training or technology to exceed expectations. A survey can be deployed to active clients, and the top 10% of clients should be asked individually to participate. Typical responses can be classified into categories (appreciation, technology, listening skills, compassion, honesty, and understanding), helping the leadership team to establish SMART goals for successful implementation.

> **VHMA PERFORMANCE DOMAIN TASK**
>
> Practice managers obtain client feedback on services.

Appreciation: Clients want to be appreciated for selecting the veterinary practice to care for their pet and for recommending new clients. Furthermore, clients want to be appreciated for the care they provide their pets. Identify areas where the practice can step up client appreciation, further driving the customer experience.

Technology: Clients want to have technology made available to them to enhance their ability to communicate with the practice, be better pet parents, and increase the efficiency of care provided for their pets. Consider true electronic medical records (not paper light), pet portals, online pharmacies, online appointment scheduling, and a practice app.

Listening Skills: Clients want team members to listen to their concerns and stories. Clients are the best source of information for diagnosing problems; they know if the pet skipped a meal, if the pet is sleeping more than usual, and any unusual activity. Team members can be poor listeners if they are simply completing tasks on a checklist. It is important to listen, remain nonjudgmental, and avoid making assumptions. Listening builds client relationships; long-lasting relationships build compliance and referrals.

Honesty: Clients want honesty. They want to hear the truth about their pet's condition and about all available treatment options, including transparency of cost. They want to know how to care for their pet in the best way possible for all life stages, including annual exams, weight management, and senior wellness.

Compassion: Clients want to know that the team cares about their pets. They want the receptionist to care when they call and the kennel attendant to care when they pick their pet up. Compassion and empathy are required, and expected, from every member of the veterinary healthcare team.

> **LEADERSHIP POINT**
>
> Compassion is displayed through expressions, tone of voice, and empathetic words.

Understanding: Clients want the team to understand their situation, whether it is financial or personal. Most clients are willing to pay for services, regardless of price, when the team meets their needs and expectations.

THE FRICTIONLESS CLIENT EXPERIENCE

People remember poor customer experiences more than they remember positive ones. In fact, according to Guy Winch, PhD (Psychology), the brain innately has a negativity bias, meaning people will more likely respond to negative experiences. That may also explain why people read positive news stories 26% less than those that cover negative topics.[1]

Friction can be defined as anything that impedes the client experience from glitches on the website to chaos at the front desk, team members seemingly rushed, or prolonged wait times. Friction can be found anywhere in the veterinary practice, and the team must consistently work to create a frictionless client experience. Evaluate the following areas in the practice, and again, put yourself in the client's shoes. Evaluate the perception the client has, including a lack of medical knowledge, but expertise in customer service.

Website

The client experience for new clients starts with the practice website. On average, users spend about 45 seconds on a webpage; much less if it is not responsive, does not appear professional, or does not contain the information they are looking for. Review the section on Websites in Chapter 12, Marketing.

Telephone

Once new and existing clients find a phone number on a mobile responsive website, they will click the link (is your practice phone number available for clients to click?) to call the practice; this is likely their next point of potential friction. In fact, many clients will choose to bypass the telephone and opt for text messaging or emailing to avoid a conversation. For those clients that do call, pay close attention to overcoming a friction-full experience.

Automation: Clients dislike automated telephone services, even though the team feels it improves service. Clients want to talk to someone when they are calling about their pet; someone that has compassion and cares about them. If they are prompted to leave a voicemail, they won't. New clients will call another practice or call the practice back. If clients do leave a voicemail, team members must call the client back as soon as possible (not at the end of the day). A client called with a concern that needs to be addressed and today's client expects an immediate response.

Answering the Phone: The human voice has four components: volume, tone, rate, and quality. The volume of the team member's voice should make listeners feel comfortable, thereby increasing the quality of the conversation. If a person's voice is too loud, listeners (in this case, clients) may pull the phone away from their ear, preventing them from hearing the entire conversation. If a receptionist's volume is too low, clients may be too embarrassed to ask for clarification on something they did not hear well. Correct volume is essential to a successful phone experience.

The tone of a voice is also referred to as *pitch*. Some speakers have a low, comforting tone, which is pleasing to clients. Others may have a high, squeaky pitch. Some clients may be unable to understand a squeaky voice and become irritated. The tone of voice used to answer the phone can give a client a lasting impression (answer the phone with a smile; the positive tone can instantly be heard). Team members should have a pleasant, confident, and understandable voice. Tones can indicate either *"I am too busy to take your call right now" or "I am at your service today; how may I help you?"* (Fig. 11.3).

The rate of speech can greatly affect a conversation. Speaking too quickly can leave the listener confused and unable to follow instructions, or with the perception that the team member is too busy to take the call. People who naturally speak fast should remind themselves to slow their speaking rate. Many older clients cannot hear well and may not be able to understand a team member who is speaking rapidly.

The quality of voice is a combination of clarity, volume, rate, and tone. Word choice and enunciation contribute to the clarity of a phone conversation. Poor word choice and enunciation devalue the professionalism of the individual and decrease the confidence the client has in the practice.

All four factors are interrelated and compound each other. Recording telephone conversations can help team members analyze what they sound like on the phone and help improve skills and telephone etiquette. Hearing one's own voice can be an eye-opener; it is difficult to correct a problem when you are not aware one exists. People are harder on themselves when they self-critique. Because tone of voice can make or break a conversation (and make or break a new client for the hospital), phone training techniques should be implemented. Phone recordings of team members should occur randomly because knowing that a recording is taking place can alter one's behavior. It is advised to let team members and clients know they may be recorded for training purposes only (some states regulate the use of phone recording).

LEADERSHIP POINT

Before a practice manager can ask the team to evaluate themselves on telephone etiquette, leadership must go first and identify their own opportunities for correction, share their opportunities and how they plan to overcome their shortcomings with the team, then ask the team for help to continue their improvement.

Team members should always answer the phone by introducing themselves: *"Good morning, ABC Animal Clinic, this is Teresa. How may I help you?"* Often, long-time clients feel guilty or embarrassed when they call and cannot identify with whom they are speaking. An introduction will eliminate confusion and begin developing a relationship.

It is important to write down the client and patient name when the caller provides it. This prevents team members from asking the client to repeat his/her name and appearing disorganized. This also allows the team member to address a client placed on hold personally when resuming the conversation. *"Thank you for holding, Mrs. Jones. Sparky's record indicates that he is due for vaccines ..."*

Guidelines and training protocols should be developed outlining what to say, and what not to say. Information conveyed using different words can have a different meaning to the caller. For example, a client may call the hospital to request an appointment, believing that Sparky's ear infection is a sudden emergency. The receptionist may respond, *"There are no appointments available until next week; however, you can come in as a walk-in and wait to be seen."* A client first hears *"we have no appointments,"* disengages in the conversation, and starts considering where else Sparky can be seen.

An improved response is *"It sounds like we need to see Sparky today, Mrs. Smith. We can accept you as a walk-in because our appointments are booked today. We will work Sparky in between appointments if you don't mind waiting."* By rewording the conversation, the client feels you have addressed her request, and the practice is willing to "fit" her in. This builds rapport and respect between the practice and the client.

Develop a list of frequently asked questions and appropriate responses (Fig. 11.4). Role-playing can facilitate genuine (and correct) responses to these potentially difficult situations. Role-playing is uncomfortable for fear that fellow team members will judge them. However, in a positive culture, team members help one another form excellent responses. Practicing (role-playing) together makes these situations more comfortable and easier to handle when presented by clients.

Team members must learn to refrain from phrases such as *"I don't know"* which implies the team member is not knowledgeable or does not care to get the correct information for the client. Instead, team members can reply, *"That is a great question, let me find out."* Rather than a hurried *"Just a second,"* a team member might say, *"Give me just a moment to get that information."* The combination of words and

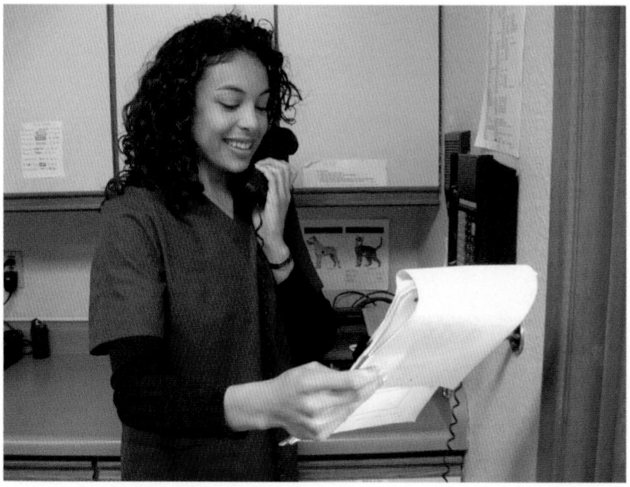

Fig. 11.3 Answering the phone with a smile projects a friendly attitude that can be detected by the listener.

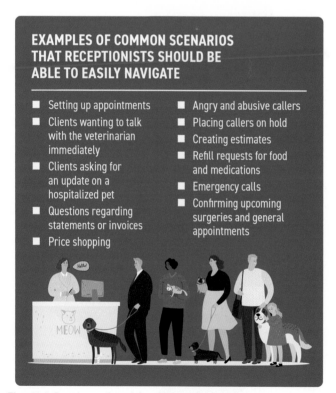

Fig. 11.4 Develop a list of frequently asked questions and appropriate responses to help the receptionist strategically navigate client conversations.

tone can have a powerful effect on clients. Phrases such as *"Absolutely!,"* *"I know how much you care,"* and *"I understand"* are powerful statements that help create empathy with clients (Fig. 11.5).

Some clients enjoy casual phone conversations with the staff. Clients enjoy talking about their pets, and veterinary professionals are ideal listeners. However, team members may need to control the conversation because another phone line is ringing, or a client is waiting at the desk to pick up a pet or check out (Fig. 11.6). A few options exist to help control conversations.

1. It is acceptable to let the client know that there is another client waiting and ask if you can call the client back in approximately 10 minutes (then provide exceptional service by calling the client back in 5 minutes).
2. Ask only closed-ended (yes or no) questions, such as *"Is Fluffy vomiting?"* or *"Does Fluffy have diarrhea?"* (Note: closed-ended questions are not ideal when taking an accurate history from clients; it is only offered as a suggestion here to help control prolonged conversations.)

Some clients may still attempt to prolong conversations, but skilled team members can get an appointment scheduled and end the conversation. With practice and role-playing, team members will learn to convey sincerity while managing these conversations.

Receptionists often hear the same questions repeatedly when answering phones. Frequently asked questions and answers can be compiled by the medical team as a guide to enhance the knowledge of the receptionist team and enable them to answer questions quickly, efficiently, and with confidence (Fig. 11.7).

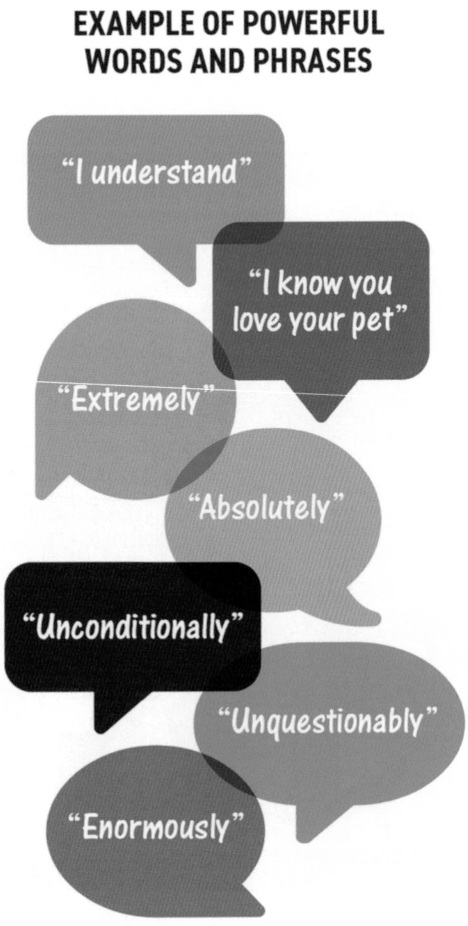
EXAMPLE OF POWERFUL WORDS AND PHRASES
"I understand"
"I know you love your pet"
"Extremely"
"Absolutely"
"Unconditionally"
"Unquestionably"
"Enormously"

Fig. 11.5 Powerful words and phrases can be used to express compassion and empathy with clients.

Triaging Phone Calls: The practice receives phone calls from clients expressing concern for their pet that don't realize that their pet is experiencing an emergency. Well-trained team members know when the pet needs to be seen immediately. Developing a list of potential emergencies with the medical team and the appropriate response for clients is essential and must be included in onboard training and continuing education events. Consider the example of a pet that is squinting the eye accommodated by drainage. Pets do not know they shouldn't scratch their eye (it hurts!), and that doing so can cause further damage. A case like this should be seen immediately, not 2 or 3 days later. See Chapter 10, Appointment Management, for more triaging tips.

Managing Multiple Phone Lines: Receptionists greet clients while they walk in and out of the practice, enter invoices or charges, and answer multiple phone lines at the same time (Fig. 11.8). In general, phones should not ring more than twice before being answered. Most clients call on cell phones (versus landlines), and the phone will ring on the client's cell phone at least once before the practice phone rings. If it has rung twice in the practice, it has rung three times for the client, and too many rings can create a negative perception for the client.

If a receptionist is with another client or on another line, it is acceptable to ask a caller to hold momentarily because another phone line is ringing. For example, *"Good morning, ABC Animal Clinic, this is Teresa. I am on the other line [or with another client], is this an emergency or are you able to hold one moment?"* Once the client answers yes (and they must be given time to answer), the team member should say, *"thank you."* This allows the receptionist to finish with the first client. Asking a client *"Are you able to hold one moment?"* does exactly that; it asks the client politely if they can hold. A short *"can you hold?"* becomes a demand, not a question.

Resume the conversation with *"Thank you for holding, how may I help you?"* If multiple lines continue ringing, a receptionist may also ask clients if a return call is possible instead of waiting on hold. *"Thank you for holding, this is Teresa. I have a client waiting for me, do you mind if I call you back in 10 minutes, so you don't have to continue to hold?"* Again, the client should be called back as soon as possible, or no more than 5 minutes later.

It is important to not leave callers on hold for more than 1 minute. Most current phone systems sound an alert after a short period; at this time clients should be told that the team member helping them would return momentarily. Do not continue to place clients on hold each time the alarm sounds. If the client will be on hold for more than 1 or 2 minutes, the client should be asked if a team member can return the call; 1 minute on hold seems like 5 minutes to a client.

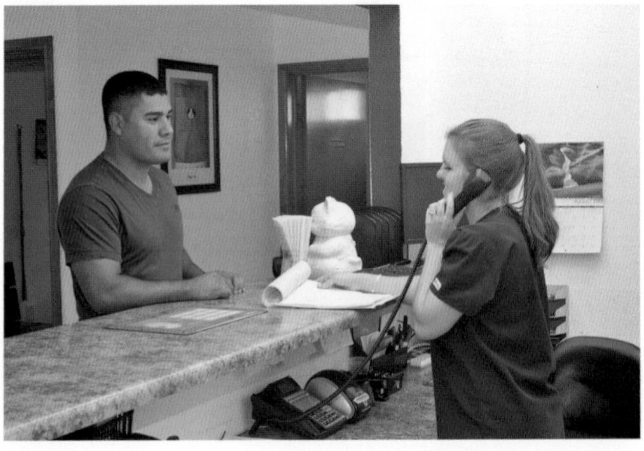

Fig. 11.6 The receptionist must be able to multitask in a friendly and polite manner.

GENERAL QUESTIONS THE RECEPTION TEAM SHOULD BE ABLE TO ANSWER

VACCINE PROTOCOLS
- How old do puppies and kittens need to be to start vaccinations?
- What vaccinations are recommended?
- What vaccinations are included?
- How often are vaccinations given?
- What is included in the initial puppy or kitten examination?
- How much do vaccinations cost?

SPAYING AND NEUTERING PETS
- How old do pets have to be to be altered?
- Do vaccinations have to be current?
- What does the surgical procedure entail?
- Is pain medication included?
- When do pets need to arrive at the practice?
- When are they usually ready to go home?
- Do they need to be held off food and water?
- How much does the procedure cost?
- What laboratory work is required? Are intravenous fluids required?

SICK PETS
- Is the pet vomiting? If yes, for how long?
- Does the pet have diarrhea? If yes, for how long?
- Does the pet have an appetite?
- Is the pet current on vaccinations?

HEARTWORM PREVENTATIVE
- What is it?
- What tests are required to start the pet on preventive?
- What products does the practice carry?
- How is it administered?
- How often is it administered?
- How much does it cost?

DIETS
- What special diets does the practice carry?
- What maintenance diets does the practice carry?
- What should I feed my pet?

FLEA AND TICK PREVENTIVE
- What diseases do fleas and ticks carry?
- Can people catch these diseases?
- What products does the practice carry?
- How are these products administered?
- How often are these products administered?
- How much do they cost?

New team members may be overwhelmed with new information. Frequently asked question sheets can help new team members answer questions almost as well as those with experience.

Fig. 11.7 The medical team can help create FAQs to help the receptionist team deliver exceptional service.

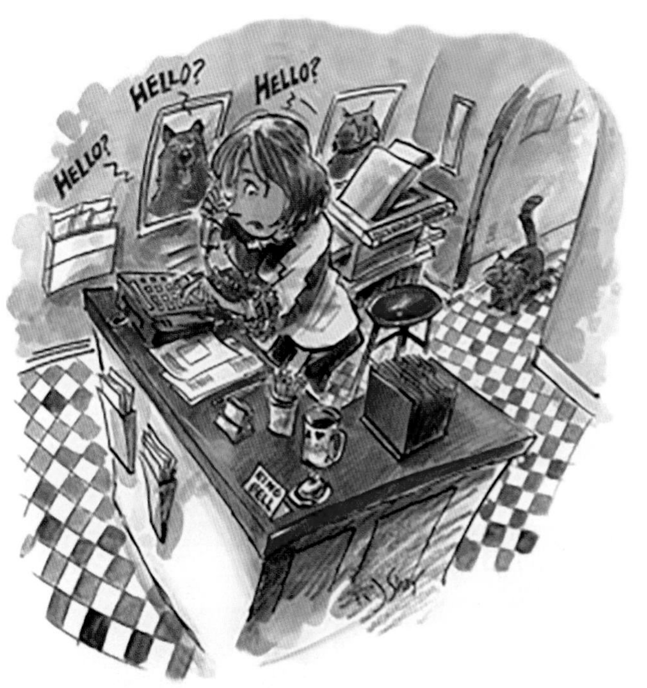

Fig. 11.8 Receptionists are responsible for many duties, including managing multiple telephone lines and greeting incoming clients.

The time a client is on hold can be valuable marketing time. Special on-hold systems can generate specific messages about the veterinary practice or diseases that may be a concern to the geographic area. Clients can listen to a variety of topics while they are on hold. This information can include practice hours, history of the veterinarians, or specialties or products that the practice offers (see Chapter 12, Marketing). If the caller has something to listen to, the wait time does not seem as long and assures the client that the phone line has not been disconnected. It can be difficult to determine whether a call has been disconnected if the line is silent, especially while on cell phones.

Cross-trained team members must help when the phone lines continue to ring; if a phone line has rung more than twice, the reception team needs help! Telephone calls are one of the first impressions made to a client, whether new or existing. If a client believes he or she was rushed through a conversation or that a call was never answered, the client may go to another practice.

LEADERSHIP POINT

Practice managers may find that all phone lines are always busy. If this is the case, it is imperative to add additional phone lines and team members to handle the call volume. Client business starts here; don't allow barriers that prevent the business from growing.

It is ideal to have a call center located separately from the reception area (Fig. 11.9), allowing receptionists to give clients their full attention as they enter and leave the practice. Mistakes are decreased when team members can concentrate on one client at a time. The team member(s) in the call center can concentrate on answering calls promptly and can review patient histories without other clients overhearing conversations. Some practice owners may argue that this will increase labor costs; however, if a receptionist can increase an average transaction by $20 by catching a missed charge or filling medication the client forgot to request, then one receptionist has covered the cost of the labor and increased the profits at the end of the day (Fig. 11.10). Ultimately, clients are satisfied and will return because they experienced superior customer service within the veterinary practice. A continued interruption in client service builds a negative perception of the practice.

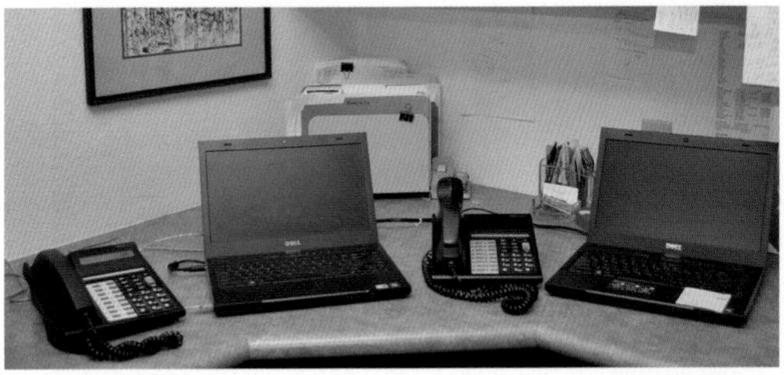

Fig. 11.9 Call centers away from the reception area allows team members to focus on the client that is in front of them.

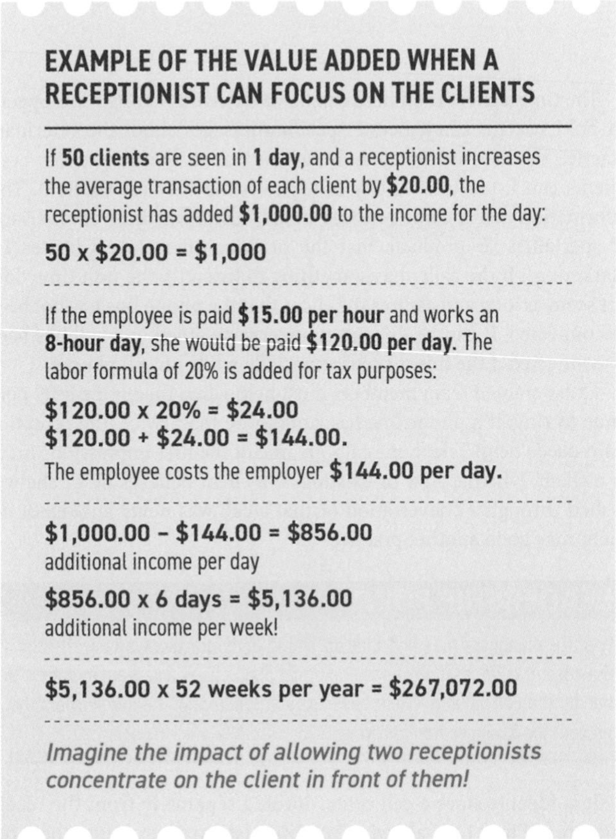
EXAMPLE OF THE VALUE ADDED WHEN A RECEPTIONIST CAN FOCUS ON THE CLIENTS
If 50 clients are seen in 1 day, and a receptionist increases the average transaction of each client by $20.00, the receptionist has added $1,000.00 to the income for the day:
50 x $20.00 = $1,000
If the employee is paid $15.00 per hour and works an 8-hour day, she would be paid $120.00 per day. The labor formula of 20% is added for tax purposes:
$120.00 x 20% = $24.00
$120.00 + $24.00 = $144.00.
The employee costs the employer $144.00 per day.
$1,000.00 - $144.00 = $856.00
additional income per day
$856.00 x 6 days = $5,136.00
additional income per week!
$5,136.00 x 52 weeks per year = $267,072.00
Imagine the impact of allowing two receptionists concentrate on the client in front of them!

Fig. 11.10 Empower the receptionist team to identify potentially missed opportunities by focusing on the client in front of them, versus multitasking across several clients.

Appointment Scheduling

Clients want to be able to book appointments on their time. They are busy and often forget to call and schedule an appointment during business hours, resulting in delayed patient care. In addition, not all appointments need a receptionist. Clients should be able to schedule appointments any time, any day, without calling the practice. Further, clients should be able to book an appointment online with a confirmed time, not wait for communication from the practice as to whether that time is in fact, available. Finally, clients should receive a text message within the hour of booking the appointment confirming the date, time, and service requested.

CRITICAL COMPETENCY: ADAPTABILITY

Being open to change and flexible work methods; the ability to adapt behavior to changing conditions or new information.

Some PIMS applications, pet portals, or communications systems allow clients to request an appointment, but the practice must reply during business hours. Additionally, some practices are hesitant to allow a third-party application to "write back to the PIMS" when booking the appointment. This system is no longer good enough to meet client expectations. Allowing the client to book directly into the PIMS without a phone call improves team efficiency by allowing them to concentrate on the clients that are in front of them at that moment. By giving clients the ability to book their own appointments and providing clients the attention they deserve while in the practice, the client experience is vastly improved. While a few cloud-based PIMS provide this service as a part of the system (at the time of publication), Vetstoria.com is the only company that directly integrates with most PIMS appointment calendars, allowing parameters to be put into place that meet practice needs. Once activated, the link should be placed at the top of the webpage, at the closing of every email, in the practice app and pet portal, and included on all reminders. Using technology like this can reduce incoming call volume by 60%.[2]

Turning Phone Calls Into Appointments: The team member answering the phone has the potential to turn every phone inquiry into a client. A friendly and genuine voice makes a potential client

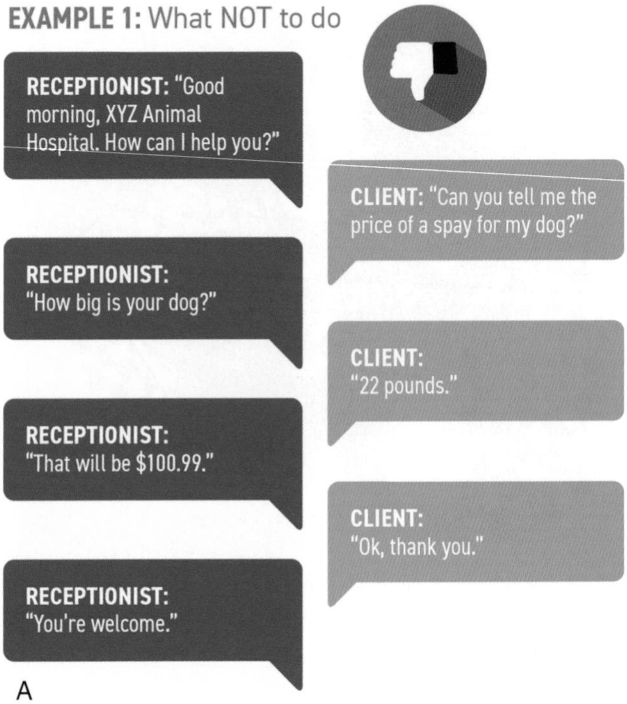
EXAMPLE 1: What NOT to do
RECEPTIONIST: "Good morning, XYZ Animal Hospital. How can I help you?"
CLIENT: "Can you tell me the price of a spay for my dog?"
RECEPTIONIST: "How big is your dog?"
CLIENT: "22 pounds."
RECEPTIONIST: "That will be $100.99."
CLIENT: "Ok, thank you."
RECEPTIONIST: "You're welcome."

A

feel comfortable and encourages the caller to ask questions. When the phone is answered in a polite, educated, and unhurried manner, the caller is inclined to ask questions and make an appointment. Ask open-ended questions to generate conversation; the more education and value a team member can provide a potential client, the more likely the practice will gain a new client. Always ask if an appointment can be made at the end of a phone conversation, and end the discussion with *"Mr. Jones, have I answered all your questions today? My name is Emma, and please call back anytime with other questions you may have."*

Anytime a client (or potential client) asks questions regarding the price of services, team members should be able to educate the client on the service itself, and "WOW!" the client with the value they will receive when coming to the practice. A client calling to obtain the price of a neuter should not just receive the dollar amount. Compare the following examples and determine which conversation is more likely to secure an appointment.

EXAMPLE 2: Add value to the conversation

RECEPTIONIST: "Good morning, XYZ Animal Hospital. How can I help you?"

CLIENT: "Can you tell me the price of a spay for my dog?"

RECEPTIONIST:"Of course I can. I need to ask a few questions, which will help me give you the best estimate. First, what is your dog's name?"

CLIENT: "Rosey."

RECEPTIONIST: "How old is Rosey, and what breed is she?"

CLIENT: "She is 6 months old and is a basset hound."

RECEPTIONIST: "Oh, bassets are so cute at this age! Tell me, how much does Rosey weigh, approximately?"

CLIENT: "22 pounds."

RECEPTIONIST: "Now that I have this information, let me give you some information about the spay procedure for Rosey, and what you can expect postoperatively. First, it is best to spay her at a young age; this will help her recover quicker and helps prevent cancer associated with heat cycles later in her life. Here at ABC Veterinary Hospital, we perform a preoperative examination and listen to her heart and lungs and look for any abnormalities that may alter our anesthesia plan. We also perform blood work, ensuring Rosey's liver and kidneys are functioning normally, as this can also alter our anesthetic plan. Each patient is different and must be evaluated as such.

Before Rosey's anesthesia, she is given pain medication and a tranquilizer to help her feel more comfortable. When Rosy is under anesthesia, we monitor her blood pressure, ECG, heart rate, respiratory rate, and temperature, among other vitals. When she awakes from anesthesia, she is kept in our recovery room with our veterinary technicians, where we continue to monitor her vitals. Rosey will go home with pain medication for you to start that evening, along with a complete set of discharge instructions. Do you have any questions about the procedure itself?"

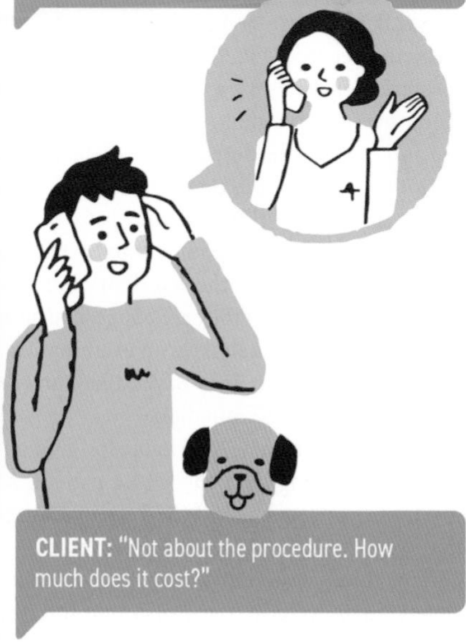

CLIENT: "Not about the procedure. How much does it cost?"

RECEPTIONIST: "The exam, blood work, preoperative pain medication, anesthesia, surgery, and pain medication for you to take home is all included in our price of $359.89. I have an appointment available for Rosey on Tuesday; would you be able to bring her in between 8 and 9 in the morning?"

B

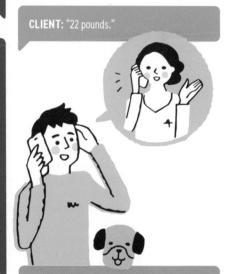

A conversation of this nature has established several points.

- A relationship has been established. The team member obtained Rosey's name, allowing it to be used in the conversation.
- The team member makes a personal comment about the breed. The comment does not have to be breed specific; it may be a comment about the pet's name or age. The point is to make a specific, positive comment about the pet itself, continuing to build the relationship.
- By explaining the procedure, the team member is showing value in the service being provided. Perhaps ABC Veterinary Clinic is more expensive than XYZ Animal Hospital; however, Carol explained why. She is also educating the client on why specific procedures are important.
- At the end of the conversation, she offers the client an appointment date right away; often team members will end a conversation with *"Would you like to make an appointment?"* This allows the client to say, *"No, I will call back later."* When a specific time slot is offered, client acceptance is much higher.

Always show value in the service being offered. Clients do not know good medicine from bad medicine, and they depend on team members to provide the education needed to make the right decision.

Practices should be able to turn 70% of phone-shopped calls into appointments. A logbook can be kept tracking incoming calls; if 70% of calls are not turned into appointments, managers should determine why and implement training to increase this number.

LEADERSHIP POINT

Potential reasons a practice may have a low percentage rate of being able to turn phone shoppers into an appointment may include a team member's tone of voice or word choice, poor explanation of services, a lack of training, an inability to answer client questions, or lack of recommending a specific time to set an appointment.

Liability of Telephone Calls: Team members can and should be held accountable for incorrect verbal communication, as misunderstood conversations can be held against the veterinarian, putting their license in jeopardy with the state veterinary medical board. Every telephone call (and text or email interaction) must be documented in the patient's record, with details regarding the conversation. Only the veterinarian should give a diagnosis or prognosis over the phone. Diagnosing over the phone by a nonveterinary staff member is inappropriate and can be considered malpractice. Phrases such as *"you may want to wait and watch," "this does not sound like an emergency,"* or *"you can just give some Pepto-Bismol if your pet is vomiting"* must never be said. If the pet happens to expire overnight, have complications, or be seen at an emergency clinic, the veterinary practice can be held liable. Always advise clients that if they are concerned about their pet's health, they should bring the animal in for an examination (and document the call in the medical record). They have called for a service; offer to solve their pet's issue with an examination.

Veterinarians can also be held liable for giving medical advice over the phone if something happens to the patient. Malpractice lawsuits may have fewer consequences if the veterinarian gives medical advice compared with staff giving advice; however, the potential still exists. Veterinarians must also remember to document the conversation immediately; many veterinarians rush into the next appointment and forget to document the conversation in the medical record.

Arriving at the Hospital: First Impressions

Clients draw preliminary opinions about a practice within the first 2 to 5 minutes of entering the building. This perception (especially if it is negative) can continue through the rest of the visit. Team members should always greet clients as they enter the practice, regardless of what other tasks they may be doing. If a team member is on the phone, acknowledging clients with a smile and a wave is acceptable. If a team member is helping another client, greet the entering client with a smile and say, *"Hello, I will be with you in a moment."* If the receptionist is working with another team member, that task should be set aside, and the client should receive the full attention of both team members.

Greeting clients by their names and addressing their pets creates a positive first impression (Fig. 11.11). This can be more difficult with first-time clients; however, clients always appreciate kind words and compliments. Try conversation starters such as *"Fluffy is such a beautiful girl,"* or *"Good morning! Thank you for bringing Fluffy in today. We're glad you're here!"* Positive comments start building a long-lasting client bond. Some clients may prefer to be addressed as Dr., Mr., or Mrs. Once the initial appointment has begun, team members may ask the new client how they wish to be addressed. A notation can be made in the record, allowing team members to address clients appropriately each time they arrive at the practice.

Controlling the Front Desk Chaos: To make a great first impression, receptionists must address any chaos happening at the front desk. Consider walking into a human practitioner's office; the phone is constantly ringing, team members appear frantic, clients are coming and going without smiles on their faces, and patients are checking their watches while they wait. What impression is made for these clients sitting in the lobby? The situation appears out of control, chaotic, and unorganized. Clients cannot see behind the scenes, but they are quick to form an overall judgment based on the first impression of chaos.

In veterinary practices, the previous scenario occurs every day; multiple phone lines ring at the same time, emergencies come in that need triaging, team members are frantic, clients appear unhappy because they have a sick pet, and wait times are long. This becomes the client's perception of the entire hospital, and a judgment forms. But chaos can be minimized at the front desk with some thoughtful planning. Consider a few of these tips:

- Place the call center elsewhere in the hospital. Allow the reception team to concentrate on the clients in front of them.
- Hire accordingly for the front office and be well-staffed for peak hours. This area makes the first impression; ensure that it runs as smoothly as possible.
- Create different spaces in the reception area for clients that are checking in and those that are checking out.

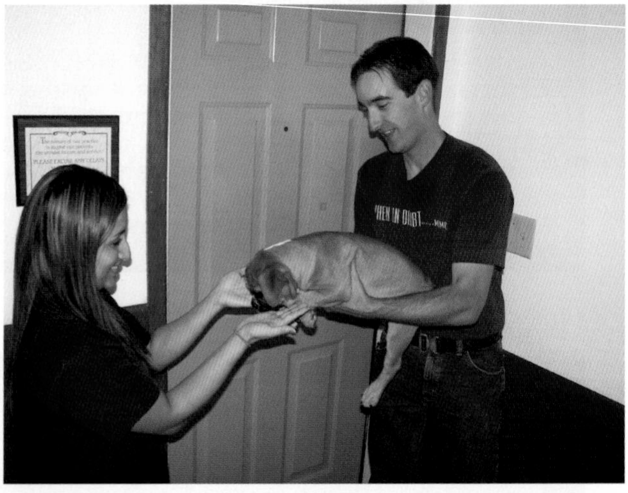

Fig. 11.11 Greeting clients at the door and addressing them by name makes them feel they are getting personalized attention.

- Review appointment times and stagger the schedule to prevent overlapping (Chapter 10, Appointments).
- Greet clients in a warm and welcoming manner, regardless of what is happening around the desk.
- Communicate with waiting clients if there are delays because of an emergency.

Chaos is sometimes unavoidable in veterinary practice, but a skilled team can control the chaos and avoid creating negative client impressions.

The first and last impression of the practice (and the client's perception) is what they will remember most. Evaluate the experience your clients are having to create a frictionless experience.

The Check-In Experience

Evaluate the check-in process in the practice. What does it "feel" like for a client? Does the team know who the client and pet are? Is the team prepared to make the client feel welcome and engage in personal conversation with the client? What can be done to make the experience simpler? Consider the tasks that must be done; verifying email and cell phone, obtaining a brief synopsis of the reason for the visit (if it was not documented previously), perhaps taking a photo of the pet, and offering the client some water, coffee, or tea as they wait. If the client called the practice to make the appointment for an ill pet and the receptionist collected notes, the details do not need to be reviewed again; a simple confirmation of the presenting complaint is fine. The client will provide the information again in the exam room with the veterinary technician and doctor (no need to tell the story 2–3 times in the same visit).

Triaging Patients: The reception team may need to triage patients when they arrive. Triage is prioritizing patients according to the severity of their conditions. If a patient arrives with an obvious medical emergency (hit by a car, dog fight, heat stroke, etc.), the pet may need to be rushed to a treatment area to be further evaluated by the team. If a client feels their pet is experiencing a medical emergency, a credentialed veterinary technician should rush to the reception area to evaluate the patient for stability. What clients consider an emergency is not always a medical emergency to team members, but the patient must be evaluated immediately. If a patient arrives with symptoms of any contagious disease, (i.e., parvo, distemper) the patient should be immediately placed in isolation or kept in the car away from other animals until an examination room is available. Cross collaboration between roles and training is required for successful triaging in the practice.

Waiting Clients: Inevitably, the appointment schedule gets backed up. Even with the best-laid plans, emergencies and walk-ins flood the practice. Team members must have a backup plan (for both entertainment and communication) for clients who may have an extended wait time.

Receptionists should constantly monitor the schedule for delays and pay attention to how long clients are waiting to be seen. Consider keeping a log so that anomalies can be addressed and corrected in the future. Statistically, client compliance drops based on how long clients wait (irritated clients are less likely to accept all recommendations). Of course, that makes sense: veterinary practices ask clients to respect the veterinarian's time and arrive for their scheduled appointments on time. If the client is late, they may be asked to wait, but if they're on time they need to be seen in an appropriate amount of time. They may have taken time off work to accommodate appointments. In the eyes of a client, if a practice asks them to respect the veterinarian's time, then the practice must respect their time. Additionally, pets are already stressed about coming in for appointments and unnecessary wait times make that worse for the patient. Running behind is sometimes inevitable. Emergencies happen and walk-ins come in at inconvenient times, but that cannot be an everyday excuse for running behind.

If a team member notes the schedule is getting backed up, call clients ahead of time and let them know of the delay. They may choose to reschedule rather than wait for a prolonged period (clients appreciate these calls). For clients that have arrived for appointments and are in an exam room, set a timer to continue checking on them every 5 minutes (5 minutes in a small room feels like 10). Communication is the key to client happiness in these situations.

Practices may consider having a tea/coffee machine for clients while they wait (Fig. 11.12). Allowing clients to select their flavor and make the brew appears to be a service bonus. Have some toys available for kids. Children get bored easily, making the wait seem even longer for their parents. Some practices may have a playroom, others may have a simple toy box in the reception area.

During wait times, team members should take the opportunity to educate clients or take them on a tour of the practice app, a pet portal, a website, or an online store, helping them become more aware of the services they can access. This is when the hospital can practice its hospitality and educational skills. Most clients don't mind a wait if they feel they are being "taken care of." What defines "taken care of"?

1. Communication. Acknowledge that there is a wait; apologize and understand the clients' frustration. Offer to reschedule if the wait is anticipated to be long.
2. Offer water, coffee, or a beverage to drink.
3. Educate the client on updates or special offers. Is it dental month? Does the practice have a new pet portal to introduce? Have they used the practice's social media? Does the client know about boarding services?
4. It is understandable If a client needs to leave their pet or reschedule; offer solutions before they become irritable. Making clients sit in an examination room alone for an extended period damages the practice brand and bond that is trying to be established (think of this as a time out; the client feels reprimanded for being on time!). If appointments are running behind, use this time to work on building the relationship.

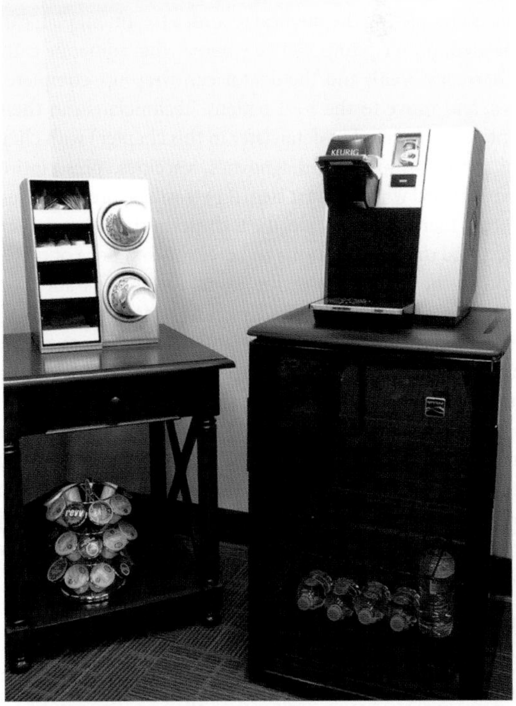

Fig. 11.12 Coffee and tea machines are a nice benefit for waiting clients.

LEADERSHIP POINT

Client behavior has changed over the past 10 years; they are no longer loyal and willing to wait an extended time to see a veterinarian. They will leave and visit another practice that respects their time.

Another tender moment is when clients bring their pets to be euthanized. This is an extremely difficult time for clients, and skilled teams make the experience less painful. The receptionist should notify team members when euthanasia is planned so everyone can be sensitive to the atmosphere of the practice (i.e., no laughing or giggling in the halls). A sign should be posted on the examination room door where the euthanasia is occurring. Consider turning off hallway lights in front of the examination room to ensure all team members are aware of the event and respond respectfully.

Take care of all business transactions for euthanasia before the procedure is performed. This includes choosing disposal options, presenting an invoice, and collecting fees. This allows a client to leave the building when they are ready, without having to stop at the reception desk on the way out.

Exam Room Experience

This experience is often friction-full for clients as they get left in rooms, can hear others talking outside the room, and their pet gets anxious waiting and sniffing "odd" smells. Evaluate this experience from both the lens of the client and the patient. What can clients see (spots of blood on the walls/ceiling, hair, and dirt among the baseboards), hear (animals recovering from anesthesia), and smell? Consider adding Fear Free® techniques to ease patient fears and help them love the veterinary practice.

Clients will tell the technician or assistant what is happening with their pet (either wellness or illness) and then repeat the same story when the doctor comes in. Add efficiency by changing this process; have the doctor and technician take the history and vitals together. To further increase efficiency, have a scribe in the room that can complete the medical record as the doctor completes the physical exam out loud, explaining what he or she is looking for during the exam. This adds value to the client, provides education, and helps the client feel more involved. As the scribe is completing the medical record, a treatment plan can be created if needed, prescriptions can be entered (that someone can prepare in the pharmacy area), and the doctor can wrap up, complete the last few notes, and move to the next patient. Technicians can then review treatment plans (covered in detail later in this chapter) with clients, gain approval for recommended diagnostics, vaccines, prescriptions, etc., and move forward with the next step. If pets will be prescribed any medication other than a parasiticide, the technician should review potential side effects and drug interactions and give the first dose of medication.

Checking the client out in the exam room adds additional efficiency measures, allowing the technicians to forward book appointments (covered in the next section) and review the invoice in detail with the client. Having a small printer (if space allows) and a credit card machine that integrates with the PIMS in the room further increases efficiency and decreases errors. If the checkout process does not occur in the exam room, the technician needs to walk the client to the reception desk and turn over the client to a receptionist by providing details of the exams and next steps (forward book appointment, etc.). The receptionist must be ready to accept the client and not appear disorganized or chaotic.

The Check-Out Experience

When clients get to this point, they are ready to leave the practice and begin to mentally check out. Waiting longer for the medical record to be completed is unacceptable and adds a level of friction for the client and pet. This is the last impression that is made on the client: it must be exceptional.

Forward Booking Appointments: When a client has been provided a service at the veterinary hospital, a follow-up appointment may be needed. Booking appointments for clients before they leave the practice is referred to as *forward booking* and is a team sport. Success starts in the exam room when the veterinarian tells the client the next appointment will be booked for them before they leave. Always forward book medical progress examinations, booster vaccines, follow-up laboratory work, and annual examinations. It is very important to schedule these appointments before accepting payment for services; once payment has been rendered, the client mentally "checks out" and is ready to leave the hospital.

Most clients return for medical progress appointments when the appointment was previously scheduled. If the patient is recovering well and the client must initiate a phone call to make an appointment, they won't. Vaccines that need boosters given within a certain time must be scheduled since most clients procrastinate and don't make the appointment on time. Although annual examinations and vaccine appointments are scheduled a year in advance, most clients adhere to the original appointment. The practice should provide clients with plenty of reminders, allowing clients to reschedule if needed. See Chapter 10 for more discussion and resources available to implement a successful forward booking program.

CRITICAL COMPETENCY: ORAL COMMUNICATION AND COMPREHENSION

The ability to express one's thoughts verbally in a clear and understandable manner, and the ability to actively listen and attend to what others are saying. Good group presentation skills are a must.

Reviewing Invoices with Owners: Whether a receptionist delivers an invoice to a client at the front desk, or a technician delivers in an exam room, the invoice should always be detailed with the owners before collecting money. The team member must be knowledgeable enough to answer questions easily to maintain the confidence of the client. Invoices should include every detail of the services provided (including items that are discounted or free). The client should be able to read the invoice (Fig. 11.13) while the team member explains the charges (Fig. 11.14).

This detailed presentation allows the client to read and understand the services and charges. The value of client service can be increased when all procedures are explained thoroughly. A less advisable conversation would be, *"Hello, Mrs. Rogers. I have Scruffy's invoice ready. The total is $398.34. How would you like to pay for that today?"* In this situation, the client does not know what she is paying for and may have sticker shock at the cost of a "simple spay." She will not perceive the value of the services her pet was provided. She may search for a cheaper clinic for her next veterinary visit. By detailing the services, you can assure the client that Scruffy was well cared for, pain relief was provided, intravenous fluids were administered, etc.; you have now illustrated the high level of care Scruffy received.

Collecting Payment: Most clients pay with debit/credit cards while a small minority pay with checks or cash (review Chapter 3, The Veterinary Team, for payment options). Having an integrated credit card swiper is integral to having decreased manual entry errors and speeds up the process for the client. The credit card invoice can be stapled to the client's invoice.

Handling Declined Transactions: If a client's credit card, check, or debit card has been declined, politely and discreetly inform the client of the decline. Ask for an alternative method of payment. Some credit cards and debit cards have a maximum charge amount per day, so the

ABC Animal Clinic
555 Uptown Circle
Anytown, MN 89000
314-134-4431

Maria Rogers
6454 Downtown Circle
Anytown, MN 89001 Account # 21312

"Scruffy" Rogers
Age: 9 years
Weight: 45#
Reminders: DHPP due 5/10/23
Rabies due 5/10/23
Heartworm Test due 5/10/23

Invoice Number: 10090
Date: 04/28/23
Dr. Nancy Bresiger

Date	Service	Unit	Extended Cost
04/28/08	Pre-Anesthetic Exam	1	0.00
04/28/08	Pre-Anesthetic Bloodwork	1	$95.99
04/28/08	CBC/Chemistry	1	
04/28/08	Electrolytes	1	
04/28/08	Pre-Anesthetic ECG	1	$49.99
04/28/08	IV Fluids – Surgery	1	$84.85
04/28/08	IV Catheter	1	
04/28/08	IV Administration Set	1	
04/28/08	Normosol 1 Liter	1	
04/28/08	General Anesthesia	1	$151.20
04/28/08	Pre-Anesthetic	1	
04/28/08	Sevoflurane	1	
04/28/08	K-9 OVH under 50#	1	$157.89
04/28/08	OVH Pack	1	
04/28/08	Suture Material	2	
04/28/08	Biohazard Fee	1	
04/28/08	Surgical Monitoring	1	
04/28/08	Post-Operative Pain Medication	1	$24.99
	Subtotal		$564.91
	Tax 6.25%		$25.10
	Invoice Total		**$590.01**

Fig. 11.13 Sample invoice.

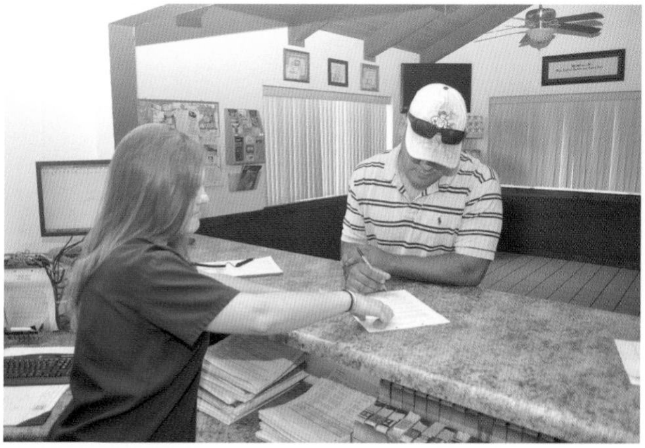

Fig. 11.14 The receptionist should review invoices with clients before accepting payment.

EXAMPLE 1: The client has arrived to pick up her pet and the receptionist greets her:

RECEPTIONIST: "Hello, Mrs. Rogers, are you here to pick up Scruffy?"

CLIENT: "Yes I am."

RECEPTIONIST: "I have her invoice ready for you. Today she had a preoperative exam at no charge; preoperative blood work for $45.99; a preoperative ECG for $49.99; and IV fluids for $54.85, which includes the IV catheter, IV administrative set, and the fluids. Her anesthesia, which included pre-operative pain medication and vital monitoring was $101.20; the ovariohysterectomy, which included the surgery pack and materials was $97.89; and her post operative pain medication which was given after surgery and for you to take home is $24.99. Scruffy's total is $398.34. Do you have any questions for me before the veterinary technician comes out to review Scruffy's post-operative instructions?

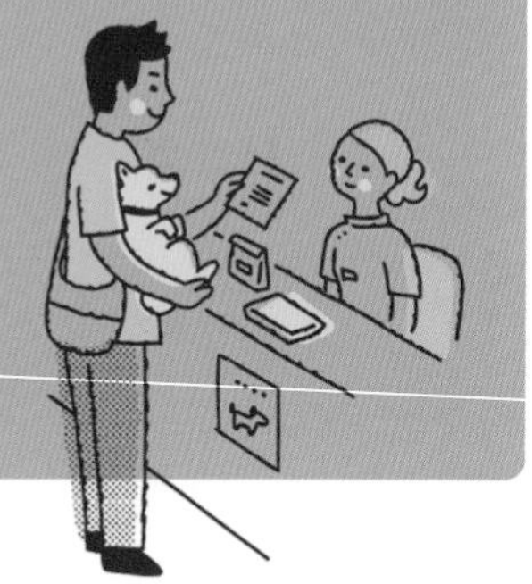

overdraft may be unintentional. Do not assume that a client has bad credit because of a refusal; there may be an innocent reason behind the decline.

Hospital policy regarding declined charges should be developed and instituted so that consistent protocol is relayed to all team members. Some practices allow a client to return to pay on the account; others may keep medication that was to be dispensed until a client can return with payment. Never keep a client's pet because of a declined payment. Practices are then responsible for the upkeep and care of the pet until the owner returns. If the pet is sick or debilitated, the owner may not return! It is also against the law in many states to hold a pet for ransom. Each state has different lien laws regarding holding pets; practice owners and managers should check with their state board of veterinary medicine for clarification.

Practice leadership is responsible for determining whether the clinic will allow clients to charge for services rendered. Every member of the team must be familiar with the policy, including the veterinarians. Practice managers and/or office managers should be the only team members allowed to approve this type of transaction. Often, veterinarians and technicians empathize with the client and wish to extend credit; unfortunately, many clients will not return to the practice to make payments. CareCredit should always be offered to clients wishing to finance services. This allows the practice to give clients an option when they may not be able to pay for services rendered (the practice will receive immediate payment, and the client can make payments to CareCredit). Not all clients can afford expensive services, so several payment options should be available so that care can be provided. Clients may elect conservative treatments because of the cost of services and should not be judged for their decisions. On the other hand, never assume clients cannot afford necessary services. Pets are often considered family members, and clients will often stretch their budget to care for them.

Help Clients Navigate to their Car: Clients may have their hands full with their pets as they leave the practice. Carry bags of food and open the door, carry an umbrella if it is raining, and offer to hold the pet while they get their keys and unlock the door. While some of these recommendations may not be applicable every time, it is the act of kindness and caring being displayed by the team member that creates a frictionless experience.

Following Up with Clients After the Visit

Checking in with clients after the visit is important, regardless of the reason for the visit. These are also known as "recalls" and should be done for every patient. Clients always have questions after their visit; connecting with them before they call the practice shows care and concern, and simply exceptional service.

Recalls can be in the form of text messages or phone calls, whichever the client prefers. Recalls are generated by the PIMS to remind the team to check on patients that have had any service performed (Fig. 11.15). Service codes should be set up to automatically generate recalls; on occasion, a manual entry will be needed when requested by the doctor. Fig. 11.16 provides ideas of when a client should be connected with to enhance the frictionless client experience.

Each day, the reception team can print the list and distribute it to the appropriate team member to complete the calls or text messages. Receptionists may be able to connect with clients for basic or routine cases, whereas the technician team will need to connect with clients on more difficult cases. On occasion, the veterinarian may want to call specific cases personally. These check-ins allow the team to follow the threads of patient care while being able to ensure that the client was satisfied with the services and answer any remaining questions. If the client has any concerns or the pet has not progressed as expected, medical progress exam appointments can be made. These check-ins must always be documented in the medical record; details of the conversation and how the pet is recovering must be recorded.

Team members must be given an appropriate amount of time to complete phone calls correctly. Often, team members are asked to make calls during a slow time in their schedule. If the slow time does not happen, then the team member is rushed, creating a poor perception for the client. The client interprets rushed calls as team members not caring and won't feel comfortable asking questions.

RECALL LIST **ABC ANIMAL CLINIC**
Printed for dates 3/3/23 - 3/3/23

Acct no	Client	Patient	Phone	Procedure	Dr
28	Sharon Bean	Miss Kitty	123-458-0901	Fe OVH	ND
17266	Steve Doolittle	Lucky	345-234-1234	K9 OVH	ND
17266	Steve Doolittle	Cookie	345-234-1234	K9 OVH	ND
3427	Desiree Cloud	Scamp	456-123-1234	Dental	SM
6785	Nancy Shade	Wheeler	123-567-8901	K9 OVH	ND

Fig. 11.15 Recall lists are generated for team members to call and check on patients.

- Puppy and kitten visits: ensure there was no vaccine reaction, and the client has no questions about behavioral or training issues
- Annual Wellness Exams
- Senior Wellness Exams
- Surgical patients - call the same night if the pet was released early, then call again 3 days later
- Hospitalized patients - call the same night, then call again 3 days later
- Pets seen for illness (vomiting/diarrhea): is it resolving not eating (is the pet eating again)
- Post lab work - call with results

Fig. 11.16 While there are many opportunities to follow up with clients after their visit, practices must identify what opportunities impact the frictionless client experience the most.

VARIOUS AREAS OF POTENTIAL FRICTION FOR CLIENTS

The perception of incompetent, annoyed, or rushed team members can bruise the experience that is trying to be created. Often, team members don't realize when they are coming across this way to clients; practice managers must be astute to the behaviors that are being demonstrated by team members and call attention (if needed) to the situation immediately. Team members cannot correct what they can't see (or feel did not display); security cameras with audio provide great training opportunities. The upcoming section on communication provides more ideas to help overcome these behaviors.

Handling Client Complaints and Grievances

Clients can be difficult depending on the day they have had, situations they are currently experiencing in their life, or a situation presented to them once they arrive at the practice. All the aforementioned reasons, except situations caused by the practice, are not a team member's fault, and actions or words displayed by the client should not be taken personally. Instead, place efforts into improving the client's day.

However, clients who are frustrated by receiving poor customer service, not feeling that they were provided the best medicine, or unintentional mistakes made by the team must be addressed immediately (and not just by the practice manager). Team members must be able to handle difficult conversations with clients when they arise. Passing upset clients to the practice manager upsets the client further.

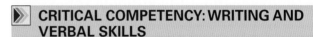

> **CRITICAL COMPETENCY: WRITING AND VERBAL SKILLS**
>
> The ability to comprehend written material easily and accurately; the ability to express thoughts clearly and succinctly in writing.

Clients may call and be upset about a specific situation (usually some type of miscommunication), but the team member handling the conversation can turn the call into a positive experience.

1. The receptionist should listen to the client.
2. Recap the conversation once the client has finished his or her portion of the conversation.
3. Identify the client's needs and provide a solution, in turn, making the client happy.

Every team member must be able to have the knowledge and autonomy to resolve situations immediately. The practice values and mission should guide what options the receptionist can provide to immediately resolve situations; if the complaint was resolved and it carried out the goals of the practice, the receptionist should not fear they will get in trouble for providing the wrong resolution. Leadership must set this up, train it, demonstrate it, and compliment every time a team member other than the practice manager must resolve situations.

It is important for team members to not become defensive when discussing complaints with clients. When team members get defensive, the intensity and emotion of the conversation rise, and clients become even more upset. Team members should immediately take the distraught or angry client to a quiet examination room, away from other clients. Emotions can be more intense when other people are around; taking clients to a quiet room can quickly diffuse the intensity. Team members should listen (and express nonverbal empathy) to what the client has to say and maintain eye contact throughout the conversation. Let the client air the complaint before asking any questions. Once the client has finished, the team member should repeat what was said, ensuring no miscommunication arises. Once the client and team member agree on the event that has occurred, the team member can offer some solutions to satisfy the client.

Often, once clients can voice their concern(s), their anger or frustration decreases a level. When they hear the concern repeated back to them and it appears the team member has understood their side of the story, the frustration level drops another level. When solutions are offered, clients feel satisfied that their problem(s) will be handled appropriately.

Solutions that may be presented to clients may be as simple as adjusting the invoice (use caution here, as most clients are not just looking for a reduction in their invoice unless an inappropriate charge was incorrectly added). Other solutions that may satisfy clients are to let them know a new policy or procedure may be enacted (because of this dilemma), that team member education will increase, and/or client education will change to prevent this scenario from occurring again. Clients are satisfied when they realize that they can make a difference. Although it may be hard for a team member to say "thank you" after a client discussion of this caliber, it is necessary; "thank you" is a powerful phrase for a client.

At times, regardless of the steps a team member has taken to calm the client, the client will remain irritable. When this happens, the team member must step aside and ask for help from another team member, practice manager, or owner to resolve the situation. Emotions, defense (nonverbal communication), and communication barriers have likely prevented client satisfaction from being accomplished. All team members must realize that arguing and defending a situation will not resolve the conflict.

VHMA PERFORMANCE DOMAIN TASK

Practice managers handle client complaints (and teach others how to, as well).

If a client becomes abusive toward a team member despite the team member having taken every step possible to calm the person, the client should be asked to leave the premises. A discussion can continue when the emotions have subsided. If a client will not leave the property when asked, the police should be called immediately. Staff and client safety should always be a concern. Today, a client cannot be trusted to not harm others. A client may be under the influence of an illegal substance or may have uncontrolled psychological issues. Once the client's emotions have subsided, a telephone call can be made by team members to find a solution to the issue at hand.

When clients present problems and complaints to team members, they should be assessed as learning experiences. What can be learned from the problem or complaint? Clients perceive actions, conversations, and procedures differently than team members do. If one client perceives an action to be a problem, other clients may as well. It is important to be proactive and prevent problems from arising, rather than being reactive and solving problems only after clients have become upset. Every team member should possess the skill and knowledge to satisfy a client whether the practice manager or owner is present or not.

Grieving clients can be difficult because they have just suffered an emotional loss much like the experience of losing a family member. Depending on the situation, clients may be in shock and disbelief; others have accepted the situation and are very emotional. Clients in shock and disbelief may be angry (the pet may have just been hit by a car, and they are angry at the driver as well as at the practice for not doing more to save their pet). In other cases, a poor prognosis may have been given for a patient, but the client believes that more could be done to save the pet. The client may leave quickly, ask for a copy of the animal's records, and go to another veterinarian for a second opinion. Team members must be empathetic with clients in this moment and understand that a traumatic situation has just occurred for the client. It should not be taken personally. Every person handles grief differently.

There is certainly a time and place to terminate clients for continued bad behavior or abuse to the staff. Evaluate the circumstances and use client termination as a last resort. Ensure the practice is doing everything possible to create a frictionless client experience first. Additionally, the client needs to know that their behavior is unacceptable (so that when they are terminated as a client, it is not a shock).

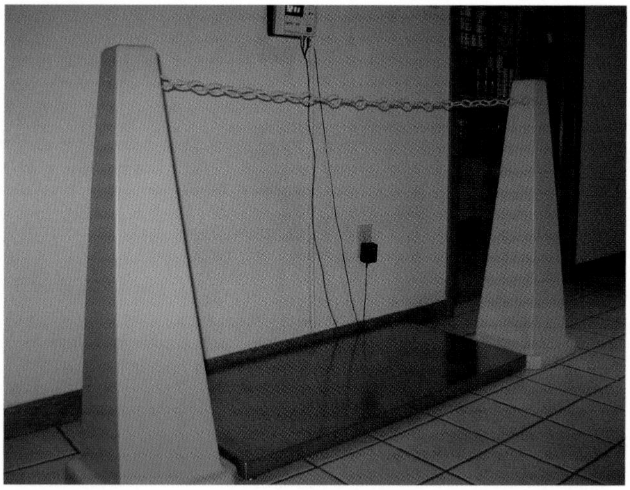

Fig. 11.17 Bright yellow barriers around the weight scale prevent clients and team members from tripping.

When the inevitable time comes, ensure the pet is not receiving emergent care. By law, the practice cannot terminate a client when the pet is receiving treatment unless the client terminates the relationship (Chapter 5, Veterinary Ethics and Legal Issues). Once treatment has been completed, print off the medical records for the client, and write a short letter to the client indicating that the service provided by your practice cannot meet the client's expectations, and another practice should be sought for veterinary care.

Client Injury While Visiting the Practice

There is always a risk of a slip and fall in the practice, presenting a significant liability. Signs must be posted when the floor is wet, and a team member should be available to direct clients around the wet area until it is dry. Clients may trip on rugs, shelving units, weight scales, or any other object that sits on the floor. Wall-to-wall carpets should not curl up at the seams, and area rugs should have antiskid material on the back to prevent tripping and slipping. Objects such as scales should have large warning barriers at the corners to prevent tripping (Fig. 11.17).

Often, team members are in shock when a client falls, and they stop and stare. Instead, team members should rush to the aide of any client who has fallen and ask if he or she feels any pain and where the pain is located. If needed, stabilize the patient in the same location until an ambulance arrives. Once the client feels stable enough to leave independently or the ambulance leaves for the hospital, pictures of the area should be taken. All team members who witnessed the accident should immediately write down the facts. If time passes before events are documented, important details may be forgotten. It is advised to call the liability insurance company to inform them of an accident in case a lawsuit is brought against the practice. Chapter 15 discusses a variety of safety issues within the practice that should be addressed.

TEAM TRAINING THAT ENHANCES THE FRICTIONLESS CLIENT EXPERIENCE

Many team members have never been in an environment where they have received communication training, been asked to view protocols through the eyes of a client, or even taken a moment to understand the client's perspective. For some extroverted personalities, these may be innate skills. Introverted personalities need the most help, and practice managers must put forth the time and energy to coach these individuals to success. Team members need coaching and will appreciate the transferable skills that they can use outside of the practice as well.

Client Communications

Communication is one of the most important aspects of working with veterinary clients. It is extremely important that clients fully understand the procedures being performed on their pets, understand lifelong healthcare needs, and be supported when the difficult time comes to say goodbye to their pet. All communications must be handled in a compassionate, empathetic, and professional manner.

> **LEADERSHIP POINT**
>
> Lack of client communication is the number one complaint to the state board of veterinary medicine.

Client communications occur in every area of the practice and can be through text, email, telehealth, phone calls, and when the client arrives at the practice. Clients must feel welcomed and comfortable in the practice environment, regardless of the type of communication.

Written communication is equally as important as verbal communication. Written communication includes client education materials, postoperative discharge instructions, posthospitalization discharge instructions, patient medical report cards, or boarding report cards (Fig. 11.18).

Components of a Message

Messages have three skill components: verbal, paraverbal, and nonverbal. Verbal skills (word choices) account for 7% of a message, paraverbal skills (the way words are spoken through pitch, enunciation, and tone) contribute 38%, and nonverbal skills (body language) are the major contributor at 55% of the message (Fig. 11.19).

It is important to remember that all messaging must be professional and done in a manner that all clients, team members, and colleagues in the industry can understand. While society has adapted to texting, using social media, and communicating in short phrases and abbreviations (LOL!), team members must remember to communicate professionally to clients when they are present, and medical entries made must use standard veterinary abbreviations.

Verbal Skills

Specific words may be chosen when talking with clients to project the professional image of the practice. For example, simple words such as "vaccinations" should be used instead of "shots," and "yes, sir" or "yes, ma'am" should be used instead of "yeah." Team members may not realize the number of times filler sounds such as "um" are used in a sentence until they are counted.

Team members should be discouraged from using phrases such as "I don't know"; "I'm not sure"; "I don't think so." Instead, phrases should be replaced with "That is a great question, let me find out!" "No, we do not accept payments" can be replaced with "we offer payment plans through an outside agency." Enhancing the staff's verbal skills will help take the veterinary practice to the next level.

Improving Verbal Image: For practice, have team members record a conversation and review the recording; listening to oneself helps team members evaluate their own communication skills. Are they professional and confident? Do they use appropriate terminology? Are they

Report Card

For ____________________ Arrival ____________________
Date ____________________ Departure ____________________

How I Ate:
_______ I devoured my food!
_______ I ate some of my food.
_______ I didn't feel like eating much.

My personality:
_______ I was very friendly.
_______ I was shy.
_______ I was quiet.
_______ I was talkative.

How I Played:
_______ I was so excited, I played like crazy.
_______ I was shy.
_______ It took me awhile to feel comfortable.
_______ I need to work on my "petiquette."

Potty Time:
_______ I went regularly.
_______ I went infrequently.

My Behavior Was:
_______ Absolutely wonderful!
_______ Better than most.
_______ Could have been better.
_______ Did my best.
_______ Forget it. I will be good next time!

Comments: ____________________

Thank you for boarding with us.

Fig. 11.18 Sample boarding report card.

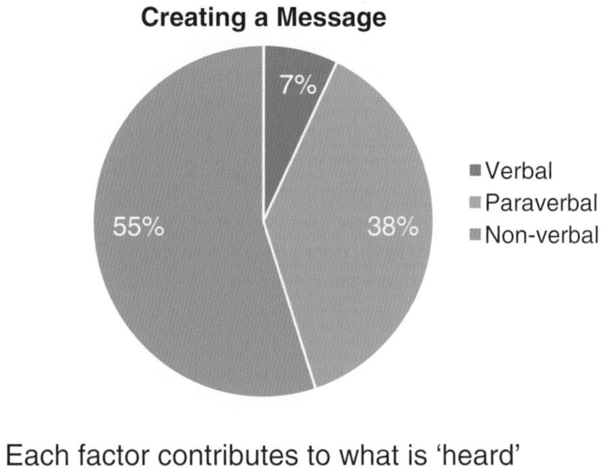

Fig. 11.19 Components of a message.

successfully leading clients through appointments? Verbal skills need to be practiced and rehearsed to improve the client experience and build trust and compliance.

Veterinary team members should role-play delivering client education topics to improve verbal word choices that contribute to improved client understanding, confidence in the speaker, and professionalism. Clients do not have the same medical knowledge as the team does; it can often feel like a foreign language. Topics that seem basic to a team member are completely foreign to a new pet owner, and the team cannot get frustrated when answering questions for clients, no matter how many times they must answer the same question. A client service manual is suggested to help new team members learn preferred answers to client questions, including correct verbiage, correct pronunciation, and the skills to respond to such questions.

Paraverbal Skills

Lower and deeper voice tones of team members are often perceived as more confident and authoritative, whereas high-pitched tones sound insecure and immature. With practice, deeper tones can be established, enhancing each team member's value. During a phone call, the first impression is made by the tone of voice and the words chosen by the team member. Practices have 10 seconds to have a positive impact on a client; when it starts with a phone call, tone of voice can make or break a new client.

Improving Paraverbal Skills: It can be difficult for one to assess their tone of voice. Most often, team members do not feel they have a rude tone of voice during a conversation (but it is easy to judge others who have a sharp tone). Team members must hear how they sound on the phone and in person to be able to adjust their tone. Voice recordings of telephone calls are a simple training method to improve paraverbal skills.

Nonverbal Skills

Nonverbal skills are visualized in a person's body language and are the main contributor to a message. Listeners subconsciously watch body language and either lean into a conversation or back away. Body posture, hand gestures, facial expressions, and eye contact are behaviors displayed in nonverbal communication and are communicated whether the person speaking is stressed, annoyed, anxious, or has a lack of confidence.

Being able to read a client's body language will increase client compliance because team members can alter their communication style based on what the nonverbal body language is saying. Trust and compliance are also built when clients can read team members.

Folded Arms: When a person has folded arms, it generally indicates that they are defensive and unwilling to accept recommendations or advice. If a client approaches a team member and the team member has folded arms, the client may feel uncomfortable asking questions (role-playing will help teach team members to unfold their arms while in the practice). A client with folded arms may be unwilling to accept recommendations and may have some underlying issues with the service being provided (Fig. 11.20A). A team member can correct this situation easily by handing the client something to hold. A brochure or a model of a joint (e.g., hip, knee, elbow) will force the person to unfold their arms; this will gradually open the lines for communication (Fig. 11.20B). Once this has occurred, the team member can continue educating the client and ask if there is any other information that the client needs. Team members should also make sure to ask if all the client's concerns have been addressed at this point.

Body Posture: The team member's body posture also sends a message to the client, either positive or negative. If a team member enters an examination room in a slouched position with their head down and shoulders sunk forward, the client will interpret that the team member lacks confidence and skill or may not enjoy their job (Fig. 11.21). Team members who are slumped are likely to have quiet voices, lack energy, and appear unmotivated, all of which highly impact a client's decision to accept recommendations. Team members that enter examination

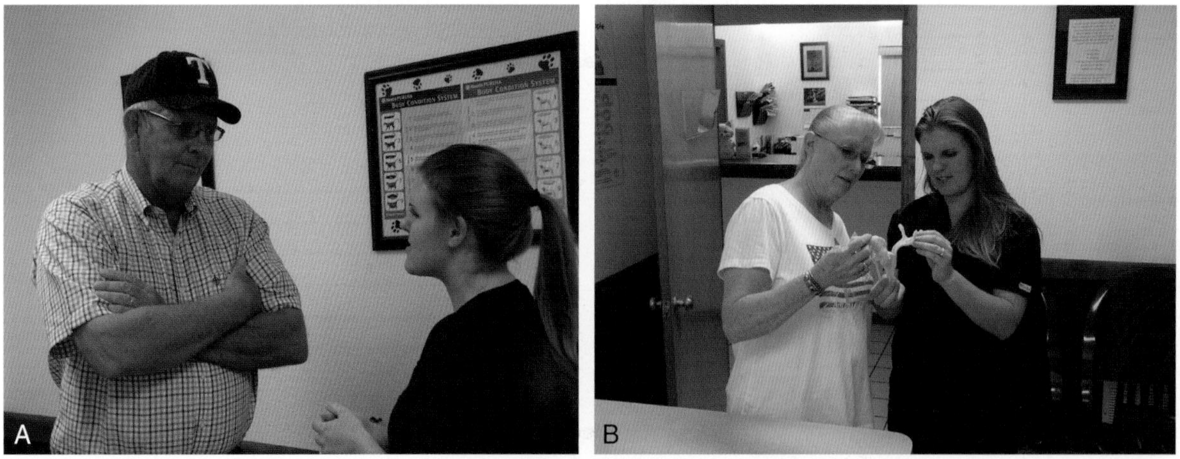

Fig. 11.20 (A) A client who has closed arms held close to the body may be defensive and unwilling to accept new information. (B) Technician educating a client by handing her a model.

rooms with their heads up, a tall body posture, and shoulders back convey confidence, excitement, and technical skill. Clients are more likely to accept recommendations that are made with positive nonverbal skills and are willing to further develop a trusting relationship with the team (Fig. 11.22).

Eye Contact and Facial Expressions: Eyes communicate a large amount of emotion, including feelings of joy, fear, confusion, sadness, or stress. Consider the subconscious activity of rolling the eyes. Many times, a person who is annoyed with a response subconsciously rolls their eyes, conveying that annoyance (words are not needed). While educating and conversing with clients, maintain eye contact to convey knowledge and confidence, leading them to accept the recommendations being provided.

Facial expressions include smiling (or lack of) and reveal happiness, anger, surprise, sadness, disgust, and or fear. Other facial expressions include eyebrow movement, which shows that the speaker is listening and understands the conversation. When one is empathetic, the eyebrows subconsciously raise, the head becomes tilted, and the listener nods their head, whereas tense eyebrows can indicate confusion.

Improving Nonverbal Skills: Characteristics associated with trust and confidence include making strong eye contact, maintaining good posture and a peppy step (showing enthusiasm and joy), and using hand gestures to help convey information. Characteristics associated with sincerity include eye contact, good posture, and alert facial expressions (nodding, tilting the head, and raised eyebrows).

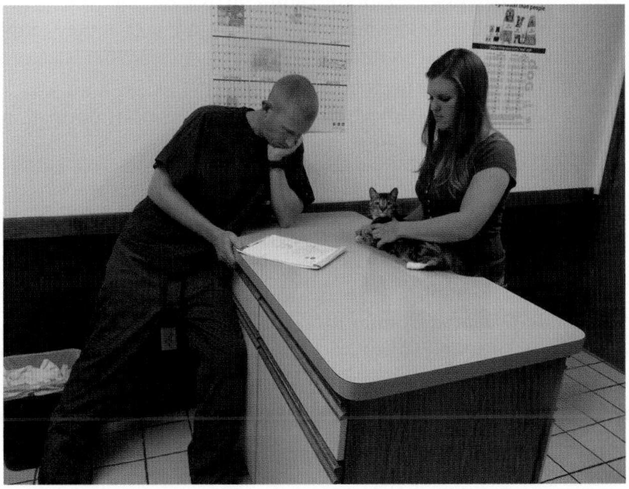

Fig. 11.21 A technician who is slumped over and not engaged appears unprofessional to clients, resulting in lower compliance rates.

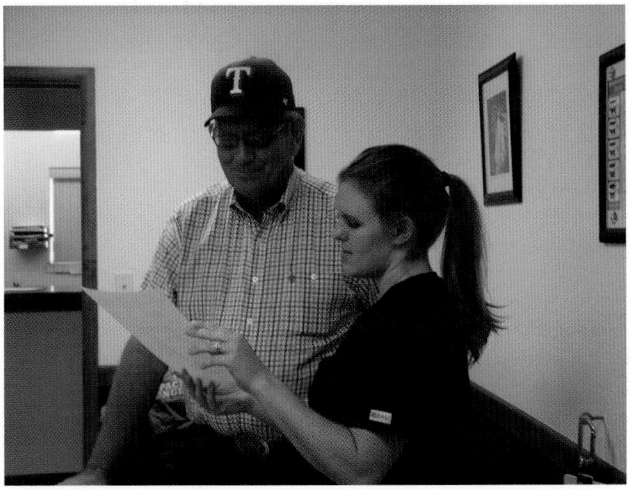

Fig. 11.22 A professional team member standing up straight with shoulders held back.

Characteristics that might break trust and confidence with a client include poor body odor (including breath, residual smell from cigarettes, and not showering), and wrinkled or stained uniforms. Often, team members do not realize they have an unpleasant body odor until something is mentioned to them. Help colleagues become aware of the odor by politely having a positive conversation with them. Eighty percent of revenue is driven by 20% of the clients. If that 20% of clients are offended by a team member's nonverbal communication, then client service will be severely impacted. Professional appearance helps increase client confidence in the veterinary team; clean, unwrinkled uniforms project confidence and credibility. This makes uniform maintenance a high priority for every team member, and practice managers must budget accordingly

The success of the veterinary practice depends on client compliance driven through client education and the acceptance of recommendations. Clients will not accept recommendations from team members that display a lack of confidence, knowledge, or belief in what they are recommending. By providing continuing education for team members, they will be able to thoroughly discuss procedures, protocols, and diseases with pride and confidence. Role-playing and posting a "word of the day" improves the knowledge, enthusiasm, and proficiency of all.

Barriers to Client Communication

Clients may display behaviors that team members should observe to help overcome any barriers a client may have. Clients may appear nervous, defensive, or embarrassed, have a language barrier, or may be hearing impaired. Team members also display behaviors, such as prejudging a client and making assumptions about what they will accept before a treatment plan is discussed. These behaviors impact compliance and the care a patient will receive. If the behaviors of a client are not addressed and become misperceived, best medicine won't be offered to the client. Team members must "listen" to the client (verbal and nonverbal) to understand the client's perspective. Once that is achieved, effective communication continues, and patients will have a higher chance of receiving the care they need.

Clients may be defensive or embarrassed when they feel they have not given their pet the best care or cannot afford the best care. Clients may have crossed arms, avoid making eye contact with team members, or only interact with the team when questions are asked. A caring, empathetic team member can easily break this barrier by finding something to compliment the pet and client on, helping the clients feel a small sense of pride and become more open to suggestions and advice.

The United States has a broad range of cultures and languages throughout regions (Northeast, Southeast, Southwest, West, Northwest) that communicate differently, have varying dialog and lingo, and values. Additionally, international cultures have settled into larger cities, bringing an unintentional language barrier and varying communication styles to veterinary practices. It is important to understand and embrace the cultural differences and elements of language to provide the best medicine to clients. Nonverbal behavior varies from culture to culture and differences can be expressed through gestures, eye contact, interpersonal distance, and touch (or lack of touch). A client with folded arms may be insecure about the situation due to cultural differences or language barriers rather than being upset; give the client something to hold while educating to improve understanding and acceptance of recommendations.

Other communication barriers come from team members. It can be extremely difficult to discuss an obese pet with an overweight owner or discuss dental disease with a client who has bad teeth. Role-playing these difficult scenarios can help team members become more comfortable with these situations. Some clients have more compassion for their pets than themselves and are willing to accept recommendations. If a pet is overweight and a walking and exercise plan is discussed, the owner may be willing to take the pet for walks as recommended (also benefits the client). The team cannot shy aware from these conversations. The pets need an advocate: that is the role of the veterinary healthcare team.

Putting It All Together

Listeners can receive confusing verbal, paraverbal, and nonverbal messages from a speaker, and when this occurs, the listener will default to the nonverbal message that is conveyed. The nonverbal communication behavior that is unintentionally displayed by team members is having decreased confidence in the recommendation that is being made. Decreased confidence may result from not understanding why the recommendation is being made, or the team member may not personally believe the "why" of the recommendation that is being made.

When clients observe team members with confidence, they begin to feel they can trust the information that has been provided to them and a relationship with that team member develops. Clients who build relationships with team members have a higher compliance and retention rate compared with those who only have a relationship with the veterinarian. Team members who are compassionate, concerned, and interested in patients come across as more confident and will stimulate clients to ask more questions. Nonveterinary team members drive passive income and should be responsible for developing 50% of the gross revenue for the practice. Team member confidence is a great asset to the practice and should be a top training priority for all employees.

When bad news must be delivered to the client, it should be relayed in a professional, tactful environment with empathy. Team members should expect clients to be sad, shocked, upset, angry, or emotional. Being prepared for these situations will help team members best support the client's needs. Many times, it is the veterinarian that will deliver the news; however, team members should always be prepared for these difficult conversations. Team members should speak slowly and listen to the client's response. Clients may not fully understand the conversation, and it may be necessary to repeat the information.

Understanding Client and Patient Needs

Team members who take the time to understand both client and patient needs will have the highest compliance acceptance rates. Many team members excel at one but not the other, and it takes time, practice, and patience to excel at both.

Understanding the diverse personalities that make up our population has long been studied for application in many industries, but this information has been lacking in the veterinary profession for years. The International Conference on Communication in Veterinary Medicine, in conjunction with Institute for Healthcare Communications, has been working to create educational programs to meet this need.

Understanding client personalities and communicating with clients based on those attributes can bring higher compliance rates to the practice. Team members may be familiar with personality tests such as the Meyers-Briggs Type Indicator, Colors, or Wheels (just to name a few). These tests certainly aid in the understanding of oneself, but often are not applied to how we understand and communicate with others. If these studies have been used within the practice, it is rare for the information to be applied to client interactions.

For the team to absorb the broad nature of personalities and communication tools, it is important that a tool be used that the team can relate to. One of the author's favorite tools (because of the ability to apply it to veterinary healthcare) is the Patterson Veterinary University Pawsonality Tool (PVU). This tool associates personality types with common dog breed attributes. It's fun for team members and highly relatable. This tool can be obtained by enrolling in a Patterson Veterinary-hosted course. For this chapter, various personalities are reviewed, providing a greater understanding of how to communicate with clients.

LEADERSHIP POINT

The Pawsonality tool also helps improve communication between team members, enhancing the culture and team dynamic in the practice.

Driver-Oriented Communication Style: A driver-oriented person is driven to achieve results. Compare this personality style with herding breeds like the Border Collie, Heeler, or Australian Shepherd. They:

- always need a job and must be in charge of something,
- are incredibly efficient with their time and expect everyone else to be as well,
- don't cut corners but will find the shortest point to connect the dots,
- are task-oriented,
- are comfortable taking risks, and
- can be identified by the following traits: talking first, talking fast, and often cutting others off.

Analytic-Oriented Communication Style: An analytic person analyzes information before making decisions and, in fact, they cannot easily make decisions without all the facts. This personality is comparable with the German Shepherd; they:

- think before they speak (must have time to process the information),
- easily overanalyze, resulting in analysis paralysis,
- are task-oriented,
- focus on perfection,
- are not comfortable with risk, and
- may be labeled as snobby or stand-offish (when they take time to analyze the situation).

Amiable-Oriented Communication Style: An amiable person is a devoted, consistent individual who avoids confrontation. Consider the Labrador Retriever for this scenario. They:

- are hard workers (often working longer hours than others),
- cooperate with the team,
- are not risk takers,
- are uncomfortable with chaos and change,
- are very relationship-oriented, and
- consider other opinion(s) and feelings before their own.

Expressive-Oriented Communication Style: Expressive people are social butterflies; they get along with everyone and have charming and charismatic personalities. The Golden Retriever is a nice example. They are:

- engaging and persuasive,
- relationship-oriented,
- great idea generators,
- excellent client educators,
- positive and enthusiastic, and
- enjoy helping others.

When reviewing these personality types, one can see why it would be advantageous to identify how clients fit into these categories. Communicating the way clients want to be communicated with is the key. It is human nature to communicate with others the way we want to be communicated with. By taking into consideration what the client's personality style may be, miscommunication and frustration may be drastically alleviated. Some examples for review:

- A Border Collie (BC or Driver) client and a Golden Retriever (GR or Expressive) team member: The BC prefers to get to the point and is efficient. The GR talks a lot, often with their hands, and adds too much fluff to the conversation. The BC gets annoyed because the GR is not getting to the point quickly. The BC rejects information being presented because of their annoyance, and the GR won't accept recommendations because there is not enough "talk."

- A German Shepherd (GS or Analytic) client and a GR team member: The GS wants facts to analyze information and needs time to process. The GR presents a charismatic story that lacks facts and talks too much. The GS becomes frustrated and can't decide (because facts weren't presented) and can't process the information when the GR won't stop talking.
- A Labrador (Lab or Amiable) client and a BC team member: The Lab makes decisions based on how it will affect their pet and others. They need the "feel good factor" to consider the options. The BC team member states facts to the Lab client, talking too quickly and without compassion. The client gets their "feelings" hurt and walks away with the impression that the BC team member doesn't care about their pet.

Client personalities can be identified rather easily when paying attention, but there can also be "mutts" with a combination of personality styles, making it hard to distinguish the correct personality. However, those clients accept various communication styles easier than a "full breed." Take the time to identify what "breed" a client is and communicate with them based on that characteristic, rather than your own. In addition, it is recommended to identify the client "breed" in the client alert section available in the PIMS.

Once a practice starts using client personality identifiers for communications, track compliance; monitoring the increased compliance will help the team understand why communicating based on client preference is a valuable tool. If the ability is available to go a step further, consider tracking compliance based on personality type, and provide further team training to those who are in the lower compliance categories. For team members familiar with the Meyers-Briggs Type Indicator, information can be extrapolated from the Extrovert/Introvert, Sensing/Intuition, Thinking/Feeling, and Judger/Perceiver categories to create additional personality profiles to enhance client communications.

Treatment Plans (Estimates)

All clients should be provided with a treatment plan/estimate of costs for procedures and services that will be performed on their pets. Treatment plans are a major part of client communications, and the failure of a practice to provide one is the most common complaint for state board investigators when clients report grievances against veterinary practices. Clients must be informed regarding the procedure(s) their pet is going to receive and the associated costs.

VHMA PERFORMANCE DOMAIN TASK

Practice managers ensure compliance with contract law as it applies to clients.

Treatment plans can be developed and preprinted for simple outpatient procedures such as yearly examinations, anal sac expressions, and nail trims, or for inpatient procedures such as routine spays, neuters, and laceration repairs. Patients being admitted to the hospital must have a detailed and customized treatment plan provided. Furthermore, two separate treatment plans should be provided for patients admitted to the hospital: a diagnostic plan and a patient treatment plan (Fig. 11.23). The diagnostic plan includes all medical services and tests needed to diagnose the problem; the treatment plan should cover all services needed to treat the patient, including medications needed when the patient is released. Templates developed in the PIMS system make this process quick and easy and usually eliminate missed charges or the need to call clients back when adjustments need to be made because a test, procedure, or medication was inadvertently missed. Additionally, the newer-based PIMS system will populate the invoice when outpatient plans are approved by the client, and patients being admitted to the hospital have their treatment/diagnostic plans autopopulated to the whiteboard. See chapter 8 for more information.

LEADERSHIP POINT

Providing two separate plans prevents the team from underestimating, missing charges, or providing an inaccurate estimate when the diagnosis changes because of test results.

Knowledgeable, empathetic team members should present treatment plans; veterinarians should be left out of financial discussions because their job is to diagnose, prescribe medications, and perform surgery, not discuss finances.

When explaining treatment plans, don't "sell services," but rather teach clients why the pet needs the recommended services. When presenting treatment plans, the team member must be able to discuss treatment options with confidence. Using models and brochures to help explain specific procedures will help clients understand what is being recommended for their pets. Along with the positive characteristics described previously, team members should stand beside the client to deliver the plan, not across the examination room table (Fig. 11.24).

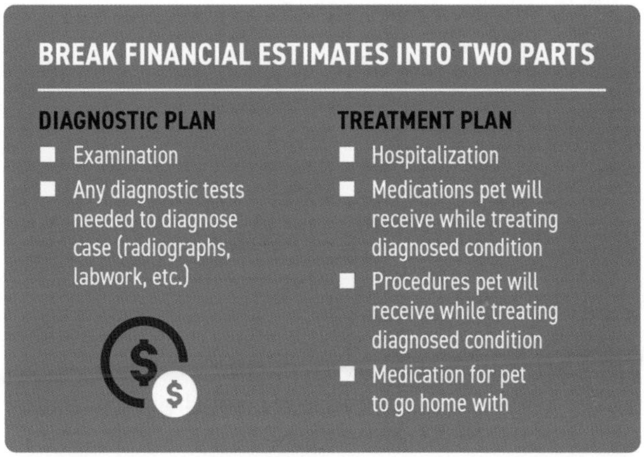

BREAK FINANCIAL ESTIMATES INTO TWO PARTS
DIAGNOSTIC PLAN
Examination
Any diagnostic tests needed to diagnose case (radiographs, labwork, etc.)
TREATMENT PLAN
Hospitalization
Medications pet will receive while treating diagnosed condition
Procedures pet will receive while treating diagnosed condition
Medication for pet to go home with

Fig. 11.23 Break financial estimates into diagnostic plans and treatment plans to improve client understanding.

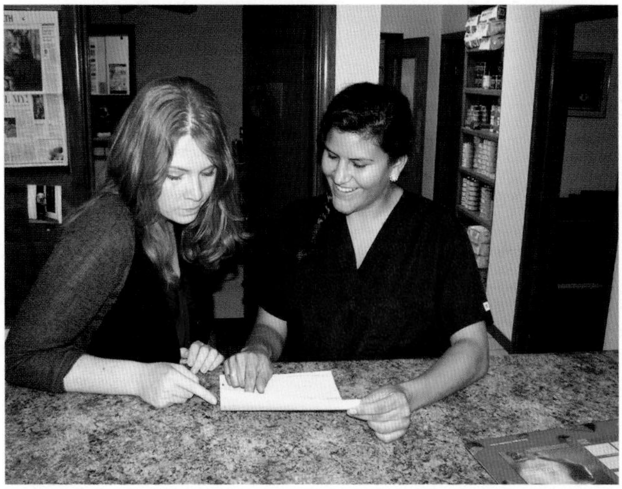

Fig. 11.24 A professional team member standing next to a client will receive better compliance when presenting a treatment plan.

The examination table is a barrier, which indirectly affects client compliance. Other barriers must also be taken into consideration, which were discussed earlier in this chapter.

Plans should persuade clients to ask questions and encourage discussions regarding the medicine their pet will be receiving. If clients do not ask questions, they may be confused or overwhelmed. This is a good time for the team member to stop and ask if they understand the procedure(s) being recommended.

Treatment plans can also initiate financial discussions about the hospital's payment policy. Some clients will need time to think about the estimate provided and may want to discuss finances with a spouse. It is advisable to discuss the treatment plan with the client and leave the examination room, giving them time to process the information. Team members can then return to the exam room after a few minutes and answer any questions the client may have. For treatment plans presented on the phone, clients may wish to call the practice back to approve or deny diagnostics after they consider the recommendations.

Once verbally approved, have clients sign the treatment plan indicating that they agree to the procedures and are financially responsible for the charges (Fig. 11.25). For hospitalized patients, clients should be updated on progress and charges on a daily (minimum) basis. Anytime additional diagnostic tests or treatments are to be added on, the client must be called for approval with an updated estimate of costs.

Managers should monitor the delivery of treatment plans and client compliance. Some team members will have exceptionally high rates of success when delivering treatment plans; others may need additional training either on medical topics or customer service skills. It is also advised to review treatment plans, ensuring they contain client-friendly words. If a client does not understand a line item, they are more likely to decline the service; for example, the word "ovariohysterectomy" should be replaced with "spay" to help gain client understanding. If the compliance rate is not being managed, it cannot be improved.

Another area to monitor is client complaints in relation to invoices. When a receptionist presents an invoice to a client that is in shock, angry at the cost, or states "that no one told them how much it would be," the treatment plan delivery process needs to be evaluated. Situations like this place the receptionist in an awkward position; they are defenseless and can only apologize. These situations are unfair to both the client and

ABC Veterinary Clinic
123 Saturn Circle
Anytown, MN 12345
(123) 456-7890

CHARGE ESTIMATION

Account: 19902
Date: 07/31/22
Page: 1

Sharon White Phone (123) 678-6789 Patient: Marshmallow

Code	Service/Item	Qty	Amount
0216	Office Call	1	$65.54
0920	IV Catheter	1	$67.90
0924	IV Fluids per Liter	2-3	$31.28-$46.92
0916	IV Care Daily	2	$68.48
909	Hospitalization Routine	1-2	$52.48-85.68
4150	Urinary Catheter	1	$55.48
0302	Anesthesia	1	$154.36
3815	General Health Profile	1	$151.24

ESIMATE TOTAL $464.76 - $695.60

THIS IS ONLY AN ESTIMATE AND DOES NOT INLCUDE SALES TAX. The actual diagnostic treatment plan may require more medications and/or procedures. The range of estimate may vary. This estimate is valid for 30 days only. I have read and understand this estimate. I understand that I must leave a deposit prior to procedure, and the balance must be paid when my pet is released from the hospital.

Signed______________________________________Date__________

Fig. 11.25 Sample estimate.

receptionist and leadership must make changes to protect the team and carry out the frictionless client experience.

When clients complain about charges, they may not fully understand the value associated with those fees. Client education techniques should be reviewed to ensure clients are being fully educated by the team when they (the client) visit the practice. For example, when a patient is hospitalized and a daily hospitalization fee applies, explain to clients what that includes that provides value: tender loving nursing care, vital checks completed multiple times in the day, wound cleaning, fluffy bedding, laundry, special food, and water. Clients value honesty, compassion, and timeliness. They want to understand the information presented to them, and without this knowledge, they will not accept the recommendations.

The Fear Free® Experience

The Fear Free® Experience enhances the value of the frictionless client experience. Consider the experience clients have when they are bringing their pets to the vet. It is usually not a frictionless experience, adding another stress level for the clients. It doesn't have to be that way. Pets should love coming to the practice; and when pets love coming to the practice, the frictionless experience just got a whole lot better!

The Fear Free® initiative was created by Dr. Marty Becker with the goal to alleviate fear, anxiety, and stress (FAS) in pets during veterinary visits, and to educate and inspire the people that care for them.

Creating a Fear Free® experience places patient care at the top of the priority list. For years, patient visits have declined, and it wasn't until recently that the cause had been identified. Pets hate coming to the vet. If pets hate coming to the vet, clients won't bring them, as they too, experience FAS. A guiding principle of Fear Free® is that pets need veterinary professionals to look after not only their physical well-being but also their emotional well-being. The focus of Fear Free® is to prevent FAS in every patient. Young and inexperienced animals may show the best response. However, Fear Free® techniques and concepts should be used with all patients, whether they are relaxed and happy to be in the practice, or afraid and displaying avoidance or aggression.

LEADERSHIP POINT

Team members appreciate and value the Fear Free® Experience. Take every opportunity to educate them on procedures that have been implemented to reduce FAS in patients and enroll them in Fear Free® courses to achieve certification.

The Fear Free® program provides tools, training, protocols, procedures, and guidelines on how to reduce FAS in patients and thus in clients and veterinary team members. Online and in-person continuing education programs are available. In addition, Fear Free® certification is available for individuals and practices. Certifications should be promoted in all marketing materials, as clients are looking for this unique service. Visit www.fearfreepets.com to enroll individuals or practices in available courses.

Understanding The Human-Animal Bond

The human-animal bond is an emotional bond that benefits both humans and animals (Fig. 11.26). Each party treats the other with mutual respect, trust, devotion, and love. To some clients, pets are their children; to others, pets are their best friends. When these connections are developed, long-lasting relationships are formed (Fig. 11.27).

This bond is strengthened by the veterinary health care team during the frictionless client experience. Each time the client visits, the bond is strengthened because the owner receives further education on how to help care for his or her pet. Team members who are empathetic

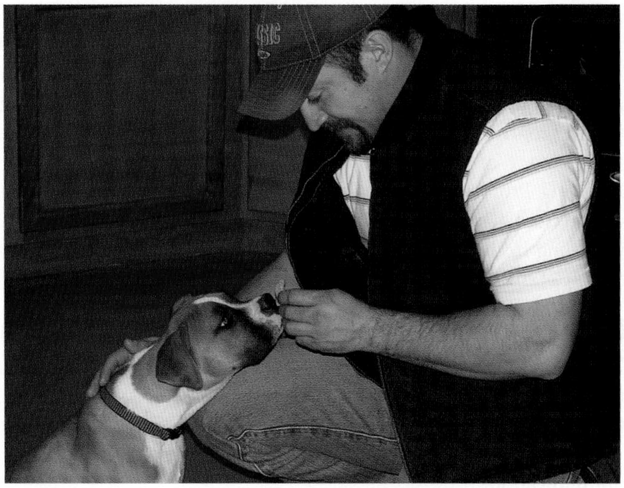

Fig. 11.26 The human-animal bond is typically a strong and long-lasting one.

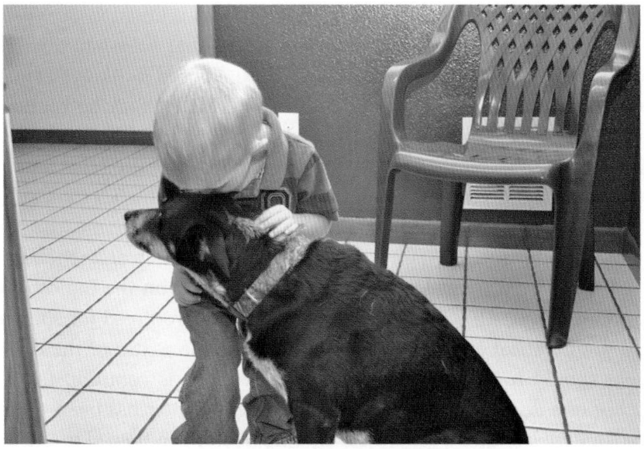

Fig. 11.27 The decision to bond with a new animal should be left to the client experiencing the loss. Bonding with a new pet should be viewed as a tribute to the love and companionship shared with the previous animal.

and encourage the human-animal bond are cherished and tend to be requested by clients. These team members are usually employed over the long term by a veterinary practice and may have the experience of seeing a pet for its first visit and following its progress until its last visit. These team members will face grieving issues with long-term clients.

Many clients do not have the support and understanding of the human-animal bond in their home or work environments. A spouse or extended family may not have the same attachment to the pet. Coworkers may not understand why the client would need to take the day off work because their pet is having surgery. The veterinary team supports this strong bond; many times, the veterinary hospital is the only place where they receive this support.

DEVELOPING THE FRAMEWORK FOR A FRICTIONLESS CLIENT EXPERIENCE

Behind every successful client experience is a team that needs operational support to help them be efficient and friendly, and can focus on client and patient needs. Therefore, the framework and operational support must be developed so that it is easy and joyful to work in the practice. The previous material covers what the experience should look like, this portion of the chapter will help a practice develop it.

Practices must be easy to do business with; digital communication is now a requirement of clients. Building and implementing technology not only contributes to the frictionless client experience but increases the efficiency of the team. Standards of Care (SOC) and Standard Operating Protocols (SOPs; also referred to as Employee Procedure Manual; see Chapter 4) build this framework; and they must be tied to everything in the practice. Client educational materials must support the SOCs, and the PIMS should be able to tie it all together.

Being Easy to Do Business with: Digital Communication

Today's client is looking for ways to easily do business with their veterinary hospital. Just like the practice, they want efficient, knowledgeable team members communicating in a method that suits the client's busy lifestyle. Practices can no longer dodge the importance of digital communication.

Emailing and Texting Etiquette

Team members must be able to write effective, professional emails, text messages, or letters for different aspects of the practice. Collection notices, vaccine reaction letters, and letters of acclimation are just a few examples that a doctor may request. Pets that have had a severe vaccine reaction in the past may have been advised by the veterinarian to avoid vaccinations in the future, and a letter may be required by the city or county as to why the client is not in compliance with the law. Airlines may require a letter of acclimation, indicating that a pet is healthy enough to fly at temperatures below 40° F or higher than 80° F.

Emails or letters should include the date, the client's name, the pet's name, and the doctor's name. The pet's species, gender, and whether it has been altered may also be required depending on the topic being communicated. All typed documents should be proofread for spelling and grammatical errors. A person other than the writer of the document should review the document for errors (it is common for the author of a document to miss errors). Once the letter has been proofread, a PDF should be generated, and the doctor can then sign the letter. The PDF should be printed for the client and made accessible to the client in their pet portal or in their practice app.

Ideally, emails should be kept short, friendly, and professional in tone. Simply state facts, leaving any emotional component out of the message. Lengthy discussions should never be conducted via email, but rather suggest having a phone call to further discuss.

When responding to a text or email, address the client by their name, answer the question(s) asked, provide recommendations, and sign the email in a professional manner. This includes the name of the team member who is responding to the message and the practice's contact information, including the web address and practice logo. Apply the same concepts to any app push notifications; any message must be professional, grammatically correct, and error-free.

Booking Appointments Online

Booking appointments online was previously covered in this chapter, but it is worth mentioning again as this is applicable to digital communication. Don't forget that action buttons must be placed at the top of every webpage, pet portal, and practice app. Additionally, a link to make an appointment should be embedded in the body of emails, text messages, and patient reminders.

> **LEADERSHIP POINT**
>
> Make it easy for clients to do business with the practice.

Requesting Medication Refills

Like booking appointments online at any time, clients want to be able to request medication refills at any time, whether they fill in-house or use an online pharmacy. No doubt, refills must be approved by the practice. However, clients refilling in-house should be able to message the practice (through text messaging, the practice portal, or the practice app) and receive a response the same day the request is submitted. If a refill cannot be granted until an exam is completed, depending on the medication, the team member may need to refill a small quantity until an exam can be scheduled. Clients appreciate this opportunity versus receiving an automatic decline. It is advised to also take the opportunity to teach why an exam or bloodwork is needed before the medication can be refilled, placing the patient's health as the main priority.

If a medication refill request is through an online pharmacy, the practice can authorize or decline the refill. A follow-up text message to the client letting them know it has been approved supports further expectational service. If a refill cannot be granted through the online pharmacy, before declining the refill, message or call the owner direct, again, focusing on why an exam or bloodwork is needed. Chapter 13, Inventory, provides detail on developing and building the practices of an online pharmacy. If a client will have multiple refills when the initial prescription order is created (thyroid medication, long-term osteoarthritis medication, etc.), place the number of available refills on the request so they can automatically be refilled. The practice will still receive notification that the order was placed and filled, but the practice does not have to approve until the number of refills runs out.

Like booking appointments, a link for medication refills should be placed at the top of the webpage, at the closing of every email, in the practice app, and pet portal, and included on all reminders.

Some practices have instituted a 24-hour turnaround time to refill prescriptions. The outstanding question is: does this really support a frictionless client experience? Does it meet client expectations to wait 24 hours? Consider when most clients request refills; they request the day they run out of medication. Refills do not take long to fill after a doctor has approved the request, so if the doctor's approving refills is slowing the process, evaluate how that can become more efficient.

Standards of Care

One of the most important aspects of veterinary medicine is the standard of care (SOC) provided to patients. Industry-acceptable SOCs must be met for every patient, or the veterinarian could be held negligent. Clients expect high standards to be met, and all patients deserve it. The veterinary team is often guilty of prejudging a client's financial situation and offering a lesser SOC. This is a big mistake and is unfair to the client and patient. Often clients will take extraordinary measures for their pets, including finding the means to pay for the best possible treatment available.

To prevent this from occurring, the practice should develop SOCs for all diseases and procedures recommended by the team. SOCs do not mandate how medicine must be practiced; rather they provide practice guidelines for treatment recommendations for every client, every time.

> **LEADERSHIP POINT**
>
> SOCs must be agreed upon by the doctor team and then implemented with staff to increase efficiency and compliance.

Benefits of SOCs include:

- New doctors will know what is expected in the care of their patients. SOCs provide guidance allowing them to feel more confident about recommendations, which encourages the client to feel better about the doctor and team caring for their pet.

- The training of new team members: Different practices have different protocols and procedures. SOCs help new team members find guidelines for treatment. The team member will know what to expect and what to recommend to clients.
- Written protocols prevent confusion or misunderstandings. When every team member knows what the protocol will be, every team member can educate every client. The client will hear a consistent message every time they call or arrive at the practice.

Developing SOCs can seem overwhelming at first but can be managed one step at a time. Start with selecting the top ten outpatient procedures (this may include the treatment of ear infections, pancreatitis, or parasite prevention). Each SOC must include:

- A general description of the condition and recommendations that will be made for any patient experiencing this condition (or disease prevention)
- Compliance protocols for the condition
- Product choices that the practice will recommend treating the patient. Because most practices carry two products to treat or prevent diseases, both should be listed.

Once those ten SOCs have been created and team members have become familiar with expectations, develop ten more SOCs (Fig. 11.28).

Because diseases and disease prevention vary (as do recommendations in different parts of the country), the SOCs will also vary in structure. Each SOC should be developed in accordance with the practices values and recommendations made by the American Animal Hospital Association (AAHA) and the American Veterinary Medical Association (AVMA). Ensure that they are simple to understand (every team member must be able to interpret the recommendations) and are reevaluated on a yearly basis. Protocols, treatments, and medications change frequently; therefore, updates are required.

Standard Operating Protocols (Employee Procedure Manual)

Chapter 4, Human Resources, covers the development, implementation, and updating of an employee procedure manual/SOP. This document should serve as the basis for training all new employees and can be tailored to the role the person is serving. This manual must reside in the practice, likely on a server that a team member can access anytime for a refresher on carrying out standard protocols. SOPs create consistency between team members, helping each anticipate the needs of others to enhance efficiency and the client experience. Like SOCs, SOPs must be updated as new procedures and protocols are implemented. Train team members accordingly and update the document residing on the server.

Client Education

Client education is central to client compliance. They must be able to understand why the procedure or service that is being recommended for their pet. Many common procedures are routine for the veterinary team, but (as stated earlier) it feels foreign to a client. Like team members, clients learn and understand information in a variety of ways. Some may learn better with visual aids such as pictures, videos, and illustrations. Others may learn better with verbal communication (Fig. 11.29).

VHMA PERFORMANCE DOMAIN TASK

The practice manager is responsible for implementing and managing client education.

Being prepared with a combination of materials will meet the needs of the clients, including literature, brochures, videos, or skeletal models when appropriate. Radiographs showing both normal and abnormal findings also help the visualize the abnormality affecting their own pet. Providing clients with materials to take home and read or view on their smartphone will increase their knowledge and trust of the veterinary practice (Fig. 11.30).

Messaging may need to be repeated several times (and in several different ways) for clients to retain the information. Studies indicate that 90% of new information learned will be lost within 30 minutes if not reinforced. Repeat, repeat, and repeat. The more times clients hear and read a message, the more they will retain the information. The receptionists, veterinary technicians, and veterinarians can reinforce consistent messages. The more consistent the message, the higher the rate of client compliance.

Educational materials that print the practice name, client, and patient names on a document titled with a specific topic or disease make the client feel like the information was personalized for them.

To help practices organize and manufacture brochures, a client education center may be developed; organizational structures such as those shown in Fig. 11.31 allow easy access to educational materials, promoting the use of such literature.

Manufacturers also provide a variety of professional posters that relate to current medical topics; these come at no charge to practices that use their products. These posters should be updated regularly to provide new information to clients each time they visit the practice.

The Role of EMR in Client Education

Electronic Medical Records that tie client education to diagnosis codes help improve the efficiency of the team tremendously. Instead of searching for educational material, the code already has the information attached. The PIMS will document the handout in the medical record, and if the practice has a pet portal or practice app that integrates with the PIMS, the handout can be accessed at any time by the client.

Discharge instructions also fall under client education; every pet being discharged from the practice must have release instructions, whether it was hospitalized, had surgery, or was just boarding. Discharge instructions are crucial and should include information about when to feed the pet, how much, exercise restriction, what medications and when to give, and if a follow-up appointment needs to be scheduled (Fig. 11.32). As with client education documents, ensure these are available in the practice app and pet portal for easy client access.

MEASURING AND MONITORING THE FRICTIONLESS CLIENT EXPERIENCE

To ensure the team is meeting client expectations, the practice must consistently ask clients for feedback, and implement changes as needed to continue improving. If you're not monitoring the process, you can't make changes that will improve the experience. Client surveys provide direct client feedback, while client retention and compliance reports are derived from the PIMS.

Client Surveys

Client surveys are extremely valuable, but only if the practice does something with the results. Surveys can be emailed or sent via text to clients and should be kept short and concise so that clients will be more likely to comply with responses. Client surveys are an easy monitoring

ABC VETERINARY HOSPITAL STANDARDS OF CARE
Non-Steroidal Anti-inflammatories

GENERAL

1. Physical exam required bi-annually.
2. Discuss alternative treatment options for pets where appropriate.
3. Explain benefits and potential side effects of NSAIDS and need for blood work screening. Provide client education handout.
4. Perform NSAID Panel to establish a baseline. Provide diagnostic interpretation PDF for client.
5. Repeat NSAID Panel 2 weeks after therapy has begun.
6. Repeat NSAID Panel every 6 months while remaining on NSAIDS
7. Set up reminder for 6-month recheck
8. Give the client a copy of all blood results in the event the patient has the need to be seen by another veterinarian while taking NSAIDS (while traveling or after hours).

FOR SURGERY PATIENTS

1. Following surgery, review discharge orders with client. This includes NSAID dosage instructions, when to give the next dose, potential side effects, and how to identify side effects. Instruct client to stop drug use and call immediately if there are any issues.
2. Provide client with handout explaining proper use of NSAIDS.
3. Call client 24-48 hours after discharge for status report, probe for indications of side effects, and answer questions.
4. When the patient returns for suture removal or recheck, probe for indications of side effects, answer questions.

FOR ACUTE PAIN PATIENTS

1. Discuss physical therapy recommendations (applying ice, massage).
2. Inform client of NSAID dosage instructions, when to give the next dose, potential side effects, and how to identify side effects. Instruct client to stop drug use and call immediately if there are any issues.
3. Provide client with handout.
4. Schedule medical progress exam in one week.

FOR CRONIC PAIN PATIENTS

1. Inform client of NSAID dosage instructions, when to give the next dose, potential side effects, and how to identify side effects. Instruct client to stop drug use and call immediately if there are any issues.
2. Provide client with drug handout.
3. Schedule reassessment with in 10-14 days. Probe for signs of adverse reaction to the drug. Adjust medication accordingly.
4. Over time, titrate the dose of NSAID to its lowest effective level and consider nutritional products and other methods to improve mobility.

	PRIMARY PRODUCT of CHOICE *(Canine)*	**SECONDARY PRODUCT of CHOICE *(Canine)***	**PRIMARY PRODUCT of CHOICE *(Feline)***
General Pain	Carprofen	Deracoxib	Onsior
Acute Pain	Carprofen	Deracoxib	Onsior
Chronic Pain	Carprofen	Deracoxib	Onsior
Post-Surgical	Carprofen +/- Tram/Gaba	N/A	Onsior

Fig. 11.28 Example of a Standard of Care.

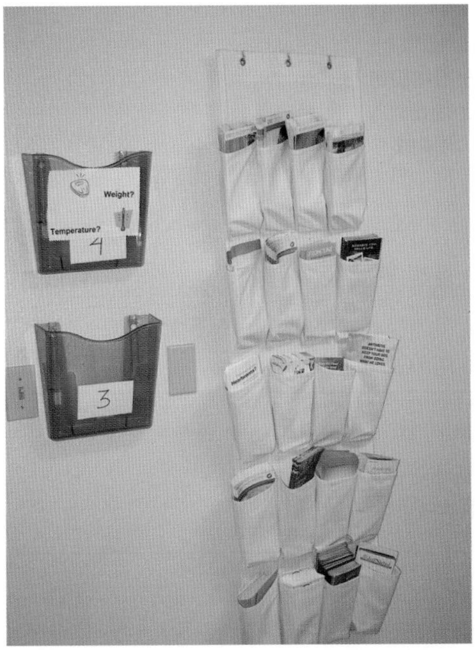

Fig. 11.29 Client education is critical in driving client compliance. Having clients grade their pets' teeth is an excellent educational tool.

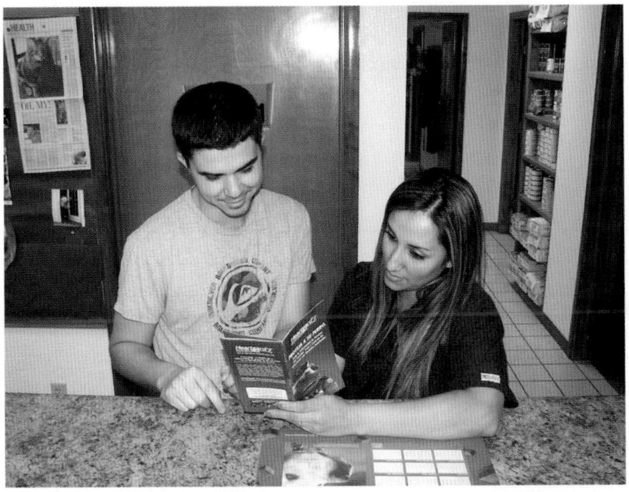

Fig. 11.30 Written information provided by the veterinary technician will increase client understanding and encourage client compliance.

solution used to assess client satisfaction and level of comfort with the services the practice provides. Survey questions should be changed every few months, which will help managers target specific areas of improvement. Providing multiple-choice questions or a number rating scale for most of the survey will contribute to a higher response rate. Survey topics are included in Fig. 11.33.

If clients are unsatisfied, practices want to be notified and given the opportunity to address the problem; unfortunately, many clients will not notify the practice; they will go to another hospital or post a negative comment online or through social media.

Handling Negative Feedback: Reading or hearing statements online that criticize the practice can be hard; practices try to provide the best service they can, and sometimes it does not meet client expectations. Negative reviews of the hospital can be posted online within minutes, and often the client hasn't taken the time to call the practice.

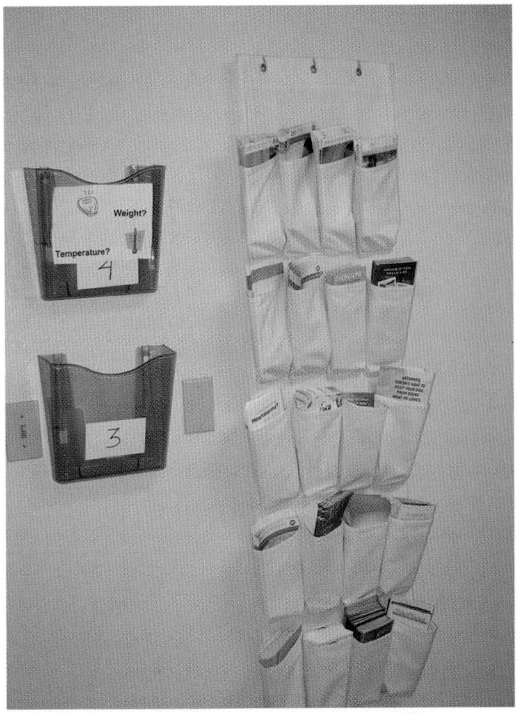

Fig. 11.31 Client education center.

These negative reviews should be addressed immediately. The recommended response to these online complaints is, *"I am so sorry you have had this experience at our hospital. Please call as soon as possible so that we can resolve this situation."* Do not attempt to defend the hospital or any actions that were taken in the response; doing so will encourage a stream of additional comments. The practice can try calling the client (if the review indicates a client name) to resolve the situation; however, most commonly online reviews are posted with usernames, and not the actual client's name. If the client does not call within a few days, add an additional reply to the complaint indicating that you welcome the opportunity to hear from them, *"We welcome the opportunity to speak with you at any time. Please give us a call at your convenience."*

If the client is reached by phone and the situation is resolved to the practice's (and the client's) satisfaction, the client may be asked to post an additional online review indicating a positive solution was reached.

Practices should always encourage clients to post positive reviews about the practice, and when they do, the practice manager should respond with a genuine comment. The more positive reviews that are posted, the less important negative reviews become. Negative reviews must still be addressed immediately, but they will be offset by clients posting about good experiences at the practice.

Practice managers must develop methods to prevent client complaints before difficult situations require resolution. Clients know what good and bad customer service is; the medicine may be spectacular, but if the customer service is poor, negative reviews will be posted.

Client Retention

Client retention is a critical element in maintaining a successful practice. A frictionless customer experience is a major factor that drives client satisfaction, resulting in returning clients and increased referrals. The veterinary team plays a significant role in building and maintaining that human-animal bond with clients starting during the first visit. Everything they do and say, how they do it and say it, and how they follow through impacts the retention rate. Reminding clients of services in the way the client wants to be reminded (postal, text, or phone call),

ABC Veterinary Clinic 555-555-5555
Dr. Roe, Dr. Morton, Dr. Larsen
Post-anesthesia Release Sheet

Please provide clean, dry bedding and a quiet place for your pet to recuperate. Please notify the hospital with any concerns.

DIET:

( ) Wait a few hours after arriving home to offer your pet water. Please give only a small amount. If no vomiting occurs, you may offer more water about an hour later. You may feed a small amount (1/4 normal amount) if water stays down.

( ) You may continue to feed your pet normally.

( ) Special diet instructions ______________________________

ACTIVITY:

( ) Restrict exercise for 1 day. NO RUNNING, JUMPING, CLIMBING OR BATHING.

( ) Restrict exercise for 7 days. NO RUNNING, JUMPING, CLIMBING OR BATHING.

( ) Other ______________________________

OTHER:

( ) Please use paper strips or pinto beans in place of litter for 7 days.

( ) Please booster vaccines in 3-4 weeks.

( ) Your pet's metabolism may permanently decrease after surgery. You may need to decrease the amount of food you feed to prevent obesity.

INCISION:

( ) Watch for swelling, redness, or drainage. Prevent scratching, rubbing, and licking of the incision. Please ask for an E-collar if you think your pet will lick the site.

( ) Ice incision for 5 minutes, 3 to 4 times daily for the first 72 hours.

MEDICATION:

( ) Give pain medication ______________________________

( ) Give antibiotics ______________________________

( ) Give other medication ______________________________

____

( ) Start medication ______________________________

FOLLOW-UP VISITS:

( ) Recheck in ________ days.

( ) There is no need to return for suture removal; the skin was closed with absorbable suture or tissue adhesive.

( ) Not necessary unless you feel there is a problem.

Comments:

Doctor ____________ Tech ____________ Client ____________ Date ____________

Fig. 11.32 Sample of discharge instructions.

CLIENT SURVEYS ARE A GOOD WAY TO DETERMINE WHETHER CLIENT NEEDS ARE BEING MET

How long was the wait time? ☐ 5 minutes or less ☐ 5 to 10 minutes ☐ Over 10 minutes

Was the team knowledgeable and able to answer questions?
☐ Yes ☐ No ☐ Most questions ☐ Not all questions

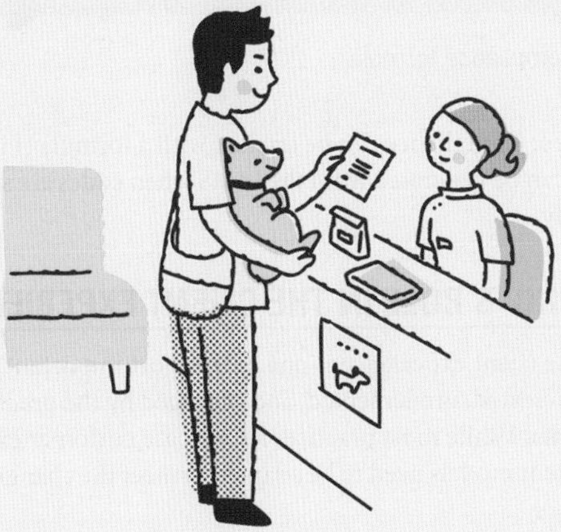

Was the veterinarian courteous and respectful? ☐ Yes ☐ No

Was the staff compassionate and caring? ☐ Yes ☐ No

Did the team listen to your concerns? ☐ Yes ☐ No

Were recommendations for treatment or care explained in an understandable manner? ☐ Yes No ☐ I have more questions

Was your pet treated compassionately? ☐ Yes ☐ No

Were costs for services explained? ☐ Yes ☐ No

Did you receive exceptional customer service? ☐ Yes ☐ No

Was the practice clean and comfortable? ☐ Yes ☐ No

Value of service: *Did you feel you received value for the cost of services.* ☐ Yes ☐ No ☐ Not sure

When a practice is focusing on obesity management, an additional question may be:

Did you receive information on activities you could do with your pet to prevent or reduce obesity? ☐ Yes No

Did you receive information on a weight management diet for your pet? ☐ Yes ☐ No

If the practice is focusing on dental disease prevention, an additional question may be:

Did you learn about methods you could do at home to help prevent gum disease in your pet's mouth? ☐ Yes ☐ No

Did you receive information on a dental cleaning for your pet? ☐ Yes ☐ No

Fig. 11.33 Example of questions that can be asked on a client survey.

and texting clients to check on patients contribute to retention, but if the experience was not great, reminders and checking on patients will do little good. It is no secret that retaining clients is much cheaper than obtaining new clients and developing their trust.

Some clients will leave a practice for reasons beyond the practice's control, such as moving, changing jobs, or the loss of a pet. Some clients may have not established a relationship with the practice and are willing to try another practice because it is closer to their home. In general, a small-animal practice will lose approximately 10% to 15% of clients each year, but a goal should be created to retain 70% to 75% over a 3-year period.

VHMA PERFORMANCE DOMAIN TASK

The practice manager monitors and manages client retention.

Client Compliance

Client compliance is defined as the percentage of clients who accept recommendations made by the veterinary health care team. Superb communication skills, reminders, recalls, education, and understanding client and patient needs are only a few areas that contribute to client compliance. The overall frictionless experience seals the deal.

Trust, satisfaction, and quality of service must be established because the veterinarian-client relationship can span a lifetime and serve a variety of pets. Positive attitudes from team members who believe in the medicine the practice provides will radiate to clients. Excellent medicine and a team-based veterinary approach provide client satisfaction and a high quality of service.

Practice managers must track compliance rates to continue growing the business. Each profit center must be analyzed, ensuring that compliance continues to grow. Areas to focus on include the dental center, surgical services, wellness visits, heartworm and flea/tick preventatives, preoperative laboratory work, or any new service center that

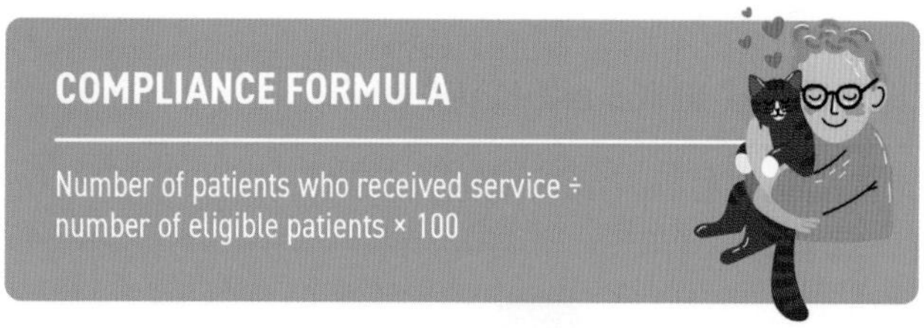

COMPLIANCE FORMULA
Number of patients who received service ÷
number of eligible patients × 100

Fig. 11.34 Compliance formula.

is being added. Compliance can be tracked with a formula (Fig. 11.34), and reports can be generated from the PIMS when codes are set up and used correctly.

LEADERSHIP'S ROLE IN THE CLIENT EXPERIENCE

Managing the client experience is one of the most important activities that must be created, implemented, and managed by the practice manager and owner. While most practices have a base customer experience in place, current models need to be adapted to meet the changing needs of clients.

Leadership must start with driving a positive, influential culture (Chapter 2) that embodies core values, a vision, and a mission statement. Regularly scheduled team meetings that are meaningful and impactful must be held in a safe environment where team members feel that they can collaborate and share ideas to achieve practice goals. Detailed training programs must be in place for every role that clearly states the expectations of the team member, and how the role contributes to strategic goal achievement.

Last but not least, leadership must view every experience in the veterinary practice from that of a client. Evaluate how easy the process is for clients to do business with the practice and if they achieve a frictionless client experience every time. PMs and owners must evaluate technology, think outside the box, and implement procedures to exceed client expectations for the long-term success of the practice.

PRACTICE MANAGER SURVIVAL CHECKLIST FOR THE CLIENT EXPERIENCE

- ☐ Identify the preferred communication methods for each client (postal, email, text message, phone call, app notification).
- ☐ Create a solid reminder system enabling postal, email, text, and app notification reminders for clients.
- ☐ Have reminders in place for annual examinations, vaccines, annual laboratory work, and chronic medication refills.
- ☐ Develop an effective recall system and allow the team adequate time to effectively connect with clients.
- ☐ Have client surveys/satisfaction tracking system in place. Evaluate results, share with the team, and improve procedures often.
- ☐ Identify and monitor key performance indicators.
- ☐ Measure client compliance
- ☐ Create a policy regarding client refunds/adjustments.
- ☐ Ensure team scheduling accommodates the busiest times.
- ☐ Develop, implement, and role-play client conflict/resolution procedures.
- ☐ Develop protocol to manage emails, text messages, practice portal, and app notifications every 15 minutes.
- ☐ Set up online review notifications with Google and Yahoo and develop a protocol to respond to both positive and negative reviews.
- ☐ Review client education protocols and ensure clients are receiving appropriate materials with each diagnosis.

REVIEW QUESTIONS

1. Why are verbal and written skills imperative in veterinary medicine?
2. What is client compliance and how can it be achieved?
3. What are the benefits of a reminder system?
4. Create a client education that improves client understanding.
5. What would be an appropriate body stance when addressing clients?
6. Why is body posture important?
7. How should an angry client be handled?
8. How can common barriers be overcome?
9. Why are estimates important?
10. How can an individual's verbal image be improved?
11. The portion of a message that involves facial expressions is:
    - **a.** Verbal
    - **b.** Paraverbal
    - **c.** Nonverbal
    - **d.** Written
12. If a client receives a confusing message, which portion of the message can they rely on for a better understanding?
    - **a.** Verbal
    - **b.** Paraverbal
    - **c.** Nonverbal
    - **d.** Written
13. The percentage of clients who accept a recommendation is known as:
    - **a.** Compliance
    - **b.** Retention
    - **c.** Turnover
    - **d.** Quantity
14. Client education should be available in which of the following forms?
    - **a.** Webpage
    - **b.** Printed material
    - **c.** Verbal education
    - **d.** Models and videos
    - **e.** All the above
15. Which team member should present treatment plans to clients?
    - **a.** Veterinarians
    - **b.** Receptionists
    - **c.** Veterinary technicians
    - **d.** B and C

REFERENCES

1. Fontanella C. What Does it Mean to offer a frictionless customer experience? HubSpot. Published January 6, 2020. Accessed September 2022. https://blog.hubspot.com/service/frictionless-customer-experience
2. Veterinary appointment scheduling software. Vetstoria. Published November 22, 2019. Accessed September 2022. https://www.vetstoria.com

ADDITIONAL READING

Finch L. *Telephone courtesy and client service*. 4th ed. Axzo Press; 2009.

Gerson RF. *Beyond customer service. Keeping clients for life*. 3rd ed. Axzo Press; 1998.

12

Marketing

LEARNING OBJECTIVES

When you have completed this chapter, you should be able to:

- Compare and contrast different methods of marketing
- Identify technology applications that apply to internal marketing
- Provide examples of unintentional marketing and explain how to overcome those examples
- Identify ways to increase search engine optimization of the practice website
- List steps to complete when responding to online reviews
- Define and provide examples of SMART goals
- Define and provide examples of a SWOT analysis

OUTLINE

KEY TERMS

Community Service
Domain Name
External Marketing
Fear Free
Hyperlinks
Internal Marketing
Marketing
On-Hold Messaging
Pet Portals
Practice App
Practice Brand
Push Notifications
ROI
SEO
SWOT Analysis
Target Marketing
Unintentional Marketing
URL
Website

VHMA PERFORMANCE DOMAINS

Veterinary Hospital Managers Association (VHMA) Performance Domains

The performance domains applicable to marketing are marketing and client relations. The practice manager is responsible for:

- Managing promotional items
- Development and management of advertising
- Website management
- Social media management
- Community service outreach management
- Monitoring client retention
- Developing and managing new client programs
- Handling client complaints
- Obtaining client feedback on services
- Development and management of reminder systems
- Managing client education

Application of VHMA Performance Domains for Practice Managers

In the marketing and client relations domain, the veterinary practice manager plans and coordinates marketing, public relations, and client service programs. In terms of marketing, the manager develops internal and external marketing plans and monitors the results of marketing efforts. The tasks related to marketing require knowledge of the principles of target marketing, market research, pricing, and product promotion. The tasks related to client services and education require knowledge of the principles and process for providing customer and personal services, including customer needs assessment and methods for evaluating customer satisfaction.

INTRODUCTION

Marketing is a critical component of practice success, and most components of marketing are completed daily without knowing that they are being carried out. Marketing is defined as the action or business of promoting and selling products or services, including market research and advertising. It includes creating, communicating, and delivering offerings that have value, also known as the client experience. Everything a practice does to create a frictionless client experience intertwines with marketing. For this chapter, we will focus on advertising the offerings that have value, since creating the value is covered in Chapter 11, Client Experience.

There are two forms of marketing that apply to the veterinary practice, and while both internal and external marketing are important, if the internal marketing strategies are not up to par, it makes no sense to spend excess money on external marketing. Internal marketing is directed toward promoting services to current clients and includes reminders, mass email communication, and the overall frictionless client experience (Fig. 12.1). External marketing includes advertising to outside resources or potential clients to continue building the business. Examples include advertising in the local newspaper or community service events. The webpage and social media serve as both internal and external examples because they provide a service to existing clients and market to potential clients.

Team members contribute to the marketing of the practice, both internally and externally, as well. Everything they do and say impacts both internal and external strategies. Internally, they impact the frictionless client experience. Externally, they advertise the veterinary hospital by wearing scrubs or polo shirts with the name of the practice outside of business hours. The bottom line is to spend more time, effort, and money on internal marketing (including the webpage) before spending money on external advertising.

EXAMPLES OF INTERNAL MARKETING

- Practice culture
- A frictionless client experience
- Recalls
- Reminders
- Client education
- Clean, updated, and pleasant-smelling office
- Team identification
- Blogs, website, and social media
- Timely replies to client requests via email, texting, pet portal or practice app messaging
- Telephone etiquette
- Client acknowledgment
- Professional appearance

Fig. 12.1 Internal marketing is directed toward current clients.

Overall, practices should have a marketing strategy that is evaluated on a yearly basis. It needs to tie to the overall strategic plan of the practice and must incorporate the vision, mission, and values (Chapter 2). Have service and sales increased with current marketing techniques? If not, where has the marketing failed? Was it an internal or external technique? Was there a decrease in the number of new clients? Practice managers must be able to track before and after results and make changes as needed (return on investment [ROI]). If one marketing technique did not work, evaluate and understand why, and adapt new strategies to achieve the strategic goals.

CRITICAL COMPETENCY: ADAPTABILITY

Practice managers must be open to change and flexible work methods and can adapt behavior to changing conditions or new information.

INTERNAL MARKETING

Practice Brand

The practice brand is an intangible and highly valuable asset that encompasses the reputation of the practice and how the practice is "identified." Successful branding takes time to develop and results in client compliance, loyalty, and retention.

Brands can also be referred to as the personality that identifies a service. Thoughts, feelings, perceptions, experiences, and attitudes contribute to brand development. If a client knows that your hospital consistently delivers quality medicine and a frictionless client experience, they are going to maintain their relationship with the hospital and continue referring friends and family (Fig. 12.2).

Positive word-of-mouth referrals are the most successful form of free marketing. The frictionless client experience drives this. By relaying the value of services to each client, they can't help but brag about the practice. Client confidence in the medical skills and professional services provided by a team is the primary gauge of value, along with friendly staff, compassion, education, and cleanliness. These all lead to a superior customer experience and client satisfaction.

A brand that is widely known in the marketplace acquires brand recognition. When brand recognition builds in communities, clients associate logos, colors, and themes with the practice. To continue developing and improving a brand, practices must be consistent in their delivery of materials (use the same colors in logo, webpage, and

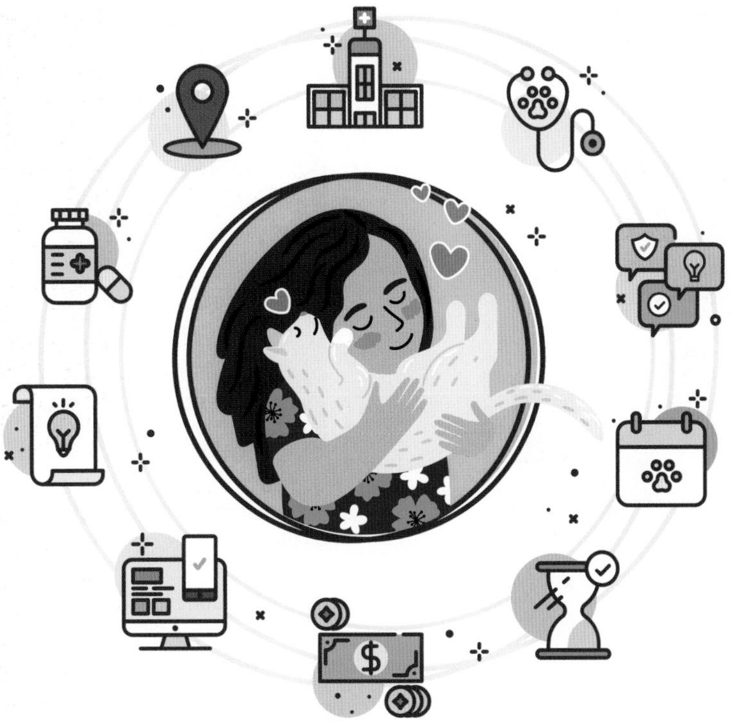

Fig. 12.2 A frictionless client experience delivers consistent high-quality medicine and customer service to every client, regardless of the situation.

client education materials) and maintain consistency in the delivery of outstanding medical and customer service. All clients must have the same standard of care offered every time they are in the practice (see Chapter 11, Standards of Care). When client experiences are negative, brand recognition suffers and word of mouth spreads.

In summary, brand recognition is driven by exceptional customer service; efficiency; excellent medicine; client education; clear, concise, and honest communication; every client receiving a treatment plan; following up with clients as promised; and the overall culture of the practice. Review Chapter 2 on Culture and the role it plays in brand recognition.

Team and Client Communication

Communication is covered extensively in Chapter 11 but is worth mentioning in marketing. Obviously, the frictionless client experience and team member experience would suffer without exceptional communication.

Team members wearing clean, wrinkle-free uniforms appear professional and approachable, which encourages clients to ask questions. Clients must be greeted upon entry and assisted when leaving. Team members wearing name tags inform the client of who they are as well as their positions within the practice.

> **LEADERSHIP POINT**
>
> Develop a culture where professionalism (appearance and attitude) is the expectation and the norm demonstrated by all team members.

Team members that establish long-term relationships with clients also promote the practice brand (Fig. 12.3). Forming relationships allows team members to address clients by name and makes the client feel important, respected, and valued. *"Good morning, Ms. Thurman. How are you and Fluffy today?"* is an excellent greeting for both the client and the pet. When the pet's name and history are addressed, the client's confidence in the practice increases, leading to better overall satisfaction with the practice.

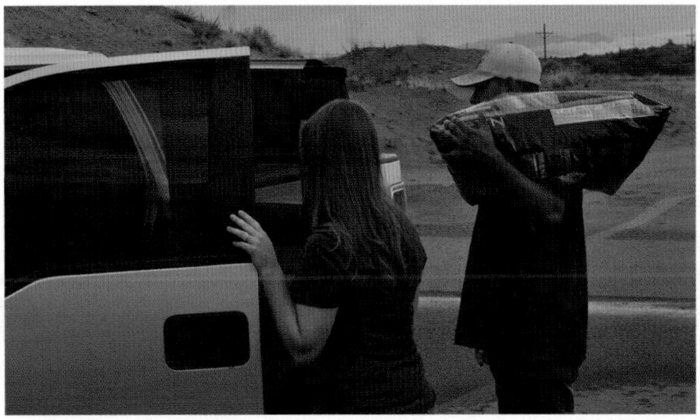

Fig. 12.3 Providing clients with consistent, exceptional service develops long-term loyalty and word-of-mouth referrals.

Creating space in the reception area to place team member names and pictures familiarizes clients with the team, as well as the role each team member plays. Veterinarians and credentialed veterinary technicians/nurses should have their appropriate credentials included, including any bachelor's or associate's degrees they may have. Practice managers should list their CVPM if they are certified (Fig. 12.4).

> **CRITICAL COMPETENCY: CREATIVITY**
>
> Practice managers must have the ability to creatively think through situations and embrace new and different ways to see opportunities by using imagination and collaboration, resulting in innovative solutions.

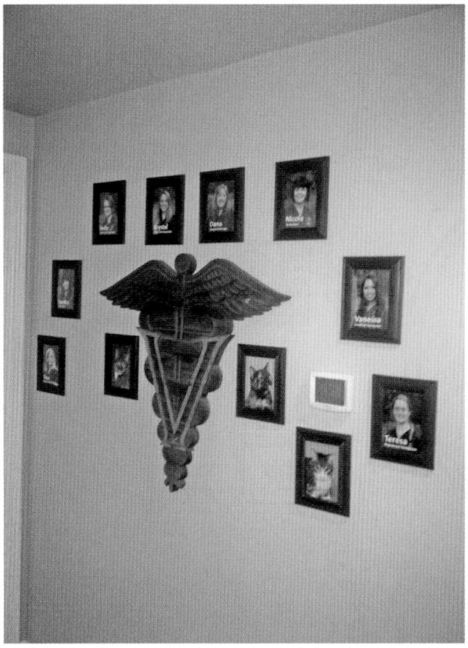

Fig. 12.4 An example of indirect marketing is placing pictures of team members on the lobby wall for clients to view. (Courtesy Ben Wilson and Star of Texas Veterinary Clinic.)

TECHNOLOGY TO SERVE CLIENT NEEDS

There are many facets of technology available to the veterinary industry that enhance internal marketing. Website development, two-way texting, pet portals, practice apps, telehealth, online pharmacy, and being able to make appointments online, are all significant contributors to internal marketing. Some PIMS integrate all these technologies for the veterinary practice, while others don't and need a third-party application to function in the digital space.

VHMA PRACTICE DOMAIN TASK

Practice managers oversee website management.

Website

Searching the Internet is the first place both existing and new clients visit when looking for veterinary information. The practice website may be the first impression a potential client has of the practice. Existing clients utilize the practice's website to look up hours of operation, who team members are, common questions they may be experiencing with their pet, and to easily make appointments or order medications. Websites must be easy to navigate, beautifully designed, and responsive so that they can be viewed on any device including cell phones and iPads.

Developing a Website

Information technology (IT) is not a strength that most practice managers or practice owners have. While IT can be considered to cover computer installment and maintenance, integration of various computer systems, and Internet connectivity, website development and maintenance can also be tied into the IT classification. What goes on the web page is a marketing initiative. Outsource website development and maintenance to a website company that does it well. They can efficiently make recommendations and designs that are appropriate for the practice but don't look like every other veterinary webpage. Use caution if using a predesigned template and ensure it does not look like other veterinary practice webpages within the community.

IMPORTANT TOPICS TO BE INCLUDED ON A WEBSITE

- Hours of operation
- Doctors
- Staff members
- Medication refills
- Schedule appointments
- Online pharmacy
- Achievements/awards
- Professional aervices offered
- Hot topics: Diseases that are prevalent in the area
- Community service
- Blogs
- Pet of the month
- Client testimonials
- Virtual tour
- Frequent forms

Fig. 12.5 A website is often the first exposure clients have to the veterinary practice. Hire the right company to develop the best first impression possible.

LEADERSHIP POINT

Opting for the cheapest version of a website will likely yield a poor perception of the practice for potential clients.

Hiring a website designer is costly and design firms should be compared before signing a contract. However, the practice website is a valuable resource, and the investment is worthwhile. In addition to reaching new clients, the practice website needs to serve the existing clientele while they are researching information for their pets. Well-designed websites generate passive revenue.

Some design companies offer complete website design and management, meaning the practices may have little or no access to the content provided. The design company handles all updates and changes (as requested by the practice), creates blogs, and drives search engine optimization. The advantage of this option is not having to worry about content management, posting, or updating. Other companies offer design and web services, and the practice manager creates content and communication with the Webmaster regularly. Another option is purchasing a complete web design and having a team member with web experience act as a webmaster for content updates and changes. Several templates are available within this option that offer user-friendly updates and changes; however, this option requires that the site be fully managed by the practice.

With any of these options, it is up to the practice to ensure that all information on the website is correct. When practice recommendations change or team members and services are added, the website must be updated. Fig. 12.5 provides examples of topics to include in website design. Content is the most important factor and should never be delegated to a webmaster without veterinary experience.

Webpages should include the same design, colors, and logo on each page (further enhancing brand recognition). The logo and clinic name should be included on the heading of each page and pages should be easy to navigate with a "back" and "home" option on each.

The home page is very important. A picture of the front of the building helps introduce the practice to potential clients and makes the practice recognizable to potential clients driving by. A welcome message should include the vision, mission, and values of the hospital, and an overview of products and services should be provided.

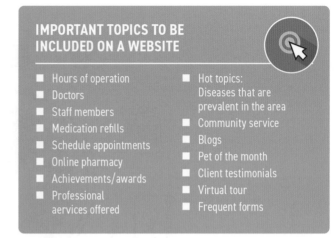

A balance of high-quality pictures and text should be used on the site. Websites with too much text will overload users and images should be strategically placed (supportive of content being covered). They should include a variety of species the practice sees while being clear and uncluttered. Low-quality pictures are often blurry when the website opens, leading visitors to a poor perception of the practice.

A web address should be secured early in the design phase. A uniform resource locator (URL) is the address of the website on the World Wide Web (www). The address is composed of letters, numbers, and periods that are unique to each site. The website address should be the name of the veterinary hospital whenever possible. For example, ABC Veterinary Hospital would ideally have a URL of www.ABCVeterinaryHospital.com. If that specific name is already used by another facility, something unique should be added to the address, such as the city where the practice is located (www.ABCVeterinaryHospitalChicago.com). Once a desired URL has been established, the domain must be secured.

Within the design software, the website should designate common keywords that are accessible to search engines on the Internet. Search engines are how consumers find information online. Keywords to consider include the name of the clinic, city, species of animals the practice treats, professional services that are available, and last names of the doctors on staff. A compilation of these words should be developed and provided to the web designer.

All websites must include email contact information; email should go to the practice manager (or designated customer service representative) to respond to any incoming inquiries immediately. The email address should be checked at least three times per day for any correspondence that may have arrived. Quick response to emails (or lack thereof) creates a lasting impression. Unanswered messages and delayed responses damage the practice's reputation.

Websites should also include hyperlinks, which are images or highlighted text on a webpage linked to other websites, or content within the same website. This allows clients to move to other locations within the website more easily, or to move to other websites that have been linked with the practice site. In addition, when relevant hyperlinks are embedded in the text content, the site's credibility with search engines increases.

CRITICAL COMPETENCY: CONTINUOUS LEARNING

Practice managers should have a curiosity for learning. Actively seeking out new information, technologies, and methods while keeping skills updated allows the application of new knowledge to the job.

Practices may wish to provide hyperlinks to local businesses that they recommend, such as groomers, pet shops, or boarding kennels. These hyperlinks must be checked regularly to ensure their viability. Search engines discredit websites that harbor invalid links, thus reducing the website's credibility with search engines.

Websites should follow a three-click rule; information that clients are looking for should be found in just three clicks. Studies suggest that the longer it takes people to find information, the less likely they are to stay on the current website. To adhere to the three-click rule, webpages should be well organized with the use of tabs on the front page, allowing quicker access to information for the reader.

Search Engine Optimization

Many owners and managers find search engine optimization (SEO) difficult to understand and underuse valuable tools available to increase the practice's visibility on the Internet. SEO is the process of affecting the visibility of a website in a search engine's search results. Example of search engines includes Google, Chrome, Safari, and Yahoo. When a client searches the Internet, they enter keywords into the search engine, which then scrolls millions of webpages that match the keywords provided (therefore keyword entry is critical when developing websites). The goal is to have the practice's website appear on the first page of results and in the top three practices listed. To achieve this goal, websites must strengthen their SEO using the following methods:

Keywords: Keywords that have been chosen for SEO should be woven into the content of the website. The more often those keywords appear within the website, the stronger the SEO.

Internal Hyperlinks: Linking to other pages within the website strengthens SEO. For example, a practice may mention digital radiography on the home page, which is then hyperlinked to another page providing the details of digital radiography.

Inbound Hyperlinks: Links from businesses drives SEO. Consider asking emergency and referral practices and the Chamber of Commerce to list the practice's website on their webpage.

External Hyperlinks: Linking to other credible websites helps strengthen SEO. Add links to reputable organizations such as the AVMA, American Animal Hospital Association, and American Association of Feline Practitioners (the links are endless). Always ensure links are viable.

Update Content Frequently: Search engines constantly look for new information; therefore, the more frequently a website is updated, the stronger the SEO.

Increased Webpage Traffic: Websites must have visitors. Without visitors, search engines find the website less credible, decreasing SEO.

Paid Space: Clinics can pay for increased search engine visibility and advertisements. Online ads can be targeted directly to consumers that search for veterinary content in the local area, or regionally.

Claim the Business: Google has the option to claim the business, update business hours, and activate the phone number so that users can simply call the practice with a click of the number. This also allows users to see where the practice is on a map.

LEADERSHIP POINT

Practice managers can drive SEO strength organically by identifying keywords that clients use to search for the practice, establishing internal hyperlinks that link the homepage to other pages within the website, and linking to credible external websites in the community.

Promoting the Website

Practices must actively work to drive site traffic. As indicated previously, increasing traffic on a website leads to a stronger search engine presence. Implement the following recommendations to increase website traffic:

Content: Build an excellent website that is easy to navigate and full of content. Consumers search the Internet for veterinary information frequently. This is an opportunity for the veterinary practice to capitalize on those searches by making sure the practice website contains useful and easy-to-find information. This starts with great web design, tabs, and an organizational structure. Consider listing the top 10 diseases the practice diagnoses and/or the top 10 procedures the practice performs and develop content and keywords about those items. Also consider having a page dedicated to each revenue center the hospital has established (rehab, pain management, orthopedic surgery, dentistry, etc.). The more content that is available for the clients, the more often they will return, therefore driving website visits.

Pet Portals: Pet portals allow clients to access their medical records at any time of the day. When portals are linked to the website (and clients continue returning to their account), the number of visits will increase.

Client Education: Provide client education documents on the top ten diseases and diagnoses made by the practice.

Preoperative Instructions: When appointments for surgery have been scheduled, clients can be directed to the website for downloadable instructions.

Client Forms: Place downloadable forms that clients will need to bring to the practice on the website.

Events: If the practice hosts events such as obesity management courses, puppy socialization dates, or open houses, an event calendar may be considered for the website. Each time an event is entered, an email can be generated and sent to clients informing them of the new event. Each time they click on the event calendar, SEO strengthens.

Practice Tour: Clients love behind-the-scenes practice tours.

Blogs: Keywords in blogs are searchable on search engines and drive traffic back to the website. Most web design companies will develop blog content for practices and post routinely.

Social Media: Post and promote social media links to any social media platforms the clinic uses.

Tasks: Appointment scheduling, medication refills, and the practice's online pharmacy are options that drive website traffic.

VHMA PRACTICE DOMAIN TASK

The Practice manager develops and manages practice promotional items.

The website address should be printed on every business item (along with contact information and logo). Business cards, brochures, and client education materials are the obvious locations for branding, but don't forget prescription labels, shopping bags, incentive items, and blogs.

Texting

Some clients love text messaging; others dislike it. The point is that team members need to ask clients how they wish to be communicated with and implement strategies to meet those needs. If texts are preferred, text messages can be sent to clients reminding them of upcoming appointments, as well as updates and pictures of their pet recovering from surgery. The practice may also send pictures of patients playing during doggy daycare. Some PIMS automatically incorporate two-way texting with clients. If that is not an option, third-party applications can integrate and provide the solution for the practice. As with any client communication, text messages should be documented in the medical record (some PIMS provides this function automatically, resulting in increased team efficiency). See Chapter 8 for more information.

LEADERSHIP POINT

Create templates of text responses for the most common questions receptionists receive; this allows them to be efficient and provide professional, error-free messages that enhance the practice brand.

Pet Portals and Practice Apps

Pet portals and practice apps increase compliance (appointments, services, and products) significantly and allow clients to view their pet's medical records, upload photos, view reminders for appointments and surgeries, make appointments, and provide the link to the online pharmacy or requesting refills in house (Fig. 12.6). Allowing clients to see their pet's medical record, laboratory work results, and radiographs contributes to the frictionless client experience that the practice should be trying to build.

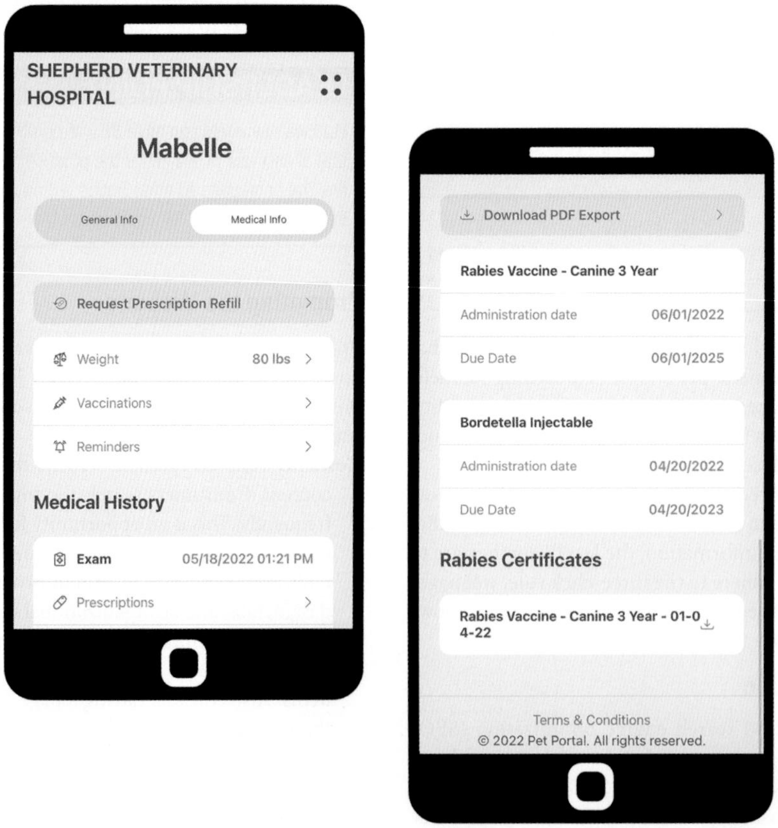

Fig. 12.6 Example of Pet Portal. (Courtesy Shepherd Software.)

Developing a customized practice app can meet the demands of clients by offering interactive communication options (Fig.12.7); consider the following options when developing an app:

- Custom branding,
- Push notifications and text messaging,
- The ability to view upcoming appointments,
- Access a pet health library, poison control, or apply for Care Credit,
- Family share (members of the same family can share the app on all mobile devices, and push notifications are then sent to all devices), and
- Rewards/loyalty program.

Push notifications are simple messages that wake up the device and alert the client with a message displayed on the home or lock screen. These instant messages remind clients to give medication (or other due services), update clients with special messages ("the practice will be closing at 3 p.m. today due to extreme weather conditions"), or provide an Amber alert for lost pets. They can also be used to notify clients when their pet is recovering from anesthesia, playing at doggy daycare, or is ready to go after a fabulous day at the spa (be sure to send pictures!). Images of laboratory results, radiographs, links to videos, or client education can also be sent to improve practice communications with the client.

Reward Programs

Rewards and loyalty programs provide a positive perception to clients by earning rewards and feeling appreciated for the money they have spent in the practice. Scientifically, feeling appreciated unlocks neuroendocrine benefits, while rewards are associated with increased oxytocin levels, both of which influence trust within the practice.[1]

Rewards programs result in clients that spend approximately $10 more per transaction when they receive a loyalty stamp, increased visits by clients when a rewards program is available, and clients that spend approximately 10% more per invoice when they are rewarded. The ROI on a loyalty program is approximately 2000%.[2]

CRITICAL COMPETENCY: ANALYTICAL SKILLS

The practice manager must have the ability to grasp complex information, analyze information and use logic to address problems accurately, quickly, and efficiently.

Online Pharmacy

The online pharmacy link should be at the top of every web page with an easy-click button. This allows clients to shop online at any time (meeting the client's need for convenience) while also feeling they can trust the products that are available on the practice's website. When products are ordered through the practice's site, they include the guarantee offered by manufacturers, just as if the products were sold in the hospital.

Online pharmacies must be marketed to the clients. Without proper marketing and promotion, clients will continue to use large competitors for their prescription medications. Track the number of requests that come in daily from large box retailers and develop protocols and client messaging to drive clients back to the practice's online pharmacy.

Having a practice online pharmacy allows the practice to consolidate inventory by not having to carry all products, resulting in

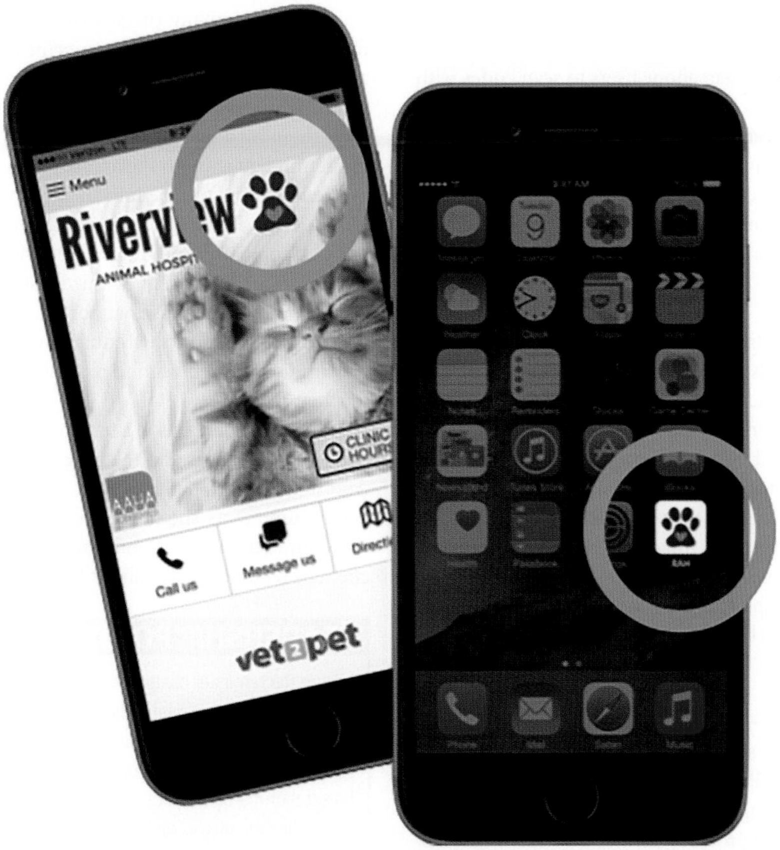

Fig. 12.7 Example of a customized veterinary practice app. (Courtesy Vet2Pet; http://www.vet2pet.com)

Fig. 12.8 Use QR codes to drive clients to the practice website, online pharmacy, or social media sites.

decreased ordering frequency and inventory-related costs (Chapter 13, Inventory).

Making Appointments Online

Just like refilling medications, clients want to be able to make appointments online, at any time day or night. Many clients get busy during regular business hours and are unable to call the practice. Clients should be able to book appointments directly into the appointment schedule and not wait for a confirmation to determine if that appointment is available. Review Chapter 12 and make this feature available on the website, in the practice portal, practice app, and in all communications sent to clients.

QR Codes

Quick response (QR) codes allow smartphone users to scan codes with their phones (Fig. 12.8). QR codes serve as a quick link feature taking users directly to the practice's website. QR codes can be generated by various companies (available online) and downloaded to use on client education materials, business cards, and medication labels. When clients need to refill a medication, they can scan the code which takes them directly to the online pharmacy or the sign-in page of the pet portal.

On-Hold Messaging

When clients are placed on hold time seems to pass slowly. When a client is on hold for 1 minute, it feels like 5 minutes! Practices can use this opportunity to entertain and educate clients while marketing products and services. Several companies produce software that can be played on a system while clients are on hold. Friendly messages can be developed specifically for the practice and include the practice name as well as the names of the doctors. New messages can then be produced on a quarterly basis and can change with the seasons. Topics may include heartworm disease, special diets, special procedures, dentals, antifreeze toxicity, chocolate toxicity, heatstroke, or plant poisonings. The choice is unlimited and innovative messaging can be created for each individual practice.

REMINDERS

Reminders are courtesy messages that remind owners their pet(s) is due for a service or a procedure. Practices may elect to send reminders for a variety of services, including yearly examinations and vaccines (based on the current vaccination protocol), senior care examinations, heartworm testing, or fecal analysis (depending on the location of the practice in the United States). Practices may also send reminders for yearly laboratory work, including testing for hypothyroidism, phenobarbital levels, or bile acids for patients that are on long-term medications that may have potential side effects if not monitored closely.

Communications can also be sent to remind clients to refill their pets' medications, including heartworm prevention and medications that treat hypothyroidism or hyperthyroidism, seizures, and allergies.

Reminders must be clear and concise and indicate what services are needed. They should state if an appointment needs to be made. Otherwise, a client may walk into the practice without an appointment, expecting to be seen for the services indicated on the card. Grammar and spelling must be correct, and the message must include a call to action. What are you asking the recipient to do when they receive the reminder?

Reminders can be sent to clients in the form of text messages, emails, postcards, or phone calls, and clients should be asked how they prefer to be communicated with and when to receive reminders. Team members should make a diligent effort to ensure that email addresses and cell phone numbers are current every time the client comes in, allowing reminders to be effective when sent through text messages or email.

For clients that have forward-booked appointments at least one month in advance of the appointment, postcards may be sent, whereas text messages and emails may be sent for an appointment less than two weeks out. A combination of postcards, emails, and text messages achieves greater results than just one format by itself. Be sure to include the link to schedule appointments in all emails and text messages, so that clients can simply book with one click.

VHMA PRACTICE DOMAIN TASK

The Practice manager develops and manages the client reminder system.

For practices utilizing postcards, it is highly recommended to outsource to a company (versus running them in-house). It is common for team members to forget to print postcards, get and apply stamps, and send them out. Additionally, they are also time-consuming and costly. An outside company can produce them at a cheaper rate and send them on a weekly basis. Weekly mailing results in clients receiving reminders close to the actual due date and reduces the large influx of clients calling to schedule an appointment when bulk reminders are sent at once. Practice managers should review reports (from the outsourced company) and internal reminder compliance reports to ensure reminders are being sent by third-party companies.

For practices that use pet portals, reminders can be customized to a particular patient, further enhancing client compliance. Clients appreciate individualized reminders that lead them to provide the best care for their pets.

Clients should receive a text to remind them of their pet's upcoming surgical procedures and the surgical protocol that should be followed. Additionally, any patients that are scheduled for lab work with special requirements should receive a text message outlining any special requirements. A link should be provided in the text message for the client to rebook if they cannot keep the appointment.

LEADERSHIP POINT

Ensure the reminder component removes deceased patients (when updated in the PIMS). It is emotionally distressing for a client to receive a reminder about a pet that has died, especially if the loss occurred at the veterinary hospital. It is not uncommon for a pet to die at home and for the owner not to inform the hospital of the death until receiving an appointment reminder. Team members should be empathetic, apologetic, and be able to guarantee that the owner will not receive further communication regarding that pet.

For reminders to work effectively, they must be linked to the correct service items in the PIMS. If reminders are not set up correctly, they will not be displayed in the client record, nor will they be deployed correctly. The reminder system should be evaluated once a year to ensure the wording that is on the reminders is accurate and meets the standard of care that the hospital has established.

DEVELOPING MARKETING THAT SUPPORTS THE FRICTIONLESS CLIENT EXPERIENCE

The frictionless client experience is driven by every person on the team, but they must be provided training and have clear expectations as to how the experience should be delivered. Each team member must understand how they contribute to the experience. But a team cannot be successful without having the base put in place first, and that starts with standard operating protocols (SOPs) and standards of care (SOCs). Everything is built around SOPs and SOCs, including the expected level of service, reminders, client education, and client communication. See Chapter 4 (SOPs) and Chapter 11 (SOCs) for more details.

Practices must develop consistent protocols and deliver the same message that is repeated several times within the same visit for the client to retain the information. This repeated message starts with the receptionist, continues with the veterinary technician, then the veterinarian, and is followed up one more time at checkout with the receptionist.

Unintentional Marketing

Unintentional marketing always occurs, whether team members or practice managers realize it or not. This unintentional marketing is marketing that represents the practice and can be detrimental if not managed daily. The following are areas within the practice significantly impact client perception:

Parking Lot: Is the parking lot appealing, or full of potholes, weeds, and trash? Are dog feces scattered about? This is an area of first impression for a client; make it a positive perception before they even walk into the practice.

Signage: Does the practice signage indicate the facility is modern and updated? Is it consistent with the vision and mission of the practice?

Smells: What does the practice smell like upon entry? Offensive smells create negative perceptions.

Audio: What do clients hear when they enter the practice? Crying dogs awaking from anesthesia? Team members yelling at boarding dogs? Team members gossiping? What does it sound like when clients call the hospital? Is the conversation rushed? Is the receptionist friendly?

Relationships: Have lasting relationships been developed with clients? Is time allotted to the team members to establish this relationship? Relationships are critical for practices; studies show consumers pay more for services based on a good relationship.

Listening: Listening to clients is a key component of effective marketing programs. If team members do not listen to clients, they will not understand their needs. This ultimately leads to client dissatisfaction and decreased compliance. Review Chapter 11 for more details on listening.

Professional, Well-Groomed Staff: Are uniforms clean, pressed, and stain-free? Are team members professional in their word choice, enunciation, and body language (Chapter 11)?

Compassion and Empathy: Do team members show compassion for pets and their parents? Is empathy demonstrated when appropriate?

> **LEADERSHIP POINT**
>
> Ask team members to evaluate the practice from the client's perspective and address the points above in a collaboration event to overcome unintentional marketing practices.

Marketing Ideas That Enhance the Frictionless Client Experience

Materials can and should be developed to further enhance the client experience. These are also known as internal marketing documents, items, and ideas that not only promote the practice brand but also provide the client value.

Creative marketing ideas can be inexpensive and offer a multitude of ways to give clients a VIP experience. Remember, it's easier (and less expensive) to increase current client visits than to reach new clients. The most effective marketing plans will focus on existing clients first. Going the extra mile in building and fostering relationships contributes to client satisfaction, loyalty, and compliance. Get creative!

Thank you cards should be sent to clients who have made referrals for new clients. Practices may send thank you cards to loyal clients for practice "anniversaries" to celebrate 5, 10, or even 20 years with the practice. Gift certificates may be awarded for special occasions to be used upon the client's next visit to the practice. Clients greatly appreciate the acknowledgment of their value and importance. It is very rare in business settings to send clients a thank you card. Stand out from the crowd!

Clients always appreciate condolence cards when they have lost a pet. The entire team can sign the card and add little notes expressing their thoughts. Special clients and clients in the top 20% of accounts should receive flowers, a plant, or perhaps a donation to a charity in the pet's name. These clients have obviously spent money helping their pets, and the practice should take the extra step to express their condolence.

In addition to condolence cards, clay paw prints or a Rainbow Bridge poem with the pets' paw print can be mailed to the owner once it dries. These caring gestures make lasting impressions on clients, and when skipped, are missed opportunities to enhance the client bond (Fig. 12.9).

A pet that has suffered and survived a traumatic experience or injury might receive a purple heart for its courage (Fig. 12.10). Purple hearts make clients feel great and are an excellent conversation piece. The practice name will be brought up in conversation when clients are asked how and why the pet received a purple heart. Pet bandannas are also relatively inexpensive to produce with custom messaging, and clients are usually excited to put them on their pets (Fig. 12.11). Purple hearts or bandannas must have the practice information on them, along with a catchy phrase such as "I survived!"

Create a client loyalty program by offering points on purchases, allowing clients to earn rewards for referrals, having regular pet wellness examinations, providing online reviews, or providing testimonials for the website or marketing materials.

Practices can initiate social media contests allowing clients to enter and win pet food, a pet goody basket, or nonveterinary items. Social media also allows subliminal client education to occur. Practice messages will be shared with client friends and followers, increasing the number of potential clients who will see practice messaging.

A weight management hall of fame can be instituted with before and after photos. A short story can be posted on the successful endeavor with both the client and the pet posing for the after photo. A weight management hall of fame can engage conversation in the reception area and can motivate other clients to enter their pets into a weight-loss program.

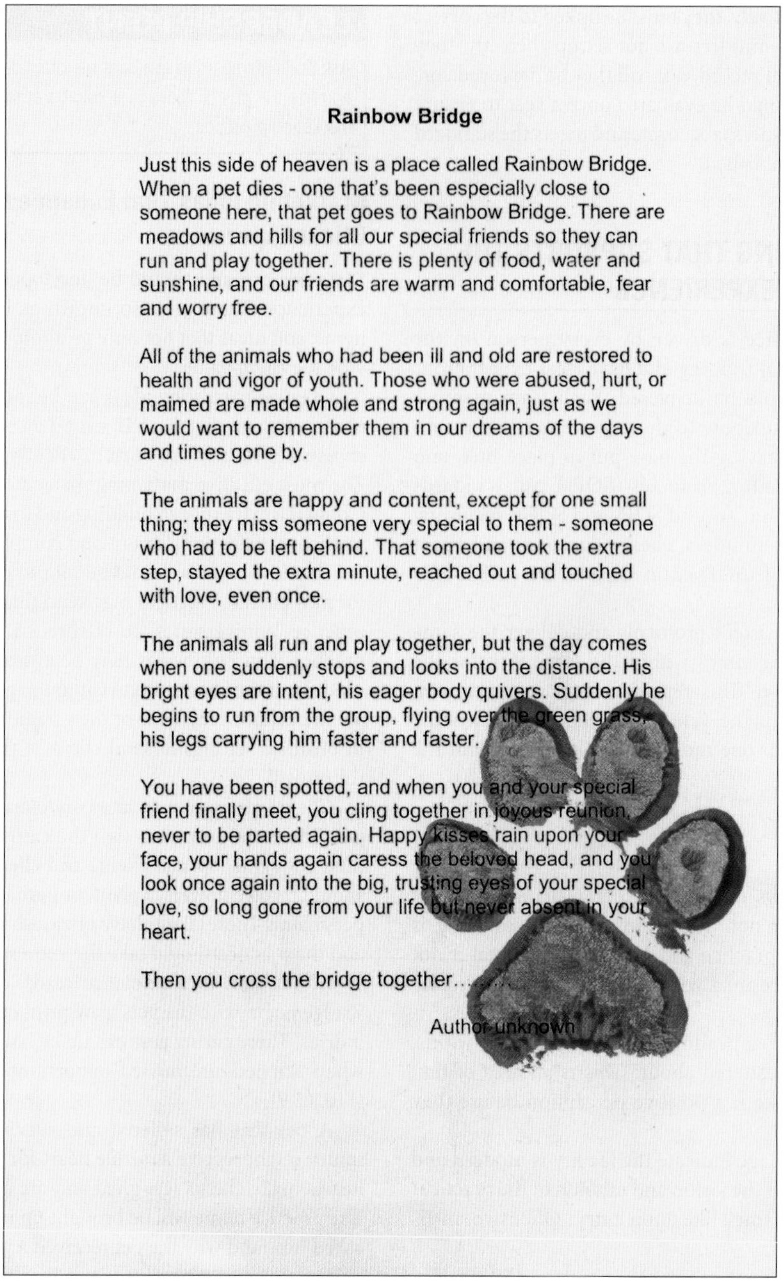

Rainbow Bridge

Just this side of heaven is a place called Rainbow Bridge. When a pet dies - one that's been especially close to someone here, that pet goes to Rainbow Bridge. There are meadows and hills for all our special friends so they can run and play together. There is plenty of food, water and sunshine, and our friends are warm and comfortable, fear and worry free.

All of the animals who had been ill and old are restored to health and vigor of youth. Those who were abused, hurt, or maimed are made whole and strong again, just as we would want to remember them in our dreams of the days and times gone by.

The animals are happy and content, except for one small thing; they miss someone very special to them - someone who had to be left behind. That someone took the extra step, stayed the extra minute, reached out and touched with love, even once.

The animals all run and play together, but the day comes when one suddenly stops and looks into the distance. His bright eyes are intent, his eager body quivers. Suddenly he begins to run from the group, flying over the green grass, his legs carrying him faster and faster.

You have been spotted, and when you and your special friend finally meet, you cling together in joyous reunion, never to be parted again. Happy kisses rain upon your face, your hands again caress the beloved head, and you look once again into the big, trusting eyes of your special love, so long gone from your life but never absent in your heart.

Then you cross the bridge together........

Author unknown

Fig. 12.9 The rainbow bridge poem with a pet's paw print is a nice way to honor a pet.

Pediatric toothbrushes can be ordered with the practice name and logo printed on the handle (Fig. 12.12). Toothbrushes can be placed in puppy and kitten kits, in dental kits, or simply given to owners when the team is talking about dental disease. Leashes can also be printed with the practice name and logo.

Luggage tags can be designed with the practice information and placed on animal carriers when pets have been dropped off. The client's name can be placed on the back of the tag and attached to the handle of the carrier. The carrier will always have identification on it when the owner returns, and the name of the practice is clearly visible for friends and family to see.

Marketing messages should be printed at the base of receipts to inform clients about important topics. The invoice in Fig. 12.13 is an example of promoting puppy classes that the practice provides.

Exam room report cards can be sent home with clients. The PIMS may autogenerate report cards or preprinted report cards can easily be marked for normal and abnormal results, with abnormal findings being summarized. Any procedures or follow-up exams that may be necessary can be prioritized for the client, indicating the most important procedure first. Report cards give clients something to take home, enabling them to review the findings with other family members to better ensure that correct information is communicated (Fig. 12.14).

If the practice does not allow clients to see their medical records, lab results, or imaging, email the owners copies of results after speaking with them. A preprinted PDF should also be sent informing the owner of which organ each test evaluates. A sheet can be included that summarizes abnormal results and follow-up instructions if applicable. Electrocardiograms, urinalysis, ultrasounds, and blood work results can all be sent to clients. This will help increase client compliance because the owner may be able to better understand the abnormal results by being able to visualize them (Fig. 12.15). If the practice has an app, push notifications can also be sent to clients that include results.

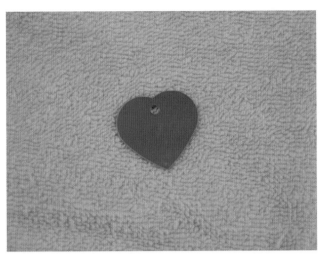

Fig. 12.10 Purple hearts can be given to pets that survived a traumatic experience.

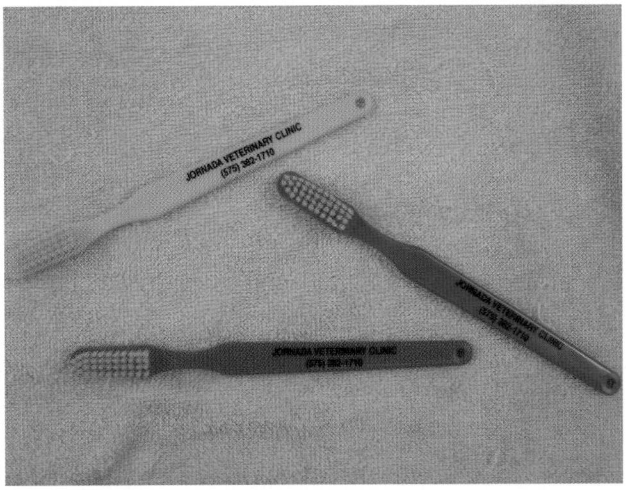

Fig. 12.12 Pediatric toothbrushes should have the practice name printed on the handle and can be given to clients when educating about dental disease.

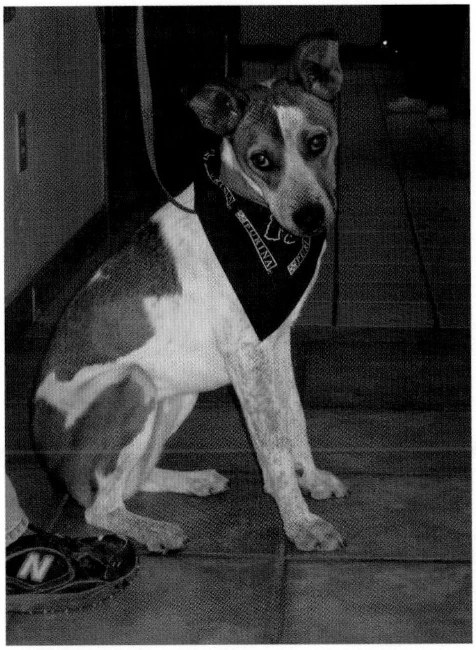

Fig. 12.11 Bandanas promote the practice and can be developed for special occasions.

To help the team be more efficient in this area, build out the PIMS, pet portals, and practice app to allow clients to automatically be able to see all results. Automate the PDF that informs owners which organs each test evaluates. See Chapter 8 on Practice Integrative Management Software for more information.

Exam room report cards and lab work summary results must have the practice name, logo, phone number, and website on the document.

Special activities and open houses that celebrate certain events can market the practice to both current and prospective clients. Open houses can be used to promote National Pet Week, National Veterinary Technician Week, the practice anniversary, the welcoming of a new doctor, or the renovation of the practice. Open houses can be simple or elaborate, depending on the budget set aside for the promotion. The American Veterinary Medical Association (AVMA), the National Association of Veterinary Technicians in America (NAVTA), and veterinary manufacturers can be contacted for more information, sponsorship, and signage to help promote the celebration. Advertising improves the success of the event.

Special events should be hosted during open houses, such as pet walks, pet shows, and presentations regarding pet health. Competitions for prizes can be developed with categories such as the cutest pet, the pet with the longest nose, or the best tricks. Simple, short talks can also be given regarding nutrition, dental care, training techniques, and/or animal behavior.

Facility cleanliness, although not often considered, is a form of indirect marketing. Facilities must be kept clean and odor free. Clients perceive value and service, along with cleanliness, as top priorities when seeking service for their pets. The same as with human healthcare, clients view veterinary practices as healthcare facilities. If a practice has heavy animal or cleaning agent odors, they may never return. Trash containers should be emptied several times a day because they are a significant contributor to odors circulating in the practice. Smaller trash cans should be used, mandating frequent emptying. Pet eliminations must be cleaned immediately, regardless of whether they occur in the reception, treatment, or kennel area. Odors circulate quickly and unfortunately, efficiently! Walls, baseboards, and door frames must be washed weekly, and pictures and fans should be dusted daily. Anatomic models must be free of dust and lint and counters clear of clutter.

Internal and indirect marketing to current clients takes many shapes and values; every facet must be explored to maximize each practice's potential. Get creative and explore what works best for the hospital, clients, and patients to take the practice to the next level.

Target Marketing

Target marketing is directed toward a specific client demographic. Marketing messaging may be developed for current clients with a special breed, species, or age of animal and/or one with a particular disease or condition (obesity, diabetes, and arthritis). Practices can easily determine the needs of this specific group of clients and develop a targeted strategy based on those results.

For example, if the practice has decided to increase dental awareness for 1 month of the year, clients with pets older than 5 years may be targeted to receive dental health information. Practice managers can create a report based on age using the PIMS that includes client names, addresses, email addresses, and pet names. The list can then

ABC Veterinary Clinic
2399 Saturn Circle
Anytown, USA 89000
555-333-1900

Maria Rogers
6454 Downtown Circle
Anytown, USA 89001

Account # 21312

"Scruffy" Rogers
Age: 9 years
Weight: 45#
Reminders: DHPP due 5/10/23
Rabies due 5/10/23
Heartworm Test due 5/10/23

Invoice Number: 10090
Date: 05/10/18
Dr. Nancy Dreamer

Date	Service	Unit	Extended Cost
05/10/18	Exam with Vaccinations	1	$62.39
05/10/18	Distemper, Adenovirus,	1	$0.00
05/10/18	Parainfluenza, Parvo	1	
05/10/18	Rabies 1 year	1	$0.00
05/10/18	Strongid	1	$5.99
05/10/18	HG Puppy Kit	1	$0.00
05/10/18	Nail Trim	1	$0.00

Subtotal	$62.39
Tax 6.25%	$ 3.90
Invoice Total	$66.29

Puppy Obedience Training Classes Begin June 15, 2023! Call to reserve your space now!

Fig. 12.13 Sample invoice with a marketing statement at the bottom.

be exported into a spreadsheet so mailing labels can be generated and affixed to postcards or an email blast can be generated. Push notifications can also be generated for specific targets through the practice app. A dental infographic will help educate clients about dental disease (Fig. 11.31), prompting them to make an appointment for an immediate dental prophylaxis.

Another way to benefit from target marketing is to stay attuned to local news. Team members should be aware of news stories regarding veterinary-related issues. For example, tick-borne diseases may be on the increase, and the media may report an increase of incidents. A push notification can be generated listing the risk factors and symptoms of tick-borne diseases and promoting tick-prevention products.

____________________'s Report Card

Owner's Name ____________________ Date ________

Vaccination Program

❑ Up to Date
❑ Vac. due: PARVO_____; DHLP-C_____; Bordetella_____; LYME_____;FCVR/C_____; Feleuk_____; FIP_____; Rabies_____
❑ Vac. given: PARVO_____; DHLP-C_____; Bordetella_____; LYME_____;FCVR/C_____; Feleuk_____; FIP_____; Rabies_____

1. Coat & Skin
❑ Appear Normal ❑ Oily ❑ Itchy
❑ Dull ❑ Shedding ❑ Parasites
❑ Scaly ❑ Matted ❑ Other ____
❑ Dry ❑ Tumors ________

2. Eyes
❑ Appear Normal ❑ Infection
❑ Discharge ❑ Cataract: L___ R ____
❑ Inflamed ❑ Other ____________
❑ Eyelid Deformities ____________

3. Ears
❑ Appear Normal ❑ Tumor: L___ R___
❑ Inflamed ❑ Excessive Hair
❑ Itchy ❑ Other ____________
❑ Mites ____________

4. Nose & Throat
❑ Appear Normal ❑ Inflamed Tonsils
❑ Nasal Discharge ❑ Enlarged Lymph Glands
❑ Inflamed Throat ❑ Other ____________

5. Mouth, Teeth, Gums
❑ Appear Normal ❑ Inflamed Lips
❑ Broken Teeth ❑ Loose Teeth
❑ Tartar Buildup ❑ Pyorrhea
❑ Tumors ❑ Other
❑ Ulcers

6. Legs & Paws
❑ Appear Normal ❑ Joint Problems
❑ Lameness ❑ Nail Problems
❑ Damaged Ligaments ❑ Other ________

7. Heart
❑ Appears Normal ❑ Slow ❑ Other____
❑ Murmur ❑ Fast ________

8. Abdomen
❑ Appears Normal ❑ Abnormal Mass
❑ Enlarged Organs ❑ Tense/Painful
❑ Fluid ❑ Other ________

9. Lungs
❑ Appear Normal ❑ Breathing Difficulty
❑ Abnormal Sound ❑ Rapid Respiration
❑ Coughing ❑ Other ________
❑ Congestion ________

10.Gastrointestinal System
❑ Appears Normal ❑ Abnormal Feces
❑ Excessive Gas ❑ Parasites
❑ Vomiting Problem ❑ Other ________
❑ Anorexia ________

11.Urogenital System
❑ Appears Normal ❑ Enlarged Prostate
❑ Abnormal Urination ❑ Mammary Tumors
❑ Genital Discharge ❑ Anal Sacs________
❑ Abnormal Testicles

12.Weight ________lbs
❑ Normal Range ❑ Thin
❑ Heavy ❑ Other ________

13.Diet
❑ Excellent ❑ Vitamins Needed
❑ Good ❑ Improvement necessary

Dogs
Last Heartworm Test
Date ________
Htwm Prevention
____
Intestinal Parasites Tested
Date ________
Flea Control
Pet ________
Yard ________
House ________

Cats
Feline Leukemia Test
Date ______ Pos Neg
Feline AIDS Test
Date ______ Pos Neg
Intestine Parasites
Checked ________
Outdoors ___ Hrs/day
Flea Control
Cat ________
Home ________
____
Drug Allergies??
____
____
____

Professional Services
____

Special Instructions/Recommendations
____

Examination Needed________ Days/Months
Next Appointment __________ @___AM/PM

Fig. 12.14 Sample examination room report card the team can fill out if the PIMS does not automatically provide one.

Other ideas include targeting allergy patients during allergy season and bringing awareness to owners of the newest dermatologic antihistamine or treatment available. Practice managers may also consider a focus on heartworm disease and offer a special on a heartworm preventive.

Target marketing can also be used when attempting to attract clients in new neighborhoods, new families moving to the area, or attendees that attended a community service event the practice hosted.

Measuring Return on Investment (ROI)

While developing target marketing plans, measuring the return on investment is critically important. Knowing how much the practice spent on a specific initiative compared to the revenue generated allows the practice manager to know if similar programs should be run in the future.

To track ROI, develop a system to monitor appointments or invoices that are a result of marketing efforts. If the clinic promoted heartworm, measure how many additional heartworm products were sold within the promotion period compared to a previous period. Did the increased revenue pay for the promotional cost? A solid marketing plan includes several deployments of emails, text messages, and push notifications. Don't forget to update the website both before and after the promotion ends.

Antispam laws and legal requirements should be reviewed before sending emails to ensure the practice is within legal boundaries.

Sharing the Plan With the Team

When a marketing initiative has been developed, all team members should be made aware of the plan and be provided examples of developed materials. If the marketing information is sent out before a team

Bloodwork Summary

Today your pet had bloodwork completed. Below is a list of the tests were completed, along with the organ or body part that is being evaluated with that test. You will also find a brief description of what may be causing the abnormality associated with that value. This is not a complete list and is just a summary. please ask our team members if you have any questions.

Pre-Anesthetic Bloodwork: An abbreviated profile that is recommended prioor to anesthesia.

Test	Organ	Common possible causes of abnormal values
BUN	Kidney	Increased = kidney disease
CREA	Kidney	Increased = kidney disease
ALT	Liver	Increased = liver disease
SGPT	Liver	Increased = liver disease
GLU	Pancreas	Increased = diabetes, stress
Total protein	Various	Decreased = protein loss; increased - dehydration; various causes
WBC	White blood cells	Increased = infection
RBC	Red blood cells	Decreased; various
HCT	RBC volume	Decreased ; Iimmune mediated tick-borne disease
platelets	Clotting function	Decreased; clotting abnormality
Urinalysis;		
Specific gravity	Kidney	Decreased; kidney disease, dehydration
WBC	Bladder	Infection
RBC	Bladder	Inflammation
Glucose	Pancreas	Diabetes
Ketones	Pancreas	Diabetes
Protein	Bladder kidney	Protein loss
pH	Bladder	Increased or Decreased; urinary stones
Crystals	Bladder	Urinary stones
Casts	Bladder kidney	
Bacteria	Bladder	Infection
ECG	Heart	Heart disease

Fig. 12.15 Summary of laboratory work results and explanation of tests.

review, a client will inevitably receive it and bring it to the attention of the staff; this is an embarrassing way for team members to find out about a marketing offer.

CRITICAL COMPETENCY: DECISION MAKING

The practice manager must be able to make good decisions based on critical thinking and problem solving and make decisions that positively impact the practice. While many alternatives are available, the PM must be able to gather and effectively analyze relevant data and choose decisively.

EXTERNAL MARKETING

For many years, human medical professionals have efficiently leveraged external marketing tools, whereas the veterinary medical community has been slow to adopt them. While competition for successful practices has risen, so has the need for effective marketing techniques. In previous years, many communities had only had one or two veterinary practices serving them, and external marketing was not necessarily needed. Today, the number of practices has increased, and working to establish a name in the community is real.

External marketing is critical in establishing the practice brand and advertising can get expensive; setting a budget and monitoring ROI is very important. Tracking all sources of new clients allows the practice manager to analyze where dollars are best spent promoting the hospital.

The key to successful external marketing is to determine prospective clients and patients and use the best method to attract them. Consistent and repetitive messaging must be used to obtain the most successful results; if the practice wishes to increase business, external marketing is required to achieve this goal. A large, professional, colorful, and modern sign that represents the practice's values and is illuminated at night is one form of external marketing (Fig. 12.16).

Ideas for External Marketing Techniques

Client Referrals: Clients bragging to friends about a positive experience they had with the practice is a form of external marketing that attracts potential clients. Referrals made by existing clients should be the largest method of attracting new clients in an established practice (if they are not, internal marketing techniques must be revisited).

Search Engine Optimization (SEO): A digital marketing technique that targets specific client parameters is critical in an external

EXAMPLES OF EXTERNAL MARKETING

- Website
- Digital advertising
- Social media
- Practice tours
- Community speaking and service events and
- Blogs
- Billboards
- Outdoor lighted building sign
- Advertising in local papers, sending mass marketing to new housing developments, marketing to families that have just moved into the target area.
- Open houses

Fig. 12.16 External marketing is intended to attract new clients to the veterinary practice.

marketing plan. Results are best seen when digital marketing programs are outsourced to the company that manages the practice website. Parameters may include targeting a specific demographic that the practice would like to gain, targeting potential clients within a set number of miles around the practice, setting up a geofence, or targeting clients that enter keywords into a search engine (puppies, kittens, vaccines, or veterinarians). These programs can get expensive, and a budget must be set and with weekly reporting determining where clients are coming from. Internet searches are their most powerful tool for attracting new clients that have just moved to the area and new pet parents that have never had a pet before. It makes sense to spend money in this area; just ensure it is well managed.

Coupons: Veterinary practices have ventured into the Groupon marketplace to access large numbers of consumers over a short period of time. Coupon offers should be considered carefully, and the practice must be prepared for an influx of new appointments quite rapidly. How many new appointments per week can the practice handle? How many new appointments in a month can the team and veterinarians accommodate? Will the practice attract the type of clientele it desires? The benefit these coupons offer is the immediate increase in foot traffic. However, keep in mind the long-term strategy is to convert "coupon" clients into long-term clients. To do this, the team must provide exceptional customer service to each new appointment scheduled. This means wait times must be short, examinations must be thorough, client education must be provided, and the value of the practice must be illustrated for every "coupon" customer. These are essentially job interviews for clients who are considering the practice's services. The practice must be spotless and odor-free, and Fear Free® techniques must be implemented so that a first-time visit doesn't become a last-time visit. This is a campaign for new business and should be treated as such. A word of caution when using coupon options: the practice may not attract the client seeking high medical standards but those looking for the best deal.

VHMA PRACTICE DOMAIN TASK

The Practice manager develops and manages advertising materials.

Yellow Page Ads: Choosing if and how to advertise in the Yellow Pages takes extra thought and consideration. Many factors should be addressed before deciding on this advertisement. What is the ROI? Is the practice gaining enough clients from the Yellow Pages to continue advertising? Be sure to ask new clients where they heard about the practice to evaluate this ROI. The cost of such ads has become greater than the ROI with the increased use of the Internet and smartphones. In fact, an overwhelming number of clients no longer use the Yellow Pages, instead using their phones to find veterinary practices. Some companies add search engine optimization to their ad, but it usually does not yield the highest results.

Newspaper Ads: How many clients (and what demographic) read the newspaper today? What is the readership of printed versus online ads? What is the visibility of ads for online versions? Some newspapers have sections available in which a practice can purchase space and submit an article educating the public about a particular disease. The ad may state to visit ABC Veterinary Hospital for more information. Other forms of advertising may include a boxed ad introducing a new veterinarian, service, or product. As with all external advertising options, evaluate the potential return on investment first.

Social Media

The term *social media* is used to apply to all social platforms, which are always changing. Twitter, Instagram, TikTok, Facebook, and YouTube are the top platforms at publication time.

Social media has become an important form of communication with clients, and just as with mobile media, supports the one-click-to-compliance theory. Previously, practices only had contact with clients once a year or when the animal was sick. Today, practices can stay connected with clients several times a week and positively influence clients with informative facts, fun trivia, and behind-the-scenes footage of the hospital.

Clients make recommendations on social media sites that attract new clients. "Thanks for taking care of Fluffy! Without you, she would have never survived!" These personal referrals are much more impactful than paid advertisements (and they are free!).

Managing Social Media: Some practices hire an outside company to act as a social media manager. Occasionally, these companies do not have veterinary experience and ultimately detract from the message trying to be delivered. The voice of the practice is no longer speaking, and practice philosophies get lost. Ideally, a practice member should be appointed (or should empower another team member that is good at social media) as a social media manager and allowed to post to the practice's social media sites (or review all messaging established by an outside company and approve before posting).

Sometimes unaccountable team members abuse the practice's social media pages and post negative comments. The practice's social media sites are for business only. Personal comments, opinions, and gaming must be saved for personal pages. A social media policy and plan must be established, along with a social media manager job description and performance evaluation.

LEADERSHIP POINT

Managing social media takes time; often time the practice manager should spend doing something else in the practice (leading people). Empower smart and accountable team members to lead SM management.

When managed correctly, social media does not have to take up a large amount of time. Once a plan has been developed, key messages, phrases, and pictures can be uploaded to platforms (Hootsuite, Zoho, Buffer) at the beginning of the quarter with scheduled release dates. In general, two to three releases per week across social media sites are acceptable. Any more than that can overwhelm clients and cause them to disengage. Pictures always increase social media traffic and must be a part of every plan.

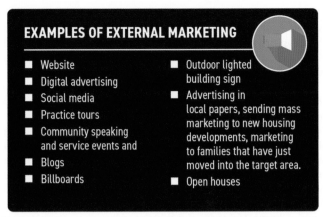

Social media reports should be monitored for valuable information. Determine what clients like and don't like and which topics drive and don't drive traffic. This helps strengthen the plan for the following quarters. Managers should also determine who follows the practice and implement strategies that target that audience. To do this, review reports provided by the social media platform and break them down to the level of detail needed, including specific demographics (age, gender, zip code, etc.).

VHMA PRACTICE DOMAIN TASK

The practice manager oversees social media (including protocol development and monitoring ROI.

Developing a Plan: A social media plan should be encompassed in the overall marketing plan the practice develops (see "Creating and Implementing a Marketing Plan" at the end of the chapter). If the practice plans to focus on wellness plans during the first quarter of 2024, the social media marketing plan should also support that initiative. Once a plan has been developed, outline the details in writing with due dates and objectives (include pictures, tag lines, and when messages will be released to the clients). Without a written plan, it may not happen!

Social Media Policy: A social media policy is a must for both clients and patients. If any pictures are taken of the client or team member pets, a social media release must be signed indicating the approval for use of the photo. The term *social media* must be used (rather than naming specific platforms such as Facebook, Twitter, etc.), because social media outlets will change over the years, and the term encompasses all platforms.

Team member social media policies are a little more complicated than the client's approval for use of pictures. Team members must understand that there are real implications for what they post (pictures and comments). Practice managers and owners cannot dictate what team members post on their personal social media sites; however, professional guidelines can be established for the practice's social media platform, and if violated, implications must occur.

LEADERSHIP POINT

Review Chapter 4 (Human Resources) for the development of a social media policy.

Practice managers can, however, mandate that pictures used for the hospital's social media platforms be taken on practice-approved cameras (never on personal cell phones) and uploaded by approved team members only. This can prevent the wrong person from uploading embarrassing or incorrect information, sharing confidential information, or posting unapproved patient pictures.

Managing Client Reviews

With the increased role of social media in everyday life, online reviews of a practice are available everywhere. Clients may upload reviews while in the examination room, especially when they are upset. It was mentioned previously that recommendations from clients are more powerful than advertising; managing reviews becomes imperative.

Practice owners and managers must set up alerts for the practice and each veterinarian in each search engine. Alerts will then be emailed when any review is posted (usually within 24 hours). Respond to positive reviews and manage negative reviews as soon as possible. Four steps should be taken to manage negative reviews.

Step One: When a negative review is posted, the initial response is typically to handle the complaint immediately; however, when an immediate response is formed, it is generally defensive and carries an authoritarian tone. Do not respond immediately. Investigate the complaint; obtain facts from the team. Take some time and create a planned response that will be perceived in a positive manner.

Step Two: Respond to the reviewer with empathy and compassion. Apologize for their experience and extend the opportunity to discuss the complaint via phone or in person. Do try and reach the client if possible. Do not attempt to solve complaints through the review; this will only ignite further negative comments.

Step Three: Promote good reviews. Ask clients to post reviews of the hospital and team members; share stories of success. The more positive reviews that appear, the lower the negative review is posted.

Step Four: Be proactive, not reactive (and this should not be considered the last step). Effective managers and leaders that form a positive culture with an excellent team prevent incidents that produce poor reviews. If negative reviews continue to be posted, the practice manager needs to take a serious look at the culture that is brewing behind closed doors. Remember, positive leadership trickles from the top down. Review Chapter 2 for techniques to create and promote a positive team.

VHMA PRACTICE DOMAIN TASK

The practice manager handles client complaints (and teaches others to as well).

Dr. Caitlyn DeWilde recently published the only book dedicated to **Social Media and Marketing for Veterinary Professionals**. This unique source is the most comprehensive resource for the veterinary team.[3]

Community Service Events

Community service events create a win-win situation for all those involved. Practice team members or owners may suggest local organizations the team can volunteer with. This is free or low-cost advertising for the practice and lets the community know that the veterinary team supports community events. This also lends to building the practice's brand and reputation.

Some ideas for participating in community service may include offering a "lump and bump" pet screening at local events. A veterinarian and technician can educate potential clients about the seriousness of lumps on pets. These are excellent places to hand out literature and educate the local community. Team members can also participate in dental screenings for pets at local events; many people do not know the significance of dental disease in their pets.

VHMA PRACTICE DOMAIN TASK

The practice manager oversees community outreach.

Attending career days at local schools is also considered a form of community service. Team members can create "kid packs" that include a surgical cap and mask as well as a business card and literature on disease risks that are high in the area. They can be placed in a bag that has the practice information printed on it. Speaking at career days can have a lasting impact on children. Showing interesting radiographs and allowing children to auscultate a dog's heart can stimulate interest and help foster their education. Community service at this level is highly gratifying.

CRITICAL COMPETENCY: ORAL COMMUNICATION AND COMPREHENSION

The practice manager must have the ability to express thoughts verbally in a clear and understandable manner, and the ability to actively listen and attend to what others are saying.

Practices may also wish to be more involved in community service events around the holidays, participating in food drives or clothing campaigns for kids, or collecting Christmas presents for an adopted family. The team may want to rally together and serve a meal at a soup kitchen, again fostering engagement with the community. Community service may not lead to advertisement of the practice directly, but indirectly team members can meet and talk with members of the community while participating, as well as being able to introduce the team from ABC Veterinary Clinic.

Client inquiry may be used to determine the effectiveness of marketing techniques. The question "How did you hear about us?" should appear on a client/patient information sheet or be included in a survey offered to clients after their first visit. This and other mechanisms can ultimately be used in an ROI analysis to help determine which marketing techniques may or may not be used in the future.

Sponsorships and Donations

Many schools, organizations, and individuals will seek donations and sponsorships for events they are holding throughout the year. Although donations to local events and organizations go to good causes, a predetermined amount should be set aside in the budget each year. Allocating the donation budget over a 12-month period will help prevent the practice from donating more than it can afford.

In exchange for sponsorships, it is reasonable to expect advertising. Some schools may place the contributor's name on a t-shirt or calendar and may recognize larger contributions at sporting events. Sponsorships are an excellent source of external marketing and build goodwill within the community.

When a donation is given to a nonprofit organization, a receipt should be generated for the practice. This receipt should be kept for year-end tax purposes. Be sure that donations and sponsorships are a budget line, ensuring the practice stays within budget.

Gift Certificates

As with donations and sponsorships, gift certificates can be provided to nonprofit charities for door prizes, raffles, or drawings. While charities are grateful for gift certificates, potential clients may or may not use the gift certificates they have won. This is a win for the practice; it develops brand recognition, shows support for the community, and they may gain a new client!

Gift certificates can be used to give away services or products. One example is to offer a gift certificate for a yearly examination and vaccines. When a client uses this certificate, he or she is likely to purchase more services or products. The new client may choose to have a heartworm test and purchase heartworm preventative while at the practice or may add a collar and a leash while checking out at the counter. Although the examination and vaccines were provided at no cost as a donation, the practice gained a client and made a profit on the additional services and products.

DEVELOPING A MARKETING PLAN

The marketing plan must achieve the practice's strategic plan and should include objectives found in the completed SWOT analysis, client reviews, and team member surveys. A strategic initiative may be to increase practice revenue year over year. Therefore, a marketing plan may focus on increasing the number of new clients and patients or improving the retention rate of current clients. Objectives will then outline initiatives that support such goals and include how each objective will be measured.

> **CRITICAL COMPETENCY: WRITING AND VERBAL SKILLS**
>
> The practice manager must have the ability to comprehend written material easily and accurately, as well as the ability to express thoughts clearly and succinctly in writing.

SWOT Analysis

A SWOT analysis evaluates the practice's strengths (S), weaknesses (W), opportunities (O), and threats (T), and helps the practice focus on initiatives that should be continued (because they are strengths) and areas that need improvement. It also helps determine what differentiates the practice from others in the area and what potential threats must be planned for to help mitigate risks. SWOT analyses are a great team-building event. Often, team members see strengths and opportunities that management overlooks (Fig. 12.17).

Strengths and weaknesses focus internally, whereas opportunities and threats focus on external factors. Keep this in mind as the team completes the analysis.

Strengths: Consider the strengths of the practice. Who makes up the team? What do clients like about the practice? What services does the hospital offer that no other hospital offers? Why do clients refer friends and family to the practice? Does the practice offer advanced technology for treatments? Does the practice work with local animal shelters or participate in community service events? Strengths are accomplishments that set the practice apart from others (and that the practice would like to brag about). The strengths that are identified will often help the practice develop marketing strategies that promote the advantages of the practice and can help overcome the weaknesses that may be determined.

Weaknesses: Weaknesses can be more difficult to assess but is an important step. Consider internal protocols that could use improvement. What do clients and team members complain most about? Why do clients leave the hospital? What do client surveys indicate? What services or technologies should the practice be utilizing or implementing that are negatively impacting business because they are not being used? Addressing weaknesses allows the practice to make sure there are no roadblocks in place that may prohibit growth and/or prohibit

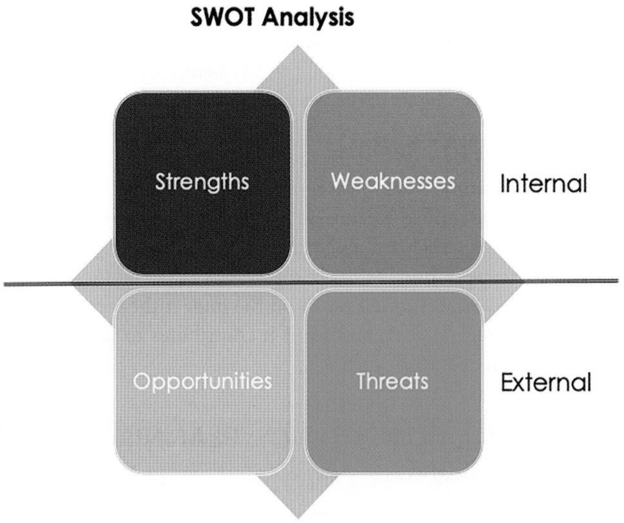

Fig. 12.17 SWOT Analyses are the first step in creating marketing and strategic plans.

marketing efforts to be effective. When weaknesses are ignored, they become larger problems. When addressed and managed, they become strengths.

LEADERSHIP POINT

Practice managers and owners should be careful not to get frustrated with weaknesses or opportunities identified by the team while completing a SWOT review. Rather, look at it as an opportunity to achieve team buy-in to improve protocols/procedures/initiatives that may already be in place, or new ideas to accelerate goal achievement.

Opportunities: Identifying opportunities is fun because it allows the team to think outside the box, be creative, and promote innovative thinking. What outside opportunities and ideas could be implemented to strengthen the client bond, retention, or compliance? Include suggestions for continuing education, current trends, social media, technology, and equipment. What resources are available in the community that could increase opportunities for the practice? Is the practice active in the community? Recognizing and acting on opportunities can take the practice to the next level.

Threats: Identifying potential threats is critical in any planning stage. While one may not be able to prevent a threat from occurring, mitigating the risk and putting a plan in place for the threat can prevent long-term damage. Consider veterinary practices that are in an area that could be impacted by a natural disaster such as fire, tornadoes, floods, or hurricanes. What threats exist? If the event happens, it is beyond the control of the practice. Therefore, business continuity plans must be established to reduce the potential loss (as much as possible). Consider the impact of the practice server that houses all data. If that is damaged during a weather event and no backup is in place, all data is lost. For this example, part of a plan would be to consider moving the server offsite, implementing data backup off-site, or moving to cloud-based PIMs. Turning the focus to client retention, consider the threat of a competitor opening a new practice across the street. While you cannot prevent the competitor from moving in, you can mitigate the risk of losing clients with appropriate planning.

Completing a SWOT analysis will help determine where marketing dollars are best spent and where improvements are needed. Ideally, efforts should be made to address detrimental weaknesses or threats before proceeding with a full marketing strategy as those weaknesses and threats could cause marketing efforts to fail. Additionally, an "A" team (that is not burned out and exhausted) that can deliver a frictionless client experience must be a top priority before new customers are targeted to become clients of the veterinary practice.

Prioritizing SWOT Results

Many ideas will come from the brainstorming session with team members (as well as identified weaknesses). Practice managers and owners should not be overwhelmed, but rather look at this as a great opportunity to continue improving the business. It is important to prioritize weaknesses and opportunities based on the impact the ideas will have in achieving strategic goals and /or if it contributes to the successful implementation of another goal.

CRITICAL COMPETENCY: PLANNING AND PRIORITIZING

Practice managers must be able to effectively manage time and workload to meet deadlines, thereby having the ability to organize work, set priorities, and establish plans to achieve goals.

After prioritizing goals, each goal must have an action plan, including who is responsible for carrying out the objectives of the goal. Goals and objectives must be specific and measurable, and the person responsible for carrying out the goal must be motivated and empowered to utilize resources outside of the practice to achieve success. Objectives can be assigned to different team members, resulting in greater goal achievement and team buy-in.

A SMART goal sheet helps define the needed elements to successfully implement the goal (Fig. 12.18). Specific (S), Measurable (M), Achievable (A), Relevant (R), and Time-bound (T) are the terms used in most SMART sheets. However, modifying the words a bit provides better results. **Specific, Measurable, Action Items/Accountability, Resources, and Timebound** is more realistic, as the goal has already been identified as being achievable and relevant (or it would not have made it through the prioritization process).

Specific defines the specific goal that is to be achieved.

Measurable identifies how the success of the goal will be measured.

Action Items/Accountability defines who will carry out the action items/objective(s) of the goal.

Resources identifies what resources will be needed to achieve and implement the goal successfully.

Timebound identifies when the goal will be achieved by and establish check-in points between the practice manager and the person accountable for achieving the set objectives.

LEADERSHIP POINT

Writing out SMART goals clarifies expectations, identifies measures that can be tracked, and sets objectives that team members can achieve (when goals have been empowered to others by leadership).

Goals and objectives will often hit snags that were not previously identified with prioritization and planning; this is normal. By critically thinking and being creative, team members can overcome snags and still implement their plans. Goals need continual assessments and change as needed to yield successful implementation.

CRITICAL COMPETENCY: CREATIVITY

Practice managers must have the ability to creatively think through situations and embrace new and different ways to see opportunities by using imagination and collaboration, resulting in innovative solutions.

METHODS OF MEASURING AND MANAGING

All goals and objectives must be measured to be managed. If one is not measuring results, changes cannot be made to yield greater results. Even revenue centers that were developed years ago and appear to have profitability need to be measured and managed. Consider the amount of change that practices had to adjust to during and after COVID. Without measuring and managing the change needed, survival would have been difficult.

Client Surveys, Compliance Reports, and ROI

While client surveys, client retention, and client compliance are topics covered in Chapter 11, they must be mentioned here. If clients are unhappy with services or technology that was implemented to achieve marketing goals, adjustments must be made. Without the client's perception, the practice will not know that the goal created a satisfaction issue.

If goals and objectives were established to help increase compliance, client satisfaction and specific compliance reports must be measured and monitored for improvement. A business cannot have a profit center that costs more than the revenue it produces, therefore, the return on investment must be examined with every implementation (Fig. 12.19).

PROJECT: Charge capture, discounts, and adjustments GOAL: Increase charge capture, decrease discounts and adjustments.	
Specific	On average, practices miss 10% of charges each year. For GCVC, YTD assumption is $144,000 per year lost revenue. Discounts for GCVC YTD are $60,000, with $20,000 in adjustments. $224,000 could be recaptured in 2023 – all improving the bottom line.
Measurable	1. Discounts decrease, monthly monitoring of total discounts and who gives discounts 2. Adjustments decrease, monthly monitoring 3. Revenue increases – measure through ACT for charge capture
Action Items	1. **Charge Capture** a. Establish group codes for the most common services. Grouped codes then autopopulate the invoice; the team member then just updates the quantity (if meds were dispensed, the pet was in the hospital, etc) b. Team enters the charges c. Train team how to use Group Codes 2. **Discounts** a. All invoice items must be entered, at full price; do not change line-item price b. Ensure that security settings are set so that price cannot be overridden. c. If a discount is to be given, use discount code. d. Create a discount budget: what is the total allowed for discounts in 2023? e. Train team on entering line items at full price and entering discount appropriately; inform team of discount budget and monitoring each month. 3. **Adjustments** a. What line items need adjustments? Should these be discounts instead? b. Develop a plan to decrease adjustments for 2023.
Resources	Cornerstone education and training
Timeline	Group codes developed by ____________; assigned to: ____________; implemented on______ Update security settings by ______________; assigned to: ______________. Discount budget created by____________; begin monitoring ____________. Adjustments plan created by ____________; begin monitoring ____________.
Projected Outcome	An additional $200,000 per year in profitability

Fig. 12.18 A chart detailing the objectives of a SMART goal can ensure each area is fully vetted to help achieve marketing goals.

Recommendation Compliance Report — **ABC Veterinary Clinic**

Period: 01/01/22 - 01/01/23

Code	Description	#of Recommendations	# of Compliances	%
R0001	Rabies	910	607	66.7
R0002	DHPP	791	298	37.67
R0003	Bordetella	126	61	48.41
R0004	Heartworm Prev	1088	544	50.00
R0005	Dental Prophylaxis	754	398	52.79
R0005	Pre Anesth BW	950	367	38.63
R0006	General Health BW	1589	1061	67.77
R0007	Senior Screening	790	421	53.29
R0008	Therapeutic Food	984	398	40.45

Fig. 12.19 Example of compliance report from a PIMS.

Some specific objectives or goals may not generate active revenue, yet they support revenue generation in another area. Websites don't generate direct, active revenue, but they attract new clients and improve active client satisfaction. The analysis should then focus on the number of visitors to the website, how long they stayed on the website, and what features they clicked on most.

IMPLEMENTING A MARKETING PLAN

It is important to remember that marketing is not a quick fix. Marketing efforts are a marathon, not a sprint and it can often take 6 to 12 months before an ROI is seen. Marketing plans take significant effort to build; however, once momentum is gained, ROI will begin to show.

The team must buy into marketing initiatives. Prepare a presentation that starts with the "why" of the plan. Identify questions that they may ask during the presentation, allowing you to be prepared and build confidence in the team. "How would this plan work? Who will measure results? Can we change if something is not working? How will we message this to clients?" It is OK to not know the answer to every question; an appropriate response would be "that is a great question that I don't know the answer to. I need your help finding the answer as we continue developing this plan." Through conversation with the team, determine tools and resources needed for success; be willing to consider and integrate their thoughts, validate their concerns, and be willing to implement suggestions.

Just like creating SMART goals, build out a detailed project timeline and break it into smaller tasks and deadlines to make it manageable. Start with the end goal date in mind and work backward. For example, consider launching a new website for the hospital. When does the website company think they will have the web page ready to deploy? Working back from that date will allow realistic timelines to be broken into smaller pieces with tasks that will need to be completed.

Set realistic goals with the marketing plan and make sure they tie directly to the strategic plan. For example, if a practice objective is to increase revenue by 10%, make sure you're measuring and monitoring things that impact revenue. Consider the number of new clients, number of invoices, average client transactions, number of appointments, compliance reports, etc. At the very least, compare results month to month.

When a specific goal is not achieving the desired result, be willing to adapt and make changes to yield successful results. Sometimes small changes can make big differences.

CRITICAL COMPETENCY: CRITICAL AND STRATEGIC THINKING

Strategic thinking and planning are essential to financial forecasting, marketing plans, and long-term plans for practice growth. Managers must have the ability to identify questions, problems, and arguments relevant to these issues and to use logic and critical reasoning to identify the strengths and weaknesses of alternative solutions or approaches to problems.

LEADERSHIP'S ROLE IN MARKETING

Just as with the Client Experience, Leadership has a large role in Marketing. The two topics are relatively entwined. Practice managers build protocols (the base of the building block) to improve the efficiency of the team and marketing plans to achieve strategic goals. Great leaders develop phenomenal culture and empower employees to help achieve goals through collaboration, participation, and the exceptional delivery of service and medicine. Veterinary medicine is a team sport. Not one person is responsible for the success; every person contributes to the success of the business! As always, leadership must communicate the results and celebrate success with the team. Receptionists drive exceptional customer service with the first and last impression. The medical team drives exceptional standards of care and consistent service. Every team member helps drive the success of the initiative when clear expectations, training, and psychologically safe environments have been created.

PRACTICE MANAGER SURVIVAL CHECKLIST FOR MARKETING

- ☐ Evaluate tasks, policies, and procedures that contribute to practice branding. Do they support the brand in the best way possible?
- ☐ Evaluate facility appearance and update often.
- ☐ Initiate continuous team training for internal marketing.
- ☐ Manage website development and evaluate for updates monthly.
- ☐ Develop methods to market the online store and monitor compliance reports.
- ☐ Develop a practice app, policies, and usage procedures, and communicate with clients consistently.
- ☐ Develop print advertisements that contribute to the practice brand and monitor ROI.
- ☐ Develop social media guidelines, policies, and procedures.
- ☐ Develop a social media manager job description and performance evaluation.
- ☐ Monitor discounts given through marketing techniques and track ROI.
- ☐ Determine community service events to participate in that enhance the practice brand and develop a return on investment.
- ☐ Measure client compliance key performance indicators relative to the current marketing plan.

REVIEW QUESTIONS

1. What is internal marketing? Give an example.
2. What is external marketing? Give an example.
3. What example can be applied to both internal and external marketing?
4. Why is a website essential in today's market?
5. What information should be included in client education materials?
6. Define practice brand.
7. What is a pet portal?
8. What is the purpose of reminders?
9. Why is indirect marketing so important?
10. What are SMART goals and why are they important?
11. What does the acronym SWOT stand for?
    a. Service with outstanding treatment
    b. Strengths, weaknesses, opportunities, and threats
    c. Service, website, office appearance, transactions
    d. None of the above
12. Which of the following is an example of internal marketing?
    a. Lectures
    b. E-newsletter
    c. Telephone etiquette
    d. Blogs
13. Which of the following can be found on a clinic's webpage?
    a. Virtual tour
    b. Appointment requests
    c. Hours of operation
    d. All the above
14. Target marketing is:
    a. directed to current clients
    b. directed to potential clients
    c. directed to patients with a particular disease or condition
    d. All the above
    e. A and C
15. What is the correct definition of SEO?
    a. The process of affecting the visibility of a website or webpage in a search engine's search results.
    b. The key terms that a search engine will use.
    c. A search engine's external hyperlinks used to promote a website.
    d. None of the above

REFERENCES

1. Tumblin D. et al. Well managed practice benchmarks, 2019. Accessed August 2022. https://www.wmpb.vet
2. Santi S. The rewards of a reward program, September 2017. VetTeamBrief. Accessed December 2022. https://files.brief.vet/migration/article/41731/the-rewards-of-a-reward-program-41731-article.pdf
3. DeWilde C. Social Media and Marketing for Veterinary Professionals. TreeFarmDogs Press; 2022.

13

Inventory Management

LEARNING OBJECTIVES

When you have completed this chapter, you should be able to:

- Develop an effective inventory system
- List methods used to maintain an appropriate amount of inventory on hand
- Define and create a central inventory location
- Define capital inventory
- Identify and use safety data sheets
- Calculate an effective price markup for products
- Describe methods used to handle expired medications

OUTLINE

KEY TERMS

Capital
Central Inventory Location
Distributor Representative
Inventory
Inventory Turns per Year
Just-in-Time Ordering
Manufacturer Representative
Markup
Order Book
Reorder Point
Reorder Quantity
Safety Data Sheet (SDS)
Turnover Rate
U.S. Food and Drug Administration (FDA)
Want List

VHMA PERFORMANCE DOMAINS

Veterinary Hospital Managers Association (VHMA) Performance Domains

Performance domains applicable to inventory management include organization of the practice and financial management. The practice manager:

- Maintains appropriate inventory systems including controlled substance ordering, tracking, security, and destruction.
- Places and tracks purchase orders for drugs, uniforms, and equipment.
- Oversees contracts for repair and maintenance of equipment, building, and grounds.
- Analyzes practice and financial reports.
- Prepares budgets and long-range fiscal plans.
- Conducts fee analysis and monitors and updates fee schedule.

Application of VHMA Performance Domains for Practice Managers

Developing efficient inventory management software improves the performance, knowledge, skills, and abilities of the practice manager by improving client service, meeting benchmarks for cost of goods performance, and improving practice profitability.

INTRODUCTION

Effective inventory controls are critical and support the overall profitability of a veterinary practice. Inventory is the second-largest expense (next to payroll); when managed correctly, it will be a profitable asset. Creating and maintaining an inventory system take continuous planning and monitoring, and when it is not properly managed, patient care suffers, revenue is lost, and clients will be inconvenienced enough to shop elsewhere.

FUNDAMENTALS OF INVENTORY

Successful inventory management results in having enough products on hand to meet client needs and not running out of products or supplies. Expired products and/or product shortages decrease profits, diminish practice efficiency, and lessen client satisfaction (Fig. 13.1). Inventory management requires a working knowledge of what each product is used for, how much product is used, how often products are sold, as well as the length of time it takes to reorder and replace products. Mastering this information makes it possible to implement an effective inventory management system that takes minimal time to oversee (Fig. 13.2).

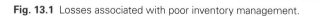

- Too much product sitting on the shelf
- Not enough product on the shelf to sell
- Frequent ordering
- Shrinkage
- Theft
- Backorders
- Expired products
- Wrong products ordered or received
- High costs of overnight shipments for products needed ASAP
- Shipping costs associated with small orders

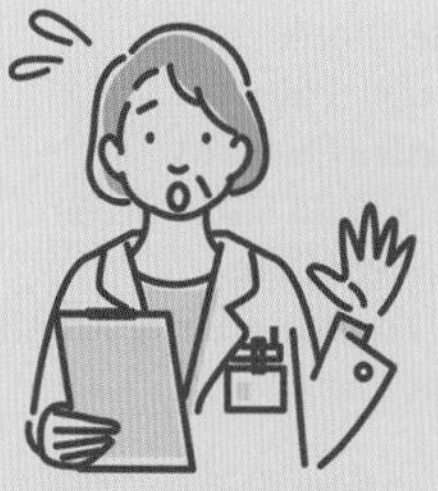

Fig. 13.1 Losses associated with poor inventory management.

- **Buy from a key distributor** to reduce shipping costs; have a secondary vendor for back up.
- **Minimize the number of times ordered** per week or month (goal: order top 20% of items monthly).
- **Evaluate soon to expire drugs monthly.** Can they be returned for credit or replaced?
- **Evaluate payment plans.** If companies offer a discount when the bill is paid by the tenth of each month, make sure the payment is made!
- **Develop** turnover rates, reorder points, and reorder quantities.
- **Limit the duplication of drugs** (package size and brand).
- **Include soft costs** (holding and ordering) when setting product pricing.
- **Maintain inventory costs** between 18% and 20% of gross revenue of the practice.

Fig. 13.2 Keys to a successful inventory management system.

Ideally, an inventory manager oversees the system and takes responsibility for errors and implements corrective changes as necessary. Under the inventory manager, duties should be broken into ordering, receiving, and reconciling. While each duty has multiple tasks associated with it, they are all linked together, creating an effective system.

One team member should oversee the ordering of all inventory items, decreasing mistakes and the potential of ordering duplicate items. Additionally, other team members know whom to contact if an item is in short supply. One person can easily organize an ordering system, which streamlines processes resulting in efficiency and satisfied clients. A fellow team member should be able to serve as backup and fill in as needed without creating a glitch in the system. Distributor and manufacturer phone numbers, account numbers, and order histories should be readily available, allowing the second team member to place orders. The front of an order book or an inventory manual is an excellent place to keep a summary of all distributors or compounding pharmacies.

A second team member should oversee receiving inventory, comparing the invoice to the order, and stocking. A third person (perhaps the inventory manager or practice manager) should be responsible for entering products into the computer and reconciling invoices. Delegating duties to different individuals will decrease the risk of internal theft.

MEETING CLIENT AND PRACTICE EXPECTATIONS

Inventory management has two very important factors: meeting client expectations by having medications available and managing the second-largest expense and revenue category of the business.

Client Expectations

Clients must be able to trust the practice to accept treatment recommendations. This trust is built through providing exceptional communications and customer service (Chapter 11, Client Experience). When trust and loyalty have been established, compliance follows. When dispensing medications to clients, team members should take time to explain the mode of action, potential side effects, and when the client should contact the practice if any complications arise. Although clients want options when filling medications, convenience is often the most important factor. If the practice has the medications available when clients are in the hospital, cost becomes secondary to convenience.

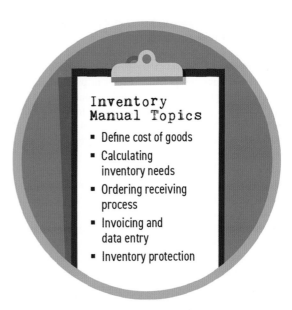

The same concept applies when clients need to refill medications: convenience is critical. The process needs to be easy and efficient. To offer more convenience to clients, the practice should consider an online pharmacy that is easy to navigate and delivers medications directly to clients' homes (see Online Pharmacy later in this chapter).

A veterinary practice mobile app (available on smartphones) can also fill this gap for clients. The practice mobile app should have two options available for refilling medication: (1) refilling and picking up orders at the practice or (2) refilling through the online store and having the medication shipped directly to the client. Customized mobile apps can even allow clients to take a picture of medications needed, select pick-up times, and add additional comments to their order. Chapter 12 Marketing, Fig. 12.7 provides more details on the development of a customized practice app.

For clients that are not comfortable using online stores or mobile apps, other options need to be considered for medication orders. Providing exceptional customer service involves knowing when clients will need medication or food refills. Most of the time, clients wait until they are out of product (or perhaps have one dose remaining) to order refills. Efficient and well-organized practices do not wait for clients to reorder but are proactive and remind clients several days to 1 week before clients need medication. For stock items, call or text the client 2 to 3 days in advance; if the product must be ordered or is specially compounded, contact the client 1 week before. Generate a recall that attaches to the client invoice, allowing this procedure to be easily implemented (and not forgotten). Once this procedure is started, it cannot be stopped without another procedure taking its place because clients will become dependent on the easy refill service provided by the practice.

Practice Expectations

An efficient inventory system should be easy to manage, also helping the practice stay on an inventory budget. To make that happen, the fundamentals must be established: turnover rates, reorder points, and quantities must be determined, and a budget must be created. Developing a successful inventory system is a marathon, not a sprint, and is constantly a work in motion. It must be fluid to adapt to change but have established protocols to maintain efficiency.

CRITICAL COMPETENCY: ADAPTABILITY

Practice managers must be open to change and flexible work methods and can adapt behavior to changing conditions or new information.

Creating an Inventory Manual

Just as an employee manual is a necessary guide for all team members, an inventory manual is also recommended. This manual can provide the guidelines that team members must follow if/when the inventory manager is absent or replaced. Fig. 13.3 provides topics that should be covered in this manual. Many team members are unaware of the "science" behind inventory and why it is so critical that the system be created and maintained. An inventory manual will provide this information and keep all team members on the same page.

LEADERSHIP POINT

Inventory manuals help the practice manager and inventory manager understand the important aspects of proper inventory management.

An organized manager must determine which technique is most effective in maintaining inventory. A variety of techniques are discussed in this chapter; however, the combination of several techniques may work better. Each practice is different, and each manager must be flexible in determining the best technique.

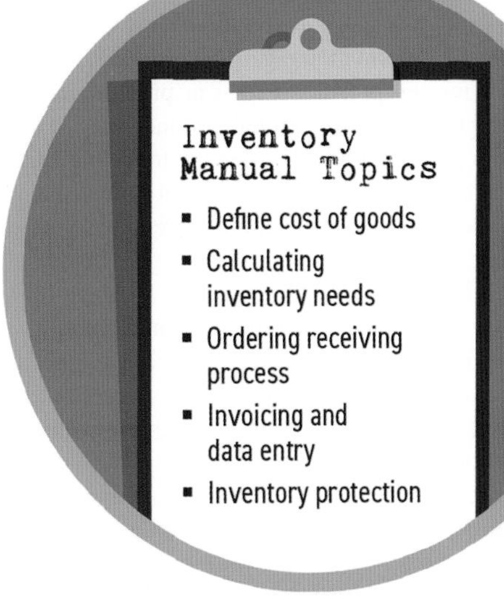
Inventory
Manual Topics
Define cost of goods
Calculating inventory needs
Ordering receiving process
Invoicing and data entry
Inventory protection

Fig. 13.3 Inventory manuals keep consistency in the inventory manager's role, should a new team member be placed in that position.

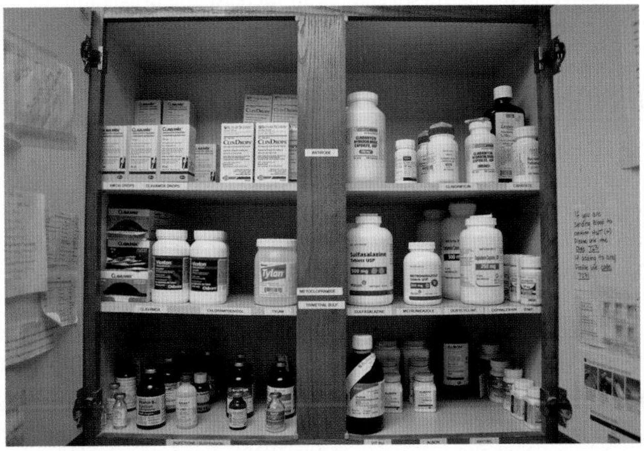

Fig. 13.4 Pharmacy organization is critical to the efficiency of a team.

Medications might be arranged in a pharmacy area and organized to help improve the efficiency of a team (Fig. 13.4). Drugs may be arranged by category, such as oral solids, oral liquids, injectable, ophthalmic, otic, and/or external topical medications. Other pharmaceuticals may be arranged by type of drug, such as tranquilizers, analgesics, cardiac, diuretics, and so forth.

VHMA PERFORMANCE DOMAIN TASK

Practice managers must develop and maintain appropriate inventory systems.

Distributor and Manufacturer Representatives

Distributor representatives work for a company that carries a full line of manufactured products ranging from pharmaceuticals to equipment and pet foods. Manufacturer representatives sell products to distributors or, in some cases, distribute products themselves. Manufacturer and distributor representatives may discuss specials with the inventory manager and educate the veterinary team when new products are launched.

Manufacturer and distributor representatives can provide team members with valuable information regarding products, and how they may increase sales for the practice. They can provide product sales histories, offering predictions for annual product usage (this is an excellent tool when preparing a budget for the following fiscal year). Representatives can be an excellent source of continuing education for team members and can provide product literature to increase the level of client education.

Caution should be used when companies have sales promotions. Some practices may not be able to sell the minimum amount of product needed to qualify for sale prices. Over purchasing products to obtain a sale price is not a good practice. The product should only be ordered when the clinic can sell through the inventory within a maximum 2-month period.

Working with a limited number of distributors and manufacturers allows larger orders to be placed at one location, usually allowing shipping and handling fees to be waived by the company. These fees are generally imposed on smaller orders and can add up quickly.

Equipment pricing should always be evaluated. One should consider if the piece of equipment will need to be installed (and by whom), what training is provided (if any), and what guarantee/warranty comes with the equipment. These factors can increase the price (and may be well worth the expense).

DESIGNING AN INVENTORY SYSTEM

The inventory component of a PIMS allows easy access from any computer (Figs. 13.5 and 13.6). This integration gives the ability to generate inventory reports, set reorder points and quantities, and (depending on the software) can place product orders for the practice. The accuracy of the reports solely depends on the setup of the system, the correct entry of the invoices, and the correct depletion of the product.

Correct categories (or departments) and codes must be set up for the PIMS to function effectively. For practices just establishing a category system and code entry, this is a simple procedure. For existing inventory systems, a code and category cleanup are highly suggested. It is advised that the categories in the PIMS match the AAHA Chart of Accounts, allowing an improved evaluation of expense versus revenue (Chapter 16, Finance). The following categories (at minimum) are recommended:

- Laboratory
- Diets
- Imaging
- Flea/tick/heartworm prevention
- Injections
- Prescription medications (pill, capsule, liquid)
- Retail/over the counter
- Medical supplies

For existing inventory systems, a code list should be printed and evaluated. Often, drugs are entered into the system multiple times under different names or are classified under the wrong category. At this point, duplicate items can be merged or reclassified (do not delete them, because this will permanently erase the history of the product from medical records). Items that are no longer in use can be placed on an inactive list (depending on the software, another term may be used), preventing that code from being used by team members.

Consolidating Inventory

Practice managers will realize that the practice carries multiple products that do the same thing. For example, a plethora of flea and tick preventatives are available, and many practices elect to carry multiple products to satisfy doctor recommendations and client needs. However, carrying too many products has a negative impact on the inventory system and cash flow of the hospital (Fig. 13.7). Ideally, practices should carry a maximum of two product options. When multiple products are carried, the following effects are seen:

- Increased dollars are spent on inventory
- Products sit on the shelf longer and have a decreased turnover rate
- Products expire and the practice loses money
- Team members need additional training for each product
- Client confusion
- Specific recommendations are not being made, ultimately decreasing client compliance

LEADERSHIP POINT

Consolidating inventory items can improve practice cash flow.

It can be difficult for veterinary team members to understand why the consolidation of products is critical; it can be even more difficult to determine which products to carry. Steps to Consolidate (Fig. 13.8):

- Produce a report for a particular category (e.g., heartworm preventative).
- Determine how many units were purchased and sold of each product in a set period.
- Determine how much of the product expired.
- Identify the top two items that were purchased and sold (without expiring) and produce a report showing profitability.
- Produce a second report, showing the losses associated with the remaining items.
- Have a doctor discussion to determine what products the practice will carry. The remaining products can be moved to the online store and still be available for clients to purchase.

Evaluating profitability is important when determining what products to carry or discontinue. If the product is not selling, it cannot be carried by the hospital. Veterinarians, owners, and practice managers must decide what top products to carry. If a specific product must be carried (i.e., medications used in emergency-only situations), a larger markup must be placed on the product to ensure that purchasing the item does not cause the practice to lose money.

CRITICAL COMPETENCY: DECISION MAKING

The practice manager must be able to make good decisions based on critical thinking and problem solving and make decisions that positively impact the practice. While many alternatives are available, the PM must be able to gather and effectively analyze relevant data and choose decisively.

Once codes and categories have been corrected and products have been consolidated, a physical count of the inventory must be completed and entered into the system. From this point forward, all invoices must be entered into the inventory system when an order is received.

Turnover Rates

Inventory managers should set goals for expected product turns per year. Turns per year is defined as the number of times a specific product turns over annually and is an efficiency ratio. The more efficiently the product turns, the higher the profitability of the item. Turnover rates determine effective reorder quantities and points and must be set for

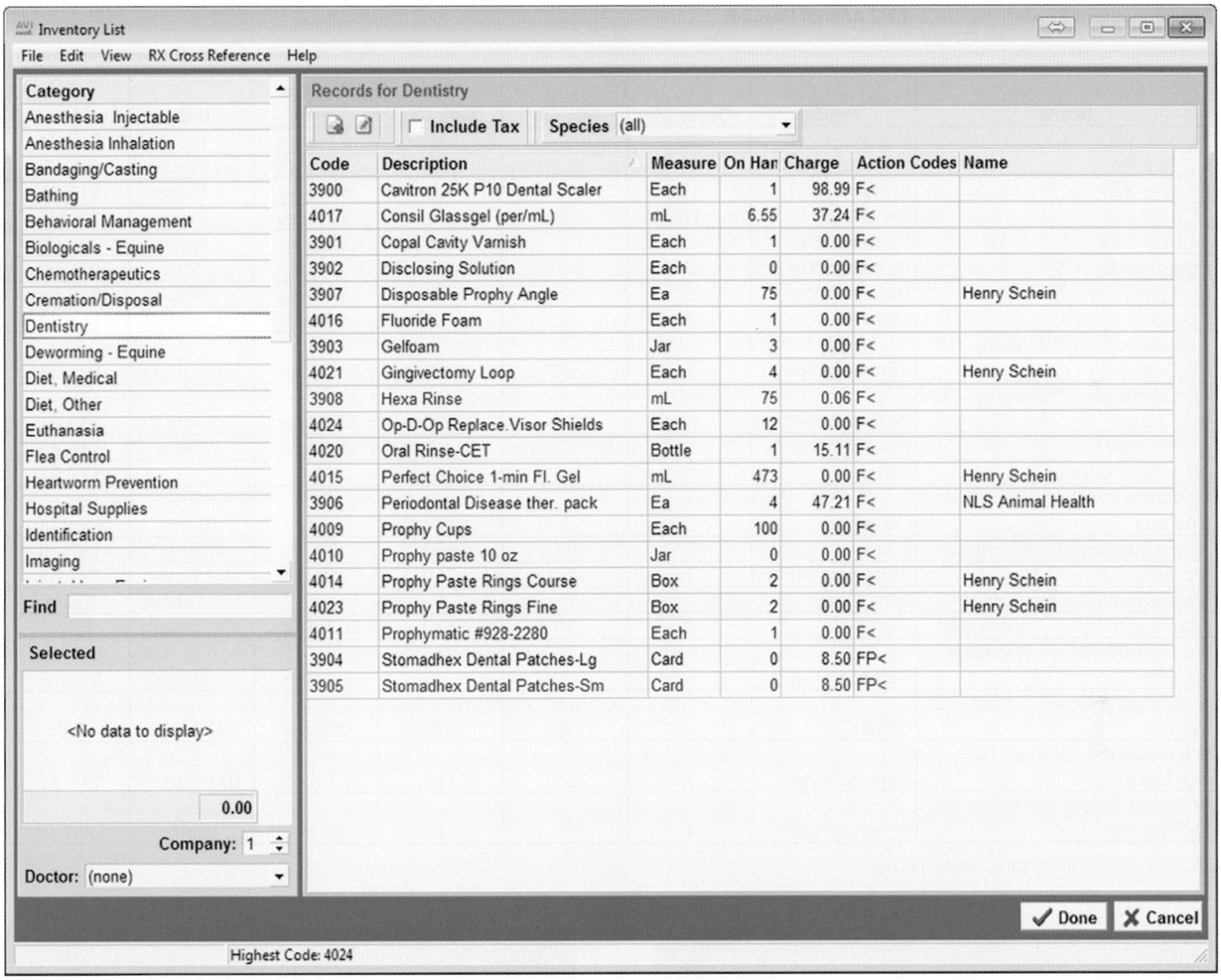

Fig. 13.5 Example of AVImark's inventory list. (Courtesy AVImark, LLC, Piedmont, Mo.)

each product based on the volume purchased and sold. Some products may have a turnover rate of 12 (very efficient and applies to high-selling items), whereas others will have a turnover rate of 6 to 10 (less efficient and would apply to lower-selling items).

The goal of developing effective turnover rates is to increase the profitability of the practice and decrease expired product, shrinkage, and soft costs (holding and ordering costs).

Statistically, 80% of income (from inventory sales) is produced from 20% of inventoried products (also known as the Pareto principle). If an inventory manager spends a consolidated amount of time managing the top 20% of inventory, higher profits will be generated because holding and ordering costs are decreased. The top 20% of items are those that produce a high level of sales or items the practice cannot function without. Examples of top items include vaccinations, flea/tick/heartworm preventatives, parvovirus stool tests, etc.

Determining Effective Turnover Rates

To determine the inventory turns per year for a specific product, the beginning inventory is added to the ending inventory and divided by two. This determines the average inventory per year. The total amount of product purchased during that period, divided by the average, yields the number of turns per year for that product (Fig. 13.9).

To determine an effective turn rate for each product, print a sales history of all inventoried items, and determine which products are in the top 20%. These items should turn 12 times per year. This means that a particular product should be ordered once a month, and when ordered, the quantity ordered should support the sales of such product for a 1-month period. Therefore, this product will be ordered 12 times during the year, resulting in a turnover rate of 12.

When ordering monthly, the costs associated with inventory management drop dramatically (also known as soft costs which will be covered later in this chapter). Products in the sales history report that produce the next 20% may have a turnover rate of 10. Any product with a turnover rate of less than 6 must be outsourced to an online pharmacy (covered later in this chapter).

Reorder Quantities

It is imperative that correct reorder quantities be determined for each product or excess product will sit on the shelf, resulting in an increase in holding costs and the potential for expiration and theft. If too little product is ordered, ordering costs increase, a product shortage occurs, and clients, patients, and team members are inconvenienced. As indicated earlier, correct reorder quantities contribute to a healthy turnover rate.

LEADERSHIP POINT

Developing and using effective reorder quantities decreases the risk of running out of inventory.

Inventory Items Report **ABC Animal Hospital**
12/31/23

Name	Vendor	Order Qty	Min Qty	Max Qty	Reorder Point	Units	Cost per Unit
E-Collar #30	Patterson Vet	20		45	5 Pieces	1 Piece	$14.01
E-Collar #8	Patterson Vet	10		13	3 Pieces	1 Piece	$6.47
E-Collar #23	Patterson Vet	10	3	15	6 Pieces	1 Piece	$11.26
E-Collar #17	Other	10	3		3 Pieces	1 Piece	$8.89
E-Collar #12	Patterson Vet	10		13	3 Pieces	1 Piece	$8.33
Fiberglass Cast 2"	Patterson Vet	3	1	4	1 Roll	1 Roll	$8.76
Fiberglass Cast 3"	Patterson Vet	5	2	7	3 Pieces	1 Piece	$10.86
Fiberglass Cast 4"	Other	3	1	5	1 Piece	1 Piece	$14.24
Acepromazine (PromAce) - 10 mg/Tablet	Patterson Vet	1	20	200	35 Tablets	100 Tablets	$24.07
Acepromazine (PromAce) - 25 mg/Tablet	Patterson Vet	1	20	200	35 Tablets	100 Tablets	$62.01
Adaptil refill	Patterson Vet	8	2	12	3 Pieces	1 Piece	$16.85
Adaptil w/ diffuser	Other	4		6	1		$19.91
Adequan Injection 100mg/ml (per mL)	Other	3	1		1 ml	10 mls	$112.00
Albon Suspension - 50 mg/ml	Other	1	200	600	200 mls	473 mls	$87.25
Albuterol Syrup - 0.4 mg/ml	Patterson Vet	1	200	750	250 mls	473 mls	$21.83
Alprazolam - 0.5 mg/Tablet	MWI					100 Tablets	$2.74
Alprazolam tabs - 1 mg/Tablet	MWI	4	30	530	30 Tablets	100 Tablets	$6.06
Alu-mend Spray on Bandage 120gm	Patterson Vet	4	2		2 Bottles	1 Bottle	$12.78
Amantadine Oral Solution - 10 mg/ml	Other	1	100	673	200 mls	473 mls	$8.08
Amantadine HCL Tab - 100 mg/Tablet	Patterson Vet	1	30	150	1 Tablet	100 Tablets	$19.95
Amikacin Sulfate (Amiglyde-V) - 250 mg/ml	Patterson Vet	1		1	12 mls	48 mls	$259.82

Fig. 13.6 Example of inventory details report.

- Shrinkage (items missing with no explanation)
- Bottles breaking
- Items expiring
- Doctors wanting to change to another product and being unable to do so because of large quantity of previous product
- Confusion among team members about the product mode of action and side effects

Fig. 13.7 Disadvantages of a large inventory.

Product	Number Purchased	Number Sold	On Shelf	Expired	Discrepancy
Prod. A	100	70	20	10	0
Prod. B	50	30	10	10	0
Prod. C	150	100	20	Unknown	30
Prod. D	780	750	20	Unknown	10

Fig. 13.8 Example of consolidating inventory.

Calculating Inventory Turns per Year

(Beginning inventory + Ending inventory) ÷ 2 =
AVERAGE INVENTORY

Total units of product purchased during measured period ÷ Average inventory = **NUMBER OF TURNS PER YEAR.**

EXAMPLE:

- Inventory for eye drops **at the beginning of the year** was 4 units.
- **Ending inventory** was 4 units.
- **Total purchased** for the year was 36.

4 (beginning units) + 4 (ending units) = 8 units.

8 units ÷ 2 = 4 (average inventory)

36 total annual products purchased ÷ 4 average inventory = **9 times turned**

This is an excellent value because the product turned 9 times!

Fig. 13.9 Example of calculating inventory turns per year.

Determining Effective Reorder Quantities

Three factors are considered when determining reorder quantities: average daily use, turnover goals, and product expiration (Fig. 13.10).

The average daily use of a product determines how many units will sell per day. Average daily use is calculated by taking the number of units sold in the year and dividing it by the number of days the practice is open in a year.

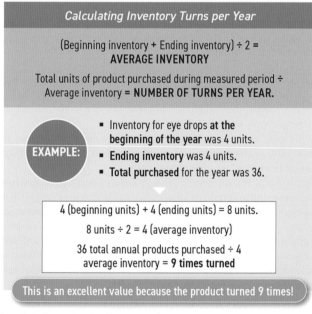

Example: A practice is open 365 days per year and sells 550 bottles of Rimadyl, 25 mg, 180 count.

- 550 units sold ÷ 365 days open = 1.5
- Rimadyl, 25 mg, 180 count, sells on an average of 1.5 bottles per day

Turnover is critical in this equation because the quantity ordered should support sales without the practice running out or having excess product.

Calculating Reorder Quantity

Average daily use × Turnover goal (in days) = **REORDER QUANTITY**

EXAMPLE:

- Heartgard Plus Small has an **average daily use of 3.5** (3.5 boxes sell daily).
- The turnover goal for this product is **12** (30 days).

3.5 (boxes daily) × 30 (turnover goal) = **105**

When this product is ordered, 105 boxes should be purchased at once (which is estimated to sell within 30 days). Because Heartgard Plus Small is supplied in 10 boxes per carton, then **11 CARTONS WOULD BE ORDERED.**

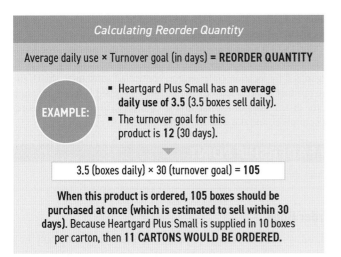

Fig. 13.10 Example of calculating inventory reorder quantities.

Product expiration is the last factor to consider. If a product is short-dated and will not sell by the end of the turnover goal, fewer quantities must be considered.

Reorder Points

Reorder points are defined as the point at which a product needs to be ordered and takes into consideration lead time and average daily use (Fig. 13.11). A reorder point is not when the product has run out!

LEADERSHIP POINT

A reorder point is not when a product has run out but the point at which a product needs to be ordered.

Determining Effective Reorder Points

Lead time is defined as the amount of time between when a product is needed and when it makes it onto the practice shelf. For example, a practice places orders on Monday and receives those orders on Tuesday. If a product is determined to be low on Wednesday, and the next order will be placed the following Monday (to be received Tuesday), then the lead time is 7 days. If a product is noted as low on Friday and the order will be placed on Monday, the lead time is 4 days.

Lead time multiplied by average daily use determines the reorder point of a product

The seasonality of certain products throughout the country may affect reorder points and reorder quantities. Potential seasonal items may include:

- Flea/tick prevention
- Heartworm prevention
- Allergy medication
- Products to treat chocolate toxicities (holidays)
- Products to treat anxiety (Independence Day, New Year's Eve)
- Products to treat ethylene glycol ingestions
- Products to treat infectious diseases that emerge seasonally (Parvo, Distemper, etc.)

Creating a list of seasonal products will help the inventory manager overcome this obstacle.

Inventory Storage

Practices that have storage space available to order bulk supplies and support a 12 times turnover rate generally have a higher profit margin than those that do not.

Calculating Reorder Points

Average daily use × Lead time = **REORDER POINT**

EXAMPLE:

- Heartgard Plus Small has an **average daily use of 3.5** (3.5 boxes sell daily).
- The lead time for this product is **4 days.**

3.5 (average daily use) × 4 days = **14**

This product must be reordered when **14 UNITS REMAIN ON THE SHELF.**

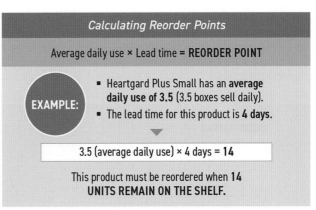

Fig. 13.11 Example of calculating inventory reorder points.

Central inventory locations store additional supplies and are generally locked, allowing limited access. Pharmacy shelves are stocked on an as-needed basis from the central inventory "closet" or "cage." Items can be checked in when they are received and checked out when a bottle is needed in the pharmacy. New items should be placed behind old items, allowing the older items to be sold first.

Practices may have one cabinet that is used for the excess product. When a bottle is emptied, the new bottle can be pulled and placed in the correct location. This can help prevent overcrowding of products in one area. Overcrowding can cause a loss of items and add to inventory discrepancies and overordering.

PREPARING ORDERS

Once inventory software has been set up correctly (codes, categories, physical inventory entered, reorder points, and reorder quantities determined), managers may learn to depend on inventory reports to help them place orders. It is advised to always double-check physical levels, ensuring the reports are accurate (human error does occur!).

LEADERSHIP POINT

Order preparation is a soft cost that must be calculated into the selling price of the item.

For practices that do not have an accurate inventory system, another method must be used to help the inventory manager to place accurate orders (it takes a team to make a system succeed).

Medical supplies can be difficult to manage with inventory software. Many procedures require supplies but do not account for the specific usage of gauze, latex gloves, syringes, and so on. Some services (such as vaccinations) can be linked to tracking syringe use, but the quantity on hand may not reflect the number of syringes used to draw blood. Physical spot-checking of these items is mandatory to ensure the practice does not run out.

Developing a Want List

A want list may be created for team members who note that a specific product is running low. A dry-erase board works well for a want list because products can be erased as soon as they arrive. A special-order board may be created for those medications that need to be custom ordered for clients; this may include compounded and/or flavored medication (Fig. 13.12). This special-order board can provide a quick reference for team members preparing the medication once it has arrived because it will have the client and pet name listed.

A spreadsheet of items needed may be developed for the inventory manager to follow while an order is being prepared. Many times, items are removed from the shelves, and team members have forgotten to write the product on the board. This spreadsheet allows a third checkpoint for inventoried items. A missing product may not be noticed until a doctor needs it. If a spreadsheet is used, low inventory can be detected earlier and the product reordered. A spreadsheet should contain the name and size of the product. It is useful to have a list of all products that should always be available.

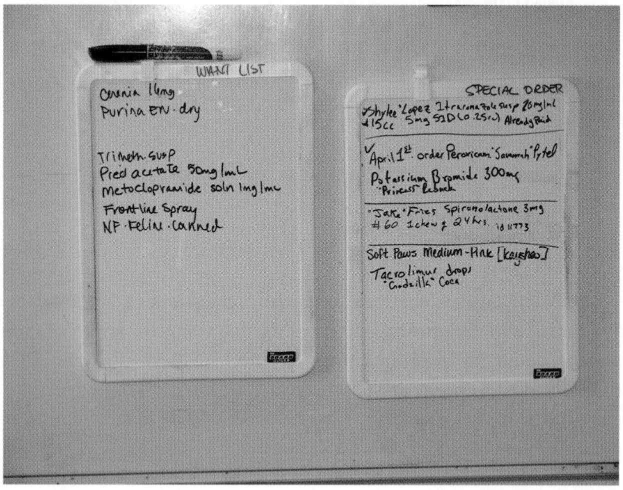

Fig. 13.12 A want list and special-order list are placed on two separate dry-erase boards.

Fig. 13.13 is an example of a spreadsheet of inventoried products for a veterinary practice. This specific practice has a pharmacy that is first organized by location (refrigerator, controlled substance, shelf); then the product is alphabetized. The quantity supplied is listed in column B, the distributor or manufacturer in column C, the quantity to reorder in column D, and the shelf life of that product in column E.

> **LEADERSHIP POINT**
>
> Train all team members to use the reorder system efficiently.

Order Book

All orders should be kept together and listed chronologically in an order book. This allows the inventory manager to see what products were ordered, how many, from which distributor or manufacturer, the date the order was placed, and the name of the representative who took the order. This is also a great history resource. To avoid order confusion, contact the same representative each time. Sales representatives become familiar with preferred products and make every effort to ensure the order is 100% satisfactory. If an item is on backorder, the representative should notify the manager. A decision can be made to order an alternative product or search for the product through another

Product	Quantity	Distributor	Reorder #	Shelf Life	Notes
FELV/FIV	30/bx	Patterson	1	30d	
General Health Profile	2/bx	Patterson	6	1d	
Heartworm 3DX	30/bx	Patterson	2	15d	
Parvo	5/box	Patterson	2	10d	
Plasma	1	ABB	1	30d	
Pre-op Profile	4/bx	Patterson	6	1d	
Apomorphine	1	VPA	5	3 mo	
Buprinex	1ml x 10vials	Covetrus	2	7d	
Butorpehnol Inj	50mg	Covetrus	1	6 mo	
Butorphenol Tabs	100	Covetrus	1	6 mo	
Diazepam	10ml; 5 vials	Covetrus	1	6 mo	
Ketamine	10ml; 5 vials	Covetrus	1	2 mo	
Hycodan	100 tabs	Covetrus	1	6 mo	
Telazol	5ml	Covetrus	5	7 d	
Activated Carcoal	1	Patterson	5	30d	
Albon	100	Zoetis	1	30d	
Amoxi Clavulanate	210	Zoetis	1	30d	
Amoxicillian	100	Patterson	1	30d	
Antirobe	100 and drops	Zoetis	1	30d	
Artifical Tears	1	Patterson	5	7 d	
Atropine Ophth	1	Patterson	2	10 d	
Barium Sulfate	1	Covetrus	1	30 d	
Benedryl Capsules	500, 1000	Covetrus	1	3 mo	
BenedrylSusp	473ml	Covetrus	1	6 mo	
Carafate	473ml	Covetrus	1	6 mo	
Cefa Drops	15ml	Covetrus	6	10 d	
Cephalexin Caps	100, 500	MWI	1	7 d	
Chlorpheniramine	1000	MWI	1	30 d	
Doxycycline	100, 500	MWI	1	7 d	
Droncit	50	MWI	1	4 mo	
Fenbendazole	Liquid or powder	MWI	1	5 mo	
Genesis	1	MWI	6	30 d	

Fig. 13.13 Example of a spreadsheet for inventoried products.

company. The backorder should be noted in the book and a notice posted for all team members.

Monthly Ordering

To decrease holding and order processing costs, the top 20% to 40% of products should be ordered monthly. Team members spend a large amount of time placing orders weekly; by ordering monthly, efficiency is gained.

Ordering monthly also improves the practice's cash flow. If a majority of inventory is ordered at the beginning of a distributor or manufacturer's billing cycle, the practice has an entire month to sell the product before a monthly invoice is produced. Spot-ordering can occur throughout the month as needed, but most ordering should occur only once a month.

Just-in-Time Ordering

Just-in-time ordering is defined as ordering a product when it is needed but before it runs out. Just-in-time ordering is needed for products that do not have a high turnover rate in the hospital but are still maintained on the shelves. Unfortunately, this method does not account for manufacturer or distributor lead times or backorders. If a product is on backorder, the inventory manager must find the product from another distributor or find a product equivalent. If a match is not available, other team members and veterinarians must be made aware of the backorder.

Just-in-time ordering is not the recommended method of inventory management. It is the primary reason practices run out of inventory and causes orders to be placed almost every day. The result is an increase in soft costs and hundreds of invoices to reconcile on a yearly basis.

LEADERSHIP POINT

Just-in-time ordering increases soft costs associated with inventory. The more time that is spent on ordering products, the higher the cost is for the clinic.

Bulk Orders

Some manufacturers offer discounts on purchasing large quantities of items. Bulk product orders can be beneficial when keeping in mind:

- Quantity is based on historic sales within the period being measured,
- The quantity ordered must sell before the delayed billing is due.
- The product cannot have a short shelf life.
- Consider year-end tax implications (cash versus accrual reporting).

To determine an effective quantity for a bulk order, a manager would consider the average daily use of the product, the number of working days in the billing period, and the percent of growth (or loss) the practice may be experiencing (Fig. 13.14).

Vetcove

Vetcove is a free platform that allows the inventory manager to compare all prices of products from various vendors at once, online, similar to Amazon, except for veterinary products and equipment only. Orders can be placed with preferred distributors or manufacturers on Vetcove, and the billing/shipping comes direct from that company. Purchase history, price savings, rebates, etc. are all available on Vetcove, and reports can be broken down by distributor, manufacturer, product, or a set period of purchase. In addition, Vetcove can integrate with the practice PIMS to autopopulate orders when they are shipped from the vendor. Vetcove significantly increases the efficiency of the inventory manager.

Calculating Bulk Orders

Average daily use × Number of working days in billing period × % of growth = **BULK ORDER**

EXAMPLE:

- Heartgard Plus Large has an **average daily use of 12** (12 boxes sell daily).
- There are **64 working days** in the billing period.
- The practice has been experiencing a steady **4% increase in business** for the year.

12 (average daily use) × 64 (days in billing period) = **768**

768 × 4% (percent of growth) = **31**

768 + 31 = **799 boxes**

FOR THIS BULK ORDER TO BE BENEFICIAL, 799 BOXES WOULD BE ORDERED. (Heartgard is sold in cartons of 10, so 80 cartons would be ordered.)

Fig. 13.14 Example of calculating bulk orders.

RECEIVING ORDERS

When a shipment is received, the receiving team member should inspect the order before it is put away. Items should be inspected for damage and compared with the invoice and order book. Quantity (e.g., number of bottles), strength of product (e.g., in milligrams or grams), and size of product (e.g., number of tablets, capsules, or milliliters) should be double-checked. Once the order accuracy has been verified (with the invoice and order book), products can be placed in the appropriate locations.

All invoices need to be reconciled against the monthly statement to ensure that no additional charges were added to the account. A manager may create an open order file. Once packing slips have been checked against the products received, these slips can be placed in an open file; the packing slips can then be reconciled with invoices received at month's end.

VHMA PERFORMANCE DOMAIN TASK

Practice managers must oversee or place and track inventory orders.

EXPIRED MEDICATIONS

The U.S. Food and Drug Administration (FDA) requires that all drugs produced be tested for efficacy and an expiration date must be printed on the label (Fig. 13.15). Once the efficacy/potency of a drug has dropped below a certain percentage, it is no longer effective. It is illegal and unethical to dispense expired drugs. Expired products must be removed from the shelves immediately and cannot be sold.

Many practices do not want to lose money associated with expired products; therefore, an effective inventory management system must be implemented to prevent medications from expiring. Inventory managers may keep a running list of products and expiration dates that can be completed each time an order is received. If a product bottle is open and getting close to expiring, a note should be made for the doctors, allowing them the opportunity to dispense the remaining product. If the bottle is not opened, the distributor or manufacturer may exchange the product at no charge. Return policies should be verified and kept on file for reference.

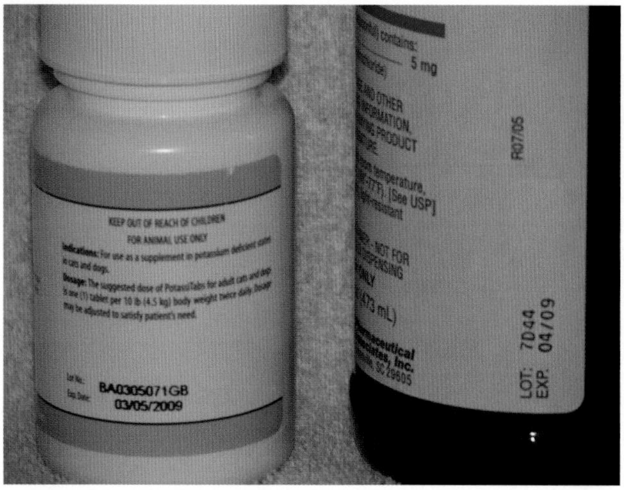

Fig. 13.15 Expired drugs cannot be sold. Inventory managers must track the expiration dates of products and dispose of expired drugs appropriately.

The U.S. Environmental Protection Agency advises against discarding products in the toilet or trash. Instead, they should be placed in a drug-neutralizing pouch. A neutralization pouch mixes the drug with warm water and activated carbon, and the active ingredient becomes neutralized, rendering it irretrievable (see Chapter 14, Fig. 14.9). The pouch can then be thrown away in the trash. Disposing of expired controlled substances is described in greater detail in Chapter 14.

Returning Products to the Distributor

For several reasons, some products may need to be returned to the distributor, including product damages or order errors. Most distributors will gladly accept returns, although some may institute a restocking or shipping fee. A call should be placed to the sales representative who may ask whether a replacement product or credit is preferred. A call tag will be sent to the practice for the item return. A call tag is an address label produced by the company to be placed on the outside of the shipment box. This label has a specific reference number so that returns can be credited to the appropriate account. Once the call tag has been received, it is important to document the product return date on the original invoice. A credit should be issued to the practice upon receipt of the product return, and a credit invoice will be generated. The credit may take a few weeks to be processed and received. Distributors and manufacturers may also take unopened bottles of recently expired product. However, instead of a credit, the product will be replaced. Each company has different policies regarding expired products, and options should be researched before ordering new products.

LEADERSHIP POINT

Be familiar with manufacturer return policies to maximize the return of expired items.

EFFECTIVE PRICING STRATEGIES

Before pricing strategies can be determined, team members must understand the replacement costs, soft costs, hard costs, and profits associated with inventory.

Replacement cost is the price a practice would pay to replace an item. The original cost associated with the product may not be the current price, or the product could have been received with free goods or bulk purchase.

- Determining reorder quantity and reorder points
- Price shopping
- Visiting with sales representatives
- Requesting an order
- Researching items to replace back orders
- Receiving and unpacking products and supplies
- Entering invoices into veterinary software
- Reconciling statements

Fig. 13.16 Fifteen to twenty percent of the cost of the product contributes to ordering costs (time spent managing inventory).

- Property tax paid on inventory value
- Insurance
- Utilities to maintain safety of product
- Shrinkage
- Pharmacy licensing/DEA fees
- OSHA training and maintenance

Fig. 13.17 Eight to fifteen percent of the cost of the product contributes to holding costs (facility-related costs to keep the product in the practice).

Calculating Soft Costs

Unit cost × (Soft cost variable percentage) + Unit cost = **SELL PRICE**

Soloxine, 0.6 mg, 250 count; unit cost $28.35

$28.35 (unit cost) × 23% = **$6.52**
(23% when inventory management is at its peak)

When inventory is being managed well and soft costs are kept to a minimum, $6.52 would be added to the original cost of $28.35

$28.35 unit cost + $6.52 soft costs =
$34.87 is the true cost of this product

When inventory is not being managed well, and soft costs are high, $9.92 would be added to the original cost of $28.35

$28.35 unit cost + $69.92 soft costs =
$38.27 is the true cost of this product

Fig. 13.18 Example of calculating soft costs.

Soft costs include holding and ordering costs and are often referred to as *hidden inventory costs*. **Ordering costs** are human resource-related and account for time spent preparing and maintaining an order (Fig. 13.16). Ordering costs account for approximately 15% to 20% of the unit cost. **Holding costs** are facility-related (Fig. 13.17) and account for approximately 8% to 15% of the unit cost. Together, ordering and holding costs account for 23% to 35% of the cost of the product (Fig. 13.18).

Soft costs can be decreased by maintaining effective turnover rates, reorder points, and reorder quantities. These will also indirectly decrease shrinkage and wastage.

Hard costs are the costs associated with paying veterinarians when they are compensated based on production. Traditionally, veterinarians are paid 10% to 25% of an item (the amount is at the discretion of the practice).

Profits must be made on inventory items; however, the profit may vary depending on the product or product category. Profit also depends on whether the item is a shopped or a competitive item. Profit goals are at least 15% to 20% of the unit costs.

LEADERSHIP POINT

Every product's selling price must include ordering costs, holding costs, profit, and hard costs (if veterinarians are paid on production).

Break-Even Analysis

To determine the lowest cost a medication can be sold for, a break-even analysis should be completed. A growing number of long-term medications, as well as heartworm and flea/tick preventives, etc., are sold through a variety of markets. Practices will want to be competitive with these products and offer low prices to clients. The following is the formula for calculating break-even costs. Break-even analysis (Fig. 13.19):

- Unit cost + hard cost + soft cost + (profit × sales price) = sales price

VHMA PERFORMANCE DOMAIN TASK

Practice managers must conduct fee analysis and monitor and update fee schedules.

Calculating Break-Even

Unit cost + Hard cost + Soft cost + (Desired profit × Sales price) = **SALES PRICE**

EXAMPLE:

OTOMAX: Unit cost = $12.28

- **Hard costs:** 15% (predetermined by practice)
- **Soft costs:** 23% (predetermined by practice)
- **Desired profit:** 20%

$12.28 x 15% (hard costs) = $1.84

$12.28 x 23% (soft costs) = $2.82

$12.28 + $1.84 + $2.82 + (20% x sales price[SP]) = $16.94

$16.94 + 0.20 SP = SP

$16.94 = SP – 0.20 SP

$16.94 = 0.80 SP

$21.18 = SP

The **absolute minimum price** this product could be sold for is **$21.18.**

Fig. 13.19 Example of calculating a break-even.

Markup

Markup is a percentage added to the cost of the unit when determining the selling price. Markup percentages can be based either on the number of inventory turns or a product category (Fig. 13.20). Products with a higher turnover rate (10× to 12×) have less markup (140%–175%); those with lower turnover rates (4× to 6×) have higher markups (200%–275%) to account for the potential expiration of product. Categories that are competitive will have a lower markup than those that are used to treat chronic conditions, cancer, etc. (Fig. 13.21).

Dispensing Fees

Dispensing fees are added after the markup has been determined. Dispensing fees cover the veterinary technician's time to count the medication, the vial used to package medication, the prescription label, and label printer wear and tear. Average dispensing fees are $10.00.[1]

Labeling Fees

Labeling fees are applied to products sold in the original container, and a team member does not have to count the medication. This fee covers the veterinary technicians' time to prepare the product, the prescription label, and label printer wear and tear. The average labeling fee is 25% to 30% of the dispensing fee.

Minimum Prescription Fees

Many practices have a minimum prescription fee that averages $13.00.[1]

Average Product Markup of In-House Inventory

Medicine	150%
Heartworm/flea tick	90%
Drugs administered	150%
Oncology drugs	150%
Drugs for chronic conditions	100%

Adapted from Tumblin, et al. Well Managed Practice Benchmarks 2017.

Fig. 13.20 Average product markup of in-house inventory.

Calculating Markup

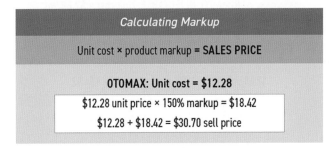

Unit cost × product markup = **SALES PRICE**

OTOMAX: Unit cost = $12.28

$12.28 unit price × 150% markup = $18.42

$12.28 + $18.42 = $30.70 sell price

Fig. 13.21 Example of calculating markup.

Injection Fees

Injections are priced differently than capsules or tablets. Injections are priced both as an inventory item and as a service item because a skilled professional must give the injection. Injection fees have similar product markup structures as tablets or capsules, with a service fee for the injection (Fig. 13.22). Injection fees range from $12.00 to $28.00 (Fig. 13.23).

LEADERSHIP POINT

Injections are priced with both an inventory cost and a service or procedure cost. The product is being used (inventory) and administered by a professional (service/procedure).

Dispensing, labeling, injection, and minimum prescription fees are hidden fees and are not detailed for clients. Clients do not understand the overhead costs associated with the veterinary practice and would question the hospital's product markup techniques.

Outsourcing Products

As stated earlier, products with a low turnover should be outsourced to the practice's online pharmacy. These are products that the practice rarely sells and often expire before the entire amount can be sold.

The practice online pharmacy should link directly to the practice website, pet portal, or practice app. Practices choose which products and prices are visible to clients. Guarantees on product and efficacy continue through the online pharmacy just as if the product were purchased from the hospital. The practice will receive an alert asking for prescription approval, and money earned from the online store is deposited into the practice checking account monthly.

Outsourcing products is an excellent way to help consolidate inventoried items, reducing the financial burden on the practice. Practices must build and manage online pharmacies to maximize this revenue stream.

Average Markup of Injectable Drugs

Chemotherapy	150%
Compounded	133%
Long term	100%
Others	150%

Fig. 13.22 Average markup of injectable drugs.

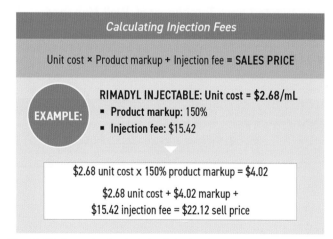

Calculating Injection Fees

Unit cost × Product markup + Injection fee = SALES PRICE

EXAMPLE:

RIMADYL INJECTABLE: Unit cost = $2.68/mL
- Product markup: 150%
- Injection fee: $15.42

$2.68 unit cost x 150% product markup = $4.02

$2.68 unit cost + $4.02 markup + $15.42 injection fee = $22.12 sell price

Fig. 13.23 Example of calculating injection fees.

ONLINE PHARMACY/STORE MANAGEMENT

Online pharmacies are a critical component of the veterinary business. Veterinary clients are looking for convenient, easy, and hassle-free ways to refill existing prescriptions and buy new products for their pets. Often, practice hours and location (or proximity to the client's home or place of employment) limit the client's ability to call the practice or stop by and pick up medication. Online pharmacies allow clients to shop when they want and have products shipped directly to their home.

Choosing an Online Pharmacy Platform

Choosing an online platform should be thoughtfully considered. It is very important for the practice to determine the most critical factors associated with the success of the revenue center. Factors and goals to consider are listed in Fig. 13.24.

Building an Online Platform

The selected vendor will build and install the practice's pharmacy platform; however, the practice will be responsible for choosing products that will be made available to clients. Some products should move from the inside pharmacy to the online platform (slow-turning products as well as those that tend to expire before the entire unit is sold). The practice should also consider offering some competitive products online as well as in the practice for client convenience. Diets and food products should also be available for online ordering. A general practice often does not have enough space to carry and turn diet products at an efficient rate. Consider carrying small bags for dispensing from the hospital, then explaining how easy refills can be ordered online with the convenience of home delivery.

Managing an Online Platform

Managing the online platform includes pricing, marketing, and measuring success. Typically, online prices will be lower than the in-house pharmacy. In-house pharmacy costs must include hard costs (product cost plus any commission paid to veterinarians), soft costs (holding

- Meeting/exceeding client expectations
- Product offerings
- Maintaining client compliance
- Personalization of the online store (matching practice website)
- Security/merchant options
- Auto-refill and reminder options
- Marketing materials
- Reporting features
- Accredited by VetVIPPS
- Pricing control
- Costs
- Billing

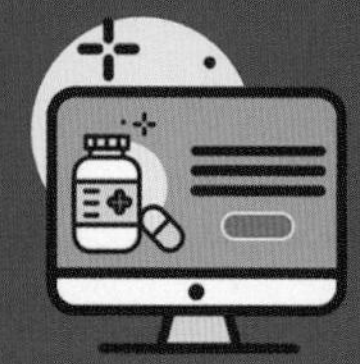

Fig. 13.24 Factors to consider when building an online pharmacy.

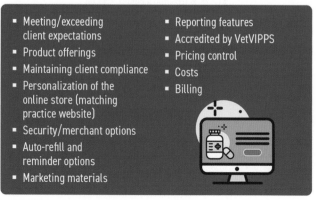

and ordering costs), plus any profit that is to be made. The online pharmacy has limited soft costs associated, mostly with the time used to manage the platform. With this pricing strategy, the online pharmacy can be competitively priced, yet still profitable.

Marketing the online pharmacy is critical; it will not market itself. Provide clear instructions to the team for when to promote, how to promote, and what to promote. Create and distribute marketing materials to clients outlining the benefits of the online pharmacy. Develop professional posters to be placed in examination rooms, brochures to be placed in puppy and kitten kits, and email messaging sent to existing clients. Identify opportunities to speak with clients and teach them how to navigate the online ordering system (Fig. 13.25).

The critical factor needed for an online pharmacy to succeed is measuring progress. Financial reports must be reviewed and analyzed, and goals must be set and achieved. It makes no sense to have a profit center that costs more than it produces. Key performance indicators (Fig. 13.26) should be reviewed and acted upon when goals are not being achieved.

VHMA PERFORMANCE DOMAIN TASK

Practice managers must analyze financial reports.

Blending In-House and Online Pharmacy Platforms

Compare blending in-house and online pharmacies the same way in-house and outside laboratories were blended years ago. Certain diagnostics needed to be performed in-house, whereas others could be outsourced for improved efficiency, cost, and results. The same applies to the pharmacy. Use each to complement the other, finding the most cost- and time-efficient benefits of both, while continuing to satisfy both client and veterinary needs.

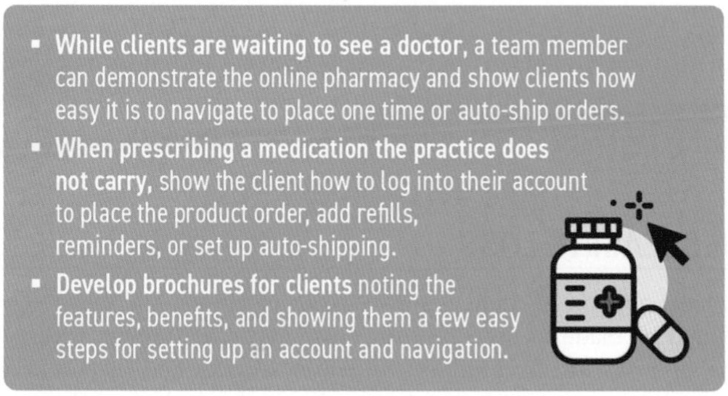

When prescribing a medication the practice does not carry, show the client how to log into their account to place the product order, add refills, reminders, or set up auto-shipping.
Develop brochures for clients noting the features, benefits, and showing them a few easy steps for setting up an account and navigation.

Fig. 13.25 Finding time to promote the practice's online pharmacy is critical.

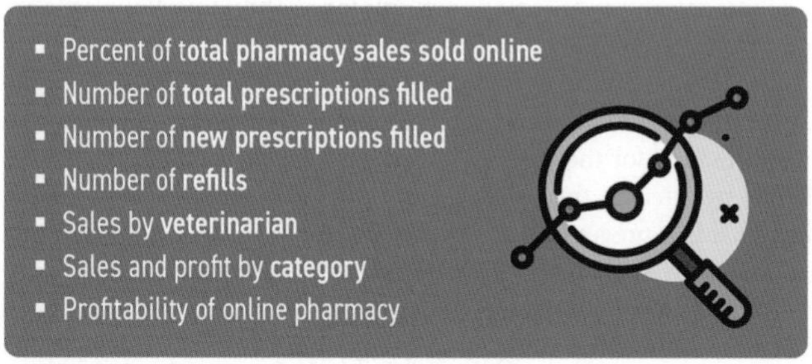
Percent of **total pharmacy sales sold online**
Number of **total prescriptions filled**
Number of **new prescriptions filled**
Number of **refills**
Sales by **veterinarian**
Sales and profit by **category**
Profitability of online pharmacy

Fig. 13.26 Examples of key performance indicators for online pharmacy management.

INVENTORY PROTECTION

Cautious measures should be in place to protect product inventory, considering that inventory is the second largest expense of the practice. The top 20% of items, which have been previously identified as Pareto's items, are the largest producing products for the hospital and should be manually counted monthly. These physical counts are then compared with computer reports. When there are discrepancies (and there will be), they must be investigated. The remaining 80% of items must also have random spot-checks, perhaps semiannually. When any item has a continued discrepancy, random spot-checks for that item should occur more frequently.

Potential Causes of Discrepancies

Shrinkage: Shrinkage is defined as the loss of product inventory. Shrinkage can be due to product expiration, theft, missed charges, or giving products away without recording the transaction. Practice managers must implement measures to decrease the shrinkage of inventoried items since this is one of the largest expenses that a veterinary hospital has.

Missed Charges: It is estimated that missed charges account for at least 10% of the gross revenue produced per year (see Chapter 16, Finance, for more information). If the practice's gross revenue is $1,000,000.00 in the fiscal year, approximately 10% (or $100,000.00) may be lost in missed charges. By managing inventory and investigating discrepancies, the practice manager should be able to determine why team members are missing charges. The practice manager should work closely with the team to improve efficiencies. Reasons for missing charges may include lack of focus, lack of training, or multitasking (creating a lack of focus). Electronic medical records that are properly set up greatly reduce unintentionally missed charges.

Incorrectly Invoiced Products: Team members may either enter the wrong product into the computer system or pull the wrong product to send home with the client.

Medical Supplies: As mentioned previously, some medical supplies are difficult to inventory, and discrepancies will likely be found. However, supplies used to run in-house laboratory work should be accountable.

Free Doses: Some promotions include free goods offered to the hospital. However, unless they are entered into the inventory system correctly, they can cause discrepancies between the physical and report counts.

In-House Use: Many inventory items are used in-house to treat patients; food is one item in this category. When items are used in this manner, they should be placed into a log or charged to an in-house account to help avoid inventory discrepancies. Errors that occur with laboratory tests could also fall into this category and should be documented.

Team members should be aware of the number of supplies they use to deliver services to clients. Dropping suture material daily can cost the practice a significant amount of money. Technicians that use a wad of gauze (instead of two to three pieces per scrub) to clean a wound increase cost. Kennel assistants that use a half gallon of bleach to clean are not only creating a safety hazard but also costing the practice money. Team meetings are a great place to analyze product use and discuss ideas to reduce loss. Once loss awareness has been established, all team members should be held accountable for proper product usage.

INVENTORY BUDGET

The goal is to keep inventory costs between 18% and 20% of revenue for the practice. If a practice generates $1 million, $180,000–$200,000 should be the set budget for inventory purchases for the year (excluding capital equipment). This contributes to successfully implementing and maintaining the larger practice budget (Chapter 16).

One could easily divide up $180,000 into 12 months, giving an equal dollar amount each month. However, most practices have some type of seasonal fluctuation based on their demographic. Dividing the total dollar amount into 12 months will make some months over budget, while others will be under budget. At the end of the year, it is still the same dollar amount.

Practice managers can also look at historical reports and determine which months are considered seasonal and allocate more dollars to those months, and fewer dollars to the slower months.

VHMA PERFORMANCE DOMAIN TASK

Practice managers must prepare budgets and long-term fiscal plans.

The trap many inventory managers fall into when a practice manager gives them a monthly spending budget, however, is that they get stuck on the set dollar amount. They fear the repercussions of going over the allotted dollar amount. Overspending is a bit more complex than just spending the dollar amount; other issues that contribute to overspending can be mitigated when the inventory management strategies discussed in this chapter are put into place. But the client and the patient are the ones that suffer when there is fear of overspending; the inventory manager may respond to doctor or client requests with "I can't order that this month, I am already over budget!"

When revenue has increased due to an increase in volume, so do inventory sales. Therefore, more money will need to be spent to replenish the supply. Along with looking at the historical perspective, consider the current revenue trend and manage 18%–20% of spend based on that.

Common reasons for going over budget:

- Inaccurate reorder points and quantities; too much product ordered at the wrong time
- Inaccurate turnover rate of a product; too much ordered that is no longer sellable/did not sell
- Bulk order placed with delayed billing
- Too many of the same products that accomplish the same thing (product consolidation)
- Employee theft
- Missed charge capture of products and services
- Inappropriate fees for services and inventory

Lessons learned from the pandemic can be applied to inventory management. A practice may have created a budget in 2020 based on 2019 numbers. Volume skyrocketed in veterinary medicine, and monthly budgets couldn't be maintained. Inventory managers had to order to keep drugs and supplies on the shelf to support revenue growth. Second, finding drugs and supplies during and post pandemic were and continue to be a challenge, and third, the prices associated with products and drugs have doubled, in some cases tripled. While most inventory managers increased prices on products when the order arrived and invoice counts were added to the PIMS, what didn't change was the price of services that use the supplies ordered on the inventory budget (suture, gauze, bandage material, etc.). The cost to deliver services dramatically increased, but the profitability of those services dropped. The result is the impact on the cost of goods sold to revenue ratio that is analyzed when reviewing practice profitability.

SAFETY DATA SHEETS

Safety data sheets (SDSs) (Chapter 15) are required for all chemical products that are sold or used within a veterinary practice. The Occupational Safety and Health Administration (OSHA) set forth standards for current practice relations. The Occupational Safety and Health Act of 1970 was enacted to ensure safe work environments for all employees. The law is based on the simple concept that all employees have the right to know about any potential hazard to which they may be exposed. Each SDS lists the potential hazards related to a substance and what protective measures can be taken if any hazard occurs.

It is the ultimate responsibility of the veterinary practice to ensure that SDSs are received every time a new product has been brought into the hospital. In addition, OSHA requires that each new SDS be posted in a highly visible area for all employees to read for 30 days before it is placed in the SDS binder. SDSs are available from either the manufacturer or the distributor, free of charge.

It is important when considering soft costs of inventoried items that the costs associated with creating and maintaining an SDS system be included.

CAPITAL INVENTORY

Capital inventory includes any equipment purchased throughout the life of the practice. Equipment includes items used to provide veterinary services, office equipment, printers, computers, filing cabinets, copy machines, etc. A running capital inventory list should be kept in a safe place and updated with any new equipment. A spreadsheet can be created that includes the equipment name, manufacturer, model number, serial number, purchase date, where the item was purchased from, and the purchase amount. If the building is vandalized or the equipment stolen, this information will be invaluable for the police report and insurance claims. Equipment purchase information is also important for tax purposes. This list is also handy when warranty information is needed. Fig. 13.27 is an example of an inventory list that has equipment purchased before the inventory manager's hire date. The cost and manufacturer of several pieces of equipment are unknown, but the fact that they are listed completes the inventory sheet.

DECREASING LOSS

A large amount of money is invested in inventory, and every effort should be made to decrease loss. Loss can occur through excess or inappropriate use of products to deliver services and inappropriate fee setting (both previously discussed), employee theft, and missed charges. Most practices don't "think" their practice is losing money, but one can't track what is not managed. Having a structured inventory system will significantly reduce loss, but even losing just 10% a year is a huge impact on raises, equipment purchases, building improvements, and overall profitability.

Employee theft can occur in a variety of ways (Chapter 16); employees can take product home with them, not charge themselves for services provided for their pet, or by giving away products to friends, aka clients, by altering the price. Ensure the PIMS security settings have been enabled, preventing anyone except the inventory manager, practice manager, or owner from altering prices. If a team member wants to give away a product, the product must be entered, then discounted. This allows the correct depletion of inventory counts, and tracks discounts being provided.

Product	Manufacture	Purchase Date/Price	Model Number	Serial Number
Anal Gland Excision Kit	Jorgenson		J-101	
Anesthesia Machine #1	Matrix		VMS	6380
Anesthesia Vaporizer #1	Cyprane LTD			300437
Anesthesia Machine #2	Matrix	24-12-2018		SN14989
Anesthesia Vaporizer #2	Vet Tech 4	12/24/18 $400.00 for both	100F	SN BASPOX7
Aspirator	Schuco Inc		130	49500008498
Autoclave	Tuttanauer	04/02/20, $2600.	2340M	2110582
Bird Scale	Pelouze		PE5	
Camera	HP	April 2023 $177.52	Photosmart 320	CN318111DG
Cast Cutter	Stryker		9002-210	8H8
Cautery Unit	Jorgenson		J313	
Centrifuge	Damon/IEC Division		MB	2513
Centrifuge	Stat-o-spin	3/14/20 $1026.83	V0901.22	607V90111962
Centrifuge (lab)	Vulcon Tech		C56C	6840
Clippers	DVM	12/15/21 91.00		
Clippers Cordless	Butler		78400-01A	
Clippers Cordless	Butler		78400-01A	
Clippers Cordless	Butler		78400-01A	
Credit Card Terminal				
Credit Card Terminal				SN 207-397-407
Copier			PC 940	NVX37080
Dental Machine	Delmarva			C028-647
Doppler, BP	Hadeco	11/2021, $800.00		SN-00090054
Doppler Probe	Jorgenson			
Doppler Ultra Sound			4070	
Dremel Unit	Craftsman		5 Speed	
ECG PAM	Technology Transfer	12/10/21, $2775.	VM8000	SN V04408
ECG Printer PAM	Technology Transfer	10-12-2000	930	1029
ECG Biolog	QRS Diagnostic	9/2021; $2735		2004-054237
ECG Printer Biolog		Came with Biolog	Brother HL-2070N	U61230M5J5
Glucometer	Walgreens			RHW4E23Ft
Home Again Scanner	Schering Plough			SN 070535
Hair Dryer				
ECG Surgery	KENZ	GW Gift		9509-2815
IDEXX Electrolytes	IDEXX	Aug. 2020		U15.9976
IDEXX Procyte	IDEXX	June 2021;	93-30002-01	DXBP005586
IDEXX Server			PCNE	H1BFQ91
IDEXX Printer			HP Deskjet 5650	MY45F4NOHI

Fig. 13.27 Sample capital inventory spreadsheet.

Both paper medical record practices and those with paper-light electronic medical records (EMRs) have found that travel sheets are an excellent way to decrease missed charges (Fig. 13.28). A travel sheet lists the most common procedures provided and products carried out in the practice. The travel sheet is attached to the medical record and travels with it throughout the day (or in the case of (EMRs), travels with the patient). When a service is performed, the procedure is then circled or highlighted on the sheet (Fig. 13.29). In multiple-doctor practices, it is advisable to use a specific-colored highlighter for each veterinarian. The receptionist can then be sure to add charges under that specific doctor (this is imperative when veterinarians are paid on production). When the medical record is complete, the receptionist can enter the charges and double-check the record against the travel sheet, looking for any missed charges.

For those who wish to save paper, travel sheets can be laminated and reused. Simply place them in a pile and clean them at the end of the day.

In a recent study, 40% of cases evaluated had missed charges, resulting in an average of $50 per case difference for inpatients, and $23.33 for outpatient services (Well Managed Practice Benchmarks 2017). Fecal smears, heartworm tests, and nail trims are often forgotten. Practices should audit a minimum of 20 records (per day) as a review for lost charges. Almost every record will have at least one item that was not charged. It is imperative to implement procedures to help control loss through missed charges (see Chapters 8, 9, and 14 for additional supporting details).

LEADERSHIP'S ROLE IN INVENTORY MANAGEMENT

Inventory management is a task that can empower a responsible team member, allowing the practice manager to focus on leading the team while the owner veterinarian sees clients and patients. However, that does not remove the responsibility of the practices' largest asset away from either role. Overall, the PM and owner are responsible for inventory; therefore, developing a team member to lead it (and implemented all points included in this chapter) successfully is critical.

PMs and owners must track monthly KPIs (and investigate questionable results immediately), reconcile invoices monthly into the appropriate chart of accounts, oversee spot and cycle counts, develop, manage, and promote the online pharmacy, and oversee capital equipment.

If KPIs are not being met, the PM must meet with the inventory manager and identify what factors may be misaligned (pricing, markup, client discounts, giving products away, embezzlement, etc.) and create goals for the inventory manager to achieve.

Client Number______________ Client Name____________________Pet___________Doctor________

DISCOUNTS	GROOMING	LAB SERVICES	LAB SERVICES
0107 Monthly Special	0506 Beak Trim- Small	3505 ACTH Stim	3821 T-4 Equilibrum Dialysis
0108 Senior Wellness	0508 Beak Trim- Large	3515 Automimmune Profile	3820 T-4 Dogs
Senior Citizen	0510 Nail Trim	3520 Avian Comp Profile	3822 T-4 Cats
	0512 Nail Trim- Exotic	3526 Avian Post Purchase	3830 Tick Born Dz Panal
OFFICE CALL	0514 Wing Trim- Small	3535 Bile Acids	4141 Tonopen
0214 Brief Office Call	0516 Wing Trim- Large	3611 BIPS	3850 Urinalysis- In house
0216 Regular Office Call	0520 Trim Teeth	3621 Blood Pressure	3855 Urinalysis-Lab
0219 Well K-9/Fe Exam	0518 Pluck ears	3560 CBC/Diff	3880 Urinalysis-SG
0222 Exotics Exam-Reg	0502 Medicated Bath	3580 Coagulation Profile	3854 Urinalysis Sediment
0220 Exotics Exam-Brief	0501 Shave Cat	3770 Chemistry #1	3853 Urinalysis-Stick
226 Exam w/ vaccines		3775 Chemistry >2	3852 Urinalysis- Yearly Exam
0228 Pre-Op Exam	**DENTAL**	3590 Culture and Sensitivity	3860 Vaginal Smear
0232 Recheck N/C	0702 Sm Normal Prophy	3605 Cytology In house	**CLINICAL PROCEDURES**
0234 Recheck	0704 Lg Normal Prophy	3593 Cytology-Lab	4005 Abdominocentesis
0109 Health Certificate	0701 Feline Normal Prophy	3610 DTM	4010 Anal Sac Expression
0106 Int'l Health Certificate	0706 Severe Periodontal Dz	3615 Ear Mite Check	4015 Anal Sac recheck
0104 Duplicate Rabies Tag	0710 Follow-Up	3620 Ear Smear	4020 Artifical Insemination
	0714 Tooth Ext. Minimum	3631 Electrolytes	4025 Bandage Wound Sm
FELINE VACCINES	0716 Tooth Ext. Moderate	3603 EKG	4030 Bandage Wound Med
0608 FVRCP Booster	0718 Tooth Ext. Extensive	3626 EKG >1 per day	4035 Bandage Wound Lg
0612 FVRCP 1 year	0712 Dental Sutures	3628 EKG Senior Wellness	3085 Cast
0609 FVRCP 3 year		3630 EKG Repeat	4050 Clean Ears
0613 FELV Booster	**HOSPITALIZATION**	3641 Ehrlicia Canis PCR	4055 Clip/Clean Wound Sm
0610 FELV 1 year	0902 Board-Canine	3655 Fecal-Direct	4060 Clip/Clean Wound Med
0611 FVRCP/FELV	0904 Board-Feline	3660 Fecal Flotation/Smear	4065 Clip/Clean Wound Lg
0607 Rabies **Only** Fe -1 yr	0903 Overnight Board, Sx	3665 Fecal- Recheck	4070 Corneal Stain (1)
0618 Rabies Feline 1 year	0906 Day Board/Obsvtn	3675 FELV Snap Test	4071 Corneal Stain (2)
0605 Feline Yearly Exam	907 Hospital Day	3685 FELV/FIV Snap Test	4080 Enema
0621 Feline Sr Wellness	0908 Hospital Overnight	4081 Fine Needle Aspirate	4083 Flush Anal Glands
	909 Hospital Day w/ IV	3695 Fungal Serology	4085 Flush ears (1)
PET WEIGHT__________	0910 Hospital Weekend	3815 General Health Profile	4090 Flush ears (2)
	0912 Hospital Exotic	3710 Heartworm SNAP	4095 Flush Nasal Duct
CANINE VACCINES	911 O2 Therepy Half Day	3715 Heartworm Difil	4105 Home Again Implant
0603 Parvo	0914 O2 Therepy Full Day	3705 HCT/TP	4110 Pass Stomach Tube
0615 Bordetella	0916 IV Care Daily	3720 Histopath	4130 Semen Collection/Eval
0616 DHPP Booster	0918 IV Care Intensive	3725 Histopath Additional	7002 Splint-Small
0602 DHPP 1 year	0920 IV Catheter	3730 Histopath Derm	5126 Re-Splint Small
0617 DHPP 3 year	0922 IV Catheter, 2nd	3731 Histopath-Bone Decal	7001 Splint-Medium
0604 Rabies Canine 1 year	0924 IV Fluids per Liter	3527 Mammalian Comp Prof	5131 Re-Splint Medium
0601 Rabies 3 year	0926 IV Fluids One time	0438 Necropsy In house	7000 Splint-Large
0690 Canine Yearly Exam	0928 Fluid Additives	0436 Necropsy NMDL	5136 Re-Splint-Large
0620 Canine Sr Wellness	0925 IV Fluids Hetastarch	0441 Necropsy Avian-NMDL	4140 Thoracocentesis
0606 Rattlesnake Vaccine	0930 SQ Fluids Once	3745 Parvovirus Snap Test	4145 Transtracheal Wash
0619 Lepto	0932 SQ Fluids Per Day	3750 Phenobarb Levels	4150 Urinary Catheter
	0934 SQ Fluids Exotic	3749 Platelet Count	
ANESTHESIA	0936 SQ Fluids Disp.	3601 Pre-Op EKG	**EUTHANASIA**
0302 Anesthesia	938 SQ Fluids No Tech/Dr.	3755 Pre-Op Profile	WT_____
0304 Extended		3785 Reptile Std. Profile	Dog_____ Cat_____
0306 Short	**RADIOLOGY**	3786 Reptile Comp Profile	Mass Cremation
0308 Local	4125 Radiographs	3795 Schirmer Tear Test	Private Cremation
0310 Tranquilization	4126 Radiographs-dental	3805 Skin Scrape	402 Exotic
0316 Geriatric Anesthesia			
SURGICAL PROCEDURES	4405 Feline Neuter	**CONSULTS**	**INJECTIONS**
4205 Abcess Debride	4410 Feline Neuter/Declaw	202 Cardiology	
4210 Amputate Limb Sm	4420 Feline OVH	213 Repeat EKG	**# of ML________**
4215 Amputate Limb Lg	4425 Feline OVH In heat	204 Internal Medicine	
4220 Amputate Digit	4430 Feline OVH Pregnant	206 Miscellaneous	1220 Amiglyde #1
4225 Amputate Tail	4435 Feline OVH Declaw	208 OFA	1225 Amiglyde >1
4235 Ant. Cruc. Repair	4441 FHO Feline	210 Radiology	1256 Baytril 100mg/ml
4240 Aural Hematoma-K-9	4442 FHO Canine	212 Shipping	1255 Baytril 22.7mg/ml
4341 Aural Hematome-Fe	4455 Growth Removal SM		1265 Cephazolin
4245 Biopsy - Wedge	4460 Growth Removal MED	**HEARTWORM MEDICATION**	1270 Cephazolin >1
4250 Biopsy - Punch	4465 Growth Removal LG	HG Small #________	1281 Cortrosyn
4246 Biopsy - Bone	4470 Growth Removal >1	HG Medium #________	1289 Dexameth 2mg/ml
4260 C-Section	4480 Hernia Repair Inguinal	HG Large #________	1290 Dexameth 4mg/ml
4265 C-Section w/ OVH	4485 Hernia Repair Abdom	HG Feline 0-5# #6	1305 Diphenhydramine
4270 Canine Neuter <50	4490 Hernia Repair Diaphm.	HG Feline 5-15# #6	Ivomec
4275 Canine Neuter >50	4495 Hernia Repair Umbil.		1335 Immiticide
4285 Canine OVH <50	4505 Patellar Luxation #1	Revolution Feline	1390 Methyl Pred Acetate
4290 Canine OVH 50-99	4510 Patellar Luxation #2	Revolution Canine	1410 Pred Acetate
4272 Canine OVH >100	4511 Prostatic Wash		1417 Solu-delta Cortef 100mg
4295 Canine OVH/Heat	4515 Puppy Dewclaws Each	Frontline Feline	1418 Solu-delta Cortef 500mg
4305 Canine OVH/Preg	4520 Puppy Tail Docks Each	Frontline Canine	1430 Torbugesic
4236 Cranial Cruc. SM (1)	4525 Pyometra w/ OVH	Frontline In Hosp Use	
4238 Cranial Cruc. LG (1)	4530 Rabbit Neuter		**E-COLLAR**
4237 Cranial Cruc. SM (2)	4535 Rabbit OVH	**POST OP PAIN MEDS**	
4239 Cranial Cruc. LG (2)	4540 Staple Wound per staple	Rimadyl 25mg	**N/C ITEMS**
4315 Cherry Eye Repair 1	4545 Stenotic Nares Repair	Rimadyl 75mg	818 HG SM
4320 Cherry Eye Repair 2	4550 Suture Wound SM	Rimadyl 100mg	822 HG M
4325 Cryptorchid Fe-Flank	4555 Suture Wound MED	Metacam	826 HG LG
4330 Cryptorchid Fe-Abdm	4560 Suture Wound LG	Buprinex	2790 Strongid
4345 Cryptorchid K-9 Abdm	4575 Third Eyelid Flap	Tramadol	510 Nail Trim
4340 Cryptorchid K-9 Flank			
4350 Cystotomy			
4355 Debride wound			
4360 Declaw/Tendonectomy			
4365 Dewclaw Unjointed #1			
4370 Declaw Jointed #1			
4375 Drain Placement			
4385 Entropion per lid			
4390 Exploratory			
4395 Eye Enucleation			

Fig. 13.28 Sample of an outpatient travel sheet.

CLIENTS LAST NAME: ____________________ **WORKING DIAGNOSIS:** __________

PET NAME ____________________ **PRIMARYDOCTOR** ____________________

DATE:	8AM	9	10	11	12	1	2	3	4	5	6	7	8
FEED													
WATER													
WALK/LITTER													
TEMPERATURE													
WEIGHT													
APPETITE?													
ATTITUDE?													
URINE?													
BM OR DIARRHEA													
VOMIT?													

OFFICE CALL
0214 Brief Office Call
0216 Regular Office Call
0222 Exotics Exam-Reg
0220 Exotics Exam-Brief
0232 Recheck N/C
0234 Recheck

FELINE VACCINES
0608 FVRCP Booster
0612 FVRCP 1 year
0609 FVRCP 3 year
0613 FELV Booster
0610 FELV 1 year
0611 FVRCP/FELV
0618 Rabies Feline 1 year
0605 Feline Yearly Exam
0621 Feline Sr Wellness

CANINE VACCINES
0603 Parvo
0615 Bordetella
0616 DHPP Booster
0602 DHPP 1 year
0617 DHPP 3 year
0604 Rabies Canine 1 year
0601 Rabies 3 year
0690 Canine Yearly Exam
0620 Canine Sr Wellness
0606 Rattlesnake Vaccine
0619 Lepto

HOSPITALIZATION
0902 Board-Canine
0904 Board-Feline
0903 Overnight Board, Sx
0906 Day Board/Obsvtn
907 Hospital Day
0908 Hospital Overnight
909 Hospital Day w/ IV
0910 Hospital Weekend
0912 Hospital Exotic
911 Oxygen Therepy Half Day
0914 0xygen Therepy Full Day
0916 IV Care Daily
0918 IV Care Intensive
0920 IV Catheter
0922 IV Catheter, 2nd
0924 IV Fluids per Liter
0926 IV Fluids One time
0928 Fluid Additives
0925 IV Fluids Hetastarch
0930 SQ Fluids Once
0932 SQ Fluids Per Day
0934 SQ Fluids Exotic
0936 SQ Fluids Disp.

RADIOLOGY
4125 Radiographs

CONSULTS
202 Cardiology
213 Repeat EKG
204 Internal Medicine
210 Radiology

LAB SERVICES
3611 BIPS
3621 Blood Pressure
3560 CBC/Diff
3770 Chemistry #1
3775 Chemistry >2
3590 Culture and Sensitivity
3605 Cytology In house
3610 DTM
3615 Ear Mite Check
3620 Ear Smear
3631 Electrolytes
3603 EKG
3626 EKG >1 per day
3655 Fecal-Direct
3660 Fecal Flotation/Smear
3675 FELV Snap Test
3685 FELV/FIV Snap Test
4081 Fine Needle Aspirate
3815 General Health Profile
3710 Heartworm SNAP
3705 HCT/TP
3745 Parvovirus Snap Test
3750 Phenobarb Levels
3601 Pre-Op EKG
3755 Pre-Op Profile
3795 Schirmer Tear Test
3805 Skin Scrape
0000 T-4

LAB SERVICES
0000 Urinalysis
3860 Vaginal Smear

CLINICAL PROCEDURES
4005 Abdominocentesis
4010 Anal Sac Expression
0000 Bandage Wound
3085 Cast
4050 Clean Ears
4055 Clip/Clean Wound Sm
4060 Clip/Clean Wound Med
4065 Clip/Clean Wound Lg
4070 Corneal Stain (1)
4071 Corneal Stain (2)
4080 Enema
4083 Flush Anal Glands
4085 Flush ears (1)
4090 Flush ears (2)
4110 Pass Stomach Tube
7002 Splint-Small
5126 Re-Splint Small
7001 Splint-Medium
5131 Re-Splint Medium
7000 Splint-Large
5136 Re-Splint-Large
4140 Thoracocentesis
4145 Transtracheal Wash
4150 Urinary Catheter

E-COLLAR

Fig. 13.29 Sample of an inpatient travel sheet.

PRACTICE MANAGERS SURVIVAL CHECKLIST FOR INVENTORY MANAGEMENT

- ☐ Develop/update job description for inventory manager.
- ☐ Develop/update performance expectations for inventory manager.
- ☐ Develop/maintain inventory budget.
- ☐ Compare income to expense and benchmark against industry standards.
- ☐ Train staff on proper inventory maintenance protocol.
- ☐ Develop/maintain inventory procedural manual.
- ☐ Determine turnover rates, reorder points, and reorder quantities for all products.

- ☐ Consolidate products, maintaining one primary product and one backup product for each category.
- ☐ Develop a procedure for expired products (sealed and unsealed).
- ☐ Develop a procedure to return goods to the manufacturer/ distributor for credit.
- ☐ Develop ordering, receiving, and stocking procedures.
- ☐ Develop procedures for special orders.
- ☐ Develop protocol to enter invoices upon receiving of product and update pricing.
- ☐ Determine/update dispensing and labeling fees.
- ☐ Develop bulk purchasing policy.
- ☐ Implement and maintain cycle counts and year-end inventory.
- ☐ Implement discrepancy/variance procedures.
- ☐ Maintain equipment inventory spreadsheet (including purchase date, price, warranty details, and serial model number).
- ☐ Develop online store protocol, including developing, updating, managing, and promoting.
- ☐ Develop a set time to allow inventory managers to place orders and maintain the inventory system effectively.

REVIEW QUESTIONS

1. Why should the inventory manager see distributor and manufacturer representatives?
2. What is the goal of an inventory system?
3. Why should a "want list" be developed?
4. What is an order book?
5. What is an SDS?
6. What is capital inventory?
7. What does an inventory manager do with expired medications?
8. What minimum percentage should products be marked up to break even?
9. What are some losses associated with poor inventory control?
10. How many times should inventory be turned over per year?
11. Improving profits in the primacy revenue center can be accomplished by:
    - **a.** Determining and using effective turnover rates
    - **b.** Determining and using effective reorder points
    - **c.** Determining and using effective reorder quantities
    - **d.** All the above
    - **e.** None of the above
12. Price shopping for inventory items is a cost-effective method to reduce cost of goods.
    - **a.** True
    - **b.** False
13. To help reduce soft costs, orders for top-producing items should be placed:
    - **a.** Weekly
    - **b.** Semimonthly
    - **c.** Monthly
    - **d.** As needed
14. Consolidating inventory reduces profits.
    - **a.** True
    - **b.** False
15. To calculate the *least* cost that can be charged, a practice must determine:
    - **a.** Turnover rate
    - **b.** Break-even cost
    - **c.** Markup
    - **d.** Soft cost

REFERENCES

1. Tumblin D., et al. *Well managed practice benchmarks*, 2019. Accessed August 20 22. https://www.wmpb.vet.

RECOMMENDED READING

Heinke MM. *Practice made perfect: a guide to veterinary practice management.*. 2nd ed. AAHA Press; 2012.

14

Controlled Substances

LEARNING OBJECTIVES

When you have completed this chapter, you should be able to:

- Define controlled substances
- Identify drugs available for use in the veterinary practice
- Explain the importance of logging all drugs used
- Discuss the importance of managing controlled substances
- Discuss methods used to inventory controlled substances
- Describe methods used to order controlled substances for a veterinary practice
- Identify appropriate documents to order Schedule II drugs
- List the process used to report the loss of controlled substances

OUTLINE

KEY TERMS

Controlled Substance
Controlled Substances Act
DEA Form 222
Schedule II
Schedule III
Schedule IV
Schedule V
U.S. Drug Enforcement Administration (DEA)

VHMA PERFORMANCE DOMAINS

Veterinary Hospital Managers Association (VHMA) Performance Domains

The performance domain applicable to controlled substances is the organization of the practice. Practice managers are responsible for maintenance of medical record systems and inventory controls including controlled substance ordering, tracking, security, and destruction.

Application of VHMA Performance Domains for Practice Managers

The tasks in this domain require a working knowledge of veterinary medical terminology, requirements for common veterinary practice procedures (treatment and surgical protocols), and regulatory compliance.

INTRODUCTION

Controlled substances are drugs with a high abuse potential that must be regulated to help prevent abuse. Controlled substances are labeled with the letter "C" and a Roman numeral indicating the applicable schedule (Fig. 14.1). The Controlled Substances Act of 1970 was passed to reduce drug abuse by restricting certain substances with a high abuse potential. The act was established and is controlled by the U.S. Drug Enforcement Administration (DEA) and provides approved means for proper manufacturing, distribution, dispensing, and use through licensed handlers.

SCHEDULES OF DRUGS

A controlled substance (CS) will have a "C" clearly marked on the bottle, with a notation next to it indicating what schedule that drug is in. Drugs are classified into five schedules according to their abuse potential. CSs include opiates (narcotics); barbiturates; hallucinogens (e.g., ketamine); amphetamines; and other addictive and habituating drugs. Class I drugs have the highest abuse potential; therefore, medical use of these substances is not legal in the United States. Drugs such as lysergic acid diethylamide (LSD) and heroin are examples of CSs in Class I. Class II drugs produce severe psychological and physical dependencies and include drugs such as morphine, oxymorphone, and pentobarbital. Table 14.1 lists drugs and their schedules.

Individual states can also place drugs on the CS list. For example, phenylpropanolamine may be classified as controlled in some states and not others.

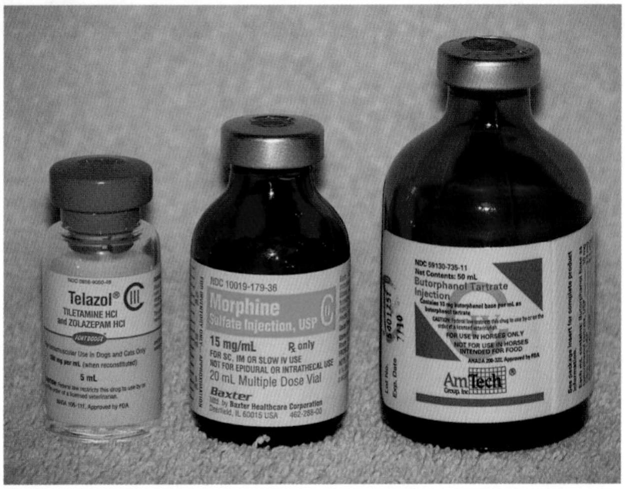

Fig. 14.1 Controlled substances are labeled with a "C" and a Roman numeral.

LEADERSHIP POINT

Any pharmaceutical with a "C" on the label is considered a controlled substance.

If veterinarians write CS prescriptions for clients, a pharmacy can only fill a 30-day supply for classes III, IV, or V. Those prescriptions can have five refills available within 6 months, at which time a new prescription must be submitted to the pharmacy. Class II drugs can only be filled for 30 days and must have a new prescription submitted every 30 days; no refills are allowed on the original script (Table 14.2).

The DEA supplies veterinarians with Form 222 to order Class II drugs, which, once completed, is then submitted to manufacturers or distributors to place orders for Schedule II drugs. Morphine, oxymorphone, and hydrocodone are examples of drugs that require DEA Form 222. As of October 2021, triplicate 222 forms are no longer valid and have been replaced with single-page forms. Veterinary practices can also sign up for electronic or digital certificates (CSOS) to order Schedule II drugs from their distributor. The CSOS program allows for secure electronic CS orders to be placed without the DEA 222 form. Each purchaser must enroll with the DEA to acquire a CSOS digital certificate. DEA practitioners that are enrolled in the CSOS program can:

- Order all classes of controlled substances online
- Order just in time, as distributors can easily verify information
- Reduce the number of ordering errors
- Increase the accuracy of orders and decrease paperwork

The CSOS Registration Authority requires a photocopy of a letter granting Power of Attorney (PoA) for all applicants requesting a CSOS Signing Certificate. The letter must include the name and address of the practice, the DEA registration number for which the PoA is being granted, a brief statement expressing that the PoA for CS is being granted to the attorney-in-fact by an authorized party, the name and signature of the PoA, name and signature of the granting PoA, the signatures of two witnesses, and the date that the PoA is granted (Fig. 14.2). A PoA can be rescinded at any time.[1]

TABLE 14.1 Federal Controlled Substance Schedule.

Schedule	Abuse Potential	Dispensing Limits	Restrictions	Examples
I	Highest	Research only	DEA Form 222 required	LSD, heroin
II	High	Written prescription, no refills	DEA Form 222 required	Oxymorphone, morphine, pentobarbital, fentanyl, Hycodan, hydromorphone, methadone, oxycodone
III	Less than II	Written prescription; can refill five times	DEA number	buprenorphine, ketamine, Telazol, anabolic steroids
IV	Low	Written prescription; can refill five times	DEA number	Diazepam, phenobarbital, alprazolam, lorazepam, midazolam
V	Low	No DEA limits	DEA number	Lomotil, Robitussin AC

TABLE 14.2 Summary of Controlled Substances Act Requirements.

	Schedule II	Schedule III and IV	Schedule V
Registration	Required	Required	Required
Receiving records	Order forms (DEA Form 222)	Invoices, readily retrievable	Invoices, readily retrievable
Prescriptions	Written prescriptions (see exceptions[a])	Written, oral, or fax	Written, oral, fax, or over the counter[b]
Refills	No	No more than 5 within 6 months	As authorized when prescription is issued
Distribution between registrants	Order forms (DEA Form 222)	Invoices	Invoices
Security	Locked cabinet or other secure storage	Locked cabinet or other secure storage	Locked cabinet or other secure storage
Theft or significant loss	Report and complete DEA Form 106	Report and complete DEA Form 106	Report and complete DEA Form 106

Note: All records must be maintained for 2 years unless the state requires a longer period.
Exceptions: A facsimile prescription serves as the original prescription when issued to residents of long-term care facilities, hospice patients, or compounded IV narcotic medications.
[a]Emergency prescriptions require a signed follow-up prescription.
[b]Where authorized by state-controlled substances authority.

Power of Attorney for DEA Forms 222 and Electronic Orders

(Name of registrant) ________________________________

(Address of registrant) ________________________________

____

(DEA registration number) ________________________________

I, ________________________ (name of person granting power), the undersigned, who am authorized to sign the current application for registration of the above-named registrant under the Controlled Substances Act or Controlled Substances Import and Export Act, have made, constituted, and appointed, and by these presents, do make, constitute, and appoint ________________________ (name of attorney-in-fact), my true and lawful attorney for me in my name, place, and stead, to execute applications for Forms 222 and to sign orders for Schedule I and II controlled substances, whether these orders be on Form 222 or electronic, in accordance with 21 U.S.C. 828 and Part 1305 of Title 21 of the Code of Federal Regulations. I hereby ratify and confirm all that said attorney must lawfully do or cause to be done by virtue hereof.

__________________________(Signature of person granting power)

I, ________________________ (name of attorney-in-fact), hereby affirm that I am the person named herein as attorney-in-fact and that the signature affixed hereto is my signature.

__________________________(Signature of attorney-in-fact)

Witnesses:

1. __________________________ (Signature of witness)

2. __________________________ (Signature of witness)

Signed and dated on __________________________ (current date).

Notice of Revocation – to be completed only when Power of Attorney is revoked

The foregoing power of attorney is hereby revoked by the undersigned, who is authorized to sign the current application for registration of the above-named registrant under the Controlled Substances Act or the Controlled Substances Import and Export Act. Written notice of this revocation has been given to the attorney-in-fact _________ this same day.

__________________________ (Signature of person revoking power)

Witnesses:

1. __________________________ (Signature of witness)

2. __________________________ (Signature of witness)

Signed and dated on __________________________ (current date).

Fig. 14.2 Example of a Power of Attorney as required by the DEA.

CRITICAL COMPETENCY: ADAPTABILITY

Practice managers must be open to change and flexible work methods and can adapt behavior to changing conditions or new information.

Paper or electronic forms must be filled out without error in the drug name, strength, or quantity. Any errors may void the form, and the distributor or manufacturer will be unable to fulfill the order. The signature and license must match those on file, or the order will be denied. Just as the DEA and State Board of Pharmacy are strict with veterinarians, they are just as strict (if not more so) with distributors and manufacturers.

Paper 222 forms must be secured and accounted for. Each form has a number associated with it, and any missing forms must be reported to the DEA field office ASAP.

Five areas must be focused on when managing CSs: registration, security and protection, record keeping, reporting of losses, and substance disposal.

VHMA PERFORMANCE DOMAIN TASK

Veterinary practice managers maintain appropriate inventory systems including controlled substance ordering, tracking, security, and destruction.

REGISTRATION

All veterinarians are required to have a DEA license to purchase or write prescriptions for CSs. Associate veterinarians are allowed to dispense a product from the hospital inventory without a DEA license (depending on the state). Some states require that veterinarians also hold a secondary CS state license to be able to prescribe CS. Therefore, DVMs that reside in those states must have both the DEA and state CS licenses.

The complication lies in the fact that the DEA allows an associate veterinarian to dispense, but not prescribe, a CS. If a patient of an associate veterinarian needs a prescription for phenobarbital to be filled at a local pharmacy, the owner DVM (or DEA licensee) must write the script for the patient. However, a valid patient relationship may not exist with this client. Therefore, it is advised that all DVMs within the practice register for a DEA license to prevent these issues from arising.

The owner of the practice can order CSs to be kept in the hospital and is responsible for protecting and accounting for all drugs dispensed. If any discrepancy occurs, the owner is held accountable and can have their DEA license revoked by the DEA as well as the state. To monitor inventory closely, it is critical that all drugs are accounted for on a frequent basis. More details are provided in the record-keeping section of this chapter.

Veterinarians are required to submit Form 224 to the DEA for the application for a Controlled Substance License. Form 223 is then issued to the veterinarian and must be posted within the facility, easily accessible, and available for inspection at any time. Form 224a must be submitted every 3 years to renew the CS license.

Some states also have a prescription monitoring plan, in which drugs dispensed must be immediately reported to the state pharmacy board. Each state varies in its requirements and procedures; visit the appropriate state board of pharmacy for more details.

SECURITY AND PROTECTION

The DEA is stringent on the regulations that practices must follow to keep drugs safe and secure.

VHMA PRACTICE DOMAIN TASK

Veterinary practice managers must understand and ensure compliance with the DEA and state and local agencies.

Employers are required to take "reasonable guard" when hiring new team members. The first part of this requirement relates to personnel with access to the drugs. Employees should undergo background checks and drug testing before employment. Practices may also wish to implement a drug-free workplace, in which random drug tests are completed on all employees. This helps the practice take reasonable guard from hiring and employing risky people.

Team members that have access to the CSs (this should be limited to a few) must be held accountable. Signature cards should be kept on file for those removing and logging drugs (allowing a comparison of signatures if ever needed).

LEADERSHIP POINT

Employers are required to take reasonable guard when hiring new team members.

All CSs that are kept in the facility must be kept in a securely locked, substantially constructed cabinet or safe. The cabinet or safe must be securely bolted to the wall or floor. If the safe weighs more than 750 lbs, it can be excluded from being bolted to the floor.

Drugs in active use can be placed in a less substantially locked cabinet (hospital cabinetry) during open hours. However, these drugs must be placed back into the substantially locked cabinet at night.

Within the safe, Schedule II drugs must be kept separate from drugs classified as Schedule III, IV, or V. This separation can be a shelf or placement in a box.

RECORD KEEPING

The DEA can inspect records, invoices, inventory, and facilities that house CSs at any time. State agencies, such as the Board of Veterinary Medicine or the Board of Pharmacy, may also inspect at any time and may have stricter rules and regulations than the DEA. The agency that has more stringent regulations takes precedence. Records and invoices must be kept for a minimum of 2 years (after the date of use) for any agency to inspect.

Logs for CSs must be kept in a separate location from the drugs themselves (i.e., logs should not be placed in the safe with the drugs). In addition, Schedule II drug logs and invoices must be kept separate from Schedule III, IV, or V drug logs and invoices.

Practices that are accredited by the American Animal Hospital Association (AAHA) must use bound logs; however, the DEA will accept logs kept in binders.

Drug Logs Must Include the Following Information:

- Client name
- Client address
- Patient name
- Reason of use
- Amount of drug administered
- Inventory of drug after use
- Initials

Inventory Logs Must Include:

- Product name, strength, and count in a full bottle
- Date of purchase
- Name and address of vendor
- Date and time of inventory

- Log quantity
- Physical quantity
- Any discrepancies found
- Initials

CRITICAL COMPETENCY: COMPLIANCE

Practice managers must be reliable, thorough, and conscientious in carrying out work assignments while having an appreciation for the importance of organizational rules and policies.

According to the DEA, drug logs can be maintained on the computer, in association with practice management software. The question lies in the confidence of the reporting should the practice be audited. Consider staging an unannounced audit of the CS logs. Print all reports and count the drugs on hand. Do they match? Can the practice account for all drugs that have been purchased, administered, or dispensed during the selected audit period? Do the reports contain all the required information? If there were any questions, it would be advisable to continue maintaining paper logs until the issues can be resolved.

MANAGEMENT OF CONTROLLED SUBSTANCES

An initial inventory must be taken when the business opens, and then taken biennially thereafter (be sure to verify state requirements, which may supersede biennial inventory). However, when considering the potential losses that can (and do) occur in this area of the practice, biennial inventory is not sufficient. Practices should be able to balance their drug counts and account for every pill and milliliter of controlled substances at any time, and therefore weekly inventory may be required. If managers feel their CS logs are consistently accurate, this inventory may only need to be performed monthly. A closing inventory must also be taken if the business closes permanently.

LEADERSHIP POINT

It is advisable for practices to complete a controlled substance inventory monthly (at minimum). If the logs do not balance, increase counts to weekly until discrepancies are resolved.

Anytime a physical inventory is taken, the following information should be documented:

- Drug (name of product, strength, and number of milliliters or tablets that come in a full bottle)
- Physical count of drug
- Name of person completing the inventory
- Time of day the inventory was completed

The inventory time of day is important; if the DEA completes an audit of the facility drugs, they need to know whether drugs that were used the day of the inventory should be included in the audit.

Drugs must be balanced on a perpetual inventory balance system; this provides a running balance that can be compared with the physical inventory at any time.

A folder should be kept separate from the CS logbook to house all invoices that list controlled drugs that have been received by the clinic. Drug listings should be highlighted on the invoice, along with the assigned bottle numbers. A stock supply sheet, or closed bottle sheet, can help keep track of bottle numbers.

Fig. 14.3 shows that 12 bottles of Telazol were received on August 4, 2022. Initially, there were no bottles available for use. Once the 12 bottles were added, the initial amount became 12 bottles. The bottles were then assigned numbers 100 through 112; these were the next numbers in the sequence (99 bottles had been previously used). The stock supply list states that two team members checked out the bottles to the surgical plane on August 5th, 8th, and 10th.

Each time bottles are checked out, they must be recorded on this list and initialed by the team member removing the bottle. A form of this nature holds team members accountable and simplifies drug tracking.

Fig. 14.4 is an example of a running drug log. Notice that the bottle number, date, time, client name, patient name, initial amount, the amount used, and balance are all required entries. Each bottle should be fully accounted for before opening another bottle.

Ketamine is the drug being logged in Fig. 14.4. The initial amount and bottle number are on line 1, along with the owner's information and the amount of drug used. Each milliliter is accounted for before opening the next bottle. Bottles 1 and 3 balance well. Obviously, bottle 2 is missing 0.7 mL, which is almost 10% of the bottle. This amount of drug must be searched for; surgical records should be reviewed, and team members questioned regarding who may have pulled the drug without writing the information down. If the missing drug cannot be found, management must consider inside theft. This information must be logged and highlighted so that it may be reported as a discrepancy on the annual CS physical inventory list.

CRITICAL COMPETENCY: ANALYTICAL SKILLS

The practice manager must have the ability to grasp complex information, analyze information and use logic to address problems accurately, quickly, and efficiently.

Stock Supply List; Veterinary Controlled Substances

Date	Time	To/From	Bottle #	Initial Amount	Amt Change	Balance	Initials
04-Aug	2:00pm	DVM Res	100-112	0 Bottles	12 Bottles	12 Bottles	CS
05-Aug	8am	Sx Plain	100	12	1	11	NS
08-Aug	10:40am	Sx Plain	101	11	1	10	CS
10-Aug	2:00pm	Sx Plain	102	10	1	9	CS
				9			

Year 2022 Name of Drug: Telazol 100mg/ml, 5ml

Fig. 14.3 Sample stock supply sheet.

Veterinary Controlled Drug Log

Bottle #	Date	Time	Owners Name	Client Address	Animal Name	Initial Amount	Amt Used	Balance	Initials
1	04-Aug	8:00am	Slatery	2456 Saturn, LC	Waldo	10ml	3	7	CS
	04-Aug	8:00am	garcia	451 MacArthur, LC	Baby	7	0.5	6.5	NS
	04-Aug	8:15am	Jones	POB 1322, T or C, NM	Prancer	6.5	1	5.5	CS
	04-Aug	8:15am	Loving	9885 Saley, LC	Tootsie	5.5	0.8	4.7	CS
	05-Aug	8:15am	Pinto	134 Tres Seca, LC	Wonder	4.7	0.4	4.3	NS
	05-Aug	9:15am	Adams	14 Adams Dr, Vado, NM	Wendy	4.3	2	2.3	NS
	05-Aug	9:30am	Howard	657 Elm St, LC	Bobo	2.3	0.3	2	NS
	06-Aug	8:15am	Bush	8573 Chickory, LC	Tristen	2	2	0	CS
2	07-Aug	8:00am	Evans	30865 Stanton Dr, LC	Ashley	10	0.6	9.4	NS
	07-Aug	8:00am	Langford	POB 352, Hatch, NM	Bobby	9.4	0.7	8.7	CS
	07-Aug	8:15am	Smith	9038 Red Hawk, LC	Capser	8.7	6	2.7	CS
	08-Aug	8:15am	Howard	Rt 2 Bx 44, T or C, NM	Wimpy	2.7	2	0.7	NS
			MIA		MIA		0.7	0	CS
3	08-Aug	9:30am	Brown	34 Evelyn St, LC	Blackie	10	1	9	NS
	09-Aug	8:15am	Hyatt	465 Elder St, Mesquite	Lawrence	9	2	7	CS
	09-Aug	8:30am	Ralph	9809 Western Dr, LC	Ariel	7	2.5	4.5	CS
	09-Aug	9:00am	Jameson	920 Riley Blvd, LC	Taylor	4.5	0.5	4	HP
	09-Aug	10:15am	Lee	23 Zeplin Rd, LC	Wheeler	4	1	3	HP
	09-Aug	10:30am	West	56 Kane Dr, Anthony, NM	Katie	3	3	0	SM

Year 2022 Ketamine 100mg/ml, 10ml

Fig. 14.4 Sample running drug log.

Annual Controlled Substance Physical Inventory Year 2022

Drug and Strength	Physical Count	Running Balance	Discrepancy +/-	Percentage of Annual Use
Diazepam 5mg Tabs	152 Tabs	155 Tabs	-3	3/225 = 0.013 x 100 = 1%
Torbutrol 1mg Tabs	112 Tabs	112 Tabs	0	0
Ketamine Inj 100mg/ml	29.3ml	30ml	-0.7ml	0.7/30 = 0.02 x 100 =2.3%
Sleepaway 100mg/ml	157 ml	150ml	+7ml	N/A

Fig. 14.5 Annual controlled substance physical inventory summary.

Each drug must have an individual log for the year. Each log must be balanced to ensure all drugs that were purchased are accounted for. An annual CS physical inventory should be performed, allowing inspectors to quickly review use within the practice. Ideally, practices should inventory CSs monthly at a minimum. Human errors do occur, and team members can forget to write down substances used to treat patients in emergency situations, or during busy times at the clinic. If practices perform monthly inventories and balances of their drugs, discrepancies can be located more easily within the month, as opposed to annually or biannually as required.

To provide an annual CS physical inventory, each drug log must be finished, and a physical count of the drug must be completed. The discrepancy is the physical count minus the running balance. The percentage of annual use should be calculated by dividing the discrepancy by the total number of milliliters or tablets (whichever form the drug comes in) and multiplied by 100 to obtain a percentage. If a discrepancy is greater than 3% for the year, the loss could be considered substantial and should be reported. Fig. 14.5 uses Fig. 14.4 to calculate the annual use of ketamine. The running balance (the total milliliters that the practice has received for the year) minus the physical count (inventory performed) gives a discrepancy of −0.7 mL. Therefore 0.7 mL divided by 30 mL (the total use for the year) equals 0.02. To obtain the percentage, 0.02 is multiplied by 100. This gives an annual percentage use of 2.3%. If this number equaled 3% or higher, it would be reported to the DEA, the police department, and the state board of pharmacy.

It is expected that there will be a small amount of hub loss associated with each draw. It is advisable to ask the state veterinary inspector or the local DEA office for the best way to account for hub loss. Some departments may allow a small percentage of the total use to be written off as hub loss. If a bottle is broken, two people must initial the log indicating the broken bottle.

Loss Reporting

Theft or drug loss must be reported to the police and DEA immediately. Ongoing losses can result in loss of license and strict fines. DEA Form 106 should be filled out and forwarded to the local DEA office; another copy may have to be forwarded to the State Board of Pharmacy (Fig. 14.6). One copy should be maintained for the CS file. Verbal reports should be made to the DEA as soon as possible, followed up with a written notification within 15 days.

LEADERSHIP POINT

If a practice has not implemented measures to protect controlled substances, veterinarians can lose their DEA license.

Substance Disposal

Formerly, expired CSs had to be submitted to a reverse distributor for destruction, and the incineration records were required to be kept with the CS logs for a minimum 2-year period. Recently the DEA updated this requirement. Title 21 Code of Federal Regulations, Part 1317.10 outlines the use of DEA Form 41 (Fig. 14.7), including logging of destructed inventory, method of destruction, and two witnesses. The

DEA FORM **106**

Report of Theft or Loss of Controlled Substances

OMB No. 1117-0001 (Exp. Date 7/31/2023)

U.S. Department of Justice
Drug Enforcement Administration
Diversion Control Division

Type of Report: *(check one box only)* ☐ **New Report** ☐**Amendment Key** ***(prior report dated):*** ____________

1. **DEA Registration Number:** ____________

   Name of Business: ____________

   Address: ____________

   City: ____________ **State:** ______ **ZIP Code:** ______

   Point of Contact: ____________

   Email Address: ____________ **Phone No.:** ____________

Date of the Theft or Loss *(or first discovery of theft or loss)*: ____________ **Number of Thefts and Losses in the past 24 months:** ______

Principal Business of Registrant: ☐Pharmacy ☐Practitioner ☐Manufacturer ☐Hospital/Clinic ☐Distributor ☐NTP ☐Other (Specify) ____________

2. **Type of Theft or Loss:** -

3. **Loss in Transit.** *(*Fill out this section only if there was a loss in transit, or hijacking of transport vehicle.)*

   Name of Common Carrier: ____________

   Telephone Number of Common Carrier: ____________ Package Tracking Number: ____________

   Have there been losses in transit from this same carrier in the past? ☐ No ☐ Yes *(If yes, how many, excluding this theft or loss?)*: ______

   Was the package received and accepted by the consignee? ☐ No ☐ Yes *(If yes, the consignee is responsible for reporting the theft or loss.)*

   If the package was accepted by the consignee, did it appear to be tampered with? ☐ No ☐ Yes

   Name of Consignee / Supplier: ____________

   Enter the Name of Consignee (if reported by the supplier), or the Name of Supplier (if the package was accepted by the consignee).
   If the consignee does not have a DEA Registration Number, e.g. if this was a shipment to a patient, or a nursing home emergency kit, enter "Patient" or "Nursing Home Kit."

   DEA Registration Number of Consignee / Supplier: ____________

   Enter the DEA Registration Number of Consignee (if reported by the supplier), or DEA Registration Number of Supplier, (if the package was accepted by the consignee). If the controlled substances were shipped to a non-registrant, leave blank, unless a registered pharmacy shipped to an emergency kit held on site at a nursing home. In this case, the supplying pharmacy is required to report the theft or loss.

4. **If this was a robbery, were any people injured?** ☐ No ☐ Yes *(If yes, how many?)*: ______ Were any people killed? ☐ No ☐ Yes *(If yes, how many?)*: ______

5. **What is the total value of the controlled substances stolen or lost?: $** ____________
   (This is the amount you paid for the controlled substances, not the retail value.)

6. **Was theft reported to Police?** ☐ No ☐ Yes *(If yes, fill out the following information)*:

   Name of Police Department: ____________ Police Report number: ____________

   Name of Responding Officer: ____________ Phone No.: ____________

7. **Which corrective measure(s) have you taken to prevent a future theft or loss?**
   - ☐ Installed monitoring equipment (e.g. video camera).
   - ☐ Increased employee monitoring (e.g. random drug tests).
   - ☐ Installed metal bars or other security on doors or windows.
   - ☐ Secured Controlled Substances within safe.
   - ☐ Other (Please describe on last page).
   - ☐ Provided security training to staff.
   - ☐ Requested increased security patrols by Police.
   - ☐ Hired security guards for premises.
   - ☐ Terminated employee.

8. **Were any pharmaceuticals or merchandise taken?** ☐ No ☐ Yes *(Estimated Value)*:

Form DEA-106 Pg. 1

Fig. 14.6 DEA Form 106. (Courtesy U.S. Department of Justice, Drug Enforcement Administration, Washington, DC.)

DEA FORM **106**

Report of Theft or Loss of Controlled Substances

OMB No. 1117-0001 (Exp. Date 7/31/2023)

LIST OF CONTROLLED SUBSTANCES LOST OR STOLEN

	Trade Name of Substance or Preparation	NDC Number	Name of Controlled Substance in Preparation	Dosage Stre
Examples	**Desoxyn**	**00074-3377-01**	**Methamphetamine Hydrochloride**	**5 mg**
	Demerol	**00409-1181-30**	**Meperidine Hydrochloride**	**50 mg/ml**
	Robitussin A-C	**00031-8674-25**	**Codeine Phosphate**	**2 mg/cc**
	1.			
	2.			
	3.			
	4.			
	5.			
	6.			
	7.			
	8.			
	9.			
	10.			
	11.			
	12.			
	13.			
	14.			
	15.			
	16.			
	17.			
	18.			
	19.			
	20.			

Remarks: (Optional)

Diversion Control Divisi

Form DEA-106 Pg. 2

Fig. 14.6 *(Continued)*

DEA FORM **106**

Report of Theft or Loss of Controlled Substances

OMB No. 1117-0001 (Exp. Date 7/31/2023)

Form DEA-106 (10/23/2020) Pg. 3

LIST OF MAIL-BACK PACKAGES OR INNER LINERS LOST OR STOLE

	Mail-Back Package	Inner Liner	Unique Identification Number(s)	Size of
Examples	X		MBP1106, MBP1108 – MBP1110, MBP1112	I
		X	CRL1007 – CRL1027	15 G
		X	CRL1201	5 G
	1.			
	2			
	3.			
	4.			
	5.			
	6.			
	7.			
	8.			

Remarks: (Optional)

If you are an authorized Retail Pharmacy or Hospital/Clinic with an onsite Pharmacy and reporting a theft or loss at a Long-Term Car address of LTCF.

Name of LTCF

Address, City, State, Zip Code

Form DEA-106 Pg. 3

Fig. 14.6 *(Continued)*

DEA FORM **106** **Report of Theft or Loss of Controlled Substances**
OMB No. 1117-0001 (Exp. Date 7/31/2023)

U.S. Department of Justice
Drug Enforcement Administration
Diversion Control Division

Describe any other corrective measure(s) you have taken to prevent a future theft or loss:

Enter remarks, if required. Description of how theft or loss occurred.

The foregoing information is correct to the best of my knowledge and belief: By signing my full name in the space below, I hereby certify that the foregoing information furnished on this DEA Form 106 is true and correct, and understand that this constitutes an electronic signature for purposes of this reporting requirement only.

Signature: ______________________

Title: ______________________ Date Signed: ______________________

NOTICE: In accordance with the Paperwork Reduction Act of 1995, no person is required to respond to a collection of information unless it displays a valid OMB control number. The valid OMB control number for this collection of information is 1117-0001. Public reporting burden for this collection of information is estimated to average 20 minutes per response, including the time for reviewing instructions, searching existing data sources, gathering and maintaining the data needed, and completing and reviewing the collection of information.

Freedom of Information: Please prominently identify any confidential business information per 28 CFR 16.8(c) and Exemption 4 of the Freedom of Information Act (FOIA). In the event DEA receives a FOIA request to obtain such information, DEA will give written notice to the registrant to obtain such information. DEA will give written notice to the registrant to allow an opportunity to object prior to the release of information.

Privacy Act Information

AUTHORITY: Section 301 of the Controlled Substances Act of 1970 (PL 91-513)

PURPOSE: Reporting of unusual or excessive theft or loss of a Listed Chemical

ROUTINE USES: The Controlled Substances Act authorizes the production of special reports required for statistical and analytical purposes. Disclosures of information from this system are made to the following categories of users for the purposes stated:

A. Other Federal law enforcement and regulatory agencies for law enforcement and regulatory purposes.

B. State and local law enforcement and regulatory agencies for law enforcement and regulatory purposes.

EFFECT: Failure to report theft or loss of Listed Chemicals may result in penalties under 21 U.S.C. § 842 and § 843 of the Federal Criminal Code.

Form DEA-106 Pg. 4

Fig. 14.6 *(Continued)*

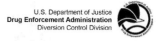

OMB APPROVAL NO. 1117-0007 Expiration Date 1/31/2024

U. S. DEPARTMENT OF JUSTICE – DRUG ENFORCEMENT ADMINISTRATION

REGISTRANT RECORD OF CONTROLLED SUBSTANCES DESTROYED

FORM DEA-41

A. REGISTRANT INFORMATION

Registered Name:	DEA Registration Number:
Registered Address:	
City: State:	Zip Code:
Telephone Number:	Contact Name:

B. ITEM DESTROYED

1. Inventory

	National Drug Code or DEA Controlled Substances Code Number	Batch Number	Name of Substance	Strength	Form	Pkg. Qty.	Number of Full Pkgs.	Partial Pkg. Count	Total Destroyed
Examples	*16590-598-60*	*N/A*	*Kadian*	*60mg*	*Capsules*	*60*	*2*	*0*	*120 Capsules*
	0555-0767-02	*N/A*	*Adderall*	*5mg*	*Tablet*	*100*	*0*	*83*	*83 Tablets*
	9050	*B02120312*	*Codeine*	*N/A*	*Bulk*	*1.25 kg*	*N/A*	*N/A*	*1.25 kg*
1.									
2.									
3.									
4.									
5.									
6.									
7.									

2. Collected Substances

	Returned Mail-Back Package	Sealed Inner Liner	Unique Identification Number	Size of Sealed Inner Liner	Quantity of Packages(s)/Liner(s) Destroyed
Examples	*X*		*MBP1106, MBP1108 - MBP1110, MBP112*	*N/A*	*5*
		X	*CRL1007 - CRL1027*	*15 gallon*	*21*
		X	*CRL1201*	*5 gallon*	*1*
1.					
2.					
3.					
4.					
5.					
6.					
7.					

Form DEA-41 *See instructions on reverse (page 2) of form.*

Fig. 14.7 DEA Form 41 Instructions. (Courtesy U.S. Department of Justice, Drug Enforcement Administration, Washington, DC.)

DEA-41 Pg. 2

C. METHOD OF DESTRUCTION

Date of Destruction:	Method of Destruction:	
Location or Business Name:		
Address:		
City:	State:	Zip Code:

D. WITNESSES

I declare under penalty of perjury, pursuant to 18 U.S.C. 1001, that I personally witnessed the destruction of the above-described controlled substances to a non-retrievable state and that all of the above is true and correct.

Printed name of first authorized employee witness:	Signature of first witness:	Date:
Printed name of second authorized employee witness:	Signature of second witness:	Date:

E. INSTRUCTIONS

1. Section A. REGISTRANT INFORMATION: The registrant destroying the controlled substance(s) shall provide their DEA registration number and the name and address indicated on their valid DEA registration, in addition to a current telephone number and a contact name, if different from the name on the valid DEA registration.
2. Section B. (1) Inventory: This part shall be used by registrants destroying lawfully possessed controlled substances, other than those described in Section B(2). In each row, indicate the National Drug Code (NDC) for the controlled substance destroyed, or if the substance has no NDC, indicate the DEA Controlled Substances Code Number for the substance; if the substance destroyed is in bulk form, indicate the batch number, if available. In each row, indicate the name, strength, and form of the controlled substance destroyed, and the number of capsules, tablets, etc., that are in a full package (pkg. qty.). If destroying the full quantity of the controlled substance, indicate the number of packages destroyed (number of full pkgs.). If destroying a partial package, indicate the partial count of the capsules, tablets, etc. destroyed (partial pkg. count). If destroying a controlled substance in bulk form, indicate that the substance is in bulk form (form) and the weight of the substance destroyed (pkg. qty.). In each row, indicate the total number of each controlled substance destroyed (total destroyed).
3. Section B. (2) Collected Substances: This part shall be used by registrants destroying controlled substances obtained through an authorized collection activity in accordance with 21 U.S.C. 822(g). In each row, indicate whether registrant is destroying a mail-back package or an inner liner. If destroying a mail-back package, enter each unique identification number separated by a comma and/or as a list in a sequential range and total quantity of packages being destroyed. If destroying an inner liner, enter each unique identification number separated by a comma and/or as a list in a sequential range based on the size of the liners destroyed and the total quantity of inner liners being destroyed. In the case of mail-back packages or inner liners received from a law enforcement agency which do not have a unique identification number or clearly marked size, include the name of the law enforcement agency and, if known, the size of the inner liner or package. DO NOT OPEN ANY MAIL-BACK PACKAGE OR INNER LINER; AN INVENTORY OF THE CONTENTS OF THE PACKAGES OR LINERS IS PROHIBITED BY LAW AND IS NOT REQUIRED BY THIS FORM.
4. If additional space is needed for items destroyed in Section B, attach to this form additional page(s) containing the requested information for each controlled substance destroyed.
5. Section C. METHOD OF DESTRUCTION: Provide the date, location, and method of destruction. The method of destruction must render the controlled substance to a state of non-retrievable and meet all applicable destruction requirements.
6. Section D. WITNESSES: Two authorized employees must declare by signature, under penalty of perjury, that such employees personally witnessed the destruction of the controlled substances listed in Section B in the manner described in Section C.
7. You are not required to submit this form to DEA, unless requested to do so. This form must be kept as a record of destruction and be available by the registrant for at least two years in accordance with 21 U.S.C. 827.

Paperwork Reduction Act Statement: The information collected on this form is necessary for DEA registrants to record controlled substances destroyed in accordance with the Controlled Substances Act (CSA). The records that DEA registrants maintain in accordance with the CSA must be kept and be available, for at least two years, for inspection and copying by officers or employees of the United States authorized by the Attorney General. 21 U.S.C. 827. DEA estimates that it will take approximately 30 minutes to complete this form, including the time for reviewing instructions, searching existing data sources, gathering and maintaining the data needed, and completing and reviewing the collection of information. The completion of this form by DEA registrants that destroy controlled substances is mandatory in accordance with 21 U.S.C. 827. Please note that an agency may not conduct or sponsor, and a person is not required to respond to, a collection of information unless it displays a currently valid OMB control number. Comments regarding this information collection, including suggestions for reducing the burden estimate, should be directed to the Drug Enforcement Administration, DEA Federal Register Representative/ODL, 8701 Morrissette Drive, Springfield, Virginia 22152.

Fig. 14.7 *(Continued)*

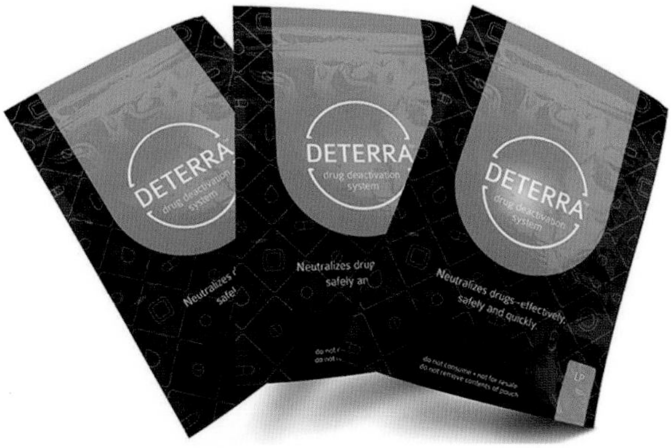

Fig. 14.8 Deterra Drug Disposal Pouches: https://deterrasystem.com

form does not have to be filed with the DEA but rather kept with the practice's CS logs.

Methods of destruction could include incineration (if the practice has direct access to incineration themselves and the drug(s) do not change hands), or drug neutralization pouches (Fig. 14.8). The activated carbon in these pouches neutralize the drug when warm water is added, in addition to preventing leaching of the drug(s) into the environment.[1]

CRITICAL COMPETENCY: CONTINUOUS LEARNING

Practice managers should have a curiosity for learning. Actively seeking out new information, technologies, and methods while keeping skills updated allows the application of new knowledge to the job.

LEADERSHIP'S ROLE IN CONTROLLED SUBSTANCES

The management of controlled substances is critical in the veterinary practice; the owner's DEA license is on the line. Therefore, while another team member may be tasked with maintaining the logs and data entry, the practice manager and owner must participate in monthly audits and reviews of records. If there are discrepancies, they must be investigated immediately. Additionally, both the PM and owner should be prepared for an audit at any time (either by DEA, the state veterinary inspector, or the state board of pharmacy). Using the forms as demonstrated in this chapter will help any leader survive an audit as it creates a clear trail of drug accountability.

PRACTICE MANAGERS SURVIVAL CHECKLIST FOR CONTROLLED SUBSTANCES

- ☐ Create a protocol to be sure all DVM DEA licenses are current and track expiration dates.
- ☐ Determine who is responsible for renewing DEA license(s).
- ☐ Post current DVM DEA licenses and monitor for expiration.
- ☐ Ensure DEA 222 forms are stored in a locked cabinet.
- ☐ Ensure prescription forms are stored in a locked cabinet.
- ☐ Make sure safes used for CSs are substantially secured.
- ☐ Ensure all inactive CSs are stored in a secured safe.
- ☐ Balance CSs monthly (at minimum).
- ☐ Develop a protocol to be sure all CS discrepancies are investigated and documented.
- ☐ Closeout CS logs on April 30 of each year.
- ☐ Confirm whether the state in which the practice resides has a prescription monitoring plan in place, and if so, confirm which CS drugs dispensed must be reported to the state.

REVIEW QUESTIONS

1. What are controlled substances?
2. What is the abuse potential of ketamine?
3. Why are log sheets required for controlled substances?
4. What is the purpose of a year-end physical inventory?
5. What is DEA Form 106 used for?
6. The class with the highest abuse potential is:
   - **a.** II
   - **b.** IV
   - **c.** V
7. DEA Form 222 is used to:
   - **a.** Register a doctor for a DEA license
   - **b.** Report lost controlled substances
   - **c.** Order Schedule II controlled substances
   - **d.** Order Schedule IV controlled substances
8. Logs should be stored in the same place as controlled substances.
   - **a.** True
   - **b.** False
9. A loss of ________ or more must be reported to the DEA.
   - **a.** 1%
   - **b.** 2%
   - **c.** 3%
   - **d.** 4%
10. A reverse distributor:
    - **a.** Sells controlled substances to veterinary hospitals
    - **b.** Incinerates expired controlled substances
    - **c.** Both above
    - **d.** Neither of the above

REFERENCES

1. Controlled substance ordering system homepage. Deaecom.gov. Accessed August 2022. https://www.deaecom.gov/poa.html

RECOMMENDED READING

Fowler W. Deterra System Deactivation of Unused Drugs: Comparison between Deterra Ingredients and Others Recommended in Federal and SmartRx Disposal Guidelines. Minnetonka, MN: Verde Environmental Technologies Inc.; 2012. Available at: https://deterrasystem.com/wp-content/uploads/2020/12/Deterra®SystemDeactivation-of-Unused-Drugs-Comparison-Between-Deterra-Ingredients-and-Others.pdf

United States Department of Justice: Drug Enforcement Administration. *Physicians manual: an information outline of the controlled substance act of 1970.* Washington, DC: Government Publishing Office; Revised 2020. Available at: https://www.deadiversion.usdoj.gov/

15

Safety in the Veterinary Practice

LEARNING OBJECTIVES

When you have completed this chapter, you should be able to:

- Identify zoonotic diseases
- Describe methods used to prevent the transmission of zoonotic diseases
- Identify the hazards associated with veterinary medicine
- List methods used to lift equipment and animals appropriately
- Define the role of the Occupational Safety and Health Administration (OSHA)
- Develop safety protocols
- Define the Right to Know
- Define employer and employee rights and responsibilities as outlined by OSHA
- Develop and implement a hospital safety manual
- Discuss and implement a training program
- Describe how to prevent fires and promote a safe working environment
- Interpret Safety Data Sheets (SDS)
- Discuss methods used to prevent the escape of animals
- Define the importance of one-way door locks
- Describe methods used to protect a computer system against embezzlement and hackers
- Describe methods used to protect the practice against theft from both employees and thieves
- Identify an effective security system for the practice
- Define perimeter lighting
- Define personal protection devices

OUTLINE

KEY TERMS

Biohazard
Carcinogen
First Notice of Accident
General Duty Clause
Hospital Safety Manual
Occupational Safety and Health Administration (OSHA)
One-Way Door Locks
OSHA 300
OSHA 300 A
Permissible Exposure Limits
Perimeter Lighting
Personal Protection Device
Personal Protective Equipment (PPE)
Safety Data Sheet (SDS)
Scavenger System
The Right to Know
Waste Anesthetic Gases
Zoonotic Disease

VHMA PERFORMANCE DOMAINS

Veterinary Hospital Managers Association (VHMA) Performance Domains

Performance domains applicable to safety in the veterinary practice include law and ethics and organization of the practice. The practice manager:

- understands and ensures compliance with OSHA and The Right to Know;
- is responsible for implementing safety regulations in accordance with local, state, and federal guidelines;
- monitors hospital violations and dangerous situations;
- ensures equipment is in safe working condition and contracts repair for maintenance when needed; and
- develops protocols for the facility (building and property) and equipment maintenance.

Application of VHMA Performance Domains for Practice Managers

Integrating the tasks required for practice safety requires knowledge of state/provincial and federal laws, legal codes, government regulations, professional standards, and agency rules. Creating a safe place for employees to work must be a high priority, and appropriate empowerment of programs to team members allows safety to become a team sport.

INTRODUCTION

Many hazards exist in a veterinary practice, and each team member must be aware of these hazards. Every employee must be proactive and prevent accidents from occurring, keeping the facility safe for all team members, patients, and clients.

In addition to avoiding workplace hazards, it is also essential to prevent the transmission of zoonotic diseases, which can spread from animal to human through various methods, depending on the disease. Team members must be aware of transmissible and take all precautions necessary to prevent transmission. Some diseases can be treated, whereas others may be fatal.

The Occupational Safety and Health Administration (OSHA) was developed in 1970 to ensure employee safety. Every employer must provide a safe working environment for all team members, and OSHA will severely penalize those that do not follow regulations. OSHA oversees all workplace hazards, including the safe use and disposal of chemicals. Each practice must have Safety Data Sheets (SDSs) available for quick reference in case any team member is exposed to a chemical hazard. SDSs provide information regarding the chemical, specifications for cleanup and exposure, as well as any special properties the chemical possesses.

Every workplace is different, therefore identifying hazards (and creating policies) at each work site is impossible for OSHA. This is where the General Duty Clause comes into play. It is the responsibility of the employer to identify hazards or potential hazards specific to their practice and to develop safety policies to reduce or eliminate the hazard. It does not matter that an OSHA policy does not exist; if there is a potential hazard, a plan must be created to inform and train the team on the hazard.

Safety manuals should be developed by all veterinary hospitals for team members. Often, a safety officer is appointed who oversees the developing, implementing, and maintaining safety manuals, allowing the practice to remain compliant with OSHA standards. Safety manuals help to create and implement a safe working environment and serve as a training tool for team members. Safety manuals are required by OSHA and must include safety plans. Accidents and emergencies will happen in the veterinary practice, and team members must be prepared to handle them.

OCCUPATIONAL SAFETY AND HEALTH ADMINISTRATION

It is the responsibility of every veterinary practice to comply with safety regulations at the local, state, and federal levels. OSHA enforces federal laws to ensure a safe workplace environment. These laws require employers to have a safety program that includes the training of employees. Both employers and employees have responsibilities that must be abided by.

Employer Responsibilities

- Provide a safe working environment
- Set and enforce safety rules
- Inform employees about the inherent risks associated with their jobs
- Provide and train on the proper use of personal protective equipment (PPE)

Employee Responsibilities

- Read OSHA's "Job Safety and Health—It's the Law" poster (Fig. 15.1)
- Comply with safety standards determined by the hospital
- Use PPE that has been provided
- Report hazardous conditions to management
- Report any injuries received and seek immediate treatment for them

VHMA PERFORMANCE DOMAIN TASK

Understand and ensure compliance with appropriate regulations at all government levels, including the OSHA Hazard Communication Standard and state and local safety regulations.

Many states also have a state-mandated OSHA program that is more stringent than federal programs. The practice should abide by whichever program is stricter.

Penalties and fines exist for those who break the law. For example, not displaying the *OSHA Job Safety and Health: It's the Law* poster carries a $7000 fine. Other willful violations can range from $5000 to $70,000.[1]

There are four sections in OSHA's compliance and safety program that must be built out by every practice: administrative tasks, facility evaluation and development of hazard communication plan, personal protection equipment (PPE) evaluation and training, and the development and implementation of a training program for all team members.

Administrative tasks include posting a fire evacuation plan, warning/hazard signs, deploying safety information to team members, hosting safety inspections, and the maintenance of training and documentation. The safety program must be in writing and placed in a central location that is always available and easily accessible to all team members.

VHMA PERFORMANCE DOMAIN TASK

Develop and manage personnel training programs and developmental programs (including safety training).

An evacuation plan should be posted for employees to see. A diagram of the practice should list potential hazards and safety equipment in each room. The diagram should include exits, circuit breakers, compressed gas cylinders, hazardous materials, and fire extinguishers. A fire evacuation plan is required for practices with ten or more employees, and although evacuation plans do not have to be posted for clients to see, it is a nice service to provide should an emergency occur.

OSHA has the right to inspect any veterinary practice. Every veterinary practice owner and/or safety officer has the right to be present for an

U.S. Department of Labor

OSHA® Occupational Safety and Health Administration

Job Safety and Health IT'S THE LAW!

All workers have the right to:

- A safe workplace.
- Raise a safety or health concern with your employer or OSHA, or report a work-related injury or illness, without being retaliated against.
- Receive information and training on job hazards, including all hazardous substances in your workplace.
- Request a confidential OSHA inspection of your workplace if you believe there are unsafe or unhealthy conditions. You have the right to have a representative contact OSHA on your behalf.
- Participate (or have your representative participate) in an OSHA inspection and speak in private to the inspector.
- File a complaint with OSHA within 30 days (by phone, online or by mail) if you have been retaliated against for using your rights.
- See any OSHA citations issued to your employer.
- Request copies of your medical records, tests that measure hazards in the workplace, and the workplace injury and illness log.

This poster is available free from OSHA.

Employers must:

- Provide employees a workplace free from recognized hazards. It is illegal to retaliate against an employee for using any of their rights under the law, including raising a health and safety concern with you or with OSHA, or reporting a work-related injury or illness.
- Comply with all applicable OSHA standards.
- Notify OSHA within 8 hours of a workplace fatality or within 24 hours of any work-related inpatient hospitalization, amputation, or loss of an eye.
- Provide required training to all workers in a language and vocabulary they can understand.
- Prominently display this poster in the workplace.
- Post OSHA citations at or near the place of the alleged violations.

On-Site Consultation services are available to small and medium-sized employers, without citation or penalty, through OSHA-supported consultation programs in every state.

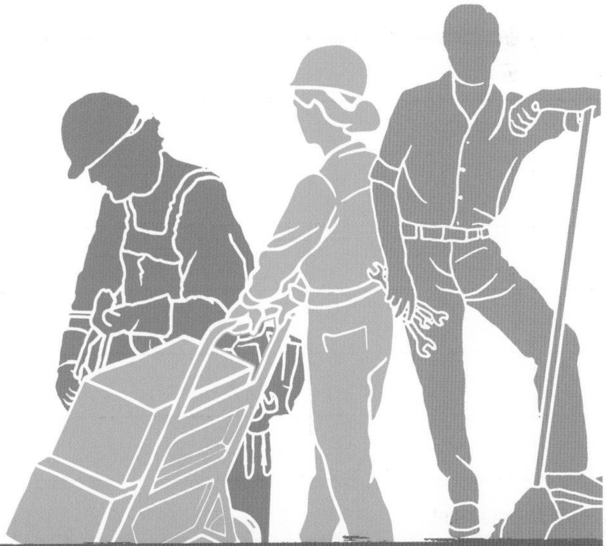

Contact OSHA. We can help.

1-800-321-OSHA (6742) • TTY 1-877-889-5627 • www.osha.gov

OSHA 3165-04R 2019

Fig. 15.1 OSHA's "Job Safety and Health It's the Law" poster. (Courtesy U.S. Department of Labor, Occupational Safety and Health Administration.)

OSHA inspection. When developing the safety manual, practice owners/managers should appoint a specific person that is to be present when an OSHA inspector arrives at the hospital. This document should be kept in the front of the safety manual, and all team members should be aware of the inspection procedure. If the owner is not present, and a representative has not been appointed, OSHA can be denied the opportunity to inspect the premises. However, if OSHA has a court order, they must be allowed to inspect the premises within 72 hours of the initial visit. Safety officers and/or owners should walk through the premises with the inspection officer; never allow an untrained team member to act as an escort.

The inspection notice must be posted on the staff bulletin board for all team members to see until the inspection has been completed. Copies of violations must be posted for at least 3 days or until the violation is corrected, whichever is longer. OSHA often returns, following up on violations that were noted on the initial inspection.

OSHA does not endorse products. Many companies use marketing tactics stating their product is "OSHA approved" when the product only meets OSHA standards. Additionally, OSHA does not "certify" personnel to teach OSHA courses to veterinary practices. Courses and trainers are considered authorized, and students receive completion cards, but anyone claiming to be OSHA certified would be mistaken (https://www.usfosha.com/osha-articles/osha-certification.aspx). In addition, safety is different in each veterinary practice; it is up to leadership to teach the veterinary team safety policies as it relates to the specific practice.

The facility evaluation and development of a hazard communication plan build out the entire safety program. To have an effective hazard safety communication plan that mitigates hazards, a facility evaluation must be completed that includes identifying physical and chemical hazards in the practice and all safety protocols, PPE, and training that mitigates each hazard identified.

PPE evaluation and training that is identified during the inspection process must be placed in both the section summarizing PPE evaluation, and with each hazard to which the PPE applies. Under OSHA guidelines, PPE must be always used (where available). This includes, but is not limited to, protective equipment for radiology, surgery, dentistry, and laboratory functions. Eyewear must be worn when performing tasks that could inflict injury to the eye, and eyewash stations must be available for team members and clients to use in case of emergency. Review all areas of the hospital; list the PPE that is available, how to use it, and when it should be used (Fig. 15.2). Train employees on each

PPE Assessment Form

Date:______________________

This inspection is a(n): [ ] Annual Inspection [ ]Follow-up Inspection [ ]Post-injury Inspection [ ] Post-change [ ] Other

Area	Description of Hazard	PPE Required	When it should it be worn?	Instructions to don and doff

Area Management:

Area 1	Lobby	Area 9	Surgery
Area 2	Reception Area	Area 10	DVMs office
Area 3	Exam Room 1	Area 11	Practice Managers Office
Area 4	Exam Room 2	Area 12	Break Room
Area 5	Exam Room 3	Area 13	Critical Care Room
Area 6	Exam Room 4	Area 14	Canine Room
Area 7	Treatment Area	Area 15	Feline Room
Area 8	Pharmacy	Area 16	Isolation Room

Fig. 15.2 Example of a personal protective equipment assessment form used to evaluate available and needed PPE for the premises. (From Occupational Safety and Health Administration, Department of Labor, Washington, DC.)

piece of PPE, then document the training with signature verification from each team member.

Development and implementation of a training program for all team members is the final build-out of the *Hazard Communication: The Right to Know* program. Team training is imperative; without proper training, safety programs are useless. It is advisable to videotape training sessions; this not only provides training information while new employees are added to the practice, but it also provides proof that a safety program exists if a complaint is ever filed against the practice. Videos may need to be updated as procedures change or equipment that pose hazardous conditions are purchased and implemented into practice protocols.

All team members must be trained on the use of the safety manual and the Right to Know standards. Further training can be tailored to specific job duties assigned to each position. For example, if the bookkeeper does not restrain pets, he or she does not need to receive training on animal restraint. However, if the receptionist occasionally restrains a patient, he or she must have training on appropriate restraint, and the practice must document this training.

When safety trainings begin, it is wise to cover the most serious hazards first while team members are paying attention. Less severe hazards can follow. Several training topics are required by OSHA, and each is covered in detail in the following sections (Fig. 15.3).

A summary of all hazardous chemicals, a workplace safety manual, and any workplace injuries and illnesses must be kept together, along with documentation of training programs, attendees, dates, and signatures. If any personal employee information is included, the entire file must be stored in a locked cabinet.

HAZARD COMMUNICATION: THE RIGHT TO KNOW

OSHA's Hazard Communication Standard—Right to Know (see Fig. 15.1)—requires that all team members who encounter hazardous materials in the workplace be aware of hazards and be instructed on how to protect themselves from said hazards (Table 15.1). This applies to all chemicals, including anesthetic gases, radiology chemicals, alcohol, and formalin. To establish compliance, a practice must have:

- a designated safety manager responsible for training all team members and ensuring the safety program meets standard requirements;
- an annual hazard-analysis inspection;
- safety plans for identified hazards;
- chemical list and safety plans for Immediately Dangerous to Life and Health (IDLH) chemicals;
- Safety Data Sheets that can be accessed by any employee at any time;
- all chemical containers are accurately labeled, including secondary containers;
- an explanation of the labeling system;
- a protocol for emergency evacuation; and
- a training program implementing the use of PPE and monitoring devices as well as the hazards of the practice, which is required for all practices with eleven or more employees.

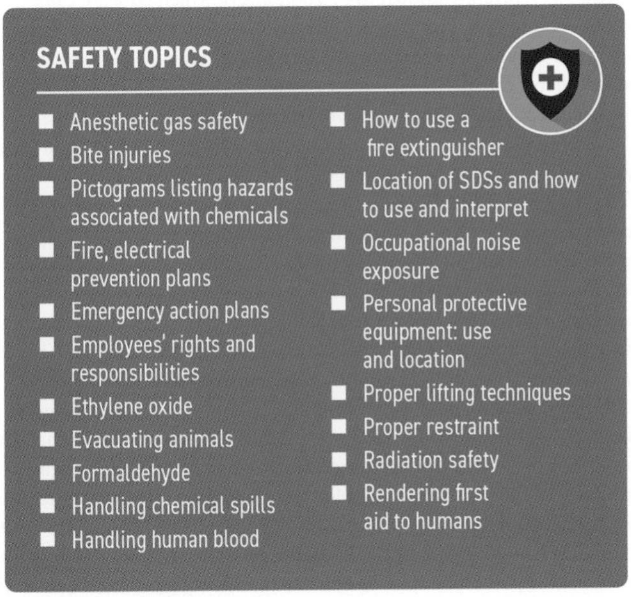
SAFETY TOPICS
Anesthetic gas safety
Bite injuries
Pictograms listing hazards associated with chemicals
Fire, electrical prevention plans
Emergency action plans
Employees' rights and responsibilities
Ethylene oxide
Evacuating animals
Formaldehyde
Handling chemical spills
Handling human blood
How to use a fire extinguisher
Location of SDSs and how to use and interpret
Occupational noise exposure
Personal protective equipment: use and location
Proper lifting techniques
Proper restraint
Radiation safety
Rendering first aid to humans

Fig. 15.3 Safety Topics.

Designating a Safety Manager

When developing the Hazard Communication plan, a safety officer must be designated. This individual will oversee several administrative duties (Fig. 15.4) and must be highly motivated and task-oriented. The safety officer should evaluate the entire facility annually and list any items that are hazardous or could become hazards in the future. Hazards include slippery floors, sharp corners, damaged radiology shielding, chemicals, biohazard containers, etc.

The safety officer must host team training events that discuss the importance of the safety plan and review the Hazard Communication Standards as well as the responsibilities of the practice and the employees. Team members should also be available to report hazards they may have developed since the annual walk-through inspection.

TABLE 15.1 Occupational hazards.

Hazard	Associated Problems	Common Solutions
Animal handling	Animal bites, zoonotic disease transmission	Proper restraint devices
Ethylene oxide	Spills, improper use	Proper safety training
Ergonomics	Back injuries	Proper lifting techniques
Facility hazards	Old lead paint, slippery tile	Update facility; nonskid shoes
Fire	Not exiting promptly and safely	Fire evacuation plan, accessible extinguishers, emergency lighting
Food	Ingestion of toxic chemicals and organisms	Separate refrigerator; no food in working areas
Housekeeping	Chemical mixing and toxicities	Do not mix cleaning products
Medical waste	Poking or cutting self with needles, glass, or blades	Appropriate use of biohazard containers
Radiology	Radiation exposure, toxic chemicals	Safety training, use of personal protective equipment; ventilate room; do not mix chemicals
Violence	Disgruntled clients or employees, angry family members, thieves	Listen to comments made by team members and clients

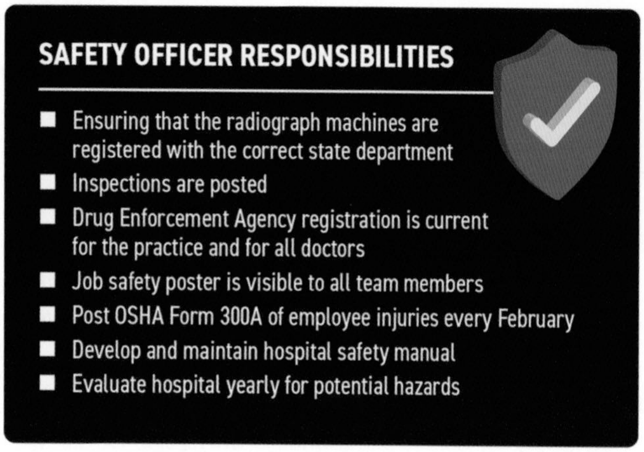
SAFETY OFFICER RESPONSIBILITIES
Ensuring that the radiograph machines are registered with the correct state department
Inspections are posted
Drug Enforcement Agency registration is current for the practice and for all doctors
Job safety poster is visible to all team members
Post OSHA Form 300A of employee injuries every February
Develop and maintain hospital safety manual
Evaluate hospital yearly for potential hazards

Fig. 15.4 Safety Officer Responsibilities.

Safety Managers should have a job description (in addition to the job description they received when they accepted employment in the practice) highlighting their responsibility as a safety manager, and practice managers should coach and guide this role as they do every other role. While the PM should not be the one to carry out this role, it should be delegated to team members who want more development opportunities, and the PM needs to oversee the program and ensure compliance is achieved. The safety manager must be trained in leadership, relationship development, adult learning theory (for effectively training others), and should be responsible for the safety training portion when team members are onboarded.

CRITICAL COMPETENCY: LEADERSHIP AND COMMUNICATION

Leadership: Practice managers must have the initiative to lead and take charge while simultaneously motivating and mobilizing others to achieve common goals.
Oral Communication and Comprehension: The practice manager must have the ability to express thoughts verbally in a clear and understandable manner, and the ability to actively listen and attend to what others are saying.
Writing and Verbal Skills: The practice manager must have the ability to comprehend written material easily and accurately, as well as the ability to express thoughts clearly and succinctly in writing.

Hazard Analysis Inspection

Every veterinary practice must perform an annual hazard inspection of the facility and update when significant building changes have been made. The updated evaluation (Fig. 15.5) must be completed and added to the safety binder outlining the hazards identified and the PPE that can be used to mitigate the risk; this analysis then creates safety and PPE plans (be sure to review plans once the annual evaluation is completed and update as needed).

Hazards can be categorized as chemical or physical. Chemical hazards will be identified by a yearly chemical hazard evaluation covered later in this chapter. Physical hazards may include animal handling, bathing, electrical and fire safety, emergency action plans, ergonomics, noise controls, and workplace violence.

When evaluating the facility, all potential hazards should be analyzed. Doors should have one-way locks, which allow clients and team members to escape from the inside at any time. Emergency lighting must be available to help guide clients and team members to exits in the event of an emergency or a power outage. Areas that should not be overlooked when evaluating the practice include but are not limited to:

- Air quality (Good flow? Even heating and cooling distribution?)
- Damaged equipment (broken rollers, exposed electrical wire, etc.)
- Distance between fire extinguishers
- Emergency lighting
- Ergonomics
- Fire alarms
- Lighting
- Proper lighting in all rooms
- Smoke alarms
- The use of extension cords
- Walking surfaces (smooth or uneven?)

VHMA PERFORMANCE DOMAIN TASK

Monitor hospital violations and dangerous situations.

The safety manager should have the entire team should participate in the annual hazard analysis. This helps the team become aware of hazards while they are being documented and encourages them to be a part of the solution created or used to mitigate the risk. Buy-in from the team is critical to reducing injuries in the practice.

CRITICAL COMPETENCY: PLANNING AND PRIORITIZING

Practice managers must be able to effectively manage time and workload to meet deadlines, thereby having the ability to organize work, set priorities, and establish plans to achieve goals.

Physical Hazards in the Veterinary Practice

Zoonotic Diseases

Zoonosis is defined as a disease that may be directly or indirectly transmitted to humans from wild or domesticated animals. More than 1400 diseases are currently known to be zoonotic, of which 60% are caused by pathogens known to cross species lines. The need to educate the public and veterinary practice team members is imperative because veterinarians may be held liable for the transmission of such diseases. Veterinarians play a vital role in public health and the control of zoonotic diseases (Table 15.2).

Veterinarians are ethically required to educate the public about zoonotic diseases. Because public health has been addressed in the American Veterinary Medical Association Code of Ethics, many state boards and regulatory agencies have mandated such education, which can leave many veterinarians liable for malpractice suits. To present a claim for malpractice, four elements must be proven: existence of a valid client-patient relationship, failure to practice the standard level of care, proximate cause, and harm that occurred to the patient because of substandard care. See Chapter 5, Veterinary Ethics and Issues, for more information on malpractice.

Once a patient has been presented to a practice for treatment, a client-patient relationship has been established. Because veterinarians have been trained in the risks and transmission of zoonotic diseases, it has become the standard of care for team members to educate the public. Therefore, if a patient with a zoonotic disease is presented for treatment, it is the obligation of the veterinary practice not only to diagnose and treat the patient but also to educate the client regarding the disease, and to recommend the client seek medical attention. If a patient has

Workplace Hazard Assessment Form

Date:____________________

This inspection is a(n): [ ] Annual Inspection [ ] Follow-up Inspection [ ] Post-injury Inspection [ ]Post-change [ ]Other

Area	Description of Hazard	Corrective Action Suggested	Corrective action taken	PPE Required	Initials

Area Management:

Area 1	Lobby	Area 9	Surgery
Area 2	Reception Area	Area 10	DVMs office
Area 3	Exam Room 1	Area 11	Practice Managers Office
Area 4	Exam Room 2	Area 12	Break Room
Area 5	Exam Room 3	Area 13	Critical Care Room
Area 6	Exam Room 4	Area 14	Canine Room
Area 7	Treatment Area	Area 15	Feline Room
Area 8	Pharmacy	Area 16	Isolation Room

Fig. 15.5 Example of a hazard analysis that should be completed on an annual basis. (From Safety and Health Administration, Department of Labor, Washington, DC.)

not been diagnosed with a zoonotic disease, it is standard of care to educate clients about potential zoonotic diseases that are present in the environmental area and advise methods of prevention, if available.

It is recommended that any new puppy or kitten brought to the practice be dewormed on the first visit. Puppies and kittens can easily transmit intestinal parasites, and this is the best opportunity to educate clients about these potential risks. If the veterinary practice initiates deworming protocols, sends clients home with materials to read, and documents the procedure in the record, it has taken the initial steps to protect itself from a lawsuit.

If a practice educates a client about the risk of contracting a zoonotic disease and advises a treatment protocol to reduce the risk of contracting that disease and the client refuses the treatment, it must be documented in the record.

Team members should receive extensive training on zoonotic diseases and precautions to take to decrease the possibility of transmissions. Employees should sign an acknowledgment indicating they have received prevention training. General cleanliness, handwashing, and the use of disinfectants are part of this training and must be implemented in the practice protocol to reduce the transmission of disease.

Disease Transmission

Understanding the mode of disease transmission is important when implementing a prevention program. Reservoirs and hosts must be considered, as these are necessary for the transmission of infectious diseases. A *reservoir* is a place where an infectious organism survives and replicates, such as within an animal or the soil. A *host* is a living organism that offers an environment for maintenance of the organism, but that may not be required for the organism's survival. Depending on the disease, the organism may be transmitted to more than one host or reservoir. Treatments are generally aimed at reservoirs and hosts of diseases when control methods are being implemented.

Direct transmission of diseases requires close contact between the reservoir of the disease and the susceptible host. Contact with infected skin, mucous membranes, or droplets from the infected animal or human can cause disease. Soil or vegetation that is contaminated also

TABLE 15.2 **Zoonotic diseases**

	Causative Organism	Small-Animal Host	Livestock Host	Wildlife Host	Mode of Transmission
Bacterial Infection					
Anthrax	*Bacillus anthracis*	Dogs	Cattle, sheep, horses, goats	Most except primates	Contact
Brucellosis	*Brucella melitensis*	Dogs	Cattle, pigs, sheep, goats	All except primates	Contact, inhalation, ingestion
Campylobacteriosis	*Campylobacter fetus*	Dogs, cats	Cattle, poultry, sheep, pigs	Rodents, birds	Ingestion, contact
Capnocytophaga infection	*Capnocytophaga canimorsus*	Dogs, cats			Bite wound
Cat scratch disease	*Bartonella henselae*	Cats			Cat bite, scratch
Erysipelas	*Erysipelothrix rhusiopathiae*		Pigs, sheep, cattle, horses, poultry	Rodents	Contact
Leptospirosis	*Leptospira* spp.	All	All	Rats, raccoons	Contact with urine or birthing fluids
Lyme disease	*Borrelia burgdorferi*	Dogs, cats	Cattle, horses	Deer, birds, rodents	Tick bite
Pasteurellosis	*Pasteurella multocida*	Dogs, cats			Bite wound
Plague	*Yersinia pestis*	Cats		Rodents, rabbits	Flea bite
Q fever	*Coxiella burnetii*		Cattle, sheep, goats	Birds, rabbits, rodents	Inhalation, milk ingestion, contact
Rat bite fever	*Streptobacillus moniliformis*			Rats	Rat bite
Salmonellosis	*Salmonella* spp.	All	All	Rodents, reptiles	Ingestion
Tetanus	*Clostridium tetani*		Horses	Reptiles	Wound
Tuberculosis	*Mycobacterium tuberculosis*	Dogs, cats	Cattle, pigs, sheep, goats, poultry	All except rodents and monkeys	Ingestion, inhalation
Tularemia	*Francisella tularensis*	All	All except horses	Rodents, rabbits	Tick bite, contact with tissue
Fungal Diseases					
Cryptococcosis	*Cryptococcus neoformans*			Birds	Contact
Ringworm	*Trichophyton* spp.	Dogs, cats	Cattle, horses, pigs, sheep	Rodents	Contact
Parasitic Infection					
Cryptosporidiosis	*Cryptosporidium parvum*		Cattle		Ingestion
Hydatid disease	Echinococcus	Dogs	Herbivores	Wolves	Ingestion
Larva migrans	*Toxocara, Ancylostoma, Strongyloides* spp.	Dogs, cats	Pigs, cattle	Raccoons	Ingestion
Scabies	*Sarcoptes scabiei*	Dogs, cats, rodents	Horses	Primates	Contact
Schistosomiasis	*Schistosoma*	Dogs, cats	Pigs, cattle, horses	Rodents	Contact
Taeniasis cysticercosis	*Taenia*		Pigs, cattle	Boars	Ingestion
Toxoplasmosis	*Toxoplasma gondii*	Cats	Pigs, sheep, goats		Ingestion
Trichinosis	*Trichinella spiralis*		Pigs	Rats, bears, carnivores	Ingestion
Rickettsial Diseases					
Psittacosis	*Chlamydophila psittaci*	Psittacine birds	Ducks, turkeys	Birds	Inhalation
Rocky Mountain spotted fever	*Rickettsia rickettsii*	Dogs		Rodents, rabbits	Tick bite

Continued

TABLE 15.2 Zoonotic diseases—Cont'd

	Causative Organism	Small-Animal Host	Livestock Host	Wildlife Host	Mode of Transmission
Viral Diseases					
Contagious ecthyma (orf)	Poxvirus	Dogs	Sheep, goats		Contact
Encephalitis (EEE, WEE)	Togavirus		Horses, poultry	Birds, rodents	Mosquito bite
Hantavirus	Hantavirus			Rodents	Contact
Lymphocytic choriomeningitis	Arenavirus	Mice			Varied
Monkeypox	Orthopoxvirus			Rodents	Contact
Newcastle disease	Paramyxovirus	Domestic birds	Poultry	Wild fowl	Contact, inhalation
Rabies	Rhabdovirus, togavirus	Almost all	Most	Most	Animal bite
Simian herpes	Herpesvirus simiae			Primates	Animal bite, direct contact
Yellow fever	Togavirus			Primates	Mosquito bite
Protozoal Infection					
Balantidiasis	*Balantidium coli*		Pigs	Rats, primates	Ingestion
Cryptosporidiosis	*Cryptosporidium* spp.	Most	Calves, sheep	Birds	Ingestion
Giardiasis	*Giardia lamblia*	Dogs, cats	Pigs, cattle	Beavers, zoo monkeys	Ingestion
Sarcocystosis	*Sarcocystis*	Dogs, cats	Pigs, cattle		Ingestion
Toxoplasmosis	*Toxoplasma gondii*	Cats, rabbits, Guinea pigs	Pigs, sheep, cattle, horses		Ingestion

EEE, Eastern equine encephalitis; *WEE*, Western equine encephalitis.

serves as a method of direct transmission. *Indirect transmission* of diseases is more complex and involves intermediaries that carry the agent of disease from one source to another. A *vector* is a living organism that transports infectious agents. A *vehicle* is the mode of transmission of an infectious agent from the reservoir to the host. Airborne transmission involves the spread of the agent through dust particles or droplet particles over long distances.

Arthropods, such as fleas, ticks, and mosquitoes, are considered vectors. They can carry an infectious agent to a susceptible host and be involved in the multiplication of organisms. They can also assist in a specific stage of development of the organism.

Food and water are vehicles for the indirect transmission of disease; both may be sources of bacterial, viral, and parasitic diseases. Foodborne diseases are acquired by the consumption of contaminated food or water and may be caused by toxins released by bacteria that are contained in the food. Parasites can also be transmitted through food, either through the ingestion of eggs or undercooked meat that contains cysts.

Control of Zoonotic Diseases

Because of the contact the veterinary team has with potentially infected pets, they may be the first to notice disease symptoms. It is important to recognize the most common threats seen in a practice's local area and to be knowledgeable about their symptoms, treatments, and prevention. Prevention programs require complete disease knowledge and how it is maintained to break the transmission cycle. Prevention of diseases may be aided by vaccinations, water filtration, and excellent hygiene skills.

People undergoing chemotherapy and/or treatment for HIV or AIDS, or those with compromised immune systems, are at particular risk of zoonotic disease. Pregnant women and individuals who have had their spleens removed are also immunocompromised and should use extra precaution when working with or around animals with zoonotic potential. Children may also be at a higher risk because they encounter contaminants in the outdoor environment.

Animal Bites

Animal bites can be a source of infection, trauma, and zoonotic diseases. An animal bite is defined as a bite wound that penetrates the skin, causing bleeding and swelling in the affected area. *Pasteurella* species are the most common bacteria present in both dog and cat bites.[2] Other bacteria that may be present in animal bites include *Staphylococcus aureus*, *Staphylococcus epidermidis*, *Streptococcus* spp., *Bacteroides* spp., *Fusobacterium* spp., and other gram-negative bacteria. In humans, these bacteria can cause fever, septicemia, meningitis, endocarditis, and septic arthritis. Any team member who is bitten by a patient should immediately wash the area with warm, soapy water for at least 5 minutes, apply a dilute povidone-iodine (Betadine) solution, and then rinse with a strong stream of water. The team member should seek medical attention, accounting for the potential risk of infection. If a team member declines medical treatment, a form should be signed and placed in the employee's medical file. This is necessary for protecting the practice in a worker's compensation case.

Animal Handling

Several safety issues are unique to veterinary hospitals, but none so much as animal behavior. Team training should focus on animal psychology and appropriate restraint. Watch the animal's body language and "listen" to the animal. Responding to the patient based on the body language presented can prevent injuries from occurring.

Restraint options fall into three categories: physical restraint (holding), chemical restraint (tranquilizers), and mechanical restraint (muzzles, bags, or blankets). When implementing Fear Free Practice techniques, chemical restraint should be administered long before mechanical restraint is even considered. See Chapters 3 (Veterinary Team) and 11 (Client Experience) for more information on Fear Free® protocols and reducing the number of team member injuries by using low-stress handling techniques.

Keep in mind that pain can cause a typically friendly dog to act out, and fear can cause even a "good dog" to bite.

Escaping Animals

Every measure should be taken to prevent the escape of an animal as the practice can be held liable. Windows should never be left open, even if there are screens on the window, as animals can go through screens. Doors should never be left open; dogs can escape from restraint or slip leashes. Any dog that is being removed from a cage or kennel should have a slip leash applied, not the owner's collar and leash, which are often too loose for appropriate control (Fig. 15.6). A slip leash tightens around the neck, preventing the dog from slipping away.

Extreme caution must be used when walking dogs outdoors. Ideally, practices should have a fenced-in area for dog walks to help prevent escapes. Again, slip leashes should be always used. Specific dogs may be denied walks based on the likelihood of them becoming scared and trying to escape. In situations such as this, the owner may be asked to come and walk the dog during the day.

When fearful animals react, the team member's safety could be jeopardized. The practice manager and safety manager must mitigate risks that place the team member's safety in jeopardy.

Feral Animals

Feral animals should always be handled with extreme caution. If an examination is necessary, they should be placed in a quiet room with no other animal access. The room should have minimal shelving and breakable items in case the animal escapes from restraint. Some feral animals can be examined with mild restraint; slow and cautious movements should be used to prevent startling the animal. If the animal escapes, it should be given time to calm down to avoid injury to the animal or team member. If this is not possible, then capture techniques will need to be used. A fish net may help capture a feral cat; a rabies pole may be needed for an aggressive dog. All precautions must be taken to avoid animal bites. Feral animals may need sedation before an examination for the safety of the staff.

Large Animals

Team members must always use caution when working with large animals and chutes. A team member's body must never be placed in a chute with an animal. The animal can be led into the chute with a rope from the outside; large animals can injure team members when there is nowhere to escape. Large animal stalls may also need to be locked, preventing the theft of patients. Large, durable locks that cannot be cut off must be used.

Bathing

Bathing and dipping patients can create a hazard; eye protection should be worn each time a bath or dip is performed. Pets tend to shake when they get wet; chemicals still present on the pet could splash into a team member's eye, causing damage. If this should occur, team members should not rub the eye(s), but rather find the nearest eyewash station and rinse the eyes for the amount of time suggested by the SDS. Dipping areas should also be well ventilated, as the fumes from many dips can be caustic.

Electrical Safety

Electrical safety in the veterinary practice generally focuses on outlets and power cords. Overloaded circuits or faulty wiring are the cause of most fires in veterinary practices (Fig. 15.7). Team members should frequently check cords for wear and tear, especially cords near patient cages. Check for crimps or breaks in the wires, either from cage doors or animal chewing.

Extension cords should only be used temporarily. If more outlets are needed, contact a certified electrician. Overloaded circuits should never be allowed. Receptacles, extension cords, surge protectors, or any plug multipliers must handle only the load they are meant to handle. Check the amperage of the equipment being used as well as the cord rating to be certain that it is not overloaded. Symptoms of electrical problems include frequently tripping circuits and lights that dim when large pieces of equipment are used.

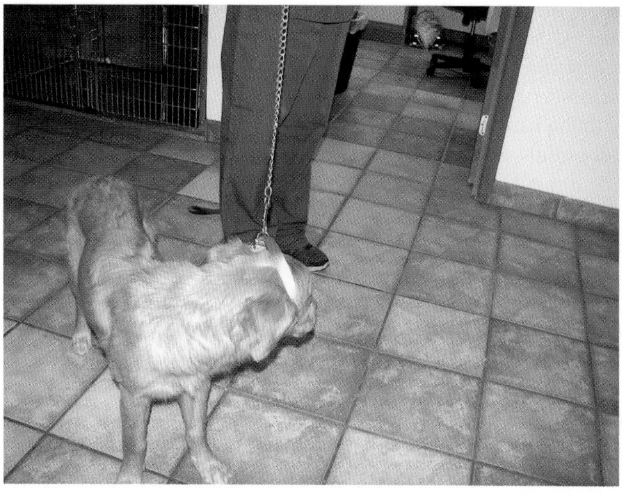

Fig. 15.6 Slip leashes should be used anytime a patient is transferred from one area of the hospital to another.

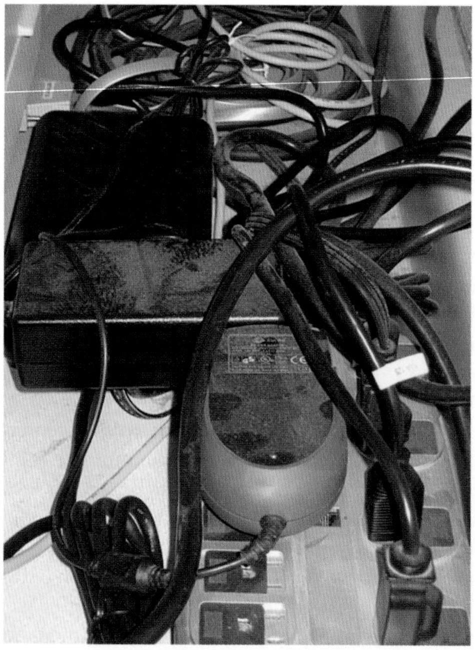

Fig. 15.7 This is an extremely unsafe electrical box with six electrical plugs.

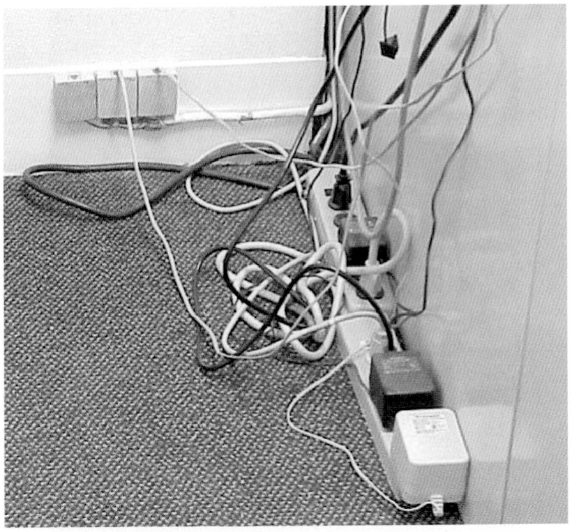

Fig. 15.8 Overloaded surge suppressors of extension cords can start a fire. (From Bassert JM, McCurnin DM: *McCurnin's clinical textbook for veterinary technicians*, ed 7, St Louis, 2010, Saunders Elsevier.)

Reviewing electrical safety should be a part of the hazard analysis completed each year (Fig. 15.8).

Emergency Action Plan

OSHA requires an emergency action plan (EAP) to be written and placed in the safety manual. The EAP must list potential reasons for an evacuation to occur and how the evacuation will be carried out. Consider the following conditions that *can* occur:

- Tornadoes
- Hurricanes
- Blizzards
- Floods
- Earthquakes
- Criminal activity
- Fire
- Explosion
- Medical emergencies (consider a client or team member having a stroke or heart attack)

> **LEADERSHIP POINT**
>
> Emergency action plans (EAPs) are a required part of a safety program to prepare the team for emergency protocols in the event of fire, tornado, blizzard, flooding, or any emergent situation that can happen in the practice.

The basic evacuation procedures should include how employees will be notified, how the emergency will be reported, where and how to exit the building, where the designated meeting place is outside of the building, and how to check in with the safety coordinator. Although not required by OSHA, EAPs should also include an evacuation plan for clients, especially those that may be visually or hearing impaired.

Patient evacuation is also important; however, team member safety cannot be compromised when there is a risk. Always leave animal rescues to properly trained professionals.

Safety coordinators should also be aware of emergency shutoff valve locations for gas, water, and electricity (where applicable).

Ergonomics

Ergonomics refers to reducing operator fatigue and discomfort through proper equipment use and the way we use our bodies. Although there are no OSHA standards regarding ergonomics, safety officers should consider any and all situations that may contribute to injuries. Employees suffering from aches and pain, caused by their environment or duties, have a higher rate of absenteeism, lower work performance, and a poor attitude due to discomfort.

> **LEADERSHIP POINT**
>
> Ergonomic injuries decrease team member productivity, accountability, and morale.

The main concern with ergonomics is back injury, though carpal tunnel syndrome is a problem for small animal surgeons and technologists who perform dental prophylaxes all day. In large animal medicine, the number one ergonomic injury is rotator cuff injury. Many people only think of computer workstations when they think of ergonomics, and veterinary hospitals have that concern as well. Often team members spend hours at a computer workstation.

Evaluate the practice for ergonomic improvements that may be made.

Fire Safety

Along with overloaded electrical circuits, items stored too close to heat sources are another common source of fires in veterinary practice. Newspapers, blankets, files, and supplies must not be stored near a furnace, water heater, or heat source, and portable heaters should never be left unattended.

Fire Prevention

Practices with 10 or more employees must have a fire prevention and response plan, which must be included in the safety manual. Fire prevention measures include a monthly walk-through of the facility. Smoke and fire alarms should be tested; if the building is equipped with a sprinkler system it should be evaluated as well. Fire extinguishers should be checked monthly for any damage or evidence of tampering. Walk-through inspections and equipment checks should be documented.

Fire Codes and Inspections

Fire codes vary by location. Each practice should become familiar with codes in its geographic area. In general, the fire department is responsible for inspections of businesses to ensure they are compliant with applicable regulations. Regulations will likely include fire extinguishers, smoke detectors, exit signs, and emergency lighting.

Exit Signs and Lighting

Signs must indicate where exits are located (Fig. 15.9). If a door looks like an exit but is not, it must be labeled "Not an Exit."

> **LEADERSHIP POINT**
>
> Doors that are not exits must be labeled "Not an Exit."

Emergency lights are required and must be tested yearly to ensure that they are working properly. Lights should be installed in locations that light the pathway to exits, as well as in locations where team members might be performing duties that could result in injury if the lighting system fails (Fig. 15.10).

Fire Extinguishers

Fire extinguishers must be located no more than 75 ft from any distance within the practice and placed 32 to 48 in above the ground surface. Along with being placed in central locations of the clinic, extinguishers should be placed near the exit doors of the practice (Fig. 15.11).

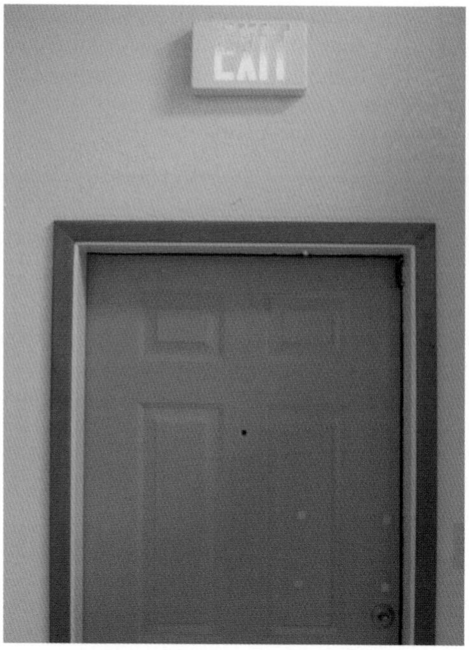

Fig. 15.9 All exits must be marked by an exit sign.

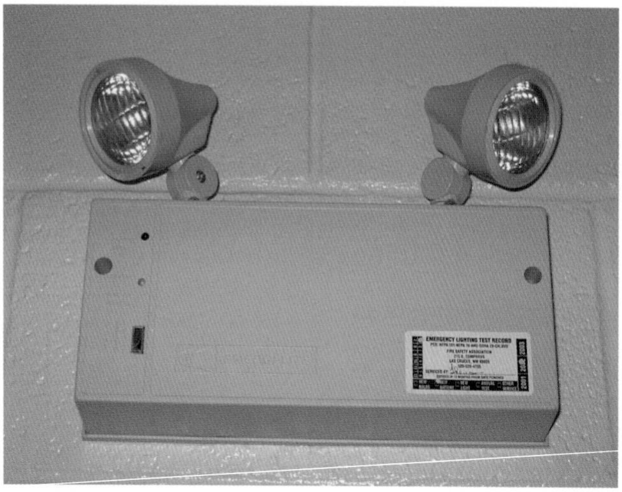

Fig. 15.10 Emergency lighting is required and must be tested on a yearly basis.

All employees must be trained in the use of a fire extinguisher. Team members should practice using extinguishers so that confident and rehearsed training can override panic in the event of an emergency. Practicing will help instill automatic reactions. Team members should remember the word "PASS" to help initiate the use of an extinguisher when needed as follows:

P = Pull the pin.
A = Aim low. Point the extinguisher to the bottom of the fire.
S = Squeeze the handle.
S = Sweep from side to side at the base of the fire until it appears to be out.

The fire department often offers complimentary instruction on fire extinguisher usage and fire safety training.

In emergency situations, employees should make sure that the fire alarm has been sounded before accessing or using fire extinguishers.

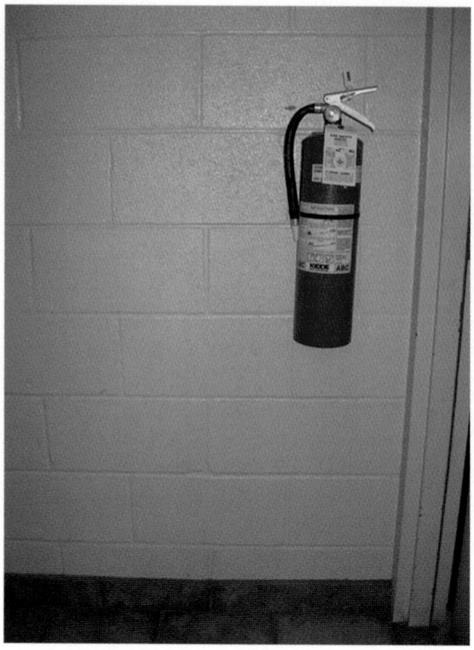

Fig. 15.11 Each team member should receive training in the use of a fire extinguisher.

Team members should never attempt to fight a fire that is larger than their immediate area, and if it is spreading, they must exit the building.

Smoke Detectors

Smoke detector batteries should be replaced annually whether a change is needed or not. Set up easy reminders in the practice appointment calendar. Monthly testing will ensure the product is in working condition.

Blocked Entries/Exits

Entries and exits must never be blocked, not even for a few minutes. In the event of a fire, anything that might obstruct emergency exits could have devastating effects.

Fire Response

The response portion of the fire safety plan should include the evacuation of employees and clients, escape routes and procedures, a process to account for all team members, and a method to report the fire. The name of the safety officer should be included as well. A fire could happen in any practice at any time. A fire could occur with no one in the building, or during the busiest time of the day. The team must be prepared to react immediately with skilled training protocols.

Fire escape drills should be a part of regular team training. At a minimum, they should be conducted once a year. The goal is to have a plan that supports order and control during emergency situations.

Indoor Air Quality

Indoor air quality is important to keep employees safe, especially those with respiratory conditions like asthma. Employees should report fumes or chemical odors immediately and let the safety officer know if they have experienced any sensitivity to fumes or odors, such as irritated nasal passages or headaches. Masks, respirators, and fume hoods should be used as needed.

The number one fume hazard in veterinary practice comes from analog radiologic processing chemicals. The exhaust fan should always be on when these are in use. Anesthetic gases are another safety issue.

Employees need to check tubing and fittings for leaks before each use. Laboratory chemicals are a third source of potential air quality problems and team members should be instructed to use a fume hood when appropriate.

Lifting

Team members should learn how to lift properly to prevent back injuries. Back injuries are the second most common job-related injury in veterinary medicine, often resulting from repeated trauma and microtears to the tissues and supporting structures in the back. Injuries can be chronic or acute; whichever the case, both can be debilitating for life. All employees must use the proper lifting techniques to prevent injuries from occurring.

Lifting must always be done with the legs rather than the back; women are especially prone to using their backs (Fig. 15.12). Team members should be aware and guide others when lifting objects to ensure the back is kept straight and the legs are used to the maximum potential. The hospital policy should require that all animals over 40 lbs. must be lifted by two team members to prevent back injuries. The practice can also obtain tables that can be raised to a variable height, either by hydraulic control or with the use of a foot pump (Fig. 15.13).

Moving Equipment

Multiple employees should assist with moving heavy equipment. More than one person must be responsible for the lifting and another team member should ensure the entryway or pathway is clear. The hospital policy should prohibit lifting anything over 40 lbs. without assistance.

Noise Hazards

Team members are often exposed to loud noises, especially in hospitals that include boarding facilities. Exposure to high levels of noise can lead to hearing deficiencies and hearing loss. Hearing must be protected, and OSHA has standard guidelines in place to do so. OSHA Standard 1910.95 requires noise measurement, noise protection, and hearing testing when noise measurement exceeds 85 dB. Noise measurement can be completed with a decibel meter and should be done at least annually, or at times when the noise level has been increased.

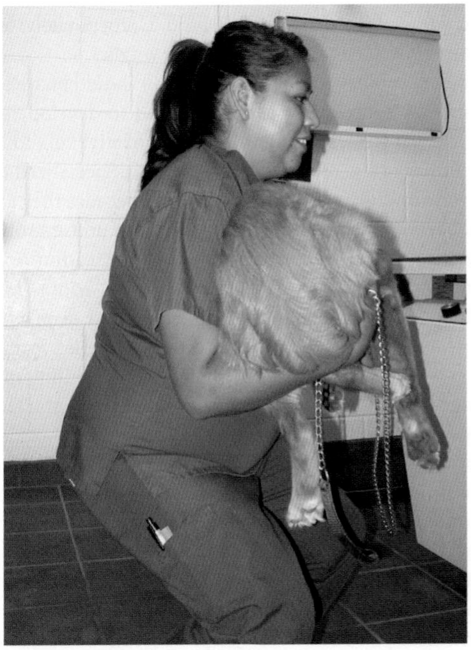

Fig. 15.12 Always lift with the legs to prevent injuries to the back.

Employee exposure to excessive noise depends on several factors, including the loudness of the noise as measured in decibels, the duration of each employee's exposure to the noise, whether employees move between work areas with different noise levels, and whether noise is generated from one or multiple sources.

Generally, the louder the noise, the shorter the exposure time before hearing protection is required. Some kennels exceed noise levels that are considered safe for short and long-term hearing of employees who are exposed.

Hearing protection should be provided to employees when exposure to loud noise occurs for prolonged periods of time. Single-use earplugs made of cotton, foam, silicone, or rubber work well when properly inserted. Preformed earplugs (Fig. 15.14) can be fitted for individuals, or earmuffs can be provided.

Noise hazard areas should be identified with signage notifying team members that hearing protection is required for prolonged exposure.

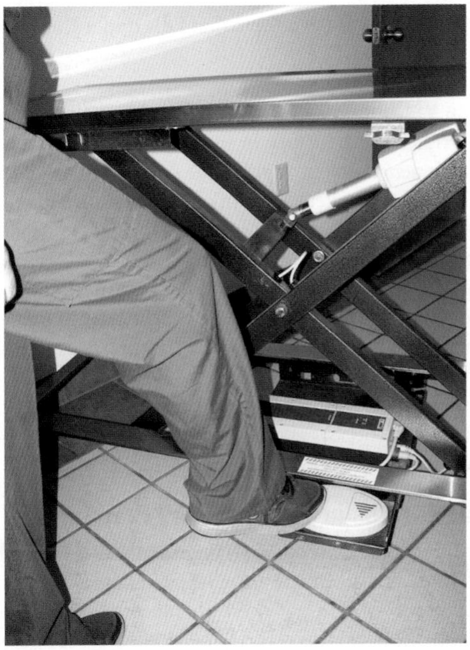

Fig. 15.13 Hydraulic tables or those with foot pumps are excellent for lifting large breed dogs.

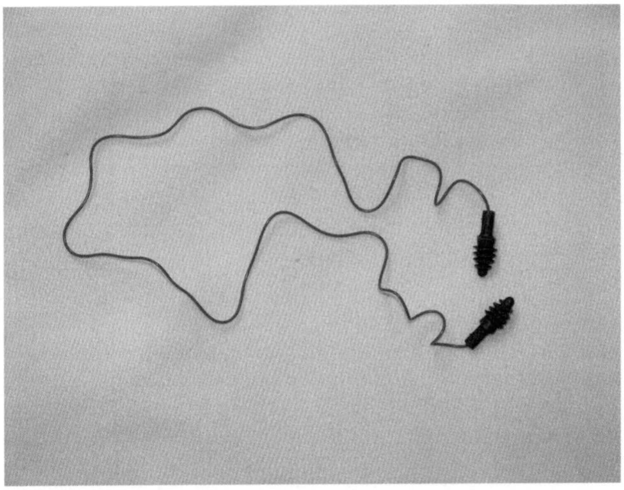

Fig. 15.14 Form-fitting earplugs should be available for team members to wear in kennel areas when sound exceeds 85 dB.

Running

Team members should never be allowed to run through the practice, regardless of how busy they are. Running increases the risk of slipping, especially on wet surfaces. An employee may have finished just mopping the floor and be placing wet floor signs; if a team member is running through the area at the same time a serious injury could occur. The same applies to horseplay while at work. Both fall under the General Duty Clause and should be forbidden and outlined in the safety manual.

Wet Floors

When floors are mopped, they become extremely slippery. "Wet floor" signage should be posted around wet areas immediately, and team members should towel dry wet areas as soon as possible. Team members and clients should be encouraged to walk around wet areas. However, the sooner floors are dry, the less likely a slip or fall will occur (Fig. 15.15). Team members are encouraged to wear nonskid shoes to help prevent slips in the veterinary practice. A wet floor is another example of a topic that falls under the General Duty Clause.

Workplace Violence

Workplace violence can happen in any veterinary practice, and OSHA includes it as a general safety topic to be addressed in the safety manual and with employees. Clients, coworkers, family, friends, drug seekers, and thieves are all potential candidates for causing violence in the workplace.

During the hazard assessment of the facility, do not forget to include potential situations that could expose team members to violence. Safety plans should identify potential threats as well as prevention and response measures.

A zero-tolerance policy for workplace violence should be developed for the protection of all team members (see Chapter 4, Human Resources).

Chemical Hazards in the Veterinary Practice

Veterinary practices have chemicals on premise that can be extremely dangerous to employees. Team members should pay special attention to these substances. Many of these chemicals are listed on OSHA's IDLH list. Chemicals in this class include (and are not limited to) ethylene oxide, formaldehyde, chemotherapy agents, and anesthetic gases.

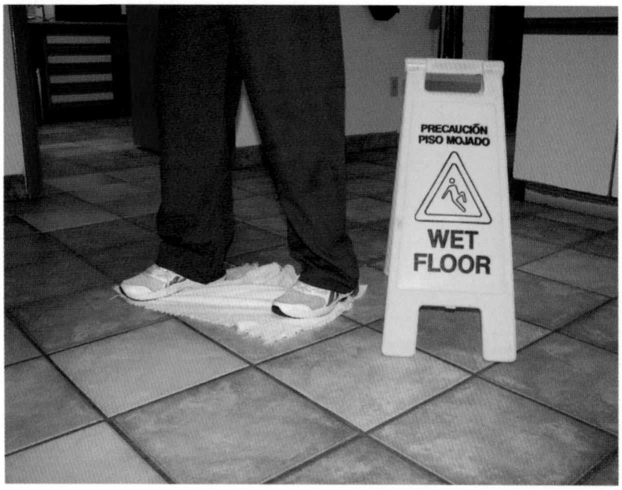

Fig. 15.15 Wet floors are always a danger. Prevent injuries by drying the floor with a towel (while a wet floor sign is posted).

View a full list of IDLH chemicals at https://www.cdc.gov/niosh/idlh/intridl4.html.

The effort involved in documenting chemical hazards in the workplace can be substantial, especially considering the number of chemicals that OSHA categorizes as hazardous. Veterinarians and team members are exposed to many chemicals with a wide range of health hazards (irritating, sensitizing, carcinogenic, etc.) and physical hazards (flammable, reactive, corrosive). Often team members take these chemicals for granted, dismissing the possibility of harming themselves while taking care of patients.

Hazardous chemicals are not limited to laboratory reagents or liquids and may include cleaning products, clerical products, or pharmaceuticals. Hazardous chemicals take many forms: liquids, solids, gases, vapors, fumes, and mists. Common chemicals used in the veterinary facility include (but are not limited to) the following:

- Alcohol (isopropyl)
- Anesthetic gases
- Antineoplastic drugs
- Povidone-iodine (Betadine)
- Bleach
- Formalin
- Glass cleaners
- Glutaraldehyde
- Room deodorizer
- Wite-Out®

Many opportunities exist for toxic exposures in veterinary practices. Chemical exposures come in the form of cleaning supplies, chemotherapy agents, and medications that are dispensed or used in the hospital for patients.

The mixing of two or more chemicals can create caustic fumes that are harmful to both team members and patients. The fumes may not seem harmful, and at times may even smell good, such as those produced when bleach and a lemon disinfectant are combined; however, prolonged exposure may be dangerous and can cause respiratory irritation.

Every team member is exposed to chemotherapy agents if they are administered in the veterinary practice (discussed in further detail later in this chapter). Many chemotherapeutic agents are expelled in the urine and feces of pets; therefore, each time the animal eliminates in the cage, some of the drug is left behind. Unfortunately, team members may be exposed to these drugs unknowingly.

Radiology developer rooms (if still in use) should be well ventilated to an outside air source. The chemicals used to develop radiographs are strong and harmful. If the developer and fixative mix for some reason, the chemical odor released can be caustic. Specialized companies should retrieve and dispose of x-ray solutions because they are an environmental hazard. This applies to both used and unused solutions.

Always remember that when handling medication, excess drug powder and residual collects on team members' hands. Medications are often handled when team members count and dispense prescriptions for owners or pull medications to treat patients. Team members must always wash their hands immediately after handling medications to avoid ingesting substances or transferring them to the face or eyes. Many drugs appear to be safe but repeated ingestion is not. Some drugs are known to have side effects. Chloramphenicol, for example, may suppress bone marrow production in some individuals. Unfortunately, this reaction does not appear for months, or even years, after exposure to the drug.

As stated in the hazard communications section, each employee must be familiar with all chemicals on the premises, know the hazards of these chemicals, and know how to protect him or herself from each hazard. Two ways to ensure this occurs are creating and maintaining a chemical inventory list and creating and maintaining Safety Data Sheets (SDSs).

Chemical Inventory List

A chemical inventory list should be completed annually (Fig. 15.16). Any time a new product is added to the hospital inventory, it should be added to this list and an SDS obtained. The new SDS sheet must also be posted in an area visible for all team members to view for 2 weeks.

Chemicals that require special attention include ethylene oxide, formaldehyde, glutaraldehyde, chemotherapeutic agents, and anesthetic gases.

Ethylene oxide is a carcinogen used for gas sterilization procedures. It is extremely important to have a safe handling protocol in place for use of this product. Only approved sterilization devices must be used with ethylene oxide, and levels should be monitored to ensure team member safety (Fig. 15.17). This chemical is highly flammable and must be used with caution.

Formaldehyde is used to fix tissue samples and is a known carcinogen. Vapors can be extremely dangerous and are known to cause cancer and loss of pregnancy. Practices should order biopsy jars that are prefilled with formalin. This prevents unnecessary exposure to team members. If gallon containers of formalin are used, the chemical should be poured into smaller containers under a fume hood that will capture the vapors. Goggles and gloves should also be worn when handling this chemical to prevent any contact.

Glutaraldehyde is a chemical used to disinfect instruments, generally in cold trays. It is an excellent fungicide and viricide but can be extremely traumatic to tissue. If glutaraldehyde is not diluted properly, it can cause tissue damage to team members and patients. Many other disinfectants provide superior protection and are much safer to use in veterinary practice.

Chemotherapeutic Agents

Practices that provide chemotherapeutic treatments to patients should strongly consider meeting the stringent standards (ventilation, isolation, PPE) before the implementation of any protocols. Safety of the team members should be the number one priority.

Every team member is exposed to chemotherapeutic agents if they are administered in the practice. Chemotherapy is composed of chemicals used to kill tumor cells; these chemicals inadvertently affect healthy cells as well. All precautions must be taken when working with these drugs (Fig. 15.18). Patients' bodily excretions, including vomitus, urine, and feces, will also contain the drugs in both metabolized and unmetabolized forms.

When prepping such drugs for administration, PPE must be worn. This includes a mask, eye protection, a disposable gown, and thick unpowdered gloves. Chemicals can be easily inhaled; therefore, a fume hood with a vent must be used during the mixing process. A mask provides some protection, but the fume hood will remove the excess aerosolized chemical. Contact lenses should not be worn at any time during the mixing and or administration of chemotherapy agents, regardless of eye protection. A disposable gown should be used and disposed of when the mixing and administration processes have been completed. Cuffs should be tucked inside gloves. Thick unpowdered gloves are required. Thin latex gloves provide less protection and powdered gloves tend to attract drug residue.

Once the entire mixing and administration process has been completed, all items including gloves, gowns, and needles must be disposed of in a yellow biohazardous waste container. The yellow container indicates that chemotherapeutic agents are inside; these containers will be incinerated separately from other biohazard containers.

Bedding used for animals receiving chemotherapy should be handled with gloves and a disposable gown for protection. Bedding must be washed separately from other bedding. It must also be washed twice with laundry detergent. Chemotherapeutic agents are released in the urine and feces of patients. Any time the bedding or kennel is contaminated, it must be treated as such, and appropriate measures must be taken to clean the area.

If a chemotherapeutic agent is spilled, team members and patients must evacuate the area. One team member should protect their exposure with a disposable gown and double gloves and place an absorbable material over the spill. Once the agent is completely absorbed, all material must be placed in a yellow biohazardous waste container. The area must be washed with 70% alcohol twice before the area can be declared safe.

Clients must also be considered when patients are receiving chemotherapy. If clients have pets at home, and the pet urinates and defecates, children may be at risk, along with their parents. Client education materials must clearly indicate the precautions that should be taken, based on the drug administered to that patient.

Anesthetic Gases

Because of their proximity to the source, veterinarians and veterinary surgical technicians are at the highest risk for overexposure to gases. Other operating room employees in the veterinary clinic are also at risk. The primary hazardous gases are nitrous oxide and halothane, which can cause congenital birth defects, loss of pregnancy, cancer, irritability, depression, and headaches.

Inhaled anesthetic agents include two different classes of chemicals: nitrous oxide and halogenated agents. Halogenated agents currently in use include halothane, enflurane, isoflurane, desflurane, and sevoflurane.

Every team member that is monitoring an anesthetized patient, whether perioperative or postoperative, must receive proper training.

Anesthesia-related training topics should include:

- depth and planes of anesthesia,
- medication's mechanism of action, side effects, and contraindications,
- proper anesthetic hose size,
- correct endotracheal tube size and proper inflation,
- anesthesia machine maintenance,
- scavenging systems,
- cleanup of liquid anesthesia spills, and
- leak-checking machine.

Anesthesia safety meetings should occur regularly to continually educate team members on the risks of anesthesia. New team members must be fully trained and made aware of the risks involved while working with anesthesia and anesthetized patients.

Some common reasons for exposure to anesthetic gases and potential preventative measures are as follows:

Improperly functioning scavenging systems: The reservoir bag should be fully collapsed to half full. If it is underfilled or overfilled, the system will not function optimally. Several scavengers exist; the practice should use the one that works best in that individual practice. Active scavengers provide the best protection; however, passive exhaust and adsorption scavenging systems are also effective means of removing gases.

The active system has some means of energetic collection. This is usually a fan enclosed in a box that creates a vacuum through a series of tubes that are connected to the patient or machine. Active scavengers may also attach directly to the machine and push the waste anesthetic gases through the system instead of producing a vacuum. Active scavengers are best for practices that handle a large volume of

Sample - Hazardous Chemicals Inventory List

Hazardous Chemical Name	Operation/Area Used	Date Brought to Site	Date Removed From Site

In accordance with 29 CFR 1910.1020(d)(1)(ii)(B), this form shall be retained for 30 years after the chemical has left the premises.

Sample Hazard Communication Program 12

Fig. 15.16 Example of a chemical inventory list that should be completed once a year in the veterinary practice. (Courtesy Occupational Safety and Health Administration, Department of Labor, Washington, DC.)

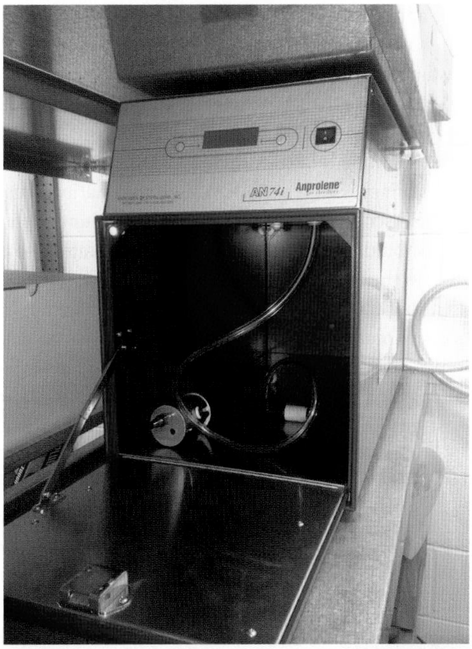

Fig. 15.17 Ethylene oxide is used in gas sterilizers and must be used with caution.

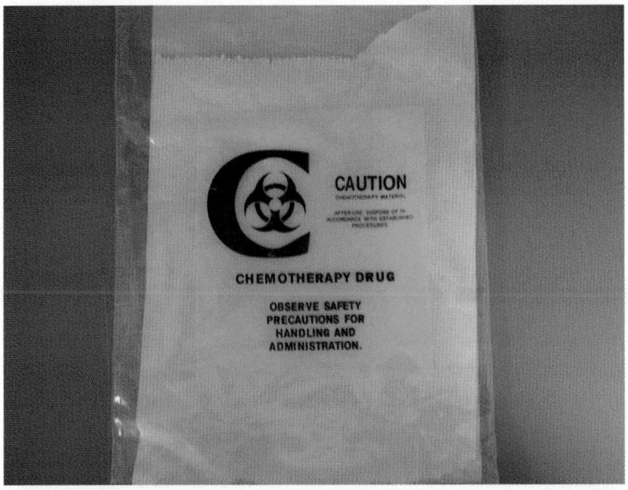

Fig. 15.18 Chemotherapeutic agents must be identified with a bright yellow label.

procedures requiring anesthesia or that perform them at various locations throughout the practice. The main disadvantage to an active scavenger system is cost. Systems can range in price from $400 to $4000, depending on the complexity of the system. Secondary disadvantages include maintenance of the machine and manual activation. Team members must turn on a switch to activate the scavenger and may forget the turn-on switch until the patient's breathing bag fails to work properly.

The passive exhaust system channels waste anesthetic gases through a tube to an acceptable location for evacuation. This system is only good for short distances because the only means of expelling the gas is the patient's lung pressure and the flow rate of gas; therefore, small or weak animals may not be able to expel gases efficiently.

The adsorption scavenger uses charcoal to remove all halogenated gases. It does not adsorb nitrous oxide. Charcoal canisters must be replaced after 20 g of adsorption and must be monitored for replacement. If canisters are not replaced, waste anesthetic gases will overflow into the room.

For the safety of both patients and team members, anesthetic machines must have adequate scavenging systems.

Improperly Fitted Endotracheal Tubes With Cuffs Inadequately Inflated: Ensure that the correct size of the endotracheal tube is selected for the patient and that the cuff is filled to an appropriate level.

Not Flushing the System With Oxygen Before Removing Patient From Machine: To help decrease waste anesthetic gases, team members should turn off the anesthesia to the patient (upon completion of a procedure), allowing the continued flow and intake of oxygen. This allows the patient to breathe off excess anesthetic gas, which circulates through the system instead of in the operating room for team members to inhale. Once the patient has received approximately 5 to 10 minutes of oxygen, it can be moved to the recovery area of the practice. "Boxing-down" patients (placing them in a sealed container with direct administration of oxygen and anesthesia) also creates waste anesthetic gases that the team inhales. Every effort should be made to use an injectable means of anesthetic induction until the patient is ready for an endotracheal tube. If a box or mask is needed, proper ventilation in the room should be mandatory.

Equipment Leaks: Machines should be inspected daily for leaks. A pressure test should be performed indicating that the machine holds pressure without leaks, the vaporizer refill lid is secure, all hoses are attached properly, and the bag does not contain a hole. Hoses and gaskets should be replaced yearly as part of an anesthetic maintenance plan, which helps prevent small, undetectable leaks. OSHA expects that practices will have professional maintenance performed on their anesthetic machines every 12 months. Some state veterinary medical boards require a professional annual inspection of all anesthetic machines.

When team members change soda lime granules on anesthetic machines, gloves should be worn. Used soda lime can be caustic to tissues.

Team members who are pregnant and required to work around anesthetic gases should wear an anesthetic monitoring badge along with proper PPE for their own safety. OSHA's exposure limit for halogenated gases (e.g., halothane, isoflurane, sevoflurane) is 2 ppm/year. Nitrous oxide's maximum exposure limit is 25 ppm/year.

If a spill of liquid anesthesia occurs, team members should be evacuated from the area. One team member using appropriate PPE should open windows and turn on exhaust fans. Cat litter can be poured over the spill. Once it has been absorbed, the litter can be swept up and disposed of. Spills may occur when the machine is being refilled or as bottles are being unpacked from a received order. All caution should be taken to prevent the inhalation of gases.

Chemical Spills

Accidents happen and spills can occur in any situation. A preparedness plan will help facilitate easy cleanup and prevent unnecessary exposure. A spill kit should be developed and maintained, and each team member must know where the kit is located. Practice using the spill kit should be included in safety training, so each member knows how to use the kit in case of emergency.

When developing a spill kit, hazardous chemicals that are kept inside the practice need to be identified. SDSs indicate the best cleanup method if a spill occurs. The information should be consolidated into an information sheet that is easy to understand. The sheet can be laminated for protection.

A spill kit should include a large plastic container to keep contents together. Contents include cat litter, a dustpan and broom, a pair of nitrile gloves, eye protection, and a laminated copy of cleanup procedures. The spill kit should be centrally located and easy to access (Fig.15.19).

Chemical Spill Cleanup Procedures

- Remove unnecessary people and pets from the area to prevent spreading and exposure to the chemical.
- Increase ventilation to the area; open windows and turn on exhaust fans and vents.
- Put on protective gloves (and gown if needed).
- Cover the spill with absorbable material; either cat litter or paper towels.
- Clean up saturated absorbent material.
- Place chemical in proper disposal container.
- Wash area with plain water and allow it to dry.
- Wash hands.
- Replace materials used in spill kit.

Eyewash Stations

Eyewash stations are required for every safety program and must be available if a team member or client gets a chemical or foreign object in the eye. Affected team members must be able to walk to an eyewash station within ten seconds of being exposed to a chemical; therefore, large practices must have more than one eyewash station.

LEADERSHIP POINT

Eyewash stations should be centrally located and easy to access at any time.

A variety of eyewash stations are available, ranging from handheld bottles to stations connected to a consistent water supply. The most common are eyewash stations that simply attach to the top of a water faucet spout and are capped until needed. When the station is needed, a lever on the station is turned to allow water pressure to dispense; water is squirted upward, allowing the employee to place their eyes in direct contact with pressurized water (Fig. 15.20). This allows the flushing of any chemical that entered the eye. Most chemicals require flushing for 5 to 10 minutes; this information can be obtained from the SDS. Water will feel uncomfortable when flushing begins, as it is not the same pH as the eye and does not have the same salt content; however, team members must understand flushing is essential to remove potentially harmful substances and objects.

Eyewash stations that are connected to a consistent water supply are ideal because they apply the same amount of pressure to the eye for a period of time. Handheld bottles (Fig. 15.21) run out of water and do not supply constant pressure. If a faucet-mounted station is used, the hot water should be disconnected to prevent further injury to the eye. Each team member should practice using the eyewash station so that all are familiar with it in the event of an emergency. Eyewash stations should be marked with a sticker or sign indicating equipment location (Fig. 15.22).

The process of maintaining the eyewash station(s) will vary depending on the type of unit; however, a log documenting the performance of weekly maintenance checks must be maintained. The American National Standards Institute (ANSI) requires a 3-minute flushing weekly.

Biohazards in the Veterinary Practice

Needles, glass, slides, surgical blades, and coverslips are all considered "sharps" and must be discarded in a biohazard or sharps container. Containers must be puncture-resistant and sealable once the container

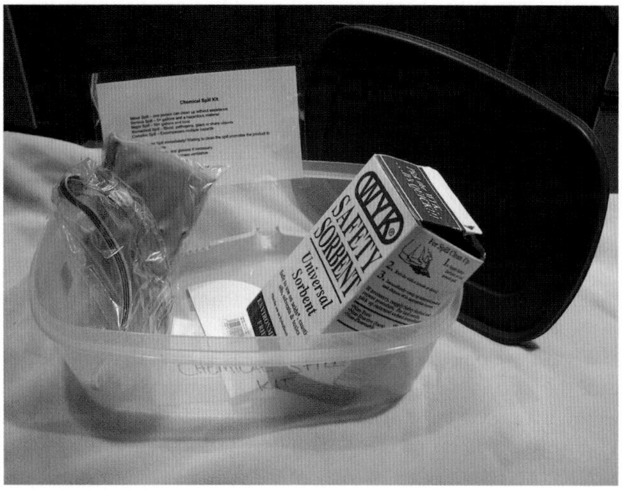

Fig. 15.19 Chemical spills kits can be purchased or created and should be located centrally within the veterinary hospital.

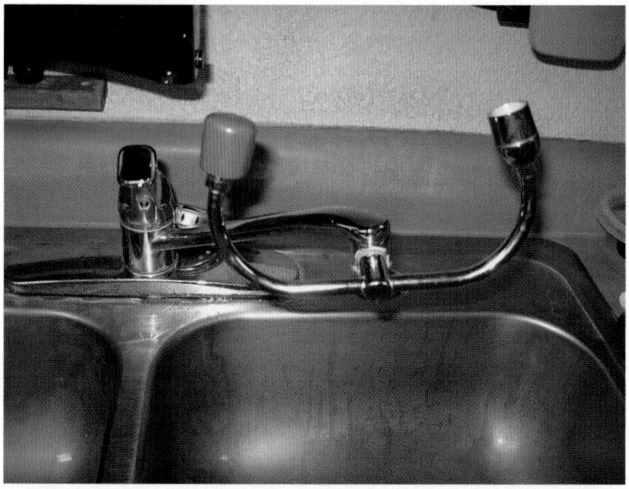

Fig. 15.20 Eyewash stations should be centrally located.

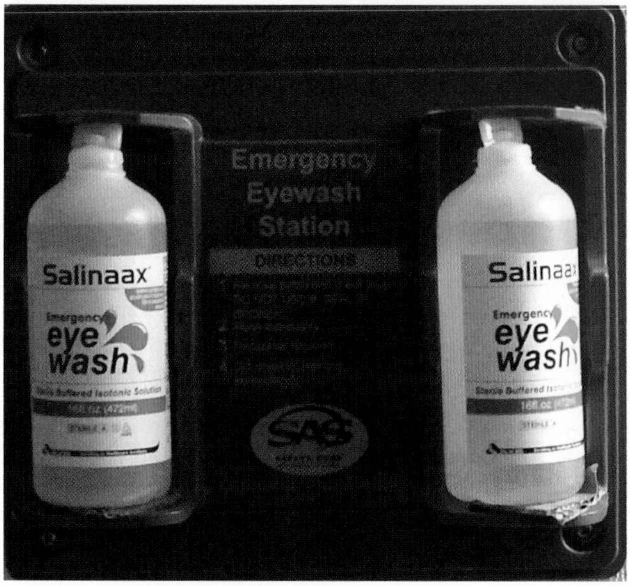

Fig. 15.21 Hand-held eyewash station.

is full. Milk jugs are not acceptable. Biohazard containers (Fig. 15.23) are red and come in a variety of sizes depending on the needs of the practice. A specialized company that incinerates the contents should pick up these containers on a regular basis. Some states may require proof of biohazard incineration; be sure to keep all receipts indicating when the biohazard container was picked up, as well as the date of incineration.

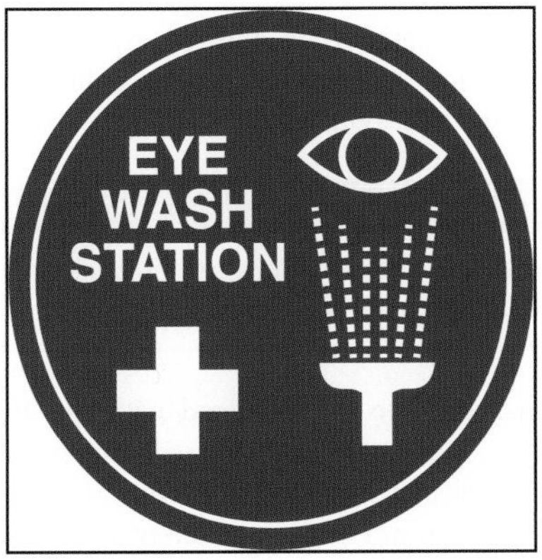

Fig. 15.22 Eyewash station sign.

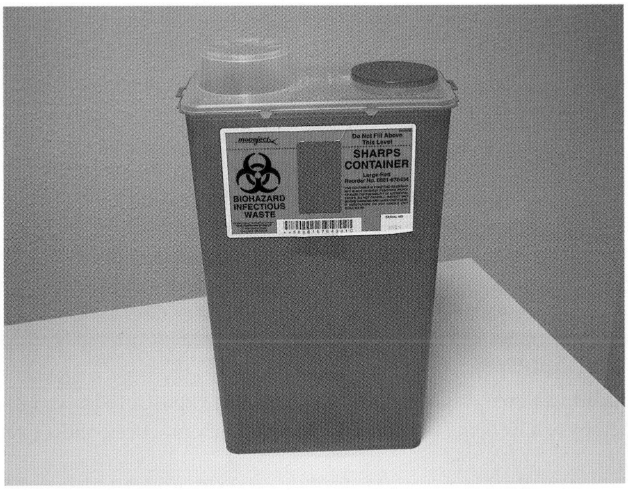

Fig. 15.23 Biohazardous waste container.

Team members must take every precaution when handling biohazard material to prevent injury or exposure to disease. Containers cannot be opened once the cap has been applied unless the plastic tabs are broken. If this happens, the container is regarded as unusable and must be emptied and discarded.

Needles should not be cut off at the tip before disposal, because this practice increases the risk of aerosolizing the contents of the needle and syringe. The entire needle must be discarded.

Practices should have two separate refrigerators labeled accordingly: one for human food and the other for biologics, laboratory tests, and drugs (Fig. 15.24). This prevents the contamination and ingestion of medical products. Team members should be encouraged to keep food, coffee, and drinks in break rooms or lounges instead of on hospital counters or examination tables. Bacteria, dirt, and residual medications reside on counters and can be easily ingested if food or drinks are placed there.

LEADERSHIP POINT

If team members are allowed to consume food on the premises, a safe environment (break room) must be provided for them to do so. This safe environment must be free of chemical and physical hazards that exist throughout the hospital (OSHA's General Duty Clause).

Radiation Safety

Radiation exposure in the practice must be taken seriously. Excess radiation causes birth defects, decreased fertility, and cancer, and every precaution must be taken to limit exposure. Team members must always wear PPE when taking radiographs. Employers who do not provide proper PPE are in violation of OSHA standards, as they are not providing a safe work environment. OSHA states that team members must be properly trained on PPE usage. Practices can include a section in their employee and safety manual that states if employees do not abide by the requirements set forth by the hospital, they can be terminated immediately for lack of or improper use of protective equipment.

Lead gloves, gowns, and thyroid collars are the minimum PPE that must be worn to take radiographs. If possible, team members should leave the room for best protection. If an animal is sedated, rice bags, sandbags, ties, and tape can be used to position the animal for the desired view, allowing team members to leave the room.

Radiographs should be collimated, preventing excess radiation exposure to team members. *Collimation* can be defined as shrinking the light source to only include the patient; this light source indicates

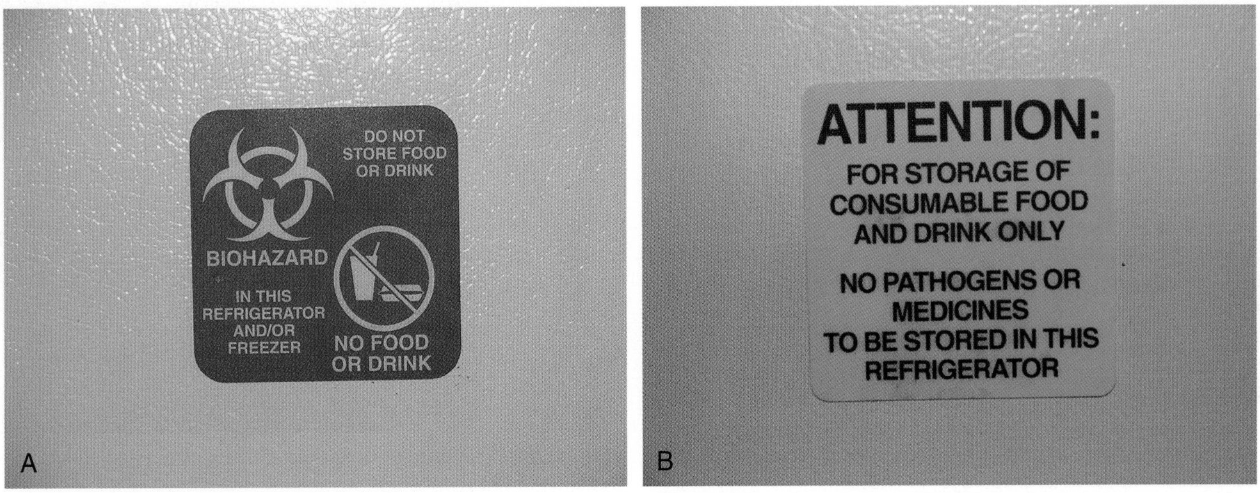

Fig. 15.24 (A) Biohazard materials, including vaccinations and tests, should never be stored with human food intended for consumptions. (B) Consumable food should never be stored with biohazard materials. Magnets can be placed on refrigerators to indicate contents.

where the radiation beam will penetrate. If excess beams miss the patient and bounce off the table, this is termed *scatter radiation*, which increases a team member's exposure to radiation.

Gloves should never be in the direct x-ray beam because radiation can penetrate lead that is cracked and/or broken. Full gloves are the only gloves that can provide protection for team members' hands. Partial gloves may make it easier to restrain pets, but the exposure to radiation increases dramatically (Fig. 15.25). Partial gloves do not meet OSHA standards. Never compromise team member safety for convenience.

LEADERSHIP POINT

Never compromise team member safety by using partial gloves for radiographs.

All PPE should be x-rayed on a yearly basis to look for cracks that may have occurred. Cracks develop when team members fold gowns, gloves, or thyroid collars instead of hanging or laying them on a flat surface. If any cracks or holes have developed, the PPE device must be replaced immediately. Radiographs should be kept for comparison from year to year.

Portable units are often found in large animal practices and can be dangerous because the x-ray beam can be pointed in any direction. A cassette-holding pole should be used to hold the cassette during the x-ray process. A gloved hand should never hold the cassette. Team members should also make sure there is not another person in the direct line of the beam, even at a distance.

Some hospitals may have their x-ray machine located in the main treatment room. Although this is not ideal, some hospitals may not be able to relocate the machine, because of structural or design challenges. It should be practice policy that unprotected team members must leave the room until the radiograph images have been captured. Scatter radiation puts unprotected team members at risk.

A dosimeter badge, used to measure radiation exposure, must be worn every time an x-ray is taken. The badges should be stored outside the room to prevent scatter radiation from affecting the badges. Badges should be worn at collar level, outside of the PPE (Fig. 15.26). Dosimeters indicate the amount of exposure the team member is receiving. Badges should be sent to a monitoring company on a monthly or quarterly basis, where a report will be generated and returned to the practice. These reports must be monitored and reviewed upon their return to check for any significant change in exposure readings. If a badge reads high, this could indicate that the x-ray machine is functioning improperly and emitting excess radiation. This is detrimental to employee safety and must be corrected immediately.

As mandated by OSHA, dosimetry reports must be kept on hand for 30 years. Team members should always have access to data regarding the amount of radiation they have been exposed to while employed at the practice (Fig. 15.27).

Veterinary staff members are allowed a maximum exposure of 5 rem/year of radiation, whereas the general public is only allowed a maximum exposure of 0.5 rem/year.

LEADERSHIP POINT

Damage to human body parts after excessive exposure to radiation is real. Always wear PPE as designated to prevent long-term health risks.

Machines may need to be registered with the appropriate state agencies annually. Most state agencies will inspect the machine(s), ensure the paperwork matches serial and model numbers, and conduct individual tests. These tests evaluate the safety of the machine and confirm it is working properly and operating in an acceptable condition. State regulations may require that inspection reports be posted in the x-ray room.

Appropriate signage must be posted outside radiology rooms.

Some states also require rights and responsibilities of both employers and employees be posted, along with a written protocol of how to take and process a radiograph.

Dental x-ray machines also emit radiation, although at smaller doses. Team members should always be at least six feet away from the head of the x-ray unit, with attention being paid to the direction in which the head is pointed (stay out of the direct line of the beam). Dosimetry badges help detect inadvertent exposure, and dental film should never be held in the patient's mouth. Gauze and positioning aids must be available to aid in obtaining dental radiographs.

Laser Safety

The human eye is vulnerable to damage when exposed to lasers. Laser therapy is now being introduced into veterinary practices, and a safety

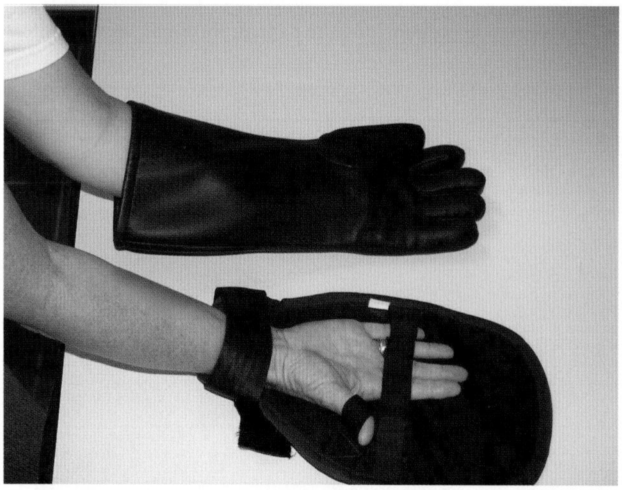

Fig. 15.25 Full x-ray gloves *(top glove)* provide complete protection, whereas partial gloves *(bottom glove)* provide minimal protection against radiation exposure (and not recommended).

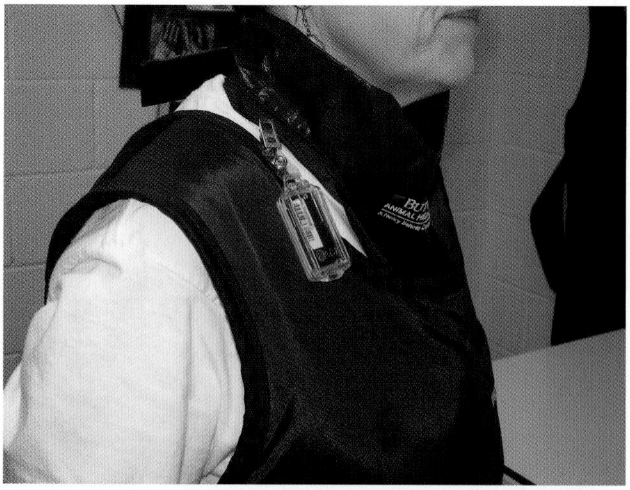

Fig. 15.26 Dosimeters monitor radiation exposure and should be worn outside of PPE.

Account Number: 0000976
Report Date: 02/13/2019
Wear Period: 01/09/2019 to 02/07/2019

ANNUAL RADIATION EXPOSURE LIMITS:

Whole body, blood forming organs	5,000 mrem/yr
Lens of eye	15,000 mrem/yr
Extremetien and skin	50,000 mrem/yr
Fetal	500 mrem/gentation period
General public	100 mrem/yr

These limits are based on USNRC Regulation Title 10, Part 20

DOSAGE LEGEND

curr - current badge reading
ytd - year-to-date accumulated dosage
the - lifetime accumulated storage

View your dosage report online & provide feedback at http://myTLDaccount.PLMedical.com

OCCUPATIONAL RADIATION DOSE RECORD — Page 1 of 1

	Name	Employee ID / DOB	Type	Badge #	Dose Equivalents (in millirem)				Comments
						Deep	Eye	Shallow	
					curr				
1	Control	-----	T		ytd				
					life				
		001			curr	18	18	18	
2	Bevery Rains	-----	T	0049402	ytd	18	18	18	
					life	421	421	409	
		002			curr	11	11	11	
3	Bernice Kim	-----	T	0103557	vtd	11	11	11	
					life	292	292	282	
		003			curr	25	32	21	
4	Alice Lynch	-----	T	0104208	ytd	25	32	21	
					lite	264	264	258	
		004			curr	MR	MR	MR	
5	Nicole Allen	-----	T	0041925	ytd	MR	MR	MR	
					life	284	284	275	
		005			curr	45	43	45	
6	Margaret Moss	-----	T	0052765	ytd	45	43	45	
					life	280	280	270	
		006			curr	MR	MR	MR	
7	Mary Williams	-----	T	0042873	ytd	MR	MR	MR	
					life	315	315	301	
		007			curr	MR	MR	MR	
8	Jeffrey Dodson	-----	T	0034456	ytd	MR	MR	MR	
					life	252	252	245	
		008			curr	101	97	98	
9	Roy Robinson	-----	T	0044819	ytd	101	97	98	
					life	255	255	246	
		009			curr	MR	MR	MR	
10	Christopher Gagne	-----	T	0083207	ytd	MR	MR	MR	
					life	242	242	234	

This report must not be used to claim product certification, approval, or endorsement by NVLAP, NIST, or any agency of the Federal Government. A copy of the PL Medical Co., LLC NVLAP certificate and scope of accreditation can be found on http://www.plmedical.com/public/Accreditation.htm.

Fig. 15.27 Example of a dosimetry report.

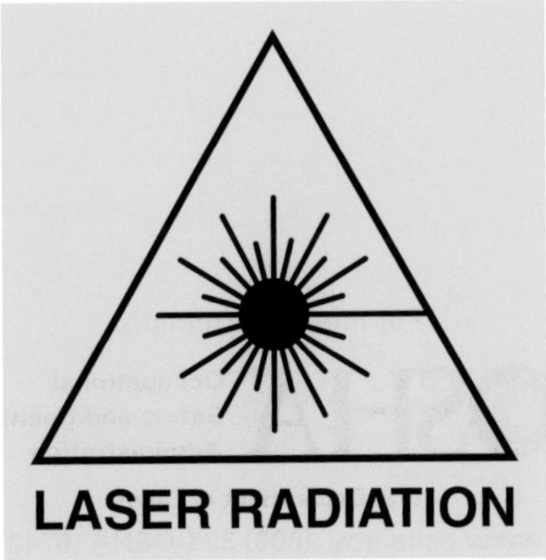

Fig. 15.28 Laser sign.

program must be implemented with this equipment to protect team members' eyes.

Lasers are classified into various levels, and include Class 1, Class 1 M, Class 2, Class 2 M, Class 3, and Class 4. Each class has its own restrictions and protection; therefore it is imperative to determine the type of laser a practice uses and develop a plan based on those risks. Protective equipment includes skin protection, protective eyewear, and laser warning signs (Fig. 15.28).

SAFETY DATA SHEETS

SDSs are fact sheets with important information and warning about hazardous chemicals (Fig. 15.29). Information included on SDSs is as follows:

- Identity of the chemical
- Physical and chemical characteristics
- Health hazards
- Permissible exposure limits
- Whether the product is a carcinogen (cancer-producing)
- Emergency first-aid procedures
- Specific hazards

SDSs must be maintained for every hazardous chemical kept in the practice. Sheets must be kept current within 3 years of the date printed on the sheet. Manufacturers and distributors provide SDSs; many are also available on a CD or their website for easy reference and printing.

OSHA allows a few SDS exemptions, meaning an SDS is not required. This includes many common items used by the practice, for example, tape, hematocrit sealer, and pens. Food and nutritional products, common household cleaning items, and drugs sold in tablet form are also exempt.

To be exempt, cleaning items must be used in the same form as in a household. For example, Windex® is commonly used to clean windows. A practice probably washes their windows at the same frequency as a homeowner, so this product is exempt. Now consider rubbing alcohol,

OSHA® QUICK CARD™

Hazard Communication Safety Data Sheets

The Hazard Communication Standard (HCS) requires chemical manufacturers, distributors, or importers to provide Safety Data Sheets (SDSs) (formerly known as Material Safety Data Sheets or MSDSs) to communicate the hazards of hazardous chemical products. As of June 1, 2015, the HCS will require new SDSs to be in a uniform format, and include the section numbers, the headings, and associated information under the headings below:

Section 1, Identification includes product identifier; manufacturer or distributor name, address, phone number; emergency phone number; recommended use; restrictions on use.

Section 2, Hazard(s) identification includes all hazards regarding the chemical; required label elements.

Section 3, Composition/information on ingredients includes information on chemical ingredients; trade secret claims.

Section 4, First-aid measures includes important symptoms/effects, acute, delayed; required treatment.

Section 5, Fire-fighting measures lists suitable extinguishing techniques, equipment; chemical hazards from fire.

Section 6, Accidental release measures lists emergency procedures; protective equipment; proper methods of containment and cleanup.

Section 7, Handling and storage lists precautions for safe handling and storage, including incompatibilities.

(Continued on other side)

For more information:

OSHA® Occupational Safety and Health Administration

U.S. Department of Labor

www.osha.gov (800) 321-OSHA (6742)

OSHA 3493-02 2012

OSHA® QUICK CARD™

Hazard Communication Safety Data Sheets

Section 8, Exposure controls/personal protection lists OSHA's Permissible Exposure Limits (PELs); Threshold Limit Values (TLVs); appropriate engineering controls; personal protective equipment (PPE).

Section 9, Physical and chemical properties lists the chemical's characteristics.

Section 10, Stability and reactivity lists chemical stability and possibility of hazardous reactions.

Section 11, Toxicological information includes routes of exposure; related symptoms, acute and chronic effects; numerical measures of toxicity.

Section 12, Ecological information*
Section 13, Disposal considerations*
Section 14, Transport information*
Section 15, Regulatory information*

Section 16, Other information, includes the date of preparation or last revision.

*Note: Since other Agencies regulate this information, OSHA will not be enforcing Sections 12 through 15 (29 CFR 1910.1200(g)(2)).

Employers must ensure that SDSs are readily accessible to employees.
See Appendix D of 29 CFR 1910.1200 for a detailed description of SDS contents.

For more information:

OSHA® Occupational Safety and Health Administration

U.S. Department of Labor

www.osha.gov (800) 321-OSHA (6742)

OSHA 3493-02-2012

Fig. 15.29 SDS descriptions. (Courtesy Occupational Safety and Health Administration, Department of Labor, Washington, DC.)

which is commonly used in both households and veterinary practices. However, the amount of alcohol used in practice is much greater than in household use; therefore, this chemical is not exempt, and an SDS must be maintained.

If tablets can be crushed or made into a dissolving solution, then an SDS must be kept onsite. Capsules, gels, and solutions are not exempt from SDS requirements.

If a chemical is no longer carried by a hospital, an SDS sheet must be maintained for 30 years after the date it is discontinued. These archived SDSs can be kept in a separate binder. OSHA mandates that each SDS for a discontinued substance contain a summary of how the product was used, where it was stored, and how long it was supplied. The reason for this mandate is that it can take as long as 30 years for personnel to see side effects from chemicals. This ensures the practice has reference material available in case this situation should arise.

SECONDARY CONTAINER-LABELING REQUIREMENTS

Part of the OSHA Hazard Communication Plan includes the development, use, and training of secondary container labeling. *Secondary container* is defined as removing any liquid from its original container and transferring it to another container. The secondary container must then be labeled to meet OSHA requirements. Fig. 15.30 outlines seven required elements that must be contained on the label. All details can be extracted from the Safety Data Sheet (SDS) sheet. It is required that the product name on the label match the product name on the SDS. It is not acceptable to make a copy of the original label and tape it on to the secondary label. Consider the following examples of chemicals that are often transferred to another container in the veterinary practice:

- Disinfectant for examination room tables
- Alcohol
- Peroxide
- Cold sterile tray disinfectant
- Surgical scrub
- Solution used to soak otoscope cones
- Solution to store mercury thermometers
- Cytology stain

Please note, the diamond labeling system once used in veterinary practice is no longer an acceptable label usage. Veterinary practices are expected to comply with GHS standards. Examples of pictograms and their interpretation can be found in Fig. 15.31.

LEADERSHIP POINT

Always label secondary bottles with proper labels. If emergency personnel enter the clinic, they should be able to immediately determine whether the chemical within the bottle is hazardous.

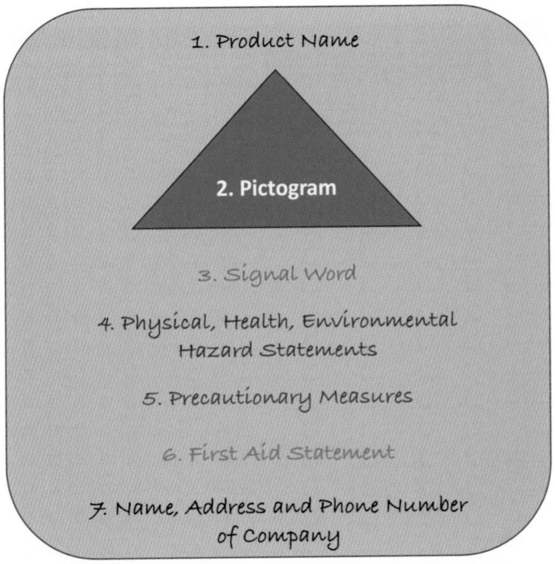

1. Product Name
2. Pictogram
3. Signal Word
4. Physical, Health, Environmental Hazard Statements
5. Precautionary Measures
6. First Aid Statement
7. Name, Address and Phone Number of Company

Fig. 15.30 Label requirements for secondary labels. (From A Guide to the GHS Classification and Labeling of Chemicals; https://www.osha.gov.)

ACCIDENT REPORTING AND INVESTIGATION

Every accident that occurs in the practice must be reported to the safety manager and/or practice manager and owner. If medical treatment is required, appropriate paperwork should be available for the employee to take to the doctor or hospital. Paperwork may include the First Notice of Accident or Injury and Illness Incident Report and/or a Workers' Compensation Insurance Claim Form. This will ensure that the employer's insurance is charged for the visit, not the team members. When the employee returns from the medical visit, paperwork should be sent to the appropriate companies, state, or local authorities. Since worker's compensation varies by state, each practice must have a full understanding of the required filing procedures.

VHMA PERFORMANCE DOMAIN TASK

Document and report accidents and file appropriate reports.

Practices with eleven or more employees must record all accidents on OSHA Form 300. Only injuries resulting in death, or the hospitalization of five or more employees, must be reported to OSHA immediately and directly. A fatality must be reported within 8 hours, and an amputation, loss of an eye, or hospitalization must be reported within 24 hours. OSHA Form 300 (Fig. 15.32) must be kept for 5 years. Because this form contains personal employee information, it should be kept in a locked cabinet.

It is imperative to investigate and document all accidents that occur. OSHA inspectors may ask for this (along with any other investigator) to obtain information for a worker's compensation claim. This information should be contained in OSHA Form 301 (Fig. 15.33).

OSHA requires form 300 A to be posted in a conspicuous place for all team members to view from February 1 to April 30 of each year. Form 300 A (Fig. 15.34) summarizes all injuries and illnesses reported from Form 300, removing all confidential information.

Beginning in 2017, OSHA required veterinary practices to submit electronic reporting of OSHA form 300 A (practices with 20–249). Forms are due March 2 of each year. Visit the OSHA Injury Tracking Website to submit practice data. The NAICS code for veterinary practices is 541940.

DEVELOPING AND IMPLEMENTING SAFETY PROTOCOLS

Now that safety hazards have been addressed, it is time to develop and implement safety protocols. All team members should practice emergency procedures to be comfortable with any situation that arises. Panic often sets in when emergencies happen. The more the hospital implements training and practice sessions the safer the team will be. Safety must be addressed at every meeting; it is taken for granted in many situations and needs to be discussed frequently. Develop the following safety protocols:

Supplies: When storing supplies, heavy items are placed on the lower shelves, along with chemicals and liquids. All chemicals must be stored in tightly sealed containers and placed below eye level in case they are spilled. Shelves should never be overweighed with products, causing them to fall on team members. If a product on an upper shelf is needed, a step stool should be used; never climb on countertops or shelves to get products.

HCS Pictograms and Hazards

Health Hazard	Flame	Exclamation Mark

• Carcinogen • Mutagenicity • Reproductive Toxicity • Respiratory Sensitizer • Target Organ Toxicity • Aspiration Toxicity	• Flammables • Pyrophorics • Self-Heating • Emits Flammable Gas • Self-Reactives • Organic Peroxides	• Irritant (skin and eye) • Skin Sensitizer • Acute Toxicity (harmful) • Narcotic Effects • Respiratory Tract Irritant • Hazardous to Ozone Layer (Non-Mandatory)
Gas Cylinder	**Corrosion**	**Exploding Bomb**
		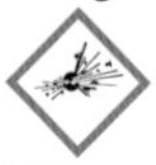
• Gases Under Pressure	• Skin Corrosion/burns • Eye Damage • Corrosive to Metals	• Explosives • Self-Reactives • Organic Peroxides
Flame Over Circle	**Environment (Non-Mandatory)**	**Skull and Crossbones**

• Oxidizers	• Aquatic Toxicity	• Acute Toxicity (fatal or toxic)

Fig. 15.31 Pictograms required for secondary labels. (Courtesy Occupational Safety and Health Administration, Department of Labor, Washington, DC.)

OSHA's Form 300 (Rev. 01/2004)

Log of Work-Related Injuries and Illnesses

Attention: This form contains information relating to employee health and must be used in a manner that protects the confidentiality of employees to the extent possible while the information is being used for occupational safety and health purposes.

Year 20__ __

U.S.Department of Labor
Occupational Safety and Health Administration

Form approved OMB no. 1218-0176

You must record information about every work-related death and about every work-related injury or illness that involves loss of consciousness, restricted work activity or job transfer, days away from work, or medical treatment beyond first aid, You must also record significant work-related injuries and illnesses that are diagnosed by a physician or licensed health care professional. You must also record work-related injuries and illnesses that meet any of the specific recording criteria listed in 29 CFR Part 1904.8 through 1904.12. Feel free to use two lines for a single case if you need to. You must complete an Injury and Illness Incident Report (OSHA Form 301) or equivalent form for each injury or illness recorded on this form. If you're not sure whether a case is recordable, call your local OSHA office for help.

Establishment name ____________

City ____________ State ____________

identify the person			Describe the case			Classify the case CHECK ONLY ONE box for each case based on the most serious outcome for that case:				Enter the number of days the injured or ill worker was:		Check the "Injury" column or choose one type of illness:					
								Remained at Work				(M)					
(A) Case no.	(B) Employee's name	(C) Job title (e.g., Welder)	(D) Date of injury or onset of illness	(E) Where the event occurred (e.g., Loading dock north end)	(F) Describe injury or illness, parts of body affected, and object/substance that directly injured or made person ill (e.g., Second degree burns on right forearm from acetylene torch)	Death (G)	Days away from work (H)	Job transfer or restriction (I)	Other record-able cases (J)	Away from work (K)	On job transfer or restriction (L)	Injury (1)	Skin disorder (2)	Respiratory condition (3)	Poisoning (4)	Hearing loss (5)	All other illnesses (6)
___	___	___	___/___ month/day	___	___	☐	☐	☐	☐	___days	___days	☐	☐	☐	☐	☐	☐
___	___	___	___/___ month/day	___	___	☐	☐	☐	☐	___days	___days	☐	☐	☐	☐	☐	☐
___	___	___	___/___ month/day	___	___	☐	☐	☐	☐	___days	___days	☐	☐	☐	☐	☐	☐
___	___	___	___/___ month/day	___	___	☐	☐	☐	☐	___days	___days	☐	☐	☐	☐	☐	☐
___	___	___	___/___ month/day	___	___	☐	☐	☐	☐	___days	___days	☐	☐	☐	☐	☐	☐
___	___	___	___/___ month/day	___	___	☐	☐	☐	☐	___days	___days	☐	☐	☐	☐	☐	☐
___	___	___	___/___ month/day	___	___	☐	☐	☐	☐	___days	___days	☐	☐	☐	☐	☐	☐
___	___	___	___/___ month/day	___	___	☐	☐	☐	☐	___days	___days	☐	☐	☐	☐	☐	☐
___	___	___	___/___ month/day	___	___	☐	☐	☐	☐	___days	___days	☐	☐	☐	☐	☐	☐
___	___	___	___/___ month/day	___	___	☐	☐	☐	☐	___days	___days	☐	☐	☐	☐	☐	☐
___	___	___	___/___ month/day	___	___	☐	☐	☐	☐	___days	___days	☐	☐	☐	☐	☐	☐
___	___	___	___/___ month/day	___	___	☐	☐	☐	☐	___days	___days	☐	☐	☐	☐	☐	☐
___	___	___	___/___ month/day	___	___	☐	☐	☐	☐	___days	___days	☐	☐	☐	☐	☐	☐
					Page totals➤	___	___	___	___	___	___	___ Injury (1)	___ Skin disorder (2)	___ Respiratory condition (3)	___ Poisoning (4)	___ Hearing loss (5)	___ All other illnesses (6)

Be sure to transfer these totals to the Summary page (Form 300A) before you post it.

Public reporting burden for this collection of information is estimated to average 14 minutes per response, including time to review the instructions, search and gather the data needed, and complete and review the collection of information. Persons are not required to respond to the collection of information unless it displays a currently valid OMB control number. If you have any comments about these estimates or any other aspects of this data collection, contact: US Department of 1.aimr, OS1-1A Office of Statistical Analysis, Room N-3644, 200 Constitution Avenue, NW, Washington, DC 20210. Do not send the completed forms to this office.

Page — of —

Fig. 15.32 OSHA Form 300. (Courtesy Occupational Safety and Health Administration, Department of Labor, Washington, DC.)

OSHA's Form 301
Injury and Illness Incident Report

Attention: This form contains information relating to employee health and must be used in a manner that protects the confidentiality of employees to the extent possible while the information is being used for occupational safety and health purposes.

U.S.Department of Labor
Occupational Safety and Health Administration

Form approved OMB no. 1218-0176

This *Injury and Illness Incident Report* is one of the first forms you must fill out when a recordable work-related injury or illness has occurred. Together with the *Log of Work-Related Injuries and Illnesses* and the accompanying *Summary*, these forms help the employer and OSHA develop a picture of the extent and severity of work-related incidents.

Within 7 calendar days after you receive information that a recordable work-related injury or illness has occurred, you must fill out this form or an equivalent. Some state workers' compensation, insurance, or other reports may be acceptable substitutes. To be considered an equivalent form, any substitute must contain all the information asked for on this form.

According to Public Law 91-596 and 29 CFR 1904, OSHA's rccordkccping rule, you must keep this forn on file fir 5 years following the year to which it pertains.

If you need additional copies of this form, you may photocopy and use as many as you need.

Completed by ____________

Title ____________

Phone ____ ____ ____ **Date** ___/___/___

Information about the employee

1) Full name ____________

2) Street ____________

City ____________ State ______ ZIP ______

3) Date of birth ___/___/___

4) Date hired ___/___/___

5) ❐ Male
❐ Female

Information about the physician or other health care professional

6) Name of physician or other health care professional ____________

7) If treatment was given away from the worksite, where was it given?

Facility ____________

Street ____________

City ____________ State ______ ZIP ______

8) Was employee treated in an emergency room?
❐ Yes
❐ No

9) Was employee hospitalized overnight as an in-patients?
❐ Yes
❐ No

Information about the case

10) Case number from the log ____________ *(Transfer the case number from the log after you record the case.)*

11) Date of injury or illness ___/___/___

12) Time employee began work ________ AM / PM

13) Time of event ________ AM / PM **Check if time cannot be determined**

14) ***What was the employee doing just before the incident occurred?* Describe the activity, as well as the tools,equipment, or material the employee was using. Be specific. Examples: "climbing a ladder while carrying roofing materials"; "spraying chlorine from hand sprayer"; "daily computer key-entry."**

15) ***What happened?* Tell us how the injury occurred. *Examples:* "When ladder slipped on wet floor, worker fell 20 feet"; "Worker was sprayed with chlorine when gasket broke during replacement"; "Worker developed soreness in wrist over time."**

16) ***What was the Injury or illness?* Tell us the part of the body that was affected and how it was affected; be more specific than "hurt," "pain," or sore." *Examples:* "strained back"; "chemical burn, hand"; "carpal tunnel syndrome."**

17) ***What object or substance directly harmed the employee? Examples:* "concrete floor"; "chlorine"; "radial arm saw." *If this question does not apply to the incident, leave it blank.***

18) ***If the employee died, when did death occur?* Date of death ___/___/___**

Public reporting burden for this collection of information is estimated to average 22 minutes per response, including time for reviewing instructions, searching existing data sources, gathering and maintaining the data needed, and completing and reviewing the collection of information. Persons are not required to respond to the collection of information unless it displays a current valid OMB control number. If you have any comments about this estimate or any other aspects of this data collection, including suggestions for reducing this burden, contact: US Department of labor, OSHA Office of Statistical Analysis. Room N-3644, 200 Constitution Avenue. NW, Washington, DC 20210. Do not send the completed forms to this office.

Fig. 15.33 OSHA Log 301. (Courtesy Occupational Safety and Health Administration, Department of Labor, Washington, DC.)

OSHA's Form 301
Summary of Work-Related Injuries and Illnesses

Year 20__ __

U.S.Department of Labor
Occupational Safety and Health Administration

Form approved OMB no. 1218-0176

All establishments covered by Part 1904 must complete this Summary page, even if no work-related injuries or illnesses occurred during the year. Remember to review the Log to verify that the entries are complete and accurate before completing this summary.

Using the Log, count the individual entries you made for each category. Then write the totals below, making sure you've added the entries from every page of the Log. If you had no cases, write "0."

Employees, former employees, and their representatives have the right to review the OSHA Form 300 in its entirety. They also have limited access to the OSHA Form 301 or its equivalent. See 29 CFR Part 1904.35, in OSHA's recordkeeping rule, for further details on the access provisions for these forms.

Number of Cases

Total number of deaths	Total number of cases with days away from work	Total number of cases with job transfer or restriction	Total number of other recordable cases
____ (G)	____ (H)	____ (I)	____ (J)

Number of Days

Total number of days away from work	Total number of days of job transfer or restriction
____ (K)	____ (L)

Injury and Illness Types

Total number of...
(M)

(1) Injuries	____	(4) Poisonings	____
(2) Skin disorders	____	(5) Hearing loss	____
(3) Respiratory conditions	____	(6) All other illnesses	____

Post this Summary page from February 1 to April 30 of the year following the year covered by the form.

Public reporting burden for this collection of information is estimated to average 58 minutes per response, including time to review the instructions, search and gather the data needed, and complete and review the collection of information. Persons arc not required to respond to the collection of information unless it displays a currently valid OMB control number. If you have any comments about these estimates or any other aspects of this data collection, contact: US Department of Labor, OSHA Office of Statistical Analysis, Room N-3644, 200 Constitution Avenue, NW, Washington, DC 20210. Do not send the completed forms to this office.

Establishment information

Your establishment name ____________

Street ____________

City ____________ State ____ ZIP ____

Industry description *(e.g., Manufacture of motor truck trailers)* ____________

Standard Industrial Classification (SIC), if known (e.g., 3715)
__ __ __ __

OR

North American Industrial Classification (NAICS), if known (e.g.,336212)
__ __ __ __ __ __

Employment information *(if you don't have these figures, see the Worksheet on the back of this page to estimate.)*

Annual average number of employees ________

Total hours worked by all employees last year ________

Sign here

Knowingly falsifying this document may result in a fine.

I certify that I have examined this document and that to the best of my knowledge the entries are true, accurate, and complete.

Company executive ____ Title

( ) ____ / /

Phone ____ Date

Fig. 15.34 OSHA Log 301. (Courtesy Occupational Safety and Health Administration, Department of Labor, Washington, DC.)

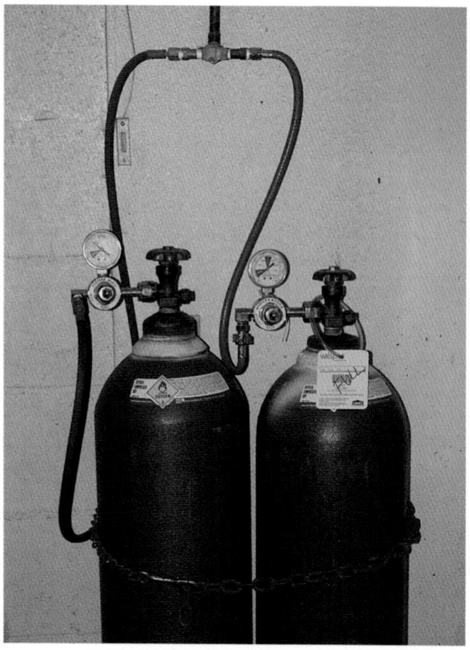

Fig. 15.35 Oxygen tanks must always be secured to a wall.

Autoclaves: Autoclaves produce intense heat and should always be properly vented before opening the door. Steam should be allowed to dissipate slowly and completely before fully opening the door. The face and hands should be kept away from both the vent and door when venting and opening the autoclave.

Oxygen Tanks: Compressed oxygen tanks must be secured in an upright position with a chain. Team members can bump into unsecured tanks and cause them to fall on a team member or to the floor (Fig. 15.35). Tanks may explode on impact, so securing tanks is essential. All tanks should be kept away from heat sources such as furnaces, water heaters, and direct sunlight.

Attire: Team members must dress appropriately for the job, as outlined in employee manuals. For safety purposes, open-toed shoes are not allowed; if team members will be working with large animals, steel-toed boots may be required. Jewelry should be kept to a minimum because long earrings and bracelets could get caught up on pets, causing injury to both team members and patients.

The Hospital Safety Manual

A hospital safety manual becomes the official safety training book and includes all materials previously discussed. Tabs can be used to separate topics allowing for easy identification:

- Administrative: name of safety officer and what to do in the event of a safety inspection
- Annual hazard analysis inspection documentation (both physical and chemical)
- Safety plans for hazards identified in the inspection (in addition to those covered in this chapter)
- Location of safety data sheets (SDS) and how to read them
- Secondary chemical labeling requirements and explanation
- Protocol for emergency evacuation (how to evacuate [varies on emergency: be specific] where to meet, etc.)
- Training program of hazards and required PPE (required for practices with 11 or more employees)
- Signatures of team members that attended training, and the dates of training (by subject)
- OSHA form 300 A (forms 300 and 301 must be locked in a file cabinet as they contain personal information)

BUILDING SAFETY AND MAINTENANCE

Practices have an ethical obligation to provide a safe and secure working environment for employees, clients, and their pets. To be safe, the building and equipment must be properly maintained, and protocols for facility maintenance must be established. Further, safety goes beyond the standard preventions for slips and falls. Security of the premises is a high priority and encompasses entrances and exits, perimeter lighting, security systems, responding to potential theft, and the safety of team members as they arrive and leave the practice.

Grounds and building maintenance contracts should be established allowing a practice manager to call a company and receive service efficiently when an issue has been identified. Additionally, having a landscape company in charge of maintaining the landscape (bushes, trees, etc.) enhances safety while also maintaining curb appeal for clients.

Contracts may be month to month (in the case of a landscaper and security systems company), include a specific number of work hours allotted to the practice per month (a contractor), or a simple retainer fee that allows efficient response. Read contracts thoroughly, consider having legal counsel review them, and research pricing with competitors annually.

Entrances and Exits

Practices should have deadbolts on all doors, and one-way locks on all doors except the main entrance. When the business is open, deadbolts must remain unlocked. One-way door locks require a key to enter the building, but clients and employees can exit anytime. The main entrance door allows clients to enter and exit as needed and a standard door lock is acceptable. All doors must be locked before the last team member leaves the premises to ensure the safety of the practice.

Entrances must be protected and always monitored. Any door other than the main entrance must be always locked. A person could enter through any unlocked door in the rear of the practice and hide until the practice closes and/or cause harm to employees. It is imperative to secure doors, and they must always remain locked from the outside. One-way door locks allow employees and clients to escape in emergency situations.

Perimeter Lighting

The practice must have excellent lighting outside of the building and in the parking lot for the protection of clients and team members (Fig. 15.36). Potential criminals may find a dark corner and wait for an employee to leave the building alone at night. The same risk should be considered for clients, who are less observant when leaving practices because they are preoccupated with their pet. Bright lights act as a deterrent to criminals and provide a safer environment.

When team members are leaving a practice, they should use the buddy system, with a minimum of two employees leaving together. If only one employee needs to leave, two others should walk the team member to his or her car, then return to the practice as the car is leaving. If team members must be at a practice alone (weekend treatments, etc.), they should be instructed never to answer the door and to park in highly visible areas. Thieves are creative at entering a business after hours, especially if they see a lone employee inside. Team members

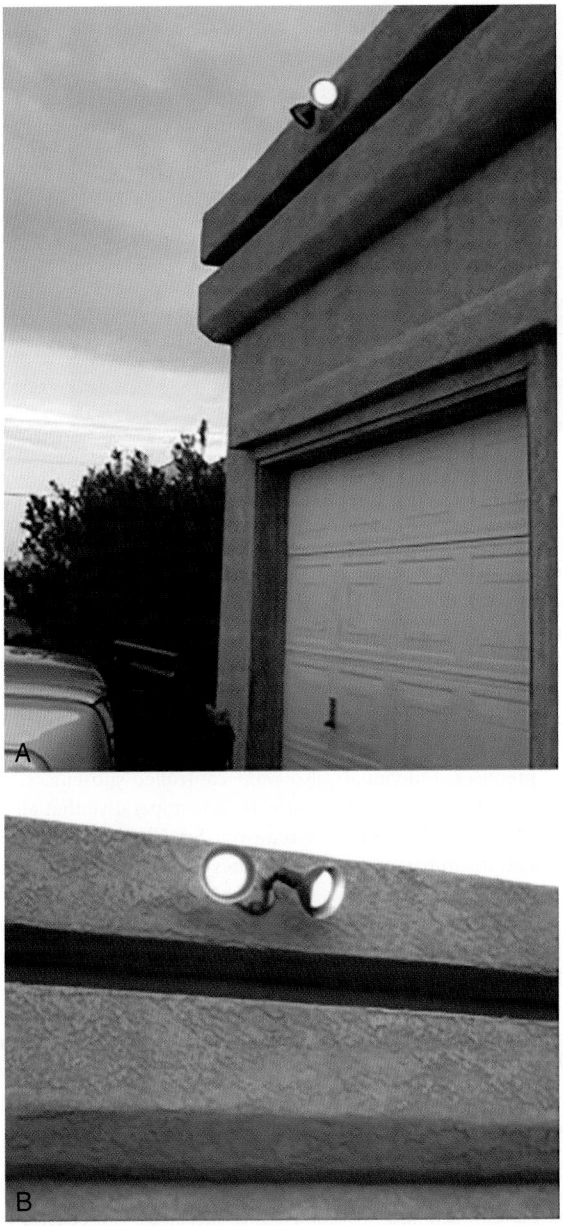

Fig. 15.36 (A and B) Perimeter lighting.

should always inspect the outside premises before leaving to ensure no one is lingering in the parking lot.

Security System

Security systems should be installed to electronically protect the premises. Sensory devices should be placed on all windows and doors; if any window or door is broken or opened after the system has been activated, an alarm will sound. Systems may also have a motion detector; once the alarm has been activated, any motion detected inside the building will trigger the alarm. Many security systems are connected to a monitoring system, which will automatically place a call to police if the alarm is triggered. Many practices have keypads at the employee entrance, allowing the alarm to be set or deactivated. Others have a badge reader and employees must swipe their badges to gain access to the building. This also allows employee monitoring during closed hours. Both devices can prevent entry to a terminated employee once their access has been deactivated.

Many security systems can send text messages or alerts to owners and practice managers regarding who has activated and deactivated the system and when. This allows the monitoring of the practice over the weekend, and notification of employees on the premises when they should not be.

Some security systems have the option of panic buttons. These buttons are excellent in the event of a robbery or assault during business hours and should be placed in the front office in a convenient, yet hidden, location. If an emergency occurs, team members can hit the panic button to automatically call 911.

Emergency and specialty practices often install entry access buzzers at their front doors, adding a second level of protection for team members. When clients arrive, they push a buzzer; the receptionist can verify the clients and allow access.

Emergency clinics must take special precautions for safety because they are open overnight and on weekends. This is a particularly easy time for criminals to target the business. Many emergency clinics have fewer employees on staff at night, and there are fewer witnesses to observe unlawful actions.

Security systems can also be linked to highly detailed security cameras and recording devices.

Cameras and Recording Devices

Cameras should be placed at entrances and exits to record activity outside of the premises, along with internal placement over cash drawers, controlled substances safes, and pharmacy, at minimum. Cameras and monitoring systems should be of high quality, allowing the practice to be able to identify facial features should the replication of images be needed. Action can be recorded on NVRs (network video recorders) or DVRs (digital video recorders), which allows more information to be stored and can be written over with the permission of the operator. Cameras can be linked through the server, allowing an owner to view actions occurring through a home computer. If a loose animal triggers the alarm, the police can be notified of the false alarm.

After Hours Emergency and Mobile Practice Safety

It is common for clinics to respond to after-hour patient emergencies. In such situations, staff members can be at increased risk for assault, and all precautions should be taken when meeting clients after hours. A technician should always respond to calls from the doctor, regardless of the time or day. Clients should be viewed through the locked entry door to visualize the pet and ensure that the client has an actual emergency.

Mobile practices are at an increased risk for robbery and assault because they do not have the same security options that are available within a building. Mobile veterinarians may carry drugs with them, along with cash, making them excellent targets for assailants. Veterinarians should always carry cell phones with emergency numbers programmed for quick access. Carrying some type of device for personal protection is recommended.

A recommended monthly meeting topic is methods of defense for violent crime or assault. It is advisable to have a local defense expert provide valuable training for the staff. Experts can locate areas of safety weakness in and around the practice and can create safety scenarios for team members to practice. The more aware team members are of a possible assault, the better they can respond.

Personal Protection Devices

Practices and mobile veterinarians should inquire with local law enforcement about the use and regulations of personal protection devices. Protection devices can cause great harm to another individual and should never be used carelessly or without training. Owners

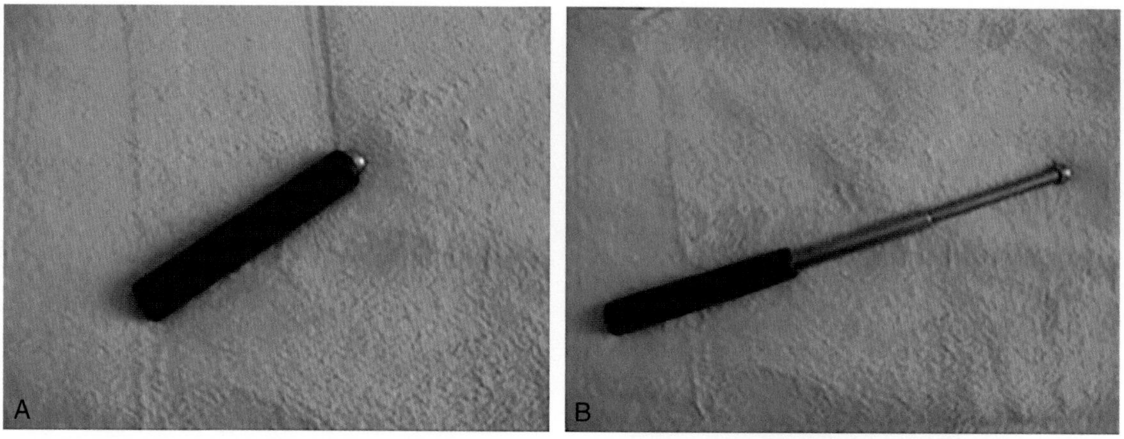

Fig. 15.37 (A) Unextended ASP Baton. (B) ASP Baton extended.

and/or hospital management must authorize the possession of personal protection devices on the premises, or the use of these devices for protection of the practice.

The ASP Tactical Baton is the most tactically sophisticated impact weapon currently available (Fig. 15.37). Easily carried and readily available, ASP batons have incredible psychological deterrence and control potential. ASP batons are small to carry, but once swung open, the baton extends immediately, providing excellent protection for an individual. ASP batons can be kept in the front office with the receptionist for defense against would-be attackers. The receptionist can swing the baton open in the event of an attack. ASP batons are also ideal for mobile veterinarians.

Mace is a brand of tear gas that is often used by police to deter potential attackers. Mace must be sprayed directly at the attacker and creates an intense burning sensation in the eyes and lungs. Mace can be extremely effective when used correctly.

Tasers are often thought of as weapons used by law enforcement to subdue those who are apprehended. Some models are also available for personal protection. A Taser is an electroshock weapon that uses electrical current to disrupt voluntary control of muscles, resulting in muscle contractions.

Both ASP batons and Tasers may require training in some states. The manufacturers of both products offer courses with certified trainers to allow individuals to become comfortable with the use of such items.

Theft

Theft can occur at any time, either by an employee or by a person who enters the building with the intent to commit a crime. Employee theft can range from embezzling cash to stealing products and/or food. Procedures must be implemented to prevent either situation from occurring. Cash transactions must be recorded immediately, both on the computer and in the client records. Receipts must be produced for clients paying with cash. End-of-day totals must match the cash in the drawer, along with all credit card and check transactions. The deposit should be double-checked by the practice manager to ensure the deposit made at the bank matches the end-of-day deposit on the computer. Any discrepancies must be investigated immediately. See Chapter 3 for more information on end-of-day reconciliation security features.

Team members purchasing products should always have an office manager enter the products or services into the computer. This ensures consistency in entering codes and determining costs/discounts. If owners, associates, or practice managers see an employee taking products out of the building without authorization or payment, the employee should be questioned immediately, not days later.

Practices must always be prepared for criminal intent and can be targeted for theft of both drugs and cash. Many practices do not keep a large amount of cash on hand, especially since the payment trend has shifted to debit cards instead of cash for payment of services. However, thieves still believe that veterinary practices hold a large amount of cash on the premises. Individuals also want controlled substances, which have a large dollar value on the streets. It is imperative that all drugs be locked in a safe that cannot be removed. See Chapter 14, Controlled Substances, for information on drug safes approved by the U.S. Drug Enforcement Administration.

If a person with criminal intent enters the practice, all money should be given to him or her from the cash drawer. Team members should not risk injury or death to themselves, clients, or other team members to protect the small amount of money that the practice has on the premises. If the thieves request drugs, give them what they want; the sooner they leave the practice, the safer the team members and clients will be. All doors should be locked, and police should be called immediately.

Any assailant descriptive information that can be provided will be helpful to the police, along with a description of the vehicle used and license plate information if visible from inside. Do not chase a criminal out of the clinic. Safety should never be compromised to gather description information.

LEADERSHIP'S ROLE IN SAFETY OF THE VETERINARY PRACTICE

Leadership has a large safety role in the veterinary practice. Appropriate behaviors must be demonstrated that support safety at all levels. While a safety program can be empowered to team members to carry out, leadership must ensure the program is complete, exceeds OSHA recommendations, and holds team members accountable for maintaining safe workplace practices. Practice managers must report injuries as required, post annual 300 forms, document training, and be prepared (with the empowered safety officer) for an unannounced inspection at any time. Additionally, PMs are tasked with maintaining facility maintenance contracts, and ensuring the perimeter of the practice is safe and maintains a high curb appeal.

PRACTICE MANAGER SURVIVAL CHECKLIST FOR SAFETY IN THE VETERINARY PRACTICE

- ☐ Evaluate the condition of PPE on a regular basis.
- ☐ Maintain current SDSs that are always accessible.
- ☐ Maintain an SDS of products no longer carried (30 years).
- ☐ Develop a document of contact numbers for all emergency situations (insurance, attorney, etc.).
- ☐ Create a safety training plan and documentation.
- ☐ Inspect fire extinguishers, eyewash stations, and sprinkler systems annually.
- ☐ Replace batteries in CO2 and smoke detectors annually.
- ☐ Post-OSHA form 300a from February 1 through April 30.
- ☐ Electronically report OSHA form 300a by March 2.
- ☐ Display OSHA 3165 poster at all times.
- ☐ Ensure doors are always locked after hours.
- ☐ Change all door locks to one-way so that employees can escape at any time but must have a key to enter.
- ☐ Create a policy regarding the distribution of keys.
- ☐ Change door locks/security codes periodically.

REVIEW QUESTIONS

1. What is a zoonotic disease?
2. How should an animal heavier than 40 lbs. be lifted onto a table?
3. What is OSHA?
4. What is the Right to Know poster?
5. What is an SDS?
6. What is the purpose of PPE?
7. When does OSHA Form 300 A have to be posted?
8. What is an eyewash station?
9. What is a biohazard material?
10. What are some hazardous chemicals used in veterinary practice?
11. Under OSHA guidelines, employees are responsible for which of the following:
    - **a.** Read the Right to Know Poster
    - **b.** Order PPE for the practice
    - **c.** Training fellow team members on the use of PPE
    - **d.** Document conditions in which PPE must be used
12. If an OSHA inspector arrives at the hospital, which of the following options should be exercised?
    - **a.** Introduce the inspector to the safety officer
    - **b.** Allow the inspection to proceed without a team member
    - **c.** Hide violations from the staff
    - **d.** Do not allow OSHA access
13. Which of the following contributes to most fires in the veterinary practice?
    - **a.** Paper files stacked up to the ceiling
    - **b.** Blankets next to a furnace
    - **c.** Overloaded electrical outlets
    - **d.** Heating units left unattended
14. Back injuries can be classified as which type of injury?
    - **a.** Physical
    - **b.** Biohazard
    - **c.** Caustic
    - **d.** Ergonomic
15. Noise protection should be provided for employees when noise levels reach which decibel level?
    - **a.** 75 dB
    - **b.** 85 dB
    - **c.** 95 dB
    - **d.** Ear protection is not required
16. What is the purpose of one-way door locks?
17. What should team members do if an armed individual enters the practice and demands money or drugs?
18. Why is exterior perimeter lighting so critical?
19. What is an ASP baton?

REFERENCES

1. OSHA.gov. Section 17, Penalties. Accessed August 2022. https://www.osha.gov/laws-regs/oshact/section_17.
2. Talan DA, et al. Bacteriologic analysis of dog and cat bites. *N Engl J Med.* 1990;340:85–92.

RECOMMENDED READING

Lappin M. General concepts in zoonotic disease control. *Vet Clin North Am.* 2005;35:1.

OSHA Publications Office. Worker's rights. OSHA 3021-02R 2023. Accessed August 2022. https://www.osha.gov/Publications/osha3021.pdf

Seibert PJ. *Be safe! A managers guide to veterinary workplace safety.* 2nd ed. AAHA Press; 2014.

Veterinary Safety & Health, CDC.gov. Published September 15, 2021. Accessed August 2022. https://www.cdc.gov/niosh/topics/veterinary/default.html.

16

Finance Management

LEARNING OBJECTIVES

When you have completed this chapter, you should be able to:

- Identify the differences between bookkeepers, accountants, public accountants, and certified public accountants
- Correlate effective key performance indicators
- Develop a practice budget
- Identify practice profit centers
- Explain insufficient funds charges
- Describe the process used to accept payments on client accounts
- Define and enforce a no-charge policy
- Calculate finance charges
- Describe the process used to collect outstanding accounts receivable effectively
- Define the Fair Debt Collection Practices Act
- Define and explain insurance policies to fellow team members and clients
- Identify the differences between hereditary and congenital conditions

OUTLINE

KEY TERMS

Accounts Payable
Accounts Receivable
Accrual Basis Accounting
Annual Deductible
Annual Payout Limit
Assets
Average Client Transaction
Balance Sheet
Benchmarking
Break-Even Analysis
Budget
Cash Basis Accounting
Cash Flow Statement
Certified Public Accountant
COGs
Collections Agency

Compliance Rate
Congenital Conditions
Deductible
Embezzlement
Exclusion
Fair Debt Collection Practices Act
Fixed Cost
Gross Revenue
Gross Profit
Hereditary Conditions
Indemnity Insurance
Key Performance Indicators
Liabilities
Profit and Loss Statement
Return on Investment
Revenue Centers
Variable Cost

VHMA PERFORMANCE DOMAINS

Veterinary Hospital Managers Association Critical Competencies

In the financial management domain, the veterinary practice manager analyzes financial reports for the practice, maintains practice financial accounts, oversees banking procedures, establishes client credit policies, conducts fee analyses, and manages the practice's payroll. In consultation with the practice owner, the manager also monitors financial trends and projections and prepares budgets.

Veterinary Hospital Managers Association Critical Competencies Knowledge Requirements

This domain requires knowledge of basic principles of financial accounting and forecasting. The manager must understand the components of a balance sheet, profit/loss accounts, and financial ratios. Knowledge of current taxation law is also needed.

INTRODUCTION

Financial planning and management are critical in small business as it leads to practice growth, improved net profits, and the ability to hire highly skilled employees with competitive wages and benefits. Merely tracking revenue and expenses has been shown by the American Veterinary Medical Association to improve net profits by $42,000.

Many owners lack the confidence and knowledge to manage finances efficiently. During the 2008 financial recession, many practices were negatively impacted. Businesses that lacked appropriate plans or had poor management structure shut their doors. Those lucky to remain open squeaked by learning a valuable lesson: without proper planning, any business can fail.

The basics of business/financial management must be considered first, allowing owners and practice managers to make wise business decisions based on data (not opinion or assumption). Key performance indicators (KPIs) are like oil in an engine. You cannot run a car engine without oil. KPIs are critical data that lead owners and practice managers to the right decisions that achieve strategic, long-term goals.

To achieve long-term goals, budgets must be created each year. Budgeting impacts the development of people (the most important asset of the practice), paying people appropriate wages, providing a frictionless client experience, providing high-level quality care to patients with working (and current) equipment, and maintaining an aesthetically pleasing, safe building that attracts clients to the business.

With budgeting comes planning for unknown emergencies (recession, fire, earthquake, tornado, pandemic) and profitability. Every business must have a reserve for the unknowns; profit needs to be planned as well. At a minimum, 10% of the profit should be reinvested back into the practice on an annual basis.

When a known profitability goal is established and known expenses are planned, appropriate product and service pricing can take be developed. Without planning, pricing is a guessing game, and most owners resort to pricing that is similar to competitors or benchmarks. Practices must use their financials to charge appropriately to achieve strategic goals that they have set forth.

Therefore, financial management is more than just creating a budget and looking at profit and loss (P&L) statements; KPIs must be monitored and managed, and changes must be implemented before financials are significantly impacted. A frictionless client experience, efficiency, and appropriate leveraging must be developed to reduce the cost of doing business. Charge capture must be a top priority and expenses must be monitored monthly. Accounts receivables must be well managed, and charity donations must be built into the budget. Finally, every team member needs to know how much it costs to run the business (open books management). The veterinary practice is a team sport, and every team member must understand how they contribute to the goals, even financial ones.

Financial terms in Fig. 16.1 will help you wrap your head around terms that are used throughout this chapter and most financial resources. Accounting and bookkeeping are closely related activities. The accounting process depends on the information produced by bookkeepers responsible for accounts payable, accounts receivable, and payroll. One or more team members may share the duties of a bookkeeper eliminating the position in smaller practices. Larger practices may employ a bookkeeper who then works with the practices accounting firm to aid in the practice's tax preparation, payroll, or benefit plans. Accountants specialize in producing and interpreting financial statements, tax planning, cash flow projections, and estate planning. The use of an accounting firm may depend on the size of the practice and the experience of the managers. Some practices may use an accountant only once a year to help prepare year-end statements and tax documents, whereas others may use an accountant monthly.

A certified public accountant (CPA) should always be considered when the practice is seeking professional accounting assistance. CPAs have extensive experience and have passed a comprehensive examination that tests their knowledge of accounting and tax principles, auditing standards, and business law. They attend yearly classes to maintain continuing education requirements and must comply with a strict code of ethics. Bookkeepers may designate themselves as "accountants," although they may not have attended college. Public accountants (PAs) may have attended college and completed a degree in accounting but not taken the CPA examination. CPAs are held to the highest standards. A CPA can ensure the practice finances are managed professionally, and ethically, and that business and tax laws are followed.

ACCOUNTING TERMS

Accrual basis method: A system that recognizes income when it is earned and expenses when they are incurred rather than when the actual cash transaction occurs.

Asset: Any property owned by a business or individual. Cash, accounts receivable, inventory, land, buildings, leasehold improvements, and tangible property are examples of assets.

Balance sheet: A financial report detailing practice assets, liabilities, and owner's equity.

Budget: An estimate of revenues and expenses for a given period.

Cash basis method: A system that recognizes income when it is received and expenses when they are paid, rather than when the income was earned, or the expense was acquired.

Cash flow statement: Report on the sources and uses of cash during a given period of time.

Equity: The rights or claims to properties. Assets = Equities + Liabilities.

Fixed cost: A cost that does not change with the variation in business. Rent, mortgage, and utility costs remain the same regardless of how busy the practice is.

Income statement: Report on financial performance that covers a period of time and reports incomes and expenses during that period. Income statements are also known as profit and loss statements.

Intangible property: Nonphysical property that has value: franchises, copyrights, client lists, goodwill, and noncompete agreements are examples of intangible property.

Key performance indicators: Statistics that can be generated from client transaction data and reviewed for performance data.

Liabilities: Obligations resulting from past transactions that require the practice to pay money or provide service. Accounts payable and taxes are examples of current liabilities.

Owner's equity: Owner's interest or claim in the practice assets.

Principal cost: Initial cost of equipment when purchased.

Profit and loss statement: Summary of the practice's income, expenses, and resulting profit or loss for a specified period of time (also known as the income statement).

Tangible property: Physical property, such as desks, chairs, equipment, computers, software, and vehicles that has value.

Transaction: A purchase that must be recorded.

Variable cost: Any cost that varies with the volume of business for the practice. The costs of medical supplies and drugs increase or decrease depending on the volume of business.

Fig. 16.1 Most common accounting/financial terms are found in this easy-access guide.

A CPA's responsibility is to produce reports for the practice; however, unless the CPA is familiar with the veterinary industry, he or she cannot determine how, when, or where the business may need improvements. It is advisable to seek out a skilled veterinary industry CPA (visit www.VHMA.org or www.VetPartners.org to view a list of professionals). Investing in a professional that understands the veterinary profession will help determine areas of improvement and make informed recommendations that benefit the practice.

CASH AND ACCRUAL BASIS ACCOUNTING

Revenue and expenses can be recorded by two different methods: cash or accrual. Which method a practice chooses is usually dictated by the need for federal or state revenue tax reporting. If revenue is measured when cash is received and expenses are measured when cash is spent, then a practice uses cash-basis accounting. Only fees paid by clients are recognized in cash-basis accounting. Therefore, outstanding accounts receivable are not included because those fees have yet to be paid by clients. Accounts payable transactions are only recorded when they have been paid for, not when they occurred.

If a practice is recording revenue and expenses while they occur, then the practice uses an accrual-basis accounting system. Practices that use an accrual basis record fees while they are earned and include outstanding accounts receivable. Accounts payable are recorded at the time of accrual, not at the time of payment.

Historically, most practices have used a cash-basis method to manage the business because it is easier to maintain and understand. When comparing the methods (cash and accrual basis), the reports will give two different pictures of the financial status of the hospital. Comparison of cash reports can provide varied results from month to month due to variations in revenue and expenses, and accrual reports are useful when reviewing a period of data as it reduces the variations seen in month-to-month reports. It is also common for a practice to use cash-based accounting to manage the business and accrual-based accounting for year-end tax reporting.

LEADERSHIP POINT

A cash-basis reporting system records when cash is received and when expenses are paid. An accrual-basis system reports when the revenue and expense occurred.

KEY PERFORMANCE INDICATORS

Accurate data is needed when compiling reports for a veterinary hospital. These metrics are also known as key performance indicators (KPIs) and should be used to monitor the practice on a monthly, quarterly, and yearly basis. Monitoring KPIs can help explain changes in financial statements and contribute to the success of the hospital. Practices should take time to determine which KPIs are important to their hospital and develop a spreadsheet to monitor changes from month to month. If KPIs are monitored monthly, negative trends can be managed more effectively (before having a significant impact on the financials). Fig. 16.2 lists some examples of KPIs a practice may wish to track. One cannot manage what one does not monitor, and it is inefficient to monitor and not manage.

EXAMPLES OF KPIs A PRACTICE MAY TRACK

- Accounts receivable summary
- Accounts payable summary
- Active clients
- Active patients
- Average client transaction
- Average doctor transaction
- Client compliance reports
- Client survey results
- Cost of goods expenses, as a percent of gross revenue
- Discounts per veterinarian
- DVM expenses, as a percent of gross revenue
- Revenue centers, as a percentage of gross revenue
- Number of active/new clients and patients
- Revenue and percent difference from previous period or year
- Staff expenses, as a percentage of gross revenue

Fig. 16.2 Common Key Performance Indicators that most veterinary practices use to track progress. One can't manage what they don't monitor!

CRITICAL COMPETENCY: CRITICAL AND STRATEGIC THINKING

Strategic thinking and planning are essential parts of financial forecasting, marketing plans, and long-term plans for the growth of the practice. Managers must have the ability to identify questions, problems, and arguments relevant to these issues and to use logic and critical reasoning to identify the strengths and weaknesses of alternative solutions or approaches to problems.

External benchmarking is the process in which a practice compares its own KPIs to others in the industry: locally, statewide, regionally, or nationally. It is important to keep in mind that KPIs can differ based on demographics, geographic location, urban versus rural setting, practice size and type, and hours of operation. Benchmarks are available from the Veterinary Hospital Managers Association (VHMA), the American Animal Hospital Association (AAHA), Well Managed Practices Benchmark Study (WMPB), and the Veterinary Management Group (VMG).

Benchmarks can also be taken from the practice's historical financial information (internal benchmarking). Both types of benchmarking must be considered when analyzing and making decisions for the practice.

LEADERSHIP POINT

Internal and external benchmarks should be evaluated together when looking for areas of opportunity in the hospital.

Accounts Receivable Summary

Accounts receivable (AR) should be monitored on an ongoing basis. A large amount of outstanding AR is detrimental to the practice and should not be greater than 1.5% of gross revenue. AR reports should break down amounts due into 0–30 days, 30–60 days, 60–90 days, and 90 days or greater overdue. Managing, monitoring, and collecting on accounts receivable is covered in more detail later in this chapter.

Accounts Payable Summary

Accounts payable reports should be monitored monthly to ensure expenses do not exceed revenue. If the practice spends more money than it generates, a serious financial deficit will result. Small practices that are relatively new may experience months with less revenue than others and should plan for variable months. Spending must decrease, inventory and waste should be closely monitored, and the fee structure and missed charges/discounts should be closely evaluated. If a line of credit is needed to keep the practice floating during the slow months, then a plan must be implemented to pay back the loan as soon as possible.

Active/New Clients and Patients per Month

The number of active clients and patients in a practice should be measured by both internal and external benchmarks. Internal benchmarks (practice numbers) should be monitored on a regular basis. External benchmarks should be used to determine where opportunities exist by a comparison of other practices in the nation or region (depending on the benchmark source). The definition of *active* may vary among benchmark resources. Identifying and comparing data for the same period is critical. If the number of active clients or patients is low, this indicates the need to review the client experience (Chapter 11), team leveraging and efficiency, and internal marketing techniques (Chapter 12). New clients and patients are critical to the long-term success of the practice; client and patient attrition normally occurs due to clients moving out of the area, changing practices, or the loss of a pet.

Average Client Transactions

Average client transactions (ACTs) include all transactions a client makes in the hospital: examinations, diagnostics, diets, and medication refills. When a client returns for a recheck, food, or medication refills, the ACT drops. Unless each transaction is monitored, practice managers may become alerted to a declining ACT. When transactions are investigated, managers can see client follow-up is the cause, and the alert is justified.

Historically, the average client transaction has been a key KPI and has been monitored to ensure that team members were making recommendations and clients were accepting them. If the average client transaction was consistently low, leaders would develop a solution to increase the low figure. Recently, ACTs have fallen out of favor because practices have focused on increasing ACTs without considering the impact of compliance (refills, medical progress exams, etc.) as well as not adding value for the client. As a result of increasing ACTs, clients had "sticker shock" from higher transactions, and consumer confidence in veterinary medicine has decreased.

ACTs can vary tremendously when comparing internal ACTs to external benchmarks because of practice size, age, demographics, and management philosophies.

Internal benchmarks and ACTs are still important because practice managers and owners need to know what is occurring in their hospital. If an ACT is declining, an investigation may be warranted; however, if the ACT is dropping because clients are following up as recommended, the investigation can cease. If the ACT is high and clients are not following up, then again, an investigation may be warranted to look for opportunities to increase compliance.

CRITICAL COMPETENCY: ANALYTICAL SKILLS

The practice manager must have the ability to grasp complex information, analyze information and use logic to address problems accurately, quickly, and efficiently.

Average Doctor Transactions

The average doctor transaction (ADT) is perhaps a better KPI than an ACT because it removes all refills of medications and food or any other nonpatient visit transactions. Average doctor transactions only consider charges that occurred during a patient visit. An ADT should be 3.5 times the cost of a regular patient examination (WMPB 2017). Many levers impact the veterinarian's ability to produce revenue and have a high average doctor transaction, including team skill, leveraging, efficiency (covered in Chapter 4, Veterinary Wage Determination), and pricing of services and products (covered later in this chapter). If the ADT is lower than benchmark numbers, start with these levers first.

Client Surveys

Client surveys are a great monitoring solution for understanding the satisfaction and level of client comfort with the services the practice provides (Chapter 12, Marketing). Client loyalty (and referrals) drive business; it is imperative to ensure that clients are satisfied and perceive the value of the service provided. Client surveys should be exported into a spreadsheet so that reports can be generated to show patterns, peaks, and areas for improvement.

VHMA PERFORMANCE DOMAIN TASK

Veterinary practice managers obtain and report client feedback on services.

Compliance Rates

Monitoring client compliance rates is useful in many ways. If clients are accepting recommendations, then the team is doing an excellent job of educating clients, and clients perceive value in the services that are being offered. Good client compliance ensures pets are getting the care they need, improves profitability, and is essential when protecting valuable long-term client relationships. It is much more cost effective to maintain existing relationships than to build new ones. Establishing new clients takes time and money. Compliance reports should include reminder compliance rates (clients booking appointments after reminders have been sent) as well as monitoring the profit centers of the practice (Chapter 11, Client Experience, and Chapter 12, Marketing).

Cost of Goods as Expenses as a Percent of Gross Revenue

Cost of goods (COGs) should be viewed in a percentage format and reviewed alongside the gross revenue. Comparing COGs percentages to external benchmarks helps practices to determine where they can improve inventory expenses and pricing. COGs are considered a variable cost, and the dollars will rise and fall based on the amount of business. If the practice is busy and buying a lot of product, the COGs expense (in dollars) will also increase; if the practice is slow and the practice is not ordering as much product, COGs (in dollars) will decrease. Therefore, percentages are imperative for comparison purposes. When using and comparing percentages, the percentage of expense to gross revenue should be relatively the same month to month (in a well-managed inventory system). If inventory is mismanaged, the percentages may remain high regardless of how busy the practice is. It is also important to compare the current percentage with historical KPIs because dramatic increases or decreases warrant an investigation (described further in the profit and loss section).

Discounts Per Veterinarian

Discounts given to clients by veterinarians must be tracked in both dollar and percentage values. Discounting, described later in this chapter, has a significant impact on the profitability of the hospital. Tracking discounts by DVM gives a better understanding of who is responsible for discounting and what is being given away.

LEADERSHIP POINT

Every team member, not just DVMs, should be held accountable for unplanned discounts given to clients.

DVM Expenses as a Percent of Gross Revenue

It is important to know how much a veterinarian "costs" the hospital in relation to how much they are producing. On average, a veterinarian should be producing five times the amount of their salary. If the veterinary expense is higher than what is being produced, alternative pay strategies (i.e., production, pro-sal) should be considered. Many factors impact the ability of DVMs to produce revenue; review veterinary wage determination in Chapter 4 for more information.

VHMA PERFORMANCE DOMAIN TASK

Veterinary practice managers develop and manage new client programs.

Revenue and Percent Difference from Previous Period or Year

It is important to analyze where the revenue is being generated from (revenue centers) and compare the difference from previous time periods. Revenue centers are defined as the areas that produce the practice revenue (professional services, pharmaceutical, lab, surgery, dental, etc.). They can be thought of as "individual businesses" within the practice and goals must be created and obtained for each "business" center, just as goals are set for the overall business. When reviewing revenue centers, reports should be viewed in dollars and percentage format. Reviewing percentages puts these numbers into perspective and gives the manager the tools to identify which revenue centers need further development, equipment, or training to increase profitability.

Taxes

Taxes must be paid on a monthly and/or quarterly basis, depending on what type of tax is due. States have various taxing strategies, and a CPA should be consulted to ensure the practice is collecting the correct tax from clients and correctly reporting each month. For example, in some states, both products and services are taxed. In other states, only products are taxed. Further, taxation on some products can vary if they are considered OTC or prescription. A CPA should evaluate the practice structure each year and provide clarity around this vague area (tax laws can change annually). Practice managers and owners need to ensure the services and inventory items in the PIMS are set to tax correctly both for collecting tax from clients and printing reports for the CPA. AVMA maintains a list of taxes imposed by the state on veterinary services, including use tax, prescription drugs and vaccines, nonprescription OTC drugs or products, taxes on veterinary services, taxes on medical equipment, and internet sales. Visit https://www.avma.org/sites/default/files/2022-07/AVMA-Sales-Tax-Chart-July-2022.pdf for annual updates.

Amounts should be calculated on the first of each month, with the scheduled dates of payment.

FINANCIAL REPORTS

Creating financial reports allows the practice to evaluate its financial status on a monthly, quarterly, and yearly basis while also being able to compare to benchmarks industry-wide. Managing finances allows trends to be monitored and changes made before a significant impact occurs.

For accurate reporting and comparison, expenses should be classified into the AAHA chart of accounts (COA). By using an industry-standard COA, practices can benchmark and find opportunities for improvement (Fig. 16.3).

> **VHMA PERFORMANCE DOMAIN TASK**
>
> Veterinary practice managers analyze practice and financial reports.

Financial reports allow a manager to recognize current problems and prevent financial problems from occurring. By recognizing issues early, problems can be resolved before they become a financial nightmare for the practice. It is essential to develop a balance sheet and profit and loss statement monthly, keeping a snapshot of the practice's finances in clear view.

> **LEADERSHIP POINT**
>
> Don't wait until year's end to review the P&L produced by the accountant for tax purposes; find trends earlier, make changes, and prevent a detrimental year-end report.

Balance Sheets

A balance sheet is referred to as the *statement of financial condition of the practice*. It summarizes the assets, liabilities, and equities of the practice. Balance sheets represent the basic accounting equation: assets = liabilities + owner equity. Assets include all things of value that the practice owns, including property, equipment, inventory, building, land, and goodwill. Liabilities include accounts payable and loans. Owner equity is the profitability of the business.

Cash Flow

Cash flow is defined as the movement of money into and out of a business, usually during a specified period. A cash flow statement provides a snapshot of the checking account with the net revenue for the period being analyzed.

Practice managers are often under the impression that the bottom line on a profit and loss statement should equal the balance in the checking account. This is untrue because several factors affect the balance, such as:

- inventory has been purchased but not yet sold,
- accounts receivable have not been settled, and
- bills have been paid but have not yet cleared the checking account.

Some practices may have cash flow issues, meaning cash is not available for accounts payable. Several reasons exist for cash flow crunches, including:

- mismanaged inventory (excess product sitting on shelves),
- mismanaged payroll (excess overtime),
- embezzlement, and
- large dividends paid to the owner(s) when revenue is low or nonexistent.

Cash flow issues need to be addressed and corrected as soon as possible to keep the practice doors open.

Profit and Loss Statements

A profit and loss statement (P&L) is a financial statement that summarizes revenue, expenses, and profits for a specific period, such as monthly, quarterly, and/or annually. These records provide information that shows the ability of a practice to generate a profit by maximizing revenue while trying to reduce expenses. P&Ls are also known as revenue statements, or revenue and expense statements.

P&L reports list revenue first followed by expenses, then profitability (revenue—expense). Entries are made in the checkbook ledger of QuickBooks (or whichever accounting software a practice uses). Entries must be entered in the correct expense category (AAHA COA) to produce accurate reports.

QuickBooks (QB) is one of the most popular accounting software programs used in the veterinary profession (although others are available that can complete the same tasks). For the sake of simplicity in this chapter, QB will be referred to.

It is particularly important to make sure that the P&L sheet is as accurate as possible, and that the proper categories within the chart of accounts are used. This allows managers to determine where inconsistencies may lie by comparing benchmarks and provides better data on how to correct any inconsistencies. The ability to manage P&Ls in house enables the manager to evaluate them monthly and make changes when needed before any negative trends have a severe impact on the practice. Understanding the chart of accounts and P&L sheets enables the accurate assessment of financials and building of budgets.

> **VHMA PERFORMANCE DOMAIN TASK**
>
> Veterinary practice managers maintain a chart of accounts.

Revenue: Revenue is recorded through deposits made to the practice (Fig. 16.4) and can be extracted from the PIMS and imported into QB. Practice managers may wish to further break down revenue into revenue centers (Fig. 16.5), allowing it to be compared to the expenses associated with that center (ensuring each center is profitable). For ease of demonstration, the figures provided list revenue for the entire year, but for proper monitoring and management, it must be broken down into a monthly basis (at minimum).

> **LEADERSHIP POINT**
>
> Detailed revenue centers on a P&L sheet allow easier comparison of expenses that are associated with each individual revenue center.

Expenses: The outflow of money (paying bills) is known as an expense and is referred to as either a fixed or variable expense.

Fixed Expenses: Fixed expenses are (in general) a set cost for the hospital; they do not change based on the amount of business produced by the hospital. Regardless of the number of clients seen, expenses such as rent/mortgage, building insurance, health insurance, internet, and telephone will remain constant.

If veterinarians are paid a salary only (no production) they are classified as a fixed expense (regardless of the number of clients seen, they will still receive the same paycheck). Medical insurance, retirement, and continuing education can either be allocated within this category or allocated to administrative costs (depending on practice preference). When comparing benchmarks, make sure to note where these expenses are placed in the benchmarks so that they do not

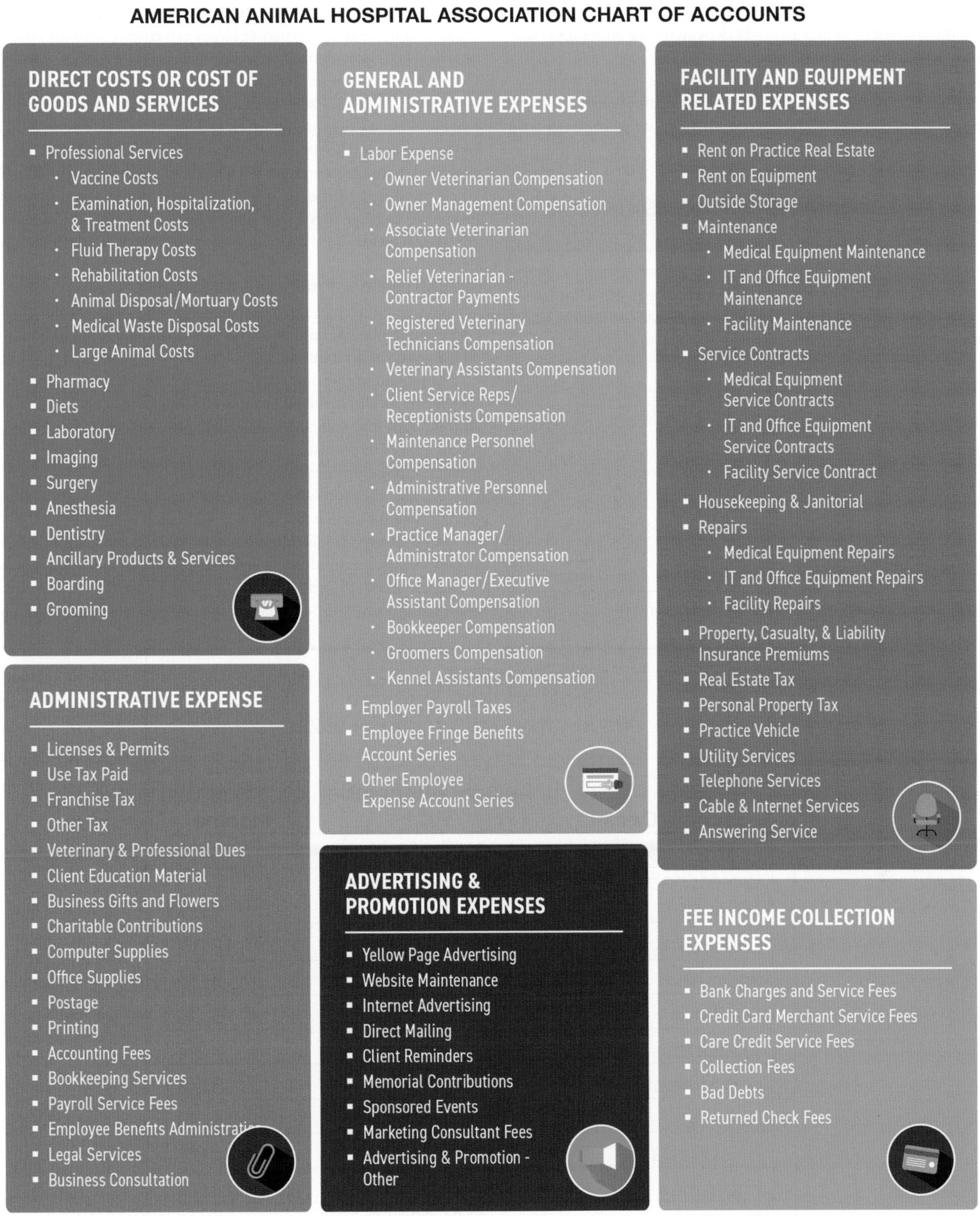

AMERICAN ANIMAL HOSPITAL ASSOCIATION CHART OF ACCOUNTS
DIRECT COSTS OR COST OF GOODS AND SERVICES
Professional Services
Vaccine Costs
Examination, Hospitalization, & Treatment Costs
Fluid Therapy Costs
Rehabilitation Costs
Animal Disposal/Mortuary Costs
Medical Waste Disposal Costs
Large Animal Costs
Pharmacy
Diets
Laboratory
Imaging
Surgery
Anesthesia
Dentistry
Ancillary Products & Services
Boarding
Grooming
ADMINISTRATIVE EXPENSE
Licenses & Permits
Use Tax Paid
Franchise Tax
Other Tax
Veterinary & Professional Dues
Client Education Material
Business Gifts and Flowers
Charitable Contributions
Computer Supplies
Office Supplies
Postage
Printing
Accounting Fees
Bookkeeping Services
Payroll Service Fees
Employee Benefits Administrat
Legal Services
Business Consultation
GENERAL AND ADMINISTRATIVE EXPENSES
Labor Expense
Owner Veterinarian Compensation
Owner Management Compensation
Associate Veterinarian Compensation
Relief Veterinarian - Contractor Payments
Registered Veterinary Technicians Compensation
Veterinary Assistants Compensation
Client Service Reps/ Receptionists Compensation
Maintenance Personnel Compensation
Administrative Personnel Compensation
Practice Manager/ Administrator Compensation
Office Manager/Executive Assistant Compensation
Bookkeeper Compensation
Groomers Compensation
Kennel Assistants Compensation
Employer Payroll Taxes
Employee Fringe Benefits Account Series
Other Employee Expense Account Series
ADVERTISING & PROMOTION EXPENSES
Yellow Page Advertising
Website Maintenance
Internet Advertising
Direct Mailing
Client Reminders
Memorial Contributions
Sponsored Events
Marketing Consultant Fees
Advertising & Promotion - Other
FACILITY AND EQUIPMENT RELATED EXPENSES
Rent on Practice Real Estate
Rent on Equipment
Outside Storage
Maintenance
Medical Equipment Maintenance
IT and Office Equipment Maintenance
Facility Maintenance
Service Contracts
Medical Equipment Service Contracts
IT and Office Equipment Service Contracts
Facility Service Contract
Housekeeping & Janitorial
Repairs
Medical Equipment Repairs
IT and Office Equipment Repairs
Facility Repairs
Property, Casualty, & Liability Insurance Premiums
Real Estate Tax
Personal Property Tax
Practice Vehicle
Utility Services
Telephone Services
Cable & Internet Services
Answering Service
FEE INCOME COLLECTION EXPENSES
Bank Charges and Service Fees
Credit Card Merchant Service Fees
Care Credit Service Fees
Collection Fees
Bad Debts
Returned Check Fees

Fig. 16.3 Standard accounting categories help practices compare practice financials to industry averages and standards. (From American Animal Hospital Association/VMG chart of accounts. https://www.aaha.org/practice-resources/aaha-benchmarking/aaha-open-standards/standard-chart-of-accounts/)

throw off the analysis. Some benchmarks allocate veterinary salaries to administrative costs, whereas others allocate them under veterinarian expenses.

Variable Expenses: Variable expenses change based on the amount of business produced by a practice. Cost of goods (COGs) is defined as the products used to produce a service for a client, or products sold to a client. Patient visits and services vary every month and so do the expenses associated with these visits. For example, a varying number of vaccines will be ordered and administered every month.

Staff payroll is typically variable, especially when seasonal staff is utilized; hence staff payroll is allocated to the variable expense category. It can be argued that in some practices staff expenses are relatively fixed; however, for comparison and analysis with benchmarks, it is referred to as a *variable expense.*

Veterinary salaries that are paid on production are variable expenses because the amount of money paid will depend on the amount of business produced in a specified period.

Profit: Profit is determined when the practice expenses are subtracted from the revenue, ideally resulting in a positive balance. If more money was spent than the revenue received, the result will be a negative balance.

CRITICAL COMPETENCY: DECISION MAKING

The practice manager must be able to make good decisions based on critical thinking and problem solving and must be able to make decisions that positively impact the practice. While many alternatives are available, the PM must be able to gather and effectively analyze relevant data and choose decisively.

ABC Veterinary Hospital
Profit and Loss Standard
January through December 2022

Ordinary Income/Expense	Jan-Dec 2022	% of Income
Income	$1,500,000	100%
Total Income	**$1,500,000**	**100%**

Fig. 16.4 Revenue summary on a profit and loss report.

Producing Monthly Profit and Loss Statements

Now that revenue and expenses have been entered into the correct categories, P&L statements can be printed. As stated earlier, P&Ls should be produced in-house every month for successful financial assessment.

In QB, the P&L statement can be generated from the "reports" menu. A detailed or summarized report can be chosen, in either cash or accrual view. The summarized report is recommended for analysis; a detailed report is recommended when looking for discrepancies. Select the option that provides expenses as a percent of revenue for ease of comparison (Fig. 16.6). This view allows both dollars and percentages to be evaluated.

Troubleshooting Profit and Loss Statements

When percentages of a category are abnormal (either internal KPI or benchmarks), a red flag should be raised, and an investigation into the discrepancy is warranted.

When managers first start to analyze data, percentages may be higher or lower than benchmarks allowing practice managers to look for changes that can be made to bring the percentages to a "normal" level. Three steps must be taken when analyzing P&Ls:

Step 1: **Look** at the percentages and compare.
Step 2: **Ask** questions about the percentages.
Step 3: **Implement** change.

First, ensure that all expenses are classified correctly with the AAHA COA, as misclassification skews percentages. Once all expenses are correctly classified, the practice manager and owner can look for opportunities to improve the percentage to get closer to the benchmark ranges.

ABC Veterinary Hospital
Profit and Loss Standard
January through December 2022

Income Center	January - December 2022	% of Income
Examination	$240,000.00	16.0%
Professional Services	$60,000.00	4.0%
Laboratory Fees	$270,000.00	18.0%
Imaging	$67,500.00	4.5%
Dentistry	$45,000.00	3.0%
Vaccines	$105,000.00	7.0%
Hospitalization	$45,000.00	3.0%
Surgery	$90,000.00	6.0%
Anesthesia	$60,000.00	4.0%
Pharmacy	$210,000.00	14.0%
Flea, Tick and HW	$135,000.00	9.0%
Diets	$75,000.00	5.0%
OTC/Retail	$30,000.00	2.0%
Boarding	$37,500.00	2.5%
Bathing/Grooming	$30,000.00	2.0%
	$1,500,000.00	**100.0%**

Fig. 16.5 Revenue detail on profit and loss report.

	April	%	May	%
Income - Total	**$150,000.00**	**100.%**	**$200,000.00**	**100**
Expenses				
Admin	$12,600.00	8.4%	$16,800.00	8.4%
Facility	$14,100.00	9.4%	$18,800.00	9.4%
DVM Salary	$22,500.00	15.0%	$30,000.00	15.0%
COG	$33,150.00	22.1%	$44,200.00	22.1%
Non-DVM Wages	$42,000.00	28.0%	$56,000.00	28.0%
DVM Prod	$15,000.00	10.0%	$20,000.00	10.0%
Expenses- Total	**$139,350.00**	**92.9%**	**$185,800**	**92.9%**
Profit	**$10,650.00**	**7.1%**	**$14,200.00**	**7.1%**

Fig. 16.6 Dollar amounts change in this monthly expense comparison, but the percentages remain the same with the increased revenue.

Dental center gross income per month	$9,989.45
Dental center, square feet used for center	100 sq ft
Annual fixed costs/sq ft (determined from P&L fixed costs: administrative, facility, and veterinary)	$190.00
Annual dental center fixed costs (100 sq ft × $190.00)	$19,000.00
Monthly dental center fixed costs (annual costs ÷ 12)	$1,583.33
Dental center variable costs	$525.39
Dental center profitability ($9,989.45 − $1,583.33 − $525.39)	**$7,880.32**

Fig. 16.7 Dental revenue profitability analysis.

The following are examples of looking at percentages, comparing them to historical numbers, and asking "why":

During the month of January, utilities were 1.3%, and for the month of February, utilities were 5%. Benchmarks show utilities should be approximately 0.7% (WMPB, 2017). Historically, the utilities for this practice average 1.2%. One might assume the winter weather has increased the cost of utilities, but when looked at by dollar amount, that increase would be too high. Therefore, the following questions would be investigated:

- Were some utility bills paid late (from January), thereby increasing February percentages?
- Did revenue drop significantly to cause this increase?
- Are more than only the practice's utility bills being paid?
- Are there maintenance issues occurring within the practice, resulting in higher percentages?
- Was an expense misclassified?

LEADERSHIP POINT

Becoming familiar with the practice's profit and loss sheet percentages will help identify areas that need immediate investigation.

A practice may also see that their COG percentage is higher (30%) than that of benchmarks (20%). To help determine why this percentage is high, a practice may look at these factors (this is not a complete list of reasons, but rather ideas to spark the investigation):

- The amount of inventory sitting on the shelves
- Potential shrinkage
- Pricing model of inventory
- Misclassified expenses
- Significant decrease in revenue

While analyzing expense opportunities is critically important, it is also important to understand how revenue impacts the expense percentages. Because many expenses are fixed expenses (the same regardless of revenue generated), a greater impact can be made by analyzing revenue opportunities (see Maximizing Revenue). Higher revenue decreases fixed expense percentages, and as you will see, missing even 10% of revenue (through lost charge capture) has a significant impact on all expenses.

Comparing Revenue and Expense Centers

It is important to be able to compare revenue and expense centers. As defined previously, revenue centers produce money for the hospital, while expense centers are expenses associated with a specific center. For example, a dental *revenue* center includes all money generated from dental prophylaxes, extractions, and dental radiographs. The dental *expense* center encompasses all inventoried items, staff time, and DVM time to produce the service. If it costs more to generate a service than the revenue produced, the center must be reevaluated for profitability.

When a center is not managed, opportunities for improvement are missed. The following information is required to evaluate the profitability of a service:

- Gross revenue per month (or year) for a specific service
- Square footage used by service
- Fixed costs per square foot (entire practice)
- Fixed costs per square foot for service
- Variable costs for service

Calculating the values in this list will determine whether a profit is being generated. For example, consider the dental center presented in Fig. 16.7. The dental center produced $9989.45 (for the month) and used 100 sq ft of the practice's total space. Fixed costs have been determined (from P&L) to be $190.00 per square foot, equaling $19,000 per year, or $1583.33 per month. Variable costs are determined to be $525.39 per month. Therefore, the center is producing a profit of $7880.32 per month.

Capital equipment used to produce services is placed in the fixed expense category of facilities and equipment and becomes a business expense (versus being allocated directly to the cost center). Service pricing (covered later in this chapter) encapsulates costs associated with facilities and equipment into an administrative cost and is shared in all charge points.

When professional services are not profitable, practice managers must consider increasing the client's cost for services, audit the potential for missed charge capture, and/or whether the service is being used to its maximum potential.

LEADERSHIP POINT

Profit centers must be analyzed for both Revenue and expenses.

Using KPIs to Analyze Data

KPIs are useful in helping to identify opportunities (or discrepancies) in reports and therefore, it is important to know the "why" behind all practice KPIs. For example, there may be a decrease in the number of clients in one month but an increase in the ADT. The increase in gross revenue and ADT may be explained if customer service initiatives were improved and the practice started focusing on developing relationships with clients. Knowing the why helps celebrate successes when initiatives have been implemented and allows the practice to continue identifying opportunities for improvements. Accurate data from KPIs is critical when making business decisions, developing a strategic plan, or adding revenue centers, and prevents decisions based on assumptions or emotions.

MAXIMIZING REVENUE

A manager is most financially effective when finding methods to maximize revenue (versus cutting expenses). There are many levers that maximize revenue; each is complex, and it can take time to see improvements. Always keep in mind that revenue is generated by every team member, regardless of their role. Having them involved in strategies and initiatives not only improves their emotional ownership of the initiative but also helps them understand the business. Team members (including associate veterinarians) have no idea that more than 80% of the revenue generated each day simply pays the expenses that run the business. See the section on open book management later in the chapter to get comfortable with sharing business data with team members.

Levers that impact revenue generation include appropriate pricing, charge capture, discounts, team leveraging and efficiency, and a frictionless client experience for existing services. Opportunities for additional revenue centers must also be evaluated, especially if the practice wishes to grow year over year (and not just from price increases).

CRITICAL COMPETENCY: CREATIVITY

Practice managers must have the ability to creatively think through situations and embrace new and different ways to see opportunities by using imagination and collaboration, resulting in innovative solutions.

Service Pricing Based on Practice Financial Data

Pricing for services must be right for the practice and the demographic of the clientele they serve. Pricing that is "right for the practice" strictly depends on the practice financial data that is found on the P&L. The P&L reveals the true cost of doing business, and the pricing strategy must use that data, along with a profitability factor, to determine appropriate pricing for clients. The bigger piece of the puzzle then relies on the demographic served by the practice: can the clients afford to pay the price that a practice must charge for a service? There is a balance, no doubt. Some service costs will be lower and can have a higher profitability associated with them, while others will be loss leaders. The practice must decide what balance works well to serve clients, covers expenses, and allows care and development of their team.

VHMA PERFORMANCE DOMAIN TASK

Veterinary practice managers conduct fee analysis and monitor and update fee schedules.

Often, practices do not know how to price services or inventory, both of which have a significant impact on the profitability of the practice. Many times, service pricing was inherited when the practice was purchased, and pricing has very minimally increased over the years. However, as the practice grows and more overhead costs are added, owners and practice managers must ensure they are charging appropriately to maximize revenue growth opportunities.

To determine how much a service costs a practice to produce, several key points must be known (Fig. 16.8A). Print a year-to-date P&L to evaluate your practice for effective pricing.

- Fixed costs of hospital per minute
- Direct costs used to produce service (inventory)
- Staff costs per minute
- Number of staff minutes used to complete the service
- DVM costs per minute
- Number of DVM minutes used to complete the service
- Desired profit

Fixed costs per minute are a total of administrative, facility, and equipment categories, along with the number of billable minutes the hospital is open.

- A hospital is open to do business for 12,000 minutes per month (to calculate this number for your practice, determine how many minutes the practice is open each day of the month).
- The P&L statement indicates that the fixed costs for the practice are $20,000 per month; $20,000 ÷ 12,000 minutes per month = $1.67.
- Fixed costs for the practice are $1.67 per minute.

Direct costs are inventoried items used to produce a service, doubled:

- Materials used to produce a service total $1.23
- $1.23 × 2 = $2.46

Staff costs per minute are determined by totaling all costs associated with paying all non-DVM staff members. This number is then divided by the billable minutes the practice is open. Taking this equation one step further, the staff costs per minute will then be multiplied by the number of non-DVM team members used to complete the procedure, along with the number of minutes it takes to complete the task.

- The P&L indicates staff costs are $17,000 per month. As indicated previously, the practice is available to produce services 12,000 minutes per month; therefore $17,000 ÷ 12,000 minutes per month = $1.42.
- Staff costs are $1.42 per minute, per staff member.

SERVICE PRICING MODEL

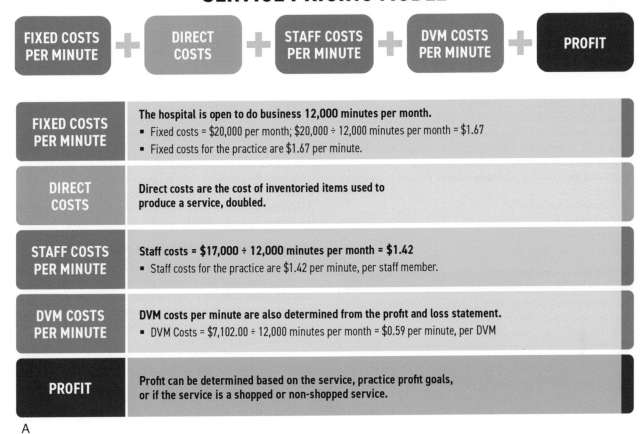

FIXED COSTS PER MINUTE + DIRECT COSTS + STAFF COSTS PER MINUTE + DVM COSTS PER MINUTE + PROFIT

FIXED COSTS PER MINUTE	**The hospital is open to do business 12,000 minutes per month.** ▪ Fixed costs = $20,000 per month; $20,000 ÷ 12,000 minutes per month = $1.67 ▪ Fixed costs for the practice are $1.67 per minute.
DIRECT COSTS	**Direct costs are the cost of inventoried items used to produce a service, doubled.**
STAFF COSTS PER MINUTE	**Staff costs = $17,000 ÷ 12,000 minutes per month = $1.42** ▪ Staff costs for the practice are $1.42 per minute, per staff member.
DVM COSTS PER MINUTE	**DVM costs per minute are also determined from the profit and loss statement.** ▪ DVM Costs = $7,102.00 ÷ 12,000 minutes per month = $0.59 per minute, per DVM
PROFIT	**Profit can be determined based on the service, practice profit goals, or if the service is a shopped or non-shopped service.**

A

PUTTING IT ALL TOGETHER

This procedure is estimated to take 10 minutes to complete.

FIXED COSTS PER MINUTE	$1.67 x 10 minutes = $16.70
DIRECT COSTS	Direct costs = $1.23 $1.23 x 2 = $2.46
STAFF COSTS PER MINUTE	1 Staff member = 5 minutes ▪ $1.42 x 5 minutes = $7.10
DVM COSTS PER MINUTE	1 DVM = 5 minutes ▪ 0.59 x 5 minutes = $2.95
PROFIT	Cost without profit: $16.70 + $2.46 + $7.10 + $2.95 = $29.21 Cost with 20% profit: $16.70 + $2.46 + $7.10 + $2.95 + $5.84 = $35.05

B

Fig. 16.8 (A) Financial data needed to create a service model specific to the practice. **(B)** Using data from the practice's financials allows accurate pricing to be determined for services provided to clients.

DVM costs per minute: P&Ls should be detailed enough to determine how much it costs to pay the veterinarian(s) monthly. For calculation purposes, if several DVMs are on staff, determine the average pay of all DVMs. The total is then divided by the number of billable minutes the hospital is open.

- The P&L indicates DVM costs are $7102 per month. As indicated previously, the practice is available to produce services 12,000 minutes per month; therefore $7102 ÷ 12,000 minutes per month = $0.59.
- DVM costs are $0.59 per minute, per DVM.

Profit can be determined based on the service, practice profitability goals, and/or if the service is a shopped or nonshopped service.

Putting It All Together: The following is an example of determining the cost of service (Fig. 16.8B):

- It is estimated that an entire procedure takes 10 minutes to complete:
- Direct cost = $1.23
- 1 staff member = 5 minutes
- 1 DVM = 5 minutes
- Desired profit = 20%
- This service should cost a client $35.05.

LEADERSHIP POINT

Don't base service pricing on benchmarks. Each practice has different costs associated with each service. Use the practice financials to establish the minimum client cost, then factor in local competitors and benchmarks.

Spot-check all services and adjust as needed. Remember, some services must have higher profitability than others to offset the loss leaders.

Keep in mind, practices cannot suddenly increase the price of services without illustrating the value of those services. Doing so will likely impart sticker shock, as indicated by the Bayer Veterinary Care Usage Study (BVCUS). Clients must understand the value of the service they are paying; if they do not perceive the value, they will decline recommendations and shop for less expensive services. Providing a frictionless client experience and developing relationships with clients prevents this scenario from occurring (Chapter 11, Client Experience).

Charging for inventory items is discussed at length in Chapter 13. Do not forget that holding and ordering costs must be assessed to prevent the practice from losing money. Additionally, shopped and nonshopped items must be considered. Shopped items will require less of a markup (or lower profitability) than nonshopped items. For example, heartworm prevention may have a 75% markup, whereas an injection may have a 200% markup. Practice managers should consider which products the practice takes a loss on and increase the profit percentage on other products to offset the difference. Additionally, outsource products to the practice's online pharmacy to reduce soft costs associated with inventory that generates less revenue.

Fees vary from laboratory to laboratory. Some laboratories may compete for the practice's business by offering special pricing on the most common profiles (ensure these tests are being selected on lab req forms and when charging clients).

Consider the following hidden costs associated with laboratory analyses and what the practice might do to recoup the lost expense:

- The time it takes the team members to obtain and prepare the samples to be shipped (use the equation to obtain service pricing to determine fixed costs per minute and staff costs per minute)
- The cost of supplies used to obtain the sample if the laboratory does not provide them. Supplies may include a syringe and needle, sampled collection tubes, formalin if purchased by the gallon, and/or slides used for cytologic analyses.
- The cost of the test
- Some laboratories may add a fuel surcharge to the monthly statement.
- Shipping fees if samples are submitted to labs other than those used for general analysis (overnight fees with FedEx or UPS)

Consider a three-DVM practice that employs 15 nonveterinary full-time staff members with:

- Fixed costs per minute of $3.92 per minute
- Staff costs of $2.82 per minute
- Two staff members taking 5 minutes to obtain the patient sample
- Assuming the laboratory provides the supplies:
  - **Fixed** costs: $3.92 × 5 = $19.60 and Staff costs: $2.82 × 5 = $5.64 × 2 = $11.28
  - Total cost to the practice: $19.60 + $11.28 = **$30.88**

It costs the practice $30.88 to obtain a patient sample (not including inventory, as the sample items had been supplied by the laboratory). According to WMPB 2017, only 31% of practices that participated in the survey charged to obtain samples (blood, urine, etc.).

Charge Capture and the Impact of Discounts

Industry standards estimate that missed charges in the veterinary practice range from 5%–10% of actual revenue. For every $1 million in revenue, $50,000–$100,000 is lost annually due to poor charge capture.[1] In a recent case study, 40% of reviewed cases had missed charges, resulting in an average of $50 per case difference for inpatient services, and $23.33 for outpatient services.[2]

Medical record audits must be completed to determine what has left the practice uncharged (Chapter 9). If a hospital produces $1,500,000.00 a year, and 10% of services and inventoried items go uncharged, the practice has lost $150,000 in profit per year! If medical record audits are not performed, a manager or owner will never recognize that money is being lost.

Identify *why* charges are being missed. Is the team understaffed? Does a team member lack focus? Do all team members understand the financial impact of missed charges?

CRITICAL COMPETENCY: LEADERSHIP

Practice managers must have the initiative to lead and take charge while simultaneously motivating and mobilizing others to achieve common goals.

To help reduce missed charges, managers may adopt several items or tasks. Travel sheets (Chapter 13, Inventory) may be used for paper and paper-light practices; electronic medical records that invoice automatically help reduce missed charges; however, if the medical record is left incomplete, charges will still be missed (review Chapter 8, PIMS, and Chapter 9, Medical Records, to learn how the proper PIMS can help eliminate lost charges). Practice managers may need to define procedures to indicate medical records must be completed before a client checks out.

When analyzing P&L statements, a loss of $200,000 can alter the percentages significantly. All managers must evaluate this area when trying to maximize revenue. In Fig. 16.9, example A represents full revenue at $1.6 million. Example B represents $200,000 of uncaptured revenue, resulting in an annual revenue of $1.4 million. Notice that while the dollars spent on expenses remain the same, the percentages dramatically change, and the result is negative profitability for the year.

Many practices do not evaluate the total dollars in discounts given to clients, nor do they review any return on investments (ROIs) from these discounts. Discounts come in two forms: managed and unmanaged. Managed discounts are those that are planned. For example: buy 11 doses and get 1 free, or give a free bottle of shampoo with every examination.

Unmanaged discounts are those that are unplanned and given because the practice "feels" it failed the client in some way. For example:

	Example A		Example B	
Income	**$1,600,000.00**	**100.0%**	**$1,400,000.00**	**100%**
Expenses				
Admin	$134,400.00	8.40%	$134,400.00	9.60%
Facility	$150,400.00	9.40%	$150,400.00	10.74%
DVM Salary	$240,000.00	15.00%	$240,000.00	17.14%
COG	$353,600.00	22.10%	$353,600.00	25.26%
Staff Wages	$448,000.00	28.00%	$448,000.00	32.00%
DVM Wages	$160,000.00	10.00%	$160,000.00	11.43%
Total	$1,486,400.00	92.90%	$1,486,400.00	106.17%
Profit	**$113,600.00**	7.10%	**($86,400.00)**	-6.17%

Fig. 16.9 Example A represents a practice that collects 100% of the Revenue produced. Example B represents a practice that has not collected all the Revenue produced and allowed $200,000 to be given away in discounts and/or missed charges. The costs to the practice remain the same; therefore, the missing $200,000 significantly affects the profit and skews the percentages.

- A veterinarian may want to continue providing the best care for a patient, but if the client can no longer afford the service, the DVM continues the treatment regardless.
- The team failed to communicate an increase in the treatment plan (estimate) with the client; the client is angry; a discount is applied to the client's account to satisfy (and maintain) the client.
- A dental procedure takes longer than expected and costs the client $1000. The DVM feels guilty and discounts the invoice instead of educating the client on why it took so long.

Unfortunately, these discounts add up. If a practice is already losing 10% of gross revenue in missed charges, how much additional revenue is lost through discounts?

There are a few steps the practice can take to better manage discounts. First, every product given away as a planned discount should be entered as a line item on the invoice (then discounted with a specific code) allowing the reporting of discounts. This also creates awareness and a sense of value for clients. Practice managers must then track discounts and evaluate the ROI. Do clients return in the future for services when discounts are offered?

LEADERSHIP POINT

Missed charges account for the loss of approximately 10% of gross revenue. For a practice that generates $1.5 million dollars, $150,000.00 is lost annually.

Unmanaged discounts have a significant impact on the practice financials, ultimately preventing the reinvested of profitability back into the health and well-being of the team or the building. While discounting will always occur, protocols can be put in place to maximize the benefit of client benefits while reducing the loss to the practice.

If client discounts are being given because of poor client experiences, then training, protocol development, leveraging, efficiency, etc. must be put into place to reduce the potential for client dissatisfaction in the future. Track reasons why an unsatisfied experience occurred and make changes as needed.

Consider developing a "discounts budget" wherein each doctor receives an annual budget for discounts they wish to give. When a DVM runs out of "discount dollars" for the year, they can no longer provide a client discount. Within the first year, discount dollars will be used rapidly. In the second year, discounts will be given more conservatively, especially as the team understands the significant impact discounts have.

CRITICAL COMPETENCY: PERSUASION

The practice manager must possess the ability to change the attitudes and opinions of others, persuade them to accept recommendations, and encourage behaviors that support practice goals.

Another potential discount solution is to build a rewards app for clients, covered in Chapter 12, Marketing. A better solution is to influence client behavior through attainable rewards versus devaluing practice services through discounting.

Managing the Frictionless Client Experience

To maximize revenue opportunities, practice managers must analyze the entire client experience (Chapter 11). When the client called the hospital to make an appointment, what did they experience? Did the client feel welcome? Did the team member answering the phone identify himself or herself? Was the client able to make a convenient appointment or was there a lengthy waiting period?

When a client enters the practice, what do they experience? Is it clean? Does it have a professional appearance? Does it smell good? Were medical records reviewed so that the team is prepared to welcome the client and patient and know what services will be needed during the visit? Preparation decreases missed opportunities for needed services and increases client compliance.

How long does the client have to wait to be seen? If appointments are running behind, how is the client notified? Review Chapter 10 for more details on appointment management. Clients who experience delayed appointments will have lower compliance.

How are treatment plans presented to the clients? Numerous studies indicate veterinarians should not be responsible for the presentation of treatment plans, and that team members should be educators to achieve the best client acceptance rates. The verbal and nonverbal skills of every team member should be optimized to increase compliance rates (Chapter 11).

How is the check-out process handled? Clients should receive a detailed, line-by-line invoice they can understand (abbreviations are not acceptable). Receptionists should explain each line to the client before reaching the final amount due. Clients must understand the value they are receiving for the price they are paying (Chapter 11).

Every client touchpoint within the practice is an opportunity to illustrate the value of services and to find opportunities for client recommendations. The most successful practices capitalize on these opportunities. A frictionless client experience is what keeps clients returning and generates referrals of friends and family to the practice. Providing excellent customer service can set the practice apart from the competition by building valuable relationships, thus enhancing compliance. Without outstanding customer service, revenue cannot be fully maximized.

Leveraging and Team Efficiency

Ensuring team members are effectively leveraged to their greatest capacity (skill set) and to the extent of their credentials (state veterinary practice act) is required to maximize revenue. It was identified in Chapter 1 that inefficiency in the team has led to team member burnout and emotional instability, ultimately resulting in a barrier to patient care. While average revenue grew in practices in 2022 by an average of 6% (resulting from price increases), the number of clients and patients seen decreased. Meanwhile, team members are still reporting a state of being understaffed and overworked. In summary, practices have become less efficient and do not utilize their staff to their fullest potential, resulting in stagnant revenue.

Proper leveraging of all team members leads to higher team member satisfaction and retention, as well as an increase in revenue. Effective leveraging means that all team members are operating at their trained skill level:

- Veterinarians diagnose, prescribe, and perform surgical procedures.
- Credentialed veterinary technicians/nurses complete all diagnostics, dental prophylaxis, treatments, surgical prep, client education, and any task as outlined by the state veterinary practice act.
- Veterinary assistants should aid in the proper restraint of patients, care of patients, and assisting credentialed veterinary technicians/nurses and doctors to complete their properly leveraged duties.

It makes no sense to hire a credentialed technician/nurse and not allow them to complete the tasks they have obtained training for. A practice would never hire a veterinarian and not let them complete surgical procedures they trained for. On the other hand, practices should not allow a veterinary assistant to complete patient care treatments without proper education and understanding of veterinary medicine (patient care is at risk with this model). The AVMA 2008 Biennial Economic Survey showed that each credentialed veterinary technician employed by a practice generated an average of $161,000 in gross revenue. After adjusting for inflation (3% compounded over 14 years), this equates to $220,000, and higher post COVID. Review Chapter 2 for the leadership's role in developing, coaching, and implementing effective leveraging and efficiency techniques.

CRITICAL COMPETENCY: PLANNING AND PRIORITIZING

Practice managers must be able to effectively manage time and workload to meet deadlines, thereby having the ability to organize work, set priorities, and establish plans to achieve goals.

Revenue Center Development and Management

Most common revenue centers were provided as examples earlier, with the context of comparing the revenue produced to the expense of the center itself. Practices should also consider which revenue centers they do not have and investigate what centers could be added to support existing revenue centers (Fig. 16.10).

Veterinarians may be recommending a needed service that cannot (currently) be provided within the practice. For example, physical therapy may be recommended often due to a high number of orthopedic surgeries. Perhaps physical therapy could be developed and offered in-house.

POTENTIAL REVENUE CENTERS

- Anesthesia
- Boarding
- Dentals
- Diets
- Examinations
- Grooming
- Hospitalization
- Laboratory
- Pharmacy
- Radiology
- Retail/OTC
- Surgery

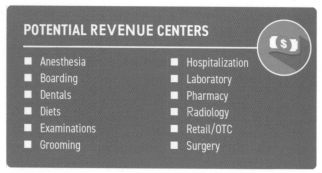

Fig. 16.10 Practice managers must manage each revenue center like a mini business within the practice; each revenue center must be monitored for revenue generated and compared to the expense of running such a center.

A practice manager/owner should build a model of what the expense center would cost to develop (equipment, space requirements, training for team members), the potential number of clients and patients it would serve, and the potential profitability of the service.

Some centers may not actually produce a profit for themselves, however, contributing to the larger profitability of another center. For example, a practice may receive more referrals for TPLO surgeries when rehabilitation is offered as a follow-up service for patients.

EXPENSE REDUCTION

Expenses should be monitored monthly, and reductions should be made whenever possible. However, as stated previously, an extensive amount of time should not be dedicated to reducing expenses. Because many expenses are fixed, revenue should be the primary focus of attention. Nonetheless, there are a few expenses that should be monitored and managed regularly:

Credit card merchant fees: Processing fees can increase every few months when contracts are amended, or additional charges are added to the practice's account. Due diligence of the manager includes consulting with the current credit card company asking where fees can be decreased and shopping around for reduced merchant fees. Although it is inconvenient to change companies every few years, it can save the practice money over the course of the year. Benchmarks show credit card fees average 1.5% of gross revenue.

Health insurance: Health insurance premiums for employees increase yearly. Insurance policies should be shopped every few years, keeping an eye on preventative health care coverage, prescriptions, and deductible costs to employees. Having an insurance agent who represents multiple companies can aid in this search.

Communications: Communications include telephone, internet, and cable. Many practices have bundled services, yet many of these bundled services are not fully utilized. Review contracts and determine whether all the services are being used; consider accepting unbundled packages for a reduced price.

Professional fees: Consider contract negotiation for payroll services, accounting, and attorney fees.

Cost of goods fees: Inventory is the second-largest expense of the hospital, and it is critically important to price shop. Some distributors are higher than others depending on the drug or supply being purchased. Vetcove (www.vetcove.com) is an easy solution for price shopping; much like Amazon, the prices of pharmaceuticals, supplies, and equipment are easy to compare. It is also critical to monitor turnover rates, reorder quantities, and reorder points; setting these points in the PIMS will significantly reduce soft costs, (known as *holding and ordering costs*), as well as shrinkage that is associated with poor inventory management. Managers must also consider product consolidation and effective pricing when reviewing effective inventory policies. Review Chapter 13 for further details.

LEADERSHIP POINT

Reduce COG expenses by implementing effective turnover rates, reorder quantities, and reorder points.

Discounts are worth mentioning again when reducing expenses. If maximum revenue is not achieved and discounts (or missed charges) are being given, expense percentages will increase (see Fig. 16.9).

Equipment: Equipment is also a price-shopped category. Consider the following components when shopping for equipment: product, warranty, installation, training, and available technical service if equipment needs servicing. Many companies offer a nice product but do not include any training for team members, installation, or servicing should the unit need it. Just because a piece of equipment is less expensive upfront does not mean it is the best piece of equipment to suit all the hospital's needs.

Payroll: When expenses are being audited for reductions, managers frequently look at lowering payroll costs. However, this can be a big mistake for many reasons. Having a lean payroll hurts the frictionless client experience. Veterinary medicine is a service-based industry, and if practices are not providing superior service, clients will go elsewhere. When team members are working at a compromised pace due to staff shortages, they do not have the time to spend developing relationships with clients (resulting in decreased client compliance, both with preventive and emergency care).

Instead of reducing payroll, consider ways to maximize payroll. Are team members being used to their fullest potential? If not, could team training be implemented to make this happen? Consider having every team member (veterinarians included) write down the duties they accomplish daily for 5 consecutive days. Managers can then compile the lists and determine how to use the staff more efficiently. Increased staff utilization prevents burnout, creates accountability, increases client compliance, and decreases staff turnover.

Let's not forget that overtime must be managed in this equation. If overtime is being charged by many team members, then the practice is likely short-staffed. Short-staffing leads to employee burnout, resulting in decreased production by the entire team. If overtime is significant, consider hiring more team members or restructuring the schedule to accommodate busy times/days in the practice.

Analyzing KPIs with payroll is useful. If the client retention and bonding rates are high, this can be attributed to an excellent team. Lower retention and compliance rates (along with new and active clients) can indicate customer service issues, resulting from a lean payroll.

Team pay wages should be analyzed on a yearly basis. Good team members cost money, and those team members produce revenue. Employees earning high wages should be performing to high expectations. Review job descriptions, employee expectations, and performance reviews in Chapter 4, Human Resources, and how to coach team members to be the best they can be in Chapter 2, Leadership.

Veterinarian salaries and/or production pay must also be analyzed. Many practices elect to pay DVMs a fixed salary. Fixed salaries are easy to calculate, and many owners feel this decreases the potential for competition among associates and charging clients for unneeded services. On the other hand, salaries can contribute to veterinarians being less motivated and not being encouraged to promote the best medicine. Comments such as "It doesn't matter to me; I get paid the same amount whether the client accepts or not" must be managed ASAP. Managers and owners may discuss a bonus or production program that facilitates the best medicine approach and breeds positive culture within the practice. Good attitudes start at the top and trickle down to team members. Doctors with a negative attitude affect the entire team.

With all the above considerations, payroll needs to be managed, but practice managers must have a full understanding of all levers impacting payroll and the implications that any decision may have on the financials of the hospital.

CRITICAL COMPETENCY: RESOURCEFULNESS

The practice manager must have the ability to understand what it takes to complete the job by applying knowledge, skills, and expertise to perform tasks quickly and efficiently.

Fraud and Embezzlement

Fraud occurs regularly in businesses globally. In fact, more than 5% of gross revenue is lost to fraud and embezzlement yearly. Unfortunately, in veterinary medicine, many owners and managers are in denial that fraud and/or embezzlement occurs in their practice. Practices are often thought of as "family-oriented" environments, and one assumes that employees working in a care-based industry are trustworthy and honest. However, an independent study completed by Marsha Henike, DVM, CVPM, CPA, reported that 67.8% of practices have been victimized by fraud or embezzlement. It is not a matter of if it will occur, it is a matter of when it will occur in most practices.

LEADERSHIP POINT

Fraud and embezzlement occur in more than 5% of small businesses per year.

Theft includes everything from inventoried items and equipment to cleaning and office supplies. In addition, time theft (i.e., employees clocking in for work but instead eating meals, taking breaks, leaving for appointments, etc. while on the clock), and cash theft (petty cash drawer, padding payroll) must also be considered.

Team members who steal from practices often '*have the opportunity to do so*'; it is the practice managers' responsibility to decrease these opportunities. A checks-and-balances system should be implemented for every area of the practice to protect the practice assets.

End-of-day reconciliation: The person taking in the payments throughout the day should not be the person to reconcile at the end of the day. Having this duty assigned to the same person allows one to alter the books and pocket cash. In addition, the employee responsible for accepting payments should not be the person making bank deposits. Practice managers must oversee all daily and monthly banking procedures, making sure to investigate any discrepancies.

VHMA PERFORMANCE DOMAIN TASK

Veterinary practice managers oversee daily and monthly banking procedures

Check machine: Consider using check machines that scan and automatically deposit funds into the practice's account, eliminating the potential for stolen checks.

Password protection in the PIMS: Only management should be allowed to delete invoices, change codes, or alter pricing.

Client credit cards: Do not retain client credit card information in client files. Many embezzlement cases are the result of stolen credit card numbers. Follow the red flags rule outlined later in this chapter.

Employee accounts: Treat employee accounts as you would a client account. A member of management must enter all products and services purchased by team members. This prevents charges from not being entered at all, or invoices from being discounted at an unauthorized rate.

Inventory: Provide spot-checking and comparisons of physical and computer inventories as outlined in Chapter 13. A large percentage of fraud cases occur when employees steal inventoried products and resell them through a variety of channels. Inventory discrepancies greater than 3%–5% must be investigated, or the door is wide open for employee theft.

Security cameras: Some leadership teams are reluctant to have security cameras in the hospital because they fear it will impact team morale. However, the benefits outweigh the risks of affecting the culture negatively through increased training opportunities (while also mitigating the risk of theft). Reactions to installing cameras may be adverse at first, but team members adjust. Review state law for camera posting requirements.

Controlled substances: Veterinary practices carry drugs that are commonly abused which places the drugs at risk for theft by team members, clients, vendors (or even strangers) if controlled substances are not secured with restricted access (Chapter 14). Discourage theft with security cameras located over controlled substance safes.

Key access: Limit the number of team members who have access to the hospital after hours. Owners may wish to install a personal security code system that tracks when each employee enters and exits the building. Unlimited, unmanaged access invites employee theft.

P&L statements: know your percentages. When a practice does not review a monthly P&L, it is hard to identify abnormal percentages. However, practice managers who analyze P&Ls (and know their percentages) will immediately notice when a category is "out of whack." Unusual percentages should be a red flag; it is much easier to investigate, assess, and solve problems when they arise than to neglect to monitor and find out months later that thousands of dollars are missing.

CRITICAL COMPETENCY: INTEGRITY

Practice managers must adhere to ethical principles and values, and be seen as honest, trustworthy, and sincere professionals (demonstrated through behaviors and words).

Decrease Practice Risk of Fraud or Embezzlement

Along with monitoring checks-and-balances systems for each area of the practice, activities that support a positive culture can be implemented to decrease the risk of fraud. Positive cultures lead to higher team member accountability, enhanced team environments, and increased staff morale, all of which decrease fraud and embezzlement in practices (and decrease employee turnover). To further decrease fraud, consider the following benefits that can be added for team members:

Pet Health Insurance: Consider adding pet health insurance as an employee benefit, allowing all team members to have access to affordable pet care. Pet health insurance is covered in detail later in this chapter.

Staff Feeding Programs: Practices managers should opt into staff feeding programs offered by various nutrition companies, allowing team members access to reduced-cost pet food, decreasing the temptation to steal food. Manufacturers also have parasiticide sampling programs for team members. Relationships must be developed with manufacturing representatives, and the product must be sold within the hospital; however, a win-win situation is produced when these programs are used.

Open Books Management System: Sharing the financial information with team members helps them understand expenses, goals, and P&L centers (covered in further detail later in this chapter.

LEADERSHIP POINT

Open-books management facilitates employee accountability and understanding of practice finances.

BUDGET CREATION

Creating a budget is critical for strategic planning and financial management. Budgets should be considered useful planning tools that help ensure the practice's success. Budgets should be created for both revenue and expenses. Revenue budgets are developed to reach strategically planned goals, whereas expense budgets track expenses and can be used to create goals to reduce costs where possible.

VHMA PERFORMANCE DOMAIN TASK

Veterinary practice managers prepare budgets and long-range fiscal planning.

Steps for Creating a Budget

It is important to ensure that the practice has an adequate program to help with the budget process. QB has an excellent program that includes a preestablished budgeting program. Microsoft Excel spreadsheets also allow data exportation into tables that create a budget. Although a basic budget could be prepared by hand, adjusting the budget, or preparing a breakdown of a yearly projection into monthly or quarterly minibudgets becomes unreasonable. Formulated spreadsheets make it easy to visualize the results of countless changes, assumptions, and trials.

Creating a Spreadsheet: The practice can easily create a spreadsheet if accounting software (such as QB) is not used. Fig. 16.11 demonstrates many columns; for this example, focus on columns 1–4. Column 1 refers to the type of expense, column 2 is the subcategory based on the chart of accounts, and column 3 is actual dollars associated with each expense category, which is linked to the formula allowing expenses to be shown as a percentage of the total practice gross revenue (column 4).

The cost of goods is shown as a percentage of gross revenue by creating a mathematical formula representing total dollars expensed, divided by total dollars of gross revenue. For example, the cost of professional services is \$98,874.32. This figure, divided by \$1.5 million = $0.066 \times 100 = 6.6\%$. Remember, to express a value as a percentage, the equation must be multiplied by 100.

The reason for this approach is to create a spreadsheet that automatically updates percentages when changes are made to the absolute values (revenue or expense). Next year, when the budget spreadsheet is updated, new data will be added. All related percentages will be calculated by the spreadsheet because of preestablished formulas.

Second, take a close look at the relation of specific expenses to gross revenue. By having a few years of data, what is normal for the practice can be compared with benchmark data. The previous year's complete financial statements plus any results from the current year of operations will be needed. Reports will need to be generated from the PIMS to help create the revenue budget.

It is critical that expenses are listed in the correct chart of accounts when they are entered. Occasionally there are inconsistencies as to how an expense is entered. Perhaps the purchase of computer-generated reminder cards was classified as office supplies in one month, computer supplies in another month, and nonmedical supplies in a third month. Refer to the AAHA Chart of Accounts for proper classification (allowing proper comparison to benchmarks).

Projected Revenue (10% Growth) Jan-Dec 2023 = $16,50,000

Projected Increase of Expenses = 4.8%

Actual 2022 Revenue: $1,500,000

Column 1	Column 2	Column 3	Column 4	Column 5	Column 6	Column 7	Column 8
Category	**Subcategory**	**2022 Actual ($)**	**2022 Actual (%)**	**4.8% Increase in Expenses (Column C x 4.8%)**	**Total $ expected annual spend**	**Expected annual % with projected revenue**	**Total $ expected monthly spend**
COGs	Professional Services Costs	$ 98,874.32	6.6	$ 4,745.97	$ 1,03,620.29	6.3%	$ 8,635.02
	Pharmacy	$ 1,01,189.23	6.7	$ 4,857.08	$ 1,06,046.31	6.4%	$ 8,837.19
	Imaging	$ 1,890.43	0.1	$ 90.74	$ 1,981.17	0.1%	$ 165.10
	Surgery	$ 2,298.94	0.2	$ 110.35	$ 2,409.29	0.1%	$ 200.77
	Dentals	$ 1,384.05	0.1	$ 66.43	$ 1,450.48	0.1%	$ 120.87
	Diets	$ 19,897.43	1.3	$ 955.08	$ 20,852.51	1.3%	$ 1,737.71
	Retail/OTC	$ 8,987.43	0.6	$ 431.40	$ 9,418.83	0.6%	$ 784.90
	TOTAL	**$ 2,34,521.83**	**15.6**	**$ 11,257.05**	**$ 2,45,778.88**	**14.9%**	**$ 20,481.57**
Administrative	Accountant	$ 7,441.82	0.5	$ 357.21	$ 7,799.03	0.5%	$ 649.92
	Advertising	$ 9,874.09	0.7	$ 473.96	$ 10,348.05	0.6%	$ 862.34
	Check Machine Fee's	$ 2,477.28	0.2	$ 118.91	$ 2,596.19	0.2%	$ 216.35
	Communications	$ 5,768.78	0.4	$ 276.90	$ 6,045.68	0.4%	$ 503.81
	Credit Card Fee's	$ 5,600.00	0.4	$ 268.80	$ 5,868.80	0.4%	$ 489.07
	Charitable Contribution	$ 3,564.60	0.2	$ 171.10	$ 3,735.70	0.2%	$ 311.31
	Client Care (Flowers)	$ 3,694.34	0.2	$ 177.33	$ 3,871.67	0.2%	$ 322.64
	Insurance - Liability	$ 6,598.00	0.4	$ 316.70	$ 6,914.70	0.4%	$ 576.23
	License	$ 2,356.03	0.2	$ 113.09	$ 2,469.12	0.1%	$ 205.76
	Office Supplies	$ 5,678.99	0.4	$ 272.59	$ 5,951.58	0.4%	$ 495.97
	Shipping	$ 2,767.34	0.2	$ 132.83	$ 2,900.17	0.2%	$ 241.68
	Taxes -Sales	$ 62,500.00	4.2	$ 3,000.00	$ 65,500.00	4.0%	$ 5,458.33
	TOTAL	**$ 1,18,321.27**	**7.9**	**$ 5,679.42**	**$ 1,24,000.69**	**7.5%**	**$ 10,333.39**
Facility	Cable/Satellite Television	$ 600.00	0.0	$ 28.80	$ 628.80	0.0%	$ 52.40
	Cell Phone	$ 2,456.87	0.2	$ 117.93	$ 2,574.80	0.2%	$ 214.57
	Electricity	$ 5,115.85	0.3	$ 245.56	$ 5,361.41	0.3%	$ 446.78
	Natural Gas/Water/Sew	$ 3,657.98	0.2	$ 175.58	$ 3,833.56	0.2%	$ 319.46
	Building Maintenance	$ 2,398.09	0.2	$ 115.11	$ 2,513.20	0.2%	$ 209.43
	Equipment Maint.	$ 1,529.88	0.1	$ 73.43	$ 1,603.31	0.1%	$ 133.61
	Equipment Purchase	$ 4,800.00	0.3	$ 230.40	$ 5,030.40	0.3%	$ 419.20
	Equipment Lease	$ 6,720.97	0.4	$ 322.61	$ 7,043.58	0.4%	$ 586.96
	Insurance- Property	$ 2,987.34	0.2	$ 143.39	$ 3,130.73	0.2%	$ 260.89
	Rent	$ 54,698.30	3.6	$ 2,625.52	$ 57,323.82	3.5%	$ 4,776.98
	TOTAL	**$ 84,965.28**	**5.7**	**$ 4,078.33**	**$ 89,043.61**	**5.4%**	**$ 7,420.30**
DVM Owner Compensation	Payroll-DVM -Owner	$ 1,25,000.00	8.3	$ 6,000.00	$ 1,31,000.00	7.9%	$ 10,916.67
	Cont Ed	$ 1,427.88	0.1	$ 68.54	$ 1,496.42	0.1%	$ 124.70
	Insurance Health	$ 4,800.00	0.3	$ 230.40	$ 5,030.40	0.3%	$ 419.20
	Insurance Workers Comp	$ -	0.0	$ -	$ -	0.0%	$ -
	sIRA	$ -	0.0	$ -	$ -	0.0%	$ -
	Taxes-Payroll	$ 8,750.00	0.6	$ 420.00	$ 9,170.00	0.6%	$ 764.17
	Unemployment	$ 1,250.00	0.1	$ 60.00	$ 1,310.00	0.1%	$ 109.17
	TOTAL	**$ 1,41,227.88**	**9.4**	**$ 6,778.94**	**$ 1,48,006.82**	**$ 0.09**	**$ 12,333.90**
DVM Non-owner Compensation	Payroll-DVM -Assoc	$ 2,02,403.24	13.5	$ 9,715.36	$ 2,12,118.60	12.9%	$ 17,676.55
	Cont Ed	$ 3,450.00	0.2	$ 165.60	$ 3,615.60	0.2%	$ 301.30
	Insurance Health	$ 9,600.00	0.6	$ 460.80	$ 10,060.80	0.6%	$ 838.40
	Insurance Workers Comp	$ 234.10	0.0	$ 11.24	$ 245.34	0.0%	$ 20.44
	sIRA	$ 2,622.40	0.2	$ 125.88	$ 2,748.28	0.2%	$ 229.02
	Taxes-Payroll	$ 8,986.76	0.6	$ 431.36	$ 9,418.12	0.6%	$ 784.84
	Unemployment	$ 1,650.87	0.1	$ 79.24	$ 1,730.11	0.1%	$ 144.18
	TOTAL	**$ 5,11,403.13**	**34.1**	**$ 24,547.35**	**$ 5,35,950.48**	**32.5%**	**$ 44,662.54**
Staff Compensation	Payroll-Non-DVM	$ 1,90,987.54	12.7	$ 9,167.40	$ 2,00,154.94	12.1%	$ 16,679.58
	Insurance-Health	$ 3,600.00	0.2	$ 172.80	$ 3,772.80	0.2%	$ 314.40
	Insurace- Wor kers Comp	$ 2,106.90	0.1	$ 101.13	$ 2,208.03	0.1%	$ 184.00
	sIRA	$ 7,756.45	0.5	$ 372.31	$ 8,128.76	0.5%	$ 677.40
	Taxes- Payroll	$ 6,678.90	0.4	$ 320.59	$ 6,999.49	0.4%	$ 583.29
	Unemployment	$ 7,176.00	0.5	$ 344.45	$ 7,520.45	0.5%	$ 626.70
	TOTAL	**$ 2,18,305.79**	**14.6**	**$ 10,478.68**	**$ 2,28,784.47**	**13.9%**	**$ 19,065.37**
	Total Expenses	**$ 11,67,517.30**	**77.8**	**$ 62,819.77**	**$ 11,42,780.48**	**69.3%**	**$ 95,231.71**
Revenue - Expenses = PROFIT		**$ 3,32,482.70**	**22.2**		**$ 5,07,219.52**	**30.7%**	**$ 42,268.29**

*Visit www.AAHA.org to download a COMPLETE COA Template. The above example is an abbreviated form for publication purposes.

Fig. 16.11 Example of a 2023 budget.

Accounting-style software programs help provide consistent classification of expenses because they retain the specific transaction. When a recurring payee is used, the software automatically classifies that payee to a specific account based on the previous transaction. Such programs quickly and easily provide P&L reports, the underlying data for the budget, after the end-of-month and checkbook reconciliation. An in-house P&L report is more than adequate for providing the historic information that forms the basis of the budget. The annual financial statements provided by an accountant do not allow the monthly assessment needed to successfully manage the business.

Third, budgeting requires the reassessment of the present fee structure, evaluation of the total gross practice revenue, and a plan of how to achieve the necessary growth to achieve the practices' strategic goal.

Budgets should be established for the entire practice, as well as for both revenue and expense segments of the practice. For example, where staffing costs have historically been higher than normal in the practice, a budget for different segments of support staff, including receptionists, technicians, and veterinarians, may be established. Likewise, mixed practices will benefit from budgeting for the different segments of the practice, which likely have different profit margins.

CRITICAL COMPETENCY: ADAPTABILITY

Practice managers must be open to change and flexible work methods and can adapt behavior to changing conditions or new information.

Revenue Prediction

A prediction of revenue for the next financial period can be determined based on historic gross revenue increases. Fig. 16.12 lists the revenue centers for 2022 (column 1), along with the practice's predicted 10% growth (column 5) for the 2023 fiscal year. ABC Animal Hospital historically has a 10% increase each year, and each revenue center's revenue is multiplied by 10% to predict the 2023 revenue. While this is a simplified version of a 10% increase in revenue, it is most likely that not all revenue centers experience growth at 10%; therefore, creating customized growth by revenue center is important (and helps when budgeting potential expenses by revenue center).

At the top of the revenue spreadsheet, enter a description, "Projected Rate of Growth." In the cell adjacent to the description, insert a percentage increase such as 5% or 10%. This number can be changed as assumptions are made regarding growth of the practice.

Revenue is projected for the following year as a formula, multiplying current revenue (column 2) by the projected rate of growth of 10% resulting in column 4. If the cells are referenced correctly, any change in the percentage growth rate changes the revenue projected for the upcoming year. Column 5 is the estimated total revenue based on a 10% increase in business.

When revenue centers have been established, changes can be identified to prevent loss or if an area needs to be capitalized on. For example, dentistry is a common revenue center in veterinary practice. To determine the percentage of profit that the dental center is contributing to the overall gross revenue, a simple equation can be used. Fig. 16.12 lists dental services as producing $45,000 for the 2022 fiscal year. The gross revenue produced was $1.5 million. The sum of $45,000 divided by $1.5 million equals 0.03. To express this number as a percentage, $0.03 \times 100 = 3\%$. Therefore 3% of gross revenue is contributed by the dental revenue center. The practice may compare this percentage to average benchmarks for dental centers and determine if changes need to be made to maximize revenue opportunities in the dental center.

Expense Prediction

There are several budgeting methods that work in veterinary practice; the "top-down" method is the most common. Expenses from the

Revenue 2022 $1,500,000				**Projected Rate of Growth 2023 = 10%**		
Column 1	Column 2	Column 3		Column 4	Column 5	Column 6
Revenue Center	Actual 2022 ($)	Actual 2022 (%)		Projected Growth of 10%	Predicted Income for 2023 ($)	Predicted Income for 2023 (%)
Examination	$ 2,40,000.00	16.0%		$ 24,000.00	$ 2,64,000.00	16%
Professional Services	$ 60,000.00	4.0%		$ 6,000.00	$ 66,000.00	4%
Laboratory Fees	$ 2,70,000.00	18.0%		$ 27,000.00	$ 2,97,000.00	18%
Imaging	$ 67,500.00	4.5%		$ 6,750.00	$ 74,250.00	5%
Dentistry	$ 45,000.00	3.0%		$ 4,500.00	$ 49,500.00	3%
Vaccines	$ 1,05,000.00	7.0%		$ 10,500.00	$ 1,15,500.00	7%
Hospitalization	$ 45,000.00	3.0%		$ 4,500.00	$ 49,500.00	3%
Surgery	$ 90,000.00	6.0%		$ 9,000.00	$ 99,000.00	6%
Anesthesia	$ 60,000.00	4.0%		$ 6,000.00	$ 66,000.00	4%
Pharmacy	$ 2,10,000.00	14.0%		$ 21,000.00	$ 2,31,000.00	14%
Flea, Tick and HW	$ 1,35,000.00	9.0%		$ 13,500.00	$ 1,48,500.00	9%
Diets	$ 75,000.00	5.0%		$ 7,500.00	$ 82,500.00	5%
OTC/Retail	$ 30,000.00	2.0%		$ 3,000.00	$ 33,000.00	2%
Boarding	$ 37,500.00	2.5%		$ 3,750.00	$ 41,250.00	3%
Bathing/Grooming	$ 30,000.00	2.0%		$ 3,000.00	$ 33,000.00	2%
	$ 15,00,000.00	**100.0%**		$ 1,50,000.00	**$ 16,50,000.00**	**100%**

Fig. 16.12 Example of predicted revenue for 2023.

previous year's budget are forwarded to the following year's budget, allowing the input of changes needed to reach the goals established for the following year. For example, the total COGs expense in Fig. 16.11 is 15.6% (column 4) of the revenue ($1.5 million) for 2022 which is then forwarded to the projected 2023 budget. Perhaps the practice wants to improve the COGs percentage for the following year; that can be changed based on the goals established for the following year's budget.

It should be remembered that gross revenue is the total money received before expenses or taxes.

The cost of supplies increases each year (which can be hard to predict) and that must be projected and budgeted. An average increase of 4.8% may cover the increase for most variable costs (keep in mind the current inflation rate) and is used in this example. Fig. 16.11, column 5 highlights the 4.8% projected increase in variable expenses for the 2023 fiscal year. If a payroll budget has been created, projected values for payroll, payroll tax, and benefit contributions may be added for a more accurate projection. The green column in Fig. 16.11 demonstrates actual expenses incurred in 2022, the blue column adds 4.8% to account for increased expenses (column 5) and calculates the new, predicted expense (column 6 [dollar amount] and 7 [percentage]), and the orange column gives the monthly projected dollar amount (column 8).

Creating an Equipment Budget: When creating a budget for equipment, two topics need to be kept in mind: the maintenance of existing equipment and the purchase of new equipment. Existing equipment may have maintenance agreements in place, and some equipment may need repairs. When purchasing new equipment, several points should be considered:

- Is the equipment for a new profit center? Establish an ROI that includes predicted practice cost, payback period, client cost, marketing plans, usage, and profitability.
- Is the equipment replacing an existing piece of equipment? Is the new piece of equipment going to provide improved, more accurate results compared with the piece it is replacing? Will there need to be an increased fee for clients?
- How will the equipment be paid for? Cash? Leasing? Financing?
- If the practice is going to finance the equipment, what is the interest rate? Can a better rate be found elsewhere?

Equipment leasing is often a purchase option because of the high cost. Finance charges and interest rates are built into the payment (but should be reviewed carefully and compared to the current rate), and balloon payments are often due at the end of the lease period. Other options include returning the equipment at the end of the lease, in which the practice will need to plan a replacement (if a piece of equipment has a short life and is replaced with an update quickly, this may be the best option). However, most pieces of equipment in veterinary medicine hold value and provide service for a long period, especially when maintenance and repair schedules are followed. Companies offer low payments that entice practices to lease equipment; however, all options should be examined before deciding. Credit lines should not be used for equipment purchases because they generally must be fully paid within a year and are better saved for emergency withdrawals if needed. Equipment loan lengths should not exceed the expected life of the piece of equipment, normally 5 to 7 years.

Determining a break-even analysis will help evaluate if an equipment purchase is right or not. The break-even point is the point at which the sales of the service will cover all costs related to the equipment, including maintenance, supplies, and the capital itself. A break-even point can be determined by dividing the total cost of the equipment by the profit of the practice. The resulting number gives the number of times the service must be performed to break even (Fig. 16.13). For example, a practice wants to purchase a digital dental radiograph unit. The unit originally costs $11,000. The practice will charge the client $88 for a set of radiographs. The cost associated with taking the

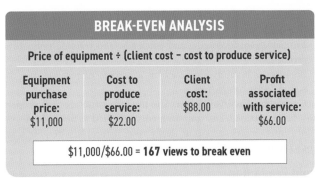

BREAK-EVEN ANALYSIS

Price of equipment ÷ (client cost - cost to produce service)

Equipment purchase price:	Cost to produce service:	Client cost:	Profit associated with service:
$11,000	$22.00	$88.00	$66.00

$11,000/$66.00 = 167 views to break even

Fig. 16.13 Use a break-even analysis when considering equipment purchases to ensure the practice will break even in a timely manner.

radiographs is $22; this includes the technician's time to take the views and the veterinarian's time to interpret the views (determine from the service pricing model previously discussed). The profit (after expenses) is $88 − $22 = $66. The break-even number (number of views needed to be charged for) is calculated as $11,000 divided by $66 equals 166.67 views; therefore 167 views must be taken (and charged for) to break even with a digital dental radiograph unit.

If an average of two dentals are completed each day, and both dentals have radiographs included, it will take 83 business days to cover the cost of the equipment.

LEADERSHIP POINT

Complete a break-even analysis before purchasing equipment.

Creating a Payroll Budget: Payroll is the largest expense in the operating budget and, depending on the practice, can be considered a variable or fixed expense. Practices that are busy year-round and have a similar payroll each period may consider payroll a fixed expense. Practices that are busy in the summer and slow in the winter should consider payroll a variable expense because it changes with the revenue of the practice. Recall that for benchmarking purposes, staff payroll is considered a variable expense.

VHMA PERFORMANCE DOMAIN TASK

Veterinary practice managers manage payroll.

To help with budget estimations, a weighted hourly wage may be used for each employee. A weighted hourly wage takes the average of a team member's pay when a raise will be expected later in the fiscal year. The original pay plus the new pay divided by 2 gives the weighted hourly wage.

Overtime pay reduces profits when not managed within a budget. Team members' schedules should be created with the intent to decrease the amount of overtime, which also contributes to the mental health and well-being of team members.

A maximum amount should be determined each year for payroll, allowing for raises, bonuses, and an allocation for new team members if needed. Raises and bonuses can be disbursed as management feels appropriate, reaching the amount set aside for the payroll budget.

If payroll costs exceed predictions, practice managers should ask "why" before simply cutting payroll to meet the budget. Reducing hours for people that produce the practice revenue is tricky; there are likely other contributing factors that need to be evaluated first:

- Did revenue significantly increase/decrease?
- Was a new veterinarian onboarded/or did a veterinarian leave?
- Was a new profit center added to the practice?

- Evaluate practice culture and the impact on the team member retention rate.
- Evaluate team leveraging and efficiency, and training/onboarding protocols.
- Be sure evaluations are based on a percent of revenue, not that actual dollar comparison.

Creating a Facility Budget: The practice structure and property must be maintained, and improvements will need to be made at some point. Emergencies can occur (leaky roof, natural disaster, etc.), and funds should be available for emergencies when needed.

Profit Prediction

Finally, profits must also be budgeted. Remaining profits may also use the top-down approach, using previous percentages in the future budget. If profits are inadequate to achieve the practice's strategic goals, additional assessments are needed and a price increase for professional services/inventory may be warranted. The goal is to obtain the necessary profit to allow adequate return on investment and reinvestment in the practice.

LEADERSHIP POINT

Profits must also be budgeted just like revenue and expenses.

In Fig. 16.11, the profits during 2022 were $332,482.70, or 22.2%. This is an average percentage (in comparison to benchmarks), and a higher goal should be set for the practice to strive for. It is advisable to reinvest at least 10% of profits back into the practice on an annual basis. This allows for the budgeting of equipment, building maintenance, upgrades, and team incentives.

Important Budgeting Tips: Creating budgets can be a trial-and-error process. Budgets are often based on assumptions and averages with the best possible information available at the time. Unpredictable events (both positive and negative) can occur and will affect projections. Natural disasters, pandemics, and wars affect the practice as well as changes within the local economy. A veterinarian may retire unexpectedly or a nearby practice may close providing an increased client base. There is no crystal ball to predict events and predicting budgets more than 2 years in advance will waste time as changes need to be made. Strategic goal achievements often take years to achieve, and yearly goals must be on track to achieve the larger goal. Don't alter strategic goals based on yearly goal misses (unless a major disaster has occurred). Instead, monitor monthly and adapt as needed to keep the goals on track.

CRITICAL COMPETENCY: CONTINUOUS LEARNING

Practice managers should have a curiosity for learning. Actively seeking out new information, technologies, and methods while keeping skills updated allows the application of new knowledge to the job.

A practice manager must plan for a learning curve when first developing a budget. Effectively collecting and adding data occurs during year 1. Tweaks will have to be made, and investigations into discrepancies will help the owner/manager understand what worked and what did not work. Year 2 will likely be more successful, with fewer tweaks needed and more goals achieved. By year 3, owners/managers should hold themselves accountable for meeting budgeted goals. Budgeting is a highly powerful tool that every practice MUST implement.

Once a budget has been created, teams can effectively look at subcategories, determine what areas are controllable, and make an impact on those areas.

It is essential to communicate the budget (and financial reports, covered in the next section, Open Books Management) to the team. Actual numbers, projections, and goals should be discussed in team meetings with updates thereafter, allowing them to be able to begin to understand the budgeting process and goals of the practice. Each team member must understand (and want to know) their role in achieving budgets and strategic goals. Goals should be celebrated when they have been achieved and brainstorming sessions with the team should be held when they are not. Teamwork goes beyond caring for patients and satisfying clients; it is also about contributing to the success of the practice. Increased profitability increases salaries for team members and allows greater reinvestment back into their practice. These factors contribute to a satisfied team that will work efficiently, intelligently, and happily because they are emotionally invested in the practice.

OPEN-BOOKS MANAGEMENT

Sharing the practice finances with team members contributes to their professional development in business acumen and increases the opportunity for them to grow their emotional investment in the growth of the business. When each team member understands the cost of doing business and the need for profitability, the team begins to work together towards a common goal. Team members only see a large amount of revenue collected daily; they never see the money paid for the expenses to run a business.

Owners and managers may start with sharing KPIs and benchmarks, slowly moving into a summarized P&L. By showing team members how the dots are connected, they understand how and why practice protocols are developed, resulting in less resistance when policies are implemented. Team members are more likely to embrace growth strategies when they understand the why and the how.

Developing goals and budgets as a team contributes to an overall positive culture within the practice, increasing accountability, productivity, and team morale.

CRITICAL COMPETENCY: ORAL COMMUNICATION AND COMPREHENSION

The practice manager must have the ability to express thoughts verbally in a clear and understandable manner, and the ability to actively listen and attend to what others are saying.

BUILDING VALUE IN THE PRACTICE

There are many factors that contribute to the valuation of a practice, and it is advisable to have the practice valued every few years, ensuring the value continues to increase. Visit www.vetpartners.com for more detailed information on obtaining a practice valuation from a professional. Practice value should consistently increase for at least 5 to 10 years prior to establishing a profitable sale.

LEADERSHIP POINT

Medical records, client retention, team member retention, building appearance, modern equipment, and financial records all contribute to the value of a practice.

Factors That Help Build Practice Value Include (But Are Not Limited To):

Medical Records: Medical records are considered in a valuation. Are recommendations being made? Are medical records complete and paperless? If recommendations are not being made (or compliance is low), the practice value decreases. Perspective buyers look for a practice that has good client compliance rates and accurate record keeping.

Clients: Client relationships fall into the category of goodwill. The practice must regularly consider what is being done to increase the goodwill value. Goodwill is driven by practice reputation. Are clients recommending friends and family? What is the client compliance rate? What is the practice doing to build and maintain the reputation of the hospital? Client feedback should be mandatory, listening to clients, and identifying and meeting their needs drives goodwill. This will keep clients returning and referring new clients to the practice. In addition, goodwill must be able to be transferred to a new owner. For example, if Smith Veterinary Hospital is strictly built around Dr. Smith (and not the team), can the goodwill be transferred? Probably not, and the value will be lowered. However, if Apple Orchard Veterinary Hospital has built its reputation on the team and all the associates (not just Dr. Larsen), that value is transferable to the new owner.

Team Members: Team members are extremely important in the value of the practice. High team member retention rates create value for the hospital; high employee turnover rates devalue the practice and are attributed to poor culture and leadership problems within the practice. See Chapter 2, Leadership, and Chapter 4, Human Resources, for opportunities to increase team member retention.

Building: The physical condition of the practice must be well maintained and visually appealing to both existing and new clients. When the facility is poorly maintained, the value of the practice will be significantly decreased. Interiors and exteriors must be evaluated frequently and updated as needed. This includes paint, signage, landscaping, parking lots, seating, examination rooms, etc. Develop a facility maintenance schedule for the hospital (Fig. 16.14).

Equipment: Equipment must be modern and suitable for producing revenue. Equipment value (and age) is included in a valuation.

Financial Records: Creating, maintaining, and analyzing financial data is critical. Prospective owners will scrutinize financial records to be sure the practice is profitable.

Revenue Centers: Revenue centers should be profitable, support standards of care, and use reliable equipment.

Profits: Profitability should increase year over year as prospective buyers will consider whether the practice has growth potential. Reinvest a minimum of 10% of the year's profits into areas that bring revenue back into the hospital. Consider team training, additional profit centers, equipment, building maintenance or upgrades, and marketing initiatives.

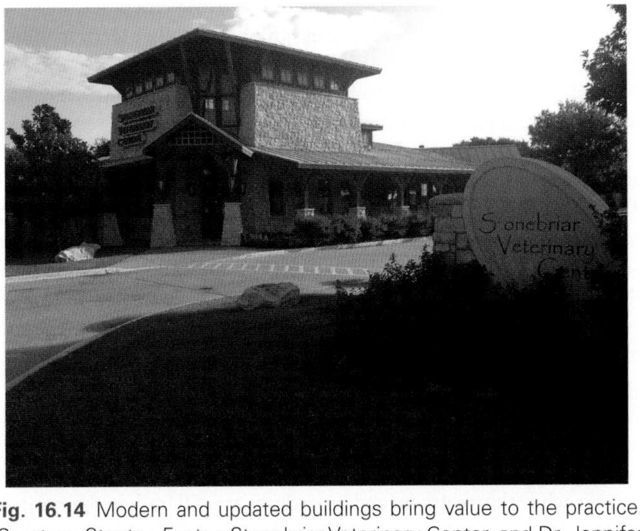

Fig. 16.14 Modern and updated buildings bring value to the practice. (Courtesy Stanton Foster, Stonebriar Veterinary Center, and Dr. Jennifer Wilcox.)

ACCOUNTS RECEIVABLE

Accounts receivable (AR) is defined as the money owed to a business for services rendered or products that are sold and not paid for at the time of service. A healthy practice allows for 1.5% to 2% of gross revenue to be allocated to accounts receivable. There will always be some clients that need to charge and will pay their balance. However, accounts receivable must be well-managed and strict protocols must be put in place. Third-party payment plans such as Care Credit should be offered in lieu of practice financing.

LEADERSHIP POINT

Accounts receivable should not be greater than 2% of gross revenue.

VHMA PERFORMANCE DOMAIN TASK

Veterinary practice managers manage accounts receivable and accounts payable.

Instituting a No-Charge Policy: To protect the practice against losses on accounts receivable, a no-charge policy should be enforced. The policy should be clearly posted for clients to see throughout the practice. Signs should read, "Full payment is required at time of service" (Fig. 16.15). Although signage is helpful, that will not be enough to discourage clients from assuming they can charge for services. Estimates/treatment/medical plans must be provided to all clients (regardless of client "status") for all services that are expected for that patient. The client should sign the estimate, which gives the practice legal documentation that the client accepted the services that the veterinary team has recommended. Payment arrangements should be discussed allowing the client to indicate how they would like to pay for services. If a pet is to be hospitalized for diagnostics and/or treatment, a 50% deposit should be collected at the time of client agreement. The deposit requirement must be communicated clearly to the client when presenting an estimate/treatment plan.

Every team member must understand and accept this policy, and it must be enforced consistently to be effective. A good policy can be both fair and compassionate.

VHMA PERFORMANCE DOMAIN TASK

Veterinary practice managers establish and enforce client credit policies.

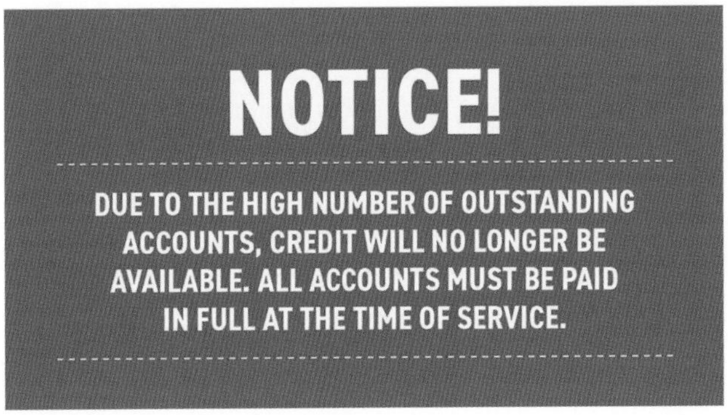

NOTICE!
DUE TO THE HIGH NUMBER OF OUTSTANDING ACCOUNTS, CREDIT WILL NO LONGER BE AVAILABLE. ALL ACCOUNTS MUST BE PAID IN FULL AT THE TIME OF SERVICE.

Fig. 16.15 Sample no-charge policy.

Third-Party Payment Plans: Many times, clients simply do not have the money to spend on their pet. Third-party payment plans allow the practice to be proactive in helping clients with financial options to care for their pet. Care Credit is a leading company in the veterinary industry, providing credit card services for clients. Clients can fill out the application in the hospital (or at home on the Internet) and be approved (or declined) within minutes of application submission. Care Credit allows clients to finance pet care costs and pay off the charges over time.

Practices also wish to establish wellness plans that allow clients to make monthly payments for pet care. The BVCUS of 2011 indicates clients would like the ability to make monthly payments for their upcoming services, and this option makes veterinary care affordable for them. See Wellness Plans at the end of this chapter.

LEADERSHIP POINT

Clients will ask for payment plans to help pay for pet care. Consider options that will be feasible for both the client and the practice.

Delinquent Checks: Checks returned for insufficient funds are a common problem for practices that do not use a check verification system, resulting in an increase in accounts receivable balances. Practices may try to collect these balances themselves or hire an outside collection agency to collect the funds. Returned check fees must be applied to the client account to recoup bank charges, lost time, and money (Fig. 16.16). If a collection agency collects the delinquent amount, service fees will be deducted from the balance once it has been collected. Most companies add a $30 service fee for returned checks. A notice indicating check return fees must be posted in a location that is clearly visible to clients.

To prevent checks from being returned for insufficient funds, consider a check machine that verifies the account and its available funds, and then automatically debits the money from the client's account and deposits it into the practice account. Check with the practice's bank first to see if this is an option and ask for references if it is not. This then eliminates the need to create a deposit slip at the end of the day (another team efficiency measure).

Held Checks: Holding checks is defined as accepting a check with the current date that the check is written but holding it for deposit until the client agrees for it to be deposited. Not only is it against the law in some states, but there is also no guarantee that the funds will be available on the day of deposit or that the client will not close the account. If a team member accidentally deposits the check early, the client will be unhappy and may try to collect returned check fees resulting from the practice's negligence. Holding checks should never be allowed.

LEADERSHIP POINT

Review state, county, and city laws regarding the acceptance of held checks and postdated checks. Some entities have banned the use of such practices.

NOTICE: By providing your check as payment, you authorize us to use information from your check to make a one time electronic fund transfer from your account.

Funds may be drawn from your account the same day, and you will not receive your check back from your bank.If payment is returned unpaid, you authorize ABC Veterinary Clinic to debit from your account, a one time electronic transfer fee of $30.00

Fig. 16.16 Sample insufficient funds notice.

Postdated Checks: Accepting postdated checks is also illegal in some states. A client that "postdates" a check date enters a future date (versus the date the transaction/payment took place). Some prosecutors will not pursue cases when a postdated check has been accepted. Check-authorizing companies will not authorize or accept postdated checks. Similar to withheld checks, funds may not be available when the check is finally deposited, or the account could be closed. Practices should not accept postdated checks.

For any check accepted, a driver's license number should be documented in case of nonpayment or a return. This allows practices to refer nonpaying clients to a collections agency to continue trying to collect the balance. If a check machine is used, a driver's license number may be required to accept the check. If local district attorney's offices prosecute stolen check writers, a driver's license may be required for prosecution. Checking driver's licenses also follows the guidelines set forth in the Red Flags Rule, verifying the presenter's identity (with the hopes of reducing fraud).

Accepting Payment on Accounts Receivable: When clients make payments to their accounts, transactions must be recorded, the transaction must be closed out, and a client receipt must be generated. Practice managers must ensure that cash payments that are received are in fact deposited, not embezzled (reduce the opportunity; see section on Fraud and Embezzlement).

Monthly Statements: After an initial invoice is generated, monthly statements should be prepared for clients who have an outstanding balance, indicating charges, payments, and the balance on their account for the month. Outstanding accounts can be difficult and time-consuming to manage, and monthly statement fees are instituted to pay for the time used to prepare and manage the accounts. A set dollar fee can be imposed, and for practices wishing to charge an additional interest rate on the outstanding balance, state laws should be consulted. Adding interest fees to client accounts encourages quicker payoffs because clients do not wish to pay additional fees.

Statement fees include time, paper, and postage along with any finance charges or interest rates. The PIMS AR component allows either a standard percentage or a set dollar amount to be selected for each statement. One or two dollars is no longer an appropriate service fee. Postage, paper, and labor preparing statements far exceed that amount.

Statements should be printed on approximately the same day each month. Having one person in charge of accounts receivable will decrease mistakes and increase the efficiency of preparing statements. For paper medical record practices, when statements are sent the team member should indicate in the medical record the date, statement fee, new balance, and the team member's initials. This allows other team members to easily access the billing fees if the client has questions regarding the account. For paperless and paper-light medical record practices, team members can refer to the transactions section of the client record.

Accounts Receivable Reporting: AR balances must be monitored and managed to be sure that every effort is made to collect these funds. The longer the receivable is unpaid, the less chance the practice has of collecting payments. Fig. 16.17 is an AR report that demonstrates the largest balance of AR is the current amount due, followed by the totals that are 90 days past due. Strategies must be implemented to prevent current amounts from rolling over to 60 and 90 days past due. The sum of $3661.32 is 90 days past due, and the AR manager must determine appropriate strategies to collect these funds as soon as possible.

Collection Procedures for Outstanding Accounts: Clients should be sent a statement immediately after the service has been performed and medications have been dispensed. Clients are more willing to pay a balance while the treatment and procedures are still fresh in their minds.

If a client is regularly making monthly payments, it is advisable to continue working with the client to collect the balance. Clients that have not made payments within 60 days should be notified of the overdue account. A handwritten note on the statement or past due sticker should be placed on the statement (Fig. 16.18). According to the Fair Debt Collection Practices Act [15 USC 1692b], stickers cannot be placed on the outside of the envelope indicating it is an attempt at debt collection.

Clients may be contacted by telephone to try to determine the client's financial status. Team members may find it difficult to collect delinquent accounts over the phone and often find the client has a negative attitude during the phone call. Team members should be trained to make these calls in a professional manner and remember not to take client frustrations personally. It is difficult for everyone to be under financial strain. Team members should maintain a friendly, helpful, and positive tone in their voices. Discussion of the patient should be avoided, keeping the conversation focused on the account collection.

Team members must verify who they are speaking with, then identify themselves. Once the client has verified themselves, the team member can continue with the goal of receiving payment. "This is Teresa with ABC Animal Clinic. I see you have a balance due on your account and was hoping I could take payment information from you today. I can gladly accept credit card payments over the phone if that is convenient?" Of course, not all phone calls will conclude with a payment being made. When the clients cannot make a payment, other arrangements must be discussed. Be prepared to offer the client a payment plan or information about third-party providers (i.e., Care Credit). If a payment plan is agreed to, determine the specific date that payment(s) will be received and advise the client that interest charges will accrue each month. Document the discussion in the medical record. A written letter to follow up on the details of the conversation should be sent to the client as a reminder of the arrangement. Clients should never be threatened, and the account should never be discussed with anyone other than the client. Messages should not be left regarding the delinquent balance; simply state the team member's name and a phone number where he or she can be reached.

Many clients have caller ID and will not answer the phone when an outstanding account or collections agent is calling. If possible, calls should be made on a blocked line eliminating the identification. Some clients still may not answer the phone, especially if they are in debt and have several businesses calling. All attempts to contact the client must be documented in the record. After several attempts have been made, a certified letter may have to be mailed, requiring that the recipient sign indicating receipt of the letter.

Clients should be informed that unpaid accounts will be sent to a collections agency and reported to credit bureaus if the practice does not receive a response by a specific date. Fig. 16.19 can be used as a guideline for developing a collection letter. Letters should be kept short and simple. Lengthy letters will be ignored by the client and may inadvertently have words or phrases that will offend the client, ultimately delaying payment.

Once team members have exhausted all legal options for collecting the outstanding balance, accounts must be turned over to a collection

Accounts Receivable Report: ABC Veterinary Hospital	
Total 0-30 days:	$4,652.79
Total 30 days Past Due:	$1,896.51
Total 60 days Past Due:	$1,455.07
Total 90 days Past Due:	$3,661.32
TOTAL ACCOUNTS RECEIVABLE	$11,665.69
Total Billing Fees:	$78.00
Total Interest Charges:	$125.49
Total Number of Statements Printed: 52	

Fig. 16.17 Sample accounts receivable report.

GUIDELINES FOR DEVELOPING AN EFFECTIVE COLLECTION LETTER

- Keep the letter brief.
- Make sure the date, amount, and client information are correct.
- Use simple words and phrases.
- Provide a specific date by which the client must respond.
- Provide a date for when a specific action will take place. For example, give the date when the account will be turned over to a collection agent.
- Be firm and polite.
- Include "thank you" at the end of the letter; this is a valuable tool in public relations.

Fig. 16.19 Client collection letters should be kept short and only contain facts.

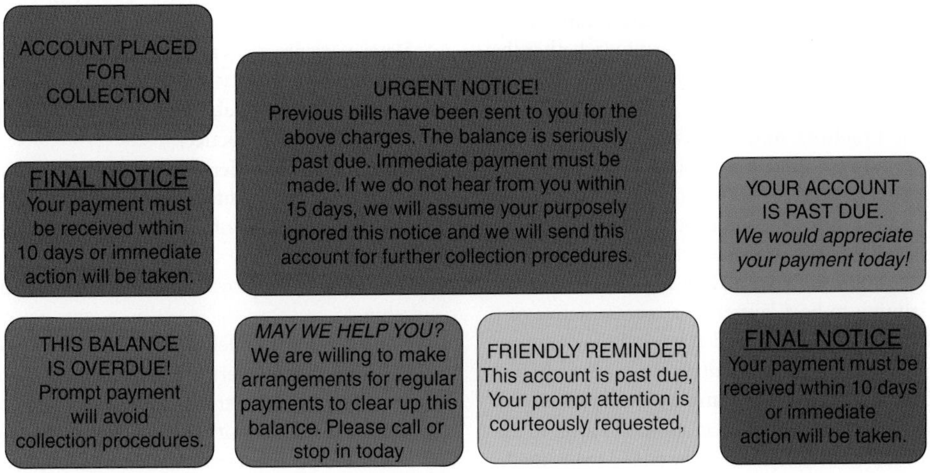
ACCOUNT PLACED FOR COLLECTION
URGENT NOTICE! Previous bills have been sent to you for the above charges. The balance is seriously past due. Immediate payment must be made. If we do not hear from you within 15 days, we will assume your purposely ignored this notice and we will send this account for further collection procedures.
FINAL NOTICE Your payment must be received wthin 10 days or immediate action will be taken.
YOUR ACCOUNT IS PAST DUE. We would appreciate your payment today!
THIS BALANCE IS OVERDUE! Prompt payment will avoid collection procedures.
MAY WE HELP YOU? We are willing to make arrangements for regular payments to clear up this balance. Please call or stop in today
FRIENDLY REMINDER This account is past due, Your prompt attention is courteously requested,
FINAL NOTICE Your payment must be received wthin 10 days or immediate action will be taken.

Fig. 16.18 Examples of late payment stickers.

VITAL INFORMATION TO PROVIDE TO A COLLECTION AGENT

- Client's full name, address, and all telephone numbers (including cell phone and work phone)
- Total balance due on account, including finance charges
- Client's occupation, if known
- Client's employment address, if known
- Client's driver's license number
- Copy of client information sheet and signature of client guaranteeing payment for services rendered

Fig. 16.20 To improve the efficiency of a collection agent/company, specific pieces of information should be submitted when each new "case" is opened.

agency (Fig. 16.20). Agencies will generally charge between 40% and 60% of the total balance that is being collected or may only charge the practice if they are able to collect (some agencies may charge an upfront, nonreturnable fee).

If the agent is unable to collect, the outstanding amount may be reported to a credit bureau or the consumer reporting agency (depending on the collection company used). A credit bureau maintains records about a person's credit and payment history. Information reported stays on the credit report for 7 years. Practices may also wish to take the client to small claims court to try and recover the owed money. Be sure to consider the amount of time to prepare for these cases and court filing costs and ensure they do not exceed the small amount owed.

LEADERSHIP POINT

When a client's account has been reported to a credit bureau, the client's credit can be affected for 7 years.

When debts have been turned over for collection the account should be flagged with a client alert, and the client should not be allowed to return for services. Clients have been known to return to the practice years later. When these clients return, it is appropriate to ask the clients to pay the previous balance before any new services are rendered.

If a practice decides not to turn an outstanding account over to a collection agent and is unable to collect the balance, it may be worthwhile to simply write off the account as bad debt. Again, the client record must be flagged so that all team members are aware of the account status. Speak with the practice's CPA to determine whether the written-off accounts need to be reported on the yearly taxes (this can depend on whether the practice reports on a cash or accrual basis).

Fair Debt Collection Practices Act: The Fair Debt Collection Practices Act of 1996 regulates collection procedures of past-due accounts. The act was passed to protect the public from unethical collection procedures and mainly applies to collection agencies. Debtors cannot be subjected to harassment, oppressive tactics, or abusive treatment. The law prohibits the collector from making any false statements to the client, such as claiming to be a lawyer or a representative of a government agency. Clients may not be called at work if the employer or client objects, or be called at inconvenient times, such as before 8 a.m. and after 9 p.m. Delinquent payments can *only* be discussed with the client named on the medical record. This is another reason to ask clients if they have a significant other that should be added to the medical record, allowing patient decisions to be made.

VHMA PERFORMANCE DOMAIN TASK

Veterinary practice managers understand and ensure compliance with legal and ethical guidelines surrounding the confidentiality of clients.

Employee Accounts Receivable: Team members are often allowed to accumulate an account balance with a veterinary practice. These accounts must be managed just the same as client accounts; if the employee resigns or is terminated, the outstanding about is incredibly difficult to collect. Not only is it an employee benefit to allow the charging of services, but practices also give team members discounts (see Chapter 4, Human Resources, and IRS regulation on fringe benefits).

LEADERSHIP POINT

An employee accounts receivable policy must be implemented and monitored; accounts should not be allowed to exceed $100.00.

When the practice discounts services and the practice carries the account balance, the practice loses money. It is in the best interest of the practice to prevent team member balances from accumulating by requiring monthly payments or implementing a no-charge policy.

Practices wishing to withdraw monthly payments from team member paychecks must check state laws, as most do not allow a withholding that exceeds the employee receiving minimum wage on their paycheck. In addition, managers must have documentation that the employee authorized each withholding (and the amount) from their paycheck.

RED FLAGS RULE

Managers must be familiar with the Red Flags Rule developed by the Federal Trade Commission (FTC) in 2010. The Red Flags Rule was established to protect against identity theft. It requires many businesses and organizations to establish an identity theft prevention program to detect the warning signs, or red flags, of identity theft in their daily operations. By identifying red flags in advance, businesses will be better equipped to spot suspicious patterns that may arise and take steps to prevent a red flag from escalating into a costly episode of identity theft.

LEADERSHIP POINT

The Red Flags Rule should be recognized in every practice, helping decrease fraud and identity theft.

Veterinary practices are not exempt from the Red Flags Rule, and it should be a top priority of every practice manager to prevent identity theft within the hospital. Consider the following guidelines to prevent identity theft in the practice:

- Do not maintain client credit numbers in files.
- Do not ask for/maintain client social security numbers in files.
- Verify the identity of clients when payment is accepted by checks or credit cards.
- Confidential employee information must be secured in a locked cabinet.
- Consider how to safely accept credit card payments over the phone, ensuring that the person providing the information has the authority to authorize the transaction.

Many cases of identity theft occur when employees steal credit card numbers and personal information from clients. Prevent security issues from affecting the hospital by implementing safe and secure policies.

CRITICAL COMPETENCY: COMPLIANCE

Practice managers must be reliable, thorough, and conscientious in carrying out work assignments while having an appreciation for the importance of organizational rules and policies.

COMPASSION ACCOUNTS

Compassion is an important aspect of the veterinary profession. Some veterinary practices have instituted a flex or indigent "compassion" account to assist with special cases in which an animal would be in danger without care and a client cannot pay. On occasion, wealthy clients want to donate money to help lower-revenue clients with pet care, and this is the perfect account to receive such donations. It allows the books to be balanced at the end of the day and generates a receipt for those who have donated. Clients must meet the requirements for team members to consider the use of this account. Team members can develop guidelines, which may include such items as owner compassion, decreased finances, exceptional pet(s), and an intense owner-patient bond. These clients will truly appreciate the services and may eventually donate back to the fund once they are economically stable. Accounts of this nature must be discussed with a CPA. State guidelines vary as to the setup and use of such accounts and may require the filing of special documents.

THE IMPACT OF PET HEALTH INSURANCE ON FINANCIAL MANAGEMENT

Pet health insurance has been available for more than 20 years but has not been a popular choice for clients until recently. Insurance allows pet owners to manage the risks of expensive health care and provide treatments they would otherwise not consider.

The standard of care and improved technology in veterinary medicine has significantly improved over the years, offering better therapeutic options for pets and a stronger human-animal bond. Pets are now living longer because veterinary health care has improved, and clients are more willing to spend additional money to treat medical conditions (Fig. 16.21). Veterinary medicine has also benefited from the progression of human medicine regarding new pharmaceuticals, disease treatments, and diagnostic equipment such as computer-based imaging. These advancements have increased the quality, quantity, and cost of veterinary care, and costs are likely to continue rising, furthering the need for pet health insurance for clients (Fig. 16.22).

Owners who have pet health insurance are more likely to accept recommendations made by the veterinary team. A study released by the North American Pet Health Insurance Association in 2016 indicated that canine pet parents spend 29% more on veterinary visits, whereas feline pet parents spend 81% more if their pet was enrolled in a pet health insurance plan. In addition, clients visit the practice 50% more often when they have a pet health insurance plan.

LEADERSHIP POINT

Owners that have pet health insurance are more likely to accept recommendations made by the veterinary team because they are better able to afford emergency situations.

It is a false perception that pet health insurance is confusing. In fact, many practices do not offer insurance to clients because they feel it will be difficult, time-consuming, and not worth the effort to manage.

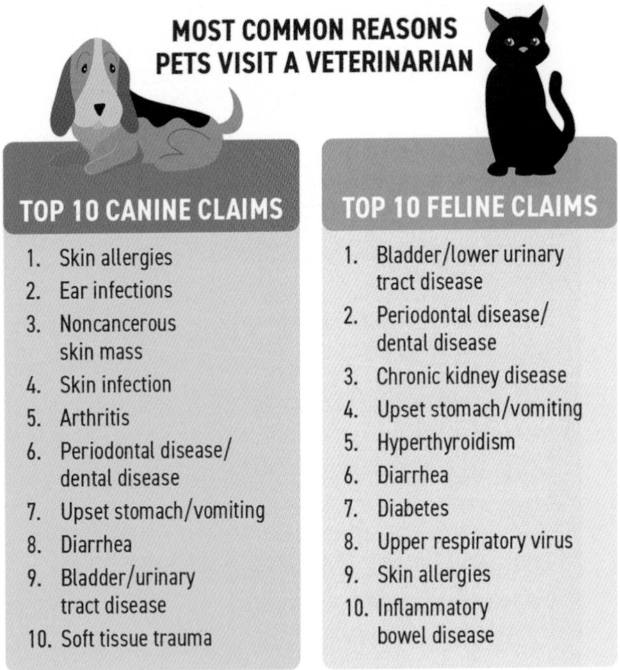
MOST COMMON REASONS PETS VISIT A VETERINARIAN
TOP 10 CANINE CLAIMS
1. Skin allergies
2. Ear infections
3. Noncancerous skin mass
4. Skin infection
5. Arthritis
6. Periodontal disease/ dental disease
7. Upset stomach/vomiting
8. Diarrhea
9. Bladder/urinary tract disease
10. Soft tissue trauma
TOP 10 FELINE CLAIMS
1. Bladder/lower urinary tract disease
2. Periodontal disease/ dental disease
3. Chronic kidney disease
4. Upset stomach/vomiting
5. Hyperthyroidism
6. Diarrhea
7. Diabetes
8. Upper respiratory virus
9. Skin allergies
10. Inflammatory bowel disease

Data reported March 2016; Nationwide Pet Health Insurance.

Fig. 16.21 The top reasons pets visit veterinarians have not changed much over the last 10 years; conditions may change ranking, but the conditions remain relatively the same.

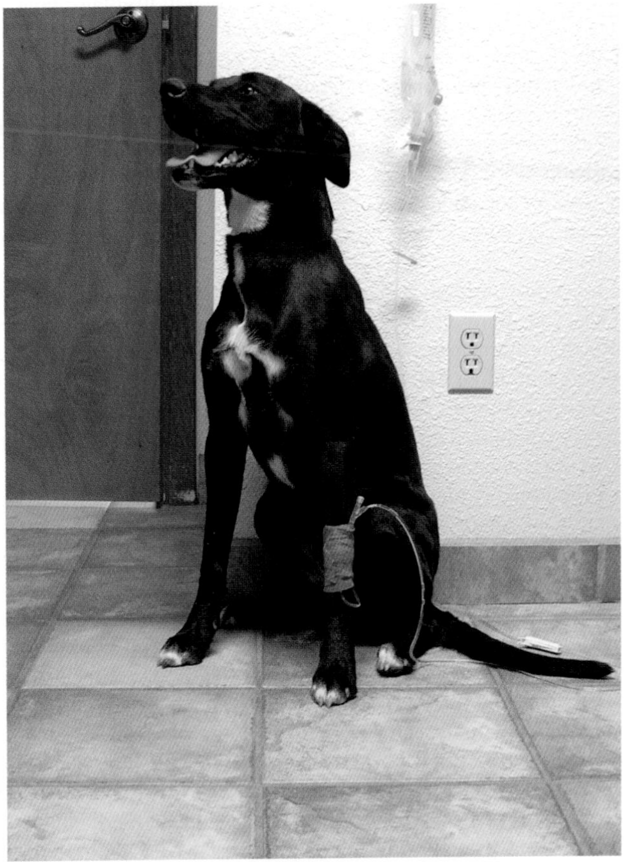

Fig. 16.22 The Standard of Care has improved over the years, resulting in an increase in the cost of veterinary care.

HELPFUL INSURANCE TERMS

Allowance: The maximum amount available for a specific diagnosis.

Annual deductible: The dollar amount the client chooses when signing up for an insurance plan. The client pays this amount before payout.

Annual payout limit: The maximum amount an insurance company will pay out on one policy, per year.

Benefit: The payment made for a specific diagnosis in accordance with an insurance plan.

Claim: A submission for a request for payment.

Copay: A specified dollar amount of covered services that is the policyholder's responsibility.

Deductible: The dollar amount an individual must pay for services before the insurance company will pay. Clients may have a choice of per-incident deductible or annual deductible.

Exclusion: A condition that is excluded from the coverage of a medical plan.

Incident: An individual accident, illness, or injury, including those that may require continual treatment until resolution.

Indemnity Insurance: A system of pet health insurance in which the client is reimbursed for services after they have been provided.

Lifetime Limit: The maximum dollar amount a company will pay out on one policy for the lifetime of the pet.

Per-Incident Deductible: The dollar amount that the policyholder is responsible for before the company will begin to pay out for each incident for which a claim form is submitted.

Per-Incident Limit: The maximum dollar amount an insurance company will pay out per incident filed.

Preexisting condition: Injury or illness contracted, manifested, or incurred before the policy effective date.

Premium: The amount paid annually or monthly for a policyholder to maintain an insurance policy.

Rider: An extension of coverage that can be purchased and added to a base medical policy.

Fig. 16.23 A quick guide to insurance terms helps the team better understand and explain to clients how pet health insurance operates.

Clients are then unaware of the benefits of such policies, and the practice loses revenue. A brief overview is provided to help team members become more familiar with the terms used in insurance policies (Fig. 16.23). Pet health insurance is a valuable resource that practices should be embracing.

Indemnity Insurance: Indemnity insurance offers compensation for treatment of injured and sick pets. Owners purchase a policy directly from a pet health insurance company and are eligible for compensation based on the care provided and policy terms. Policies are available for comprehensive illness, standard care, and accident coverage and may cover species ranging from dogs and cats to exotics and birds.

Indemnity insurance is different from insurance available for people. Indemnity insurance on the human side is generally offered through health management organizations (HMOs) or preferred provider organizations (PPOs), which are managed care organizations. Physicians are contracted to provide medical service at a set price and are then reimbursed directly by the insurance company. Pet indemnity insurance is not managed care.

Premiums: A premium is defined as the amount an owner pays monthly or annually to maintain an insurance policy for a pet. Premium amounts are affected by several factors that depend on the insurance provider, including the deductible; the copay; and the per-incident, annual, or lifetime payout limit. The cost of the premium is determined by several factors, including the species and breed of the animal, whether the pet is spayed or neutered, the age of the pet, and the geographic location of the owner in the United States. Cats tend to have lower premiums than dogs, and a Border Collie will have a lower premium than a Shar-Pei. Altered pets tend to have fewer behavioral issues and hormone-driven instincts and may have a decreased chance of developing hormone-related cancers, therefore a lower premium is likely. Owners living in rural Arizona will also have a lower premium than those who live in Los Angeles because the price of veterinary care is different in these two locations.

LEADERSHIP POINT

Insurance rates can vary by species, age, breed, and client zip code, along with selected premiums and deductibles.

Deductibles: A deductible is the amount an owner must pay before the insurance company will offer compensation. Insurance companies vary, offering either a per-incident deductible or an annual deductible. Per-incident deductibles refer to the owner paying the chosen deductible amount each time an incident occurs with the pet. An annual deductible refers to an owner paying the chosen deductible one time each year. Once the annual deductible amount has been met, the owner does not have to pay a deductible until the following year. For example, if a dog has an ear infection in March, a foreign body in June, and a fractured leg in November, and the owner chose a policy that was per-incident based, the owner will pay a deductible for each of the three claims. If the owner chose an annual deductible, he would pay the deductible amount once and would no longer be subject to a deductible for the rest of the year. Lower deductibles increase the cost of the premium, just as higher deductibles lower the premium.

Copay: A copay is the percentage that the owner is responsible for after the deductible has been met. Lower copays increase the amount of the premium and generally range from 10% to 20%. As an example, if a client's policy includes a $100 deductible and a 10% copay and the invoice balance is $4500, the owner is responsible for $540. This is calculated as follows:

- $4500 - $100 deductible = $4400 × 10% copay = $440
- $440 + $100 = $540 (client responsibility)
- $4500 - $540 = $3960 (insurance responsibility)

Annual Policy, Per-Incident, or Lifetime Limits: Some insurance companies offer clients the choice of an annual policy or a per-incident limit; others offer one or the other. Annual limits refer to the maximum amount that the insurance company will pay for a condition or illness during the policy term. Per-incident limits refer to the maximum amount an insurance company will pay each time a new problem or disease occurs. Lifetime limits refer to the maximum amount an insurance company will pay during the pet's life.

Per-incident limits can range from $1500 to $6000, but some companies do not have a per-incident limit. Annual limits range from $8000 to $20,000, allowing a larger amount for serious conditions. If a pet has been diagnosed with cancer and must undergo surgery, chemotherapy, and radiation, the invoice will likely exceed the $6000 per-incident limit. Because the cancer is classified as one incident, the maximum amount paid to the client will be the per-incident limit established in the policy. If an annual limit was chosen, the total amount paid to the client will be higher, based on the annual maximum amount established in the insurance policy. Few companies offer a lifetime limit, but if they do, it may be as high as $100,000. Policies should be examined carefully to determine which limit would meet the client's needs.

Preexisting Health Conditions: A preexisting health condition is defined as any accident or illness contracted, manifested, or incurred before the policy effective date. The pet may be enrolled; however, any preexisting condition will be excluded from coverage. It is highly recommended to enroll puppies and kittens in an insurance plan before any medical conditions arise. Some insurance companies will review preexisting conditions; if a stated condition has been diagnosed and cured, the exclusion may be waived. An example is a puppy diagnosed with gastroenteritis. If it was a one-time gastrointestinal indiscretion that was cured, a company can remove the exclusion, allowing future indiscretions to be covered.

Waiting Period: A waiting period is a period when coverage is not available and applies to the time between the submission of the application and the date the policy becomes effective. Each company varies in the length of time between application acceptance and activation. Some companies may have a 48-hour waiting period for accidents and a 2- to 4-week waiting period for a condition or illness. Any condition that occurs during the waiting period is usually considered a preexisting condition.

Hereditary and Congenital Conditions: Purebred pets that are known to have congenital and hereditary conditions may, based on company policy, also be excluded from an insurance plan. Recent veterinary books, including *Current Veterinary Therapy, Medical and Genetic Aspects of Purebred Dogs*, and the *Textbook of Small Animal Internal Medicine*, reference common congenital and hereditary conditions. A congenital condition is defined as an abnormality present at birth, whether apparent or not, that can cause illness or disease.

Congenital defects may be caused by medications administered to the mother in utero. Examples of congenital defects may include an umbilical hernia, a cleft palate, or a portosystemic shunt. The presence of a shunt may not be known until the dog matures, whereas a cleft palate is obvious immediately after birth. A hereditary condition is an abnormality that is transmitted genetically from the parent to the offspring. Examples include hip dysplasia, luxating patella, or cardiomyopathy. Some companies may also argue that some congenital defects are hereditary, thereby excluding coverage of such conditions. A portosystemic shunt is an example of a condition that may be subject to such an argument. Policies must be reviewed carefully for such exemptions.

Coverage of diseases may vary among insurance companies; a list of excluded diseases and conditions should be requested. Some companies will cover congenital conditions if they have not been previously diagnosed; others will not cover them at all. Companies that offer coverage of hereditary diseases will have higher premiums.

Chronic Conditions: Many diseases or conditions that are diagnosed will require years of care. Diabetes, Cushing disease, and Addison disease are just a few conditions that require care beyond the initial diagnosis and treatment. These conditions are known as *chronic conditions*, and some companies will only cover the initial diagnosis and treatment for the first year. Once it is time to reenroll the pet for the upcoming year, some insurance companies may consider the condition a preexisting condition and exclude it from the policy.

Exclusions: Many companies have a list of exclusions: diseases, conditions, or treatments that are excluded from policies. Frequently, behavior counseling and medications are not covered, nor are compounded medications, nutraceuticals, or diets. Exclusions should be carefully reviewed before choosing a policy.

Benefits of Pet Health Insurance

Pets can receive superior care with pet health insurance and can visit any hospital of the client's choice. If a client has an emergency at night, the client can visit the emergency hospital and have peace of mind that the expenses will be covered. If clients are traveling and need to see a veterinarian in another state, the insurance will still cover the cost of the veterinary services.

LEADERSHIP POINT

Clients with pet health insurance are more likely to follow recommended treatment plans than those who do not carry insurance policies.

Most pet insurance companies have streamlined the claims process, making it simple and hassle-free. Clients simply fill out the pet and client information, and practices fill out the form indicating the diagnosis. The veterinarian signs the claim form and either the practice or client submits it to the company by fax, email, or mail. Clients receive reimbursement within a short period. Veterinarians can practice the medicine they want; clients can choose the best options available to them. The insurance companies do not make decisions for the doctor or client; medical decisions are made between the practice and the client.

Filing a Claim

Depending on the specific insurance company, clients may be responsible for the full amount (paying the veterinary clinic at the time of service and then being immediately reimbursed by insurance) or may be responsible for their portion (and the insurance company reimburses the practice immediately). Policyholders will receive several claims forms with their packets, or they can print forms from the insurance company's website. Clients simply fill out their information, policy number, and pet information, and sign the form. It is imperative that the team member who helps the client with the claim form is knowledgeable about the pet's diagnosis. Incorrect wording and incomplete forms are the most common reason for claim payment delay. Some carriers offer a comprehensive list of diagnoses for team members to use when filling out forms. If a diagnosis has not been determined, some companies allow team members to include symptoms on the claim form. Forms should be proofread for correct wording. If multiple diagnoses are made, then all diagnoses should be listed. For example, dental prophylaxis may also find an abscessed tooth and periodontal disease; these must be written on the claim form so that the client is reimbursed for all three diseases, not just the dental procedure. Attaching a copy of the invoice and medical record will help insurance companies review the case more efficiently and will likely result in higher benefits payout. If a claim is denied, a request for review should be submitted as soon as possible. The request should provide additional information or clarification of a claim.

Making Pet Health Insurance Work for the Practice

All parties benefit from pet health insurance. Pet health insurance can ensure that pets will receive optimal, lifelong care, and veterinarians can practice cutting-edge medicine.

To successfully implement an insurance program(s) the practice should select a limited number (one or two) of insurance companies to recommend. This does not imply that the hospital will not accept other providers; it just simplifies the training for the team.

One person should be placed in charge of the selected program(s) and they should then coordinate training programs for the staff and serve as a contact person for the pet insurance company(s). Every team member, including veterinarians, must understand how insurance programs work, and how to educate clients about the benefits.

The training coordinator may place educational posters throughout the practice, brochures at the receptionist's desk, and brochures in puppy and kitten kits. When clients call for appointments, team members should ask if they have pet health insurance. Although the majority will respond "no," clients will become familiar with the phrase "pet health insurance." Once clients recognize the phrase, they may develop an interest in more information. They will look to the team for advice and recommendations, and team members can then provide education on the benefits of insurance. Pet health insurance recommendations must also be placed on the practice's website.

Once policies are in use, a team member can fill out the diagnosis and simply have the veterinarian sign the claim form. The team member may want to copy the medical record for claim purposes to ensure that the client receives the largest benefit possible. The team may want to provide exceptional service by mailing the claim form to the client, which further demonstrates the ease of filing claims.

Some claim forms are available through the PMS system. Once team members click on a claim form, the client and patient information will be automatically populated into the form. If the practice uses computerized medical records, the medical record will also be automatically uploaded with the form and sent electronically to the pet health insurance company. This will allow rapid claim processing, reimbursement of the client within a short time, and, ultimately, an increase in client satisfaction.

Recommendations to Clients

Of owners surveyed, 41% said they would purchase insurance if it were recommended by their veterinary practice (Braake). Most of the responders were younger, well-educated, and more affluent urban/suburban pet owners. Veterinary practices may target owners in this demographic with materials for pet health insurance and explain the benefits associated with policies.

LEADERSHIP POINT

A survey of owners revealed that 41% would purchase insurance if it was recommended by their veterinary practice.

Having insurance brochures at the counter for clients is another way to familiarize clients with pet health insurance. Clients can ask questions about the insurance available, and team members can provide estimates of coverage for services. Placing brochures in puppy and kitten kits as well as placing posters throughout the clinic will also increase awareness of insurance. Team members should remember the most important tip when discussing pet insurance: pet health insurance helps pay for unexpected accidents and/or illnesses. It is best to enroll pets when they are young, before the manifestation of disease or illness. Once the pet ages and health risk diagnoses are made, coverage may be limited.

Remember, 15% to 20% of the practice's active clientele generates 75% to 80% of the total practice revenue. If clients with pet health insurance spend twice that of the uninsured, then practice volume, production, revenue, and quality of medicine will dramatically increase. More active clients will spend more money and opt for specialized services.

Offering Pet Health Insurance as a Benefit

Many companies offer pet health insurance to employees as a benefit, and many veterinary clinics already discount services to team members. When pet health insurance is offered, the hospital receives the benefit. In addition, when team members insure their own pets, they understand how insurance works, thus making them valuable assets in client education. Many pet health insurance companies offer a discount to veterinary practices that wish to offer insurance as a benefit to employees.

WELLNESS PLANS

For many years, the veterinary industry relied on required vaccination protocols to bring clients into the hospital on a yearly basis. Unfortunately, when those vaccines were administered, the importance of preventive care was not relayed. The result was the decreased value of preventive care for pets. Now that many vaccines are available on a 3-year protocol, patient visits are declining, and pets are not receiving the preventive care they need to live long healthy lives.

The BVCUS of 2011 indicated that visits are decreasing for several reasons, including the fact that clients do not perceive the value of preventive care. In addition, the BVCUS indicated that 56% of cat owners and 59% of dog owners would take their pet to the veterinarian more often if they knew it would prevent problems and expensive treatments later. Further, 44% of cat owners and 46% of dog owners indicated that patient visits would increase if the veterinary office offered wellness plans with charges billed monthly.

Wellness plans are defined as evaluating all preventive recommendations that a patient would need in a 1-year period, then dividing that cost into equal monthly installments for the client. Wellness plans increase compliance and regular veterinary visits for ongoing managed care.

Components of a Wellness Plan

Most patients seen in practice are dogs and cats, and at each visit, specific recommendations are made for those patients based on their species and age group. Vaccine protocols may include an assessment of their individual environmental exposure, but, recommendations are consistent. With that in mind, wellness plans can be developed for each species and age group. A practice may consider groups for puppies, kittens, adult dogs, adult cats, senior dogs, and senior cats. Each age and species (in general) have different recommendations; additionally, while pets age, the cost of their care increases.

When creating wellness plans, the standards of care must be met; however, many clients have varying degrees of financial stability. Some clients may be able to afford the best care available and accept every recommendation made. Others may want to provide the best possible care but cannot afford all recommendations. This is an opportunity for practices to identify and meet client needs, and create various levels of plans, allowing clients to select what they can afford. Practices may consider basic, premium, and supreme plans. Clients can pick the plan most affordable to them.

Keep in mind, wellness plans are exactly that. They are used to promote the preventive care needed to maintain wellness. Wellness plans do not cover illnesses or injuries. Plans should be kept simple, easy for the staff to explain, and easy for clients to understand.

Pricing

The primary reason for developing wellness plans is to help clients budget their money to afford the services that a practice recommends. However, some clients may look for additional incentives; if they choose to sign up for a plan, is there a discount involved?

Before any discounts can be considered, practices must determine what their costs are when developing a program. Practices may wish to enlist a third party to manage their wellness plans, or they may choose to develop and manage their own. Either way, an enrollment fee must be determined, because administration costs do accumulate with these plans.

Administration costs to consider include how the plan will be implemented within the PIMS, how money will be collected from clients, how the team will be trained on the plans, how the plans will be marketed to clients, how doctors will be compensated, and how the program will be monitored for success (the following sections provide more detail on each of the mentioned topics).

In addition to administration costs, the absolute minimum of charges must be determined. In other words, if a practice wanted to offer a wellness plan at a deeply discounted price, what is the absolute minimum that could be charged while still producing a profit? Use the pricing equation earlier in this chapter to help determine real costs associated with products and services. Compare this dollar amount to a standard invoice with current charges.

Plan Development: Factors associated with plan development include those mentioned previously as well as an estimate of time for each aspect. Practices must determine which services will be provided for each species, age group, and plan (basic, premium, or supreme) (Fig.16.24).

Software Integration: Practices must consider how wellness plans will integrate with current software programs. If using a third-party provider, contact them for specifics on software integration. Practices not using a third-party provider may create a code for each wellness

KITTEN BASIC PLAN
- Physical examination (2)
- All core vaccines
- Intestinal parasite examination
- Deworming
- Nail trim
- Nutritional counseling and BCS

KITTEN PREMIUM PLAN
- Physical examination (4)
- All core vaccines
- FeLV/FIV/HWT
- Intestinal parasite examination
- Deworming
- Nail trim
- Flea/tick/HW prevention
- Nutritional counseling and BCS

KITTEN SUPREME PLAN
- Physical examination (unlimited)
- All core vaccines
- FeLV/FIV/HWT
- Intestinal parasite examination
- Deworming
- Flea/tick/HW prevention
- CBC/comprehensive chemistry profile
- Nail trim
- Nutritional counseling and BCS

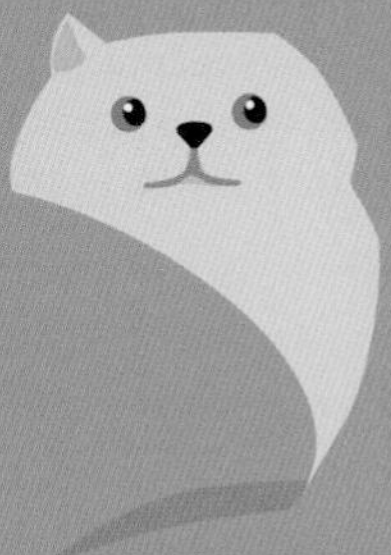

FELINE ADULT BASIC PLAN
- Physical examination (2)
- All core vaccines
- Intestinal parasite examination
- Deworming
- Nail trim
- Nutritional counseling and BCS

FELINE ADULT PREMIUM PLAN
- Physical examination (4)
- All core vaccines
- FeLV/FIV/HWT
- Intestinal parasite examination
- Deworming
- Nail trim
- Flea/tick/HW prevention
- Nutritional counseling and BCS
- Urinalysis
- Dental grade 1

FELINE ADULT SUPREME PLAN
- Physical examination (unlimited)
- All core vaccines
- FeLV/FIV/HWT
- Intestinal parasite examination
- Deworming
- Flea/tick/HW prevention
- Nail trim
- Nutritional counseling and BCS
- CBC/comprehensive chemistry profile
- Urinalysis
- Dental grade 2
- Thyroid screen
- Blood pressure

BCS, Body condition score; CB, complete blood count; FeLV, feline leukemia virus; FIV, feline immunodeficiency virus; HW, heartworm; HWT, heartworm test.

FELINE SENIOR BASIC PLAN
- Physical examination (2)
- All core vaccines
- Intestinal parasite examination
- Deworming
- Nail trim
- Nutritional counseling and BCS
- Urinalysis
- Blood pressure
- Dental grade 1

FELINE SENIOR PREMIUM PLAN
- Physical examination (4)
- All core vaccines
- FeLV/FIV/HWT
- Intestinal parasite examination
- Deworming
- Nail trim
- Flea/tick/HW prevention
- Nutritional counseling and BCS
- Urinalysis
- Blood pressure
- Thyroid screen
- Dental grade 2

FELINE SENIOR SUPREME PLAN
- Physical examination (unlimited)
- All core vaccines
- FeLV/FIV/HWT
- Intestinal parasite examination
- Deworming
- Flea/tick/HW prevention
- Nail trim
- Nutritional counseling and BCS
- CBC/comprehensive chemistry profile
- Urinalysis
- Thyroid screen
- Blood pressure
- Radiographs
- Dental grade 2

Fig. 16.24 Suggested wellness plans for different stages of a cat's life.

plan developed, and an alert can be set in the client's account indicating they have purchased a wellness plan for the year.

Client Collection: Practices must consider how they will collect money for plan installment payments. Automatic debits or credit card charges are a must, as clients may not reliably make payments. A third-party provider can be used to manage the entire program or simply just to collect payments. The benefit of a third-party collector is that credit card numbers do not have to be kept on file in the practice, violating the Red Flags Rule. In addition, if a credit or debit card is canceled, they will work to collect the funds instead of hospital personnel. Funds are then deposited into the practice account once monthly. If an account is uncollectible, the third party will notify the practice. Managers must then determine how they will manage accounts that have become uncollectible.

Educating Team Members: Team members must understand the benefits of wellness programs before client education can begin. Wellness plans promote the best possible care for patients all year long. Wellness plans drive compliance, build relationships, and encourage clients to purchase all services and products at the hospital, not at competitive locations. One thing is certain: clients who provide the best care for their pets directly decrease the compassion fatigue experienced by team members.

Educating Clients: Clients will learn about wellness programs through team members, the website, and through social media. Materials should be printed explaining the program, including the benefits of purchasing the program, including a lower cost of veterinary care.

Doctor Compensation: Determining how doctors are compensated with such programs can be challenging, especially when they are paid on a production basis. Factoring in variable compensation can increase the plan development and management costs and becomes very time-consuming during payroll periods. When managed by a third-party system, reports can be generated, reducing the number of in-house hours used to determine compensation.

Managing and Improving: Once programs have been initiated, they should be monitored for success and methods of improvement. What is the compliance rate? Which team member has the best acceptance rate? What does she do that can help other team members improve? Can marketing techniques be changed or improved? Every profit center (this is a profit center) must be managed and scrutinized regularly, ensuring the revenue produced is covering the costs associated with developing, implementing, and managing it.

LEADERSHIP'S ROLE IN FINANCE MANAGEMENT

Financial management is solely the responsibility of the practice manager and owner. While pieces may be delegated to other team members, the leadership team is responsible for strategic goal achievement. The leadership team must understand all elements of financial management and the potential impact of ALL decisions on practice finances.

Recall that financial management is more than just creating a budget and looking at profit and loss (P&L) statements; KPIs must be monitored and managed, and changes must be implemented before financials are significantly impacted. A frictionless client experience, efficiency, and appropriate leveraging must be developed to reduce the cost of doing business. Charge capture must be a top priority and expenses must be monitored monthly. Accounts receivables must be well managed, and donations to charity must be built into the budget. Finally, every team member needs to know how much it costs to run the business (open books management). The veterinary practice is a team sport, and every team member must understand how they contribute to the goals, even financial ones.

PRACTICE MANAGER SURVIVAL CHECKLIST FOR FINANCE MANAGEMENT

- ☐ Identify and monitor KPIs.
- ☐ Develop protocol and manage client discounts.
- ☐ Develop protocol and manage client account receivables.
- ☐ Develop monthly P&L statements and analyze.
- ☐ Develop/adhere to a chart of accounts.
- ☐ Ensure fee capture.
- ☐ Ensure appropriate service fee setting.
- ☐ Set goals and manage revenue centers.
- ☐ Develop/maintain budget.
- ☐ Develop accounts payable system.
- ☐ Reconcile bank statements by the first week of each month.
- ☐ Categorize credit card statements appropriately in accounting software.
- ☐ Categorize manufacturer/distributor invoices appropriately in accounting software.
- ☐ Develop an open book management/policy and share numbers with the team.
- ☐ Obtain CPA counsel that has experience in the veterinary industry for tax matters.
- ☐ Obtain financial planning counsel for retirement/investment matters.
- ☐ Ensure the practice is complying with the Red Flags Rules.
- ☐ Develop policies regarding which owner signs checks.
- ☐ Secure the organization's federal and state identification numbers in a safe, easily retrievable location.
- ☐ Determine when sales tax is reported (monthly or quarterly), and who is responsible for ensuring the report occurs.
- ☐ Determine when use tax is reported (monthly or quarterly), and who is responsible for ensuring the report occurs.
- ☐ Review sales tax-exempt status on a yearly basis.
- ☐ Annually review client pricing and determine whether/when a fee increase should occur.
- ☐ Review all insurance policies annually, and before renewal (property, professional liability, employment practices, flood, commercial auto, data breach, directors and officer's liability, health, etc.).
- ☐ Implement pet health insurance, wellness plan discussions, and promotions.

REVIEW QUESTIONS

1. Define benchmarking and describe the difference between internal and external benchmarks.
2. What is the difference between a CPA and a bookkeeper?
3. Why should a budget be created?
4. What is a variable expense? Give some examples.
5. What is a fixed cost? Give some examples.
6. Define some areas that could cause a cash flow crunch.
7. How can a practice manager increase the value of a hospital?
8. Define the Red Flags Rule and discuss why it should be implemented by the veterinary practice.

9. What is the Fair Debt Collection Practices Act and why was it established?
10. What is an insufficient funds charge?
11. What is a held check?
12. If a practice reports services when they are invoiced, they are reporting by which standard?
    a. Cash basis
    b. Accrual basis
13. Staff payroll is considered a ______ expense for benchmarking purposes.
    a. Fixed
    b. Variable
14. Accounts receivables should not exceed:
    a. 2% of gross revenue
    b. $2.00
    c. 5% of gross revenue
    d. $5.00
15. Holding checks for clients is recommended when they cannot pay for services the same day.
    a. True
    b. False
16. Which of the following is mandated by the Fair Debt Collection Act?
    a. Notification stickers can be placed on the outside of the envelope.
    b. Conversations to collect outstanding AR can be held with any of the family members residing in the home.
    c. Collection calls can only be made between 8 a.m. and 9 p.m.
    d. Clients can be threatened by withholding veterinary services.
17. Withdrawing employee accounts receivable from the employee's paycheck is an acceptable form of payment.
    a. True
    b. False
18. Third-party payment plans include:
    a. CareCredit
    b. Veterinary Pet Insurance
    c. PaymentBanc
    d. All of the above
19. Pet health insurance:
    a. Improves patient care
    b. Increases patient examinations
    c. Decreases the stop-treatment threshold
    d. A and B
20. Indemnity insurance is also known as:
    a. Managed care
    b. HMO delivered
    c. PPO delivered
    d. None of the above
21. An amount an owner pays on a monthly basis is known as a:
    a. Premium
    b. Deductible
    c. Copay
    d. All of the above
22. Wellness plans should be developed by:
    a. Species
    b. Age group
    c. Client preferences
    d. A and B
23. The purpose of Wellness Plans is to:
    a. Promote preventive care
    b. Promote all-inclusive care
    c. Promote pet health insurance
    d. None of the above

REFERENCES

1. Barnes C. *Letting your Practice Management Software for the Work for You.* Published July 2022. Accessed August 2022. Shepherd Veterinary Practice Management Software. https://www.shepherd.vet
2. Tumblin D. et al. *Well managed practice benchmarks*, 2019. Accessed August 2022. https://www.wmpb.vet

RECOMMENDED READING

Ackerman LJ. *Blackwell's five-minute veterinary practice management consult.* 3rd ed. Blackwell Publishing; 2019.

Boone D, Hauser W. *The veterinarians guide to healthy pet plans.* Lulu Publishing; 2016.

Chamblee J, Reiboldt M. *Financial management of the veterinary practice.* AAHA Press; 2010.

Kenney D. *Your guide to understanding pet health insurance.* PhiloSophia Publishing; 2009.

Santi S. *The rewards of a reward program.* Vet Team Brief. September 2017. https://files.brief.vet/migration/article/41731/the-rewards-of-a-reward-program-41731-article.pdf

Wood F. Plug the leaks in your bottom line! (Proceedings). DVM 360. Published August 1, 2009. Accessed December 2022. https://www.dvm360.com/view/plug-leaks-your-bottom-line-proceedings

17

Strategic Planning

LEARNING OBJECTIVES

When you have completed this chapter, you should be able to:

1. Define strategic planning and how it applies to the veterinary practice.
2. Differentiate between organizational design and organizational development.
3. Define learning organization.
4. Describe the importance of workforce planning and its effect on strategic goals.

OUTLINE

KEY TERMS

Business Life Cycle
Organizational Design
Organizational Development
Organizational Learning
Strategic Planning
Succession planning
SWOT Analysis
Workforce

INTRODUCTION

Strategic planning is a long-term action plan that a business puts in writing to achieve defined goals over time. Strategic planning positions the practice for success in the future and includes making decisions today to accomplish tomorrow's goals (aka the future). Future may be defined as 1, 2, or 3 years ahead of time. The pandemic taught us that detailed planning further out than 3 years may be futile, although the vision should remain intact regardless of the emergent situations that could occur.

A SWOT analysis should always be included in any strategic plan, and although threats such as the pandemic cannot be controlled, the more prepared the practice is for potential situations, the better the practice can quickly adapt. As covered in Chapter 12, Marketing, mitigating risks that threats could potentially pose are critical (for example, back-up building generators to maintain business continuity in the event of long-term power loss).

Strategic Planning starts with the vision of the owner.

- Where should the business be in X number of years?
- What needs to be accomplished to achieve the vision by each year as defined in the previous bullet point? This step needs to remain high level the details will come later.
- What monetary needs will be needed to achieve the vision?
- Establish a yearly budget for strategic achievement only. This should include revenue, expenses, and profitability expected. Again, keep this step high level, as the details will come later.
- Take the above information and develop a practice expense budget for each year established by the strategic plan (refer to Chapter 16, Finance, for expense considerations and an explanation of budget development). Don't forget to include equipment (new and maintenance of existing equipment), building maintenance, people development (continuing education, raises, bonuses, training programs, hiring, uniforms, employee benefits, etc.), IT infrastructure, marketing, cost of goods, and facility and employee safety. If the

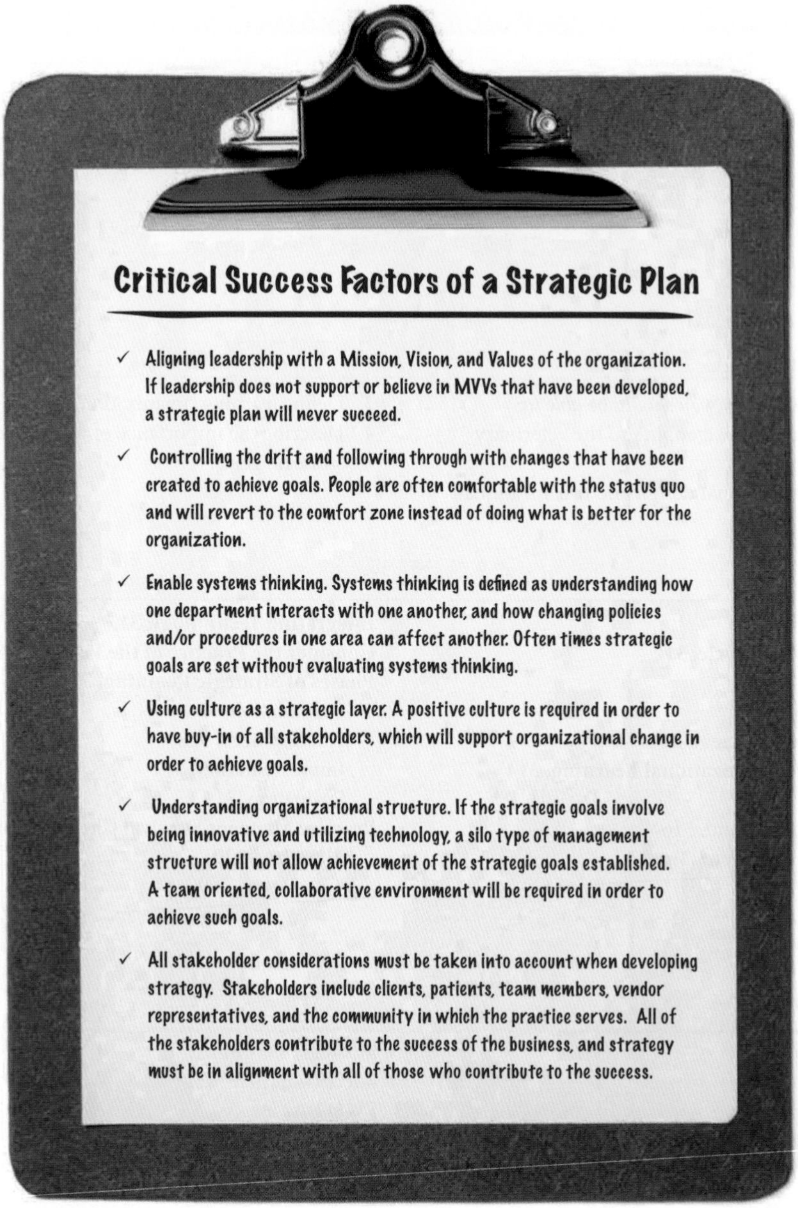

Fig. 17.1 Critical Success Factors of a Strategic Plan.

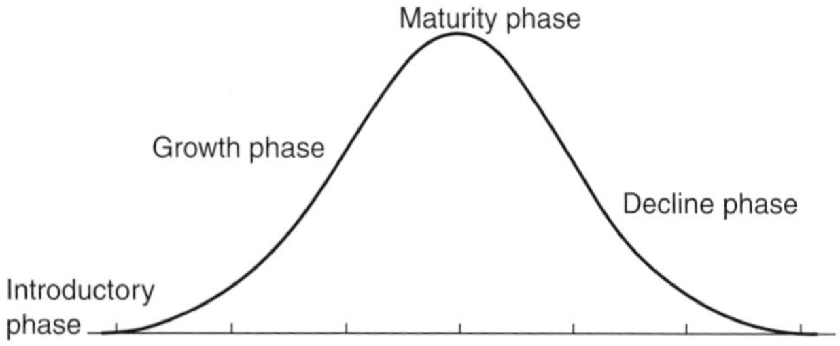

Fig. 17.2 The Business Life Cycle.

practice will be developing new revenue centers to support the strategic plan, equipment, training and development, and hiring of team members to support the revenue center should be included.

- The next step is to determine how much revenue will need to be generated to cover the expenses listed in the bullet point above, as well as achieve the profitability goal.
- Practice leadership will then need to determine how increased revenue will be achieved. Will that be through new client and patient growth, an increase in the number of revenue centers, and/or more appointments per day (e.g., increasing volume)? An overall price increase won't cut it as that will only cover expenses.

While the above bullet points cover strategic planning at a high level, it is critical to understand and incorporate the business lifecycle, organizational design, organizational development, and workforce planning (Fig. 17.1).

UNDERSTANDING THE BUSINESS LIFE CYCLE

Every business has a life cycle that should be considered, planned, and carefully watched to prevent achieving that fourth stage (decline). Therefore, the focus will be on stages one through three: introduction, growth, and maturity (Fig. 17.2).

Introductory Phase: During a business's introductory stage, vision, innovation, and energy are critical in getting the organization established and, on its way, to competing in the market successfully. This stage is usually experienced before doors are opened for business. Previously existing practices will not have an introductory stage and may have missed the importance of developing the vision, mission, and values (VMVs) for the practice. Without VMVs, the practice may have trouble achieving successful growth and scalability to achieve the maturity stage. Review Chapter 2, Leadership, for the creation of VMVs if they are not already established and implemented into daily routines.

Growth Stage: When a practice enters the growth stage, so does the demand for services, and the practice must become more disciplined and organized. At this point, efficiency and talent development typically occur. Traditionally, in veterinary medicine a starter practice has about five team members, allowing practice protocols and staff training to be implemented easily. However, many practices do not take time to create an organizational structure and planned efficiencies during this growth stage. This creates a larger problem in the maturity stage when the practice expands in both in clientele and team members. Review Chapter 2, Leadership, and Chapter 4, Human Sources, to develop the most important asset of the practice: the people. It is also important in this stage to consider how technology can help a practice become more efficient, making growth and scalability easier to achieve. Review Chapter 7 (Telemedicine), Chapter 8 (PIMS), and Chapter 11 (Client Experience) to gain ideas of how technology improves the lives of both team members and clients alike.

Maturity Stage: During the maturity stage, practices should be running proficiently in every area of the business. Prior planning and development should benefit the practice with efficiencies that support the team and patients. This stage requires leaders to manage risks, problem solve, and continuously find opportunities for growth. Efforts must be made to keep the practice culture relevant and vibrant, meeting the changing needs of the team members. Many veterinary practices struggle during this stage of the business life cycle. The practice may have experienced an increase in year-over-year revenue growth but may not be implementing infrastructure changes to support and build upon that growth rate. Often the mentality of "this is the way we have always done things" interferes with the need to challenge the status quo and improve business practices. Embracing innovation and technology and fostering employee engagement is critical during this stage. Without these, the decline stage is not far away.

In each stage of the business life cycle, businesses must evaluate the ever-changing marketplace, economy, and consumer needs, and adjust their strategic plan accordingly. In the decline stage, practices may notice the demand for services has decreased. Practices must look for methods to increase and improve efficiencies and adapt, change, or redefine themselves to stay relevant with their clients and in their communities. This requires revisiting the strategic plan and identifying where changes are required to continue competing in the profession and the marketplace. Practices that do not revitalize during the decline stage have a high risk of closing.

LEADERSHIP POINT

Prevent hitting the business life cycle decline stage by continuing to be innovative and find growth opportunities in the maturity stage.

ORGANIZATIONAL DESIGN

Organizational design is the methodology that identifies aspects of workflow, procedures, roles, and systems, and aligns them to fit current business realities and goals. In every practice, there is an owner (or multiple owners), associate veterinarian(s), practice manager, and team members. Often the roles of owner(s), associate veterinarian(s), and practice manager are unclear. The roles should be clearly defined, allowing owners to practice medicine and oversee the business, the associate veterinarians to practice medicine and understand the business, and the practice manager to manage the people and contribute to good business decisions. Great collaboration should exist among all levels of leadership, enabling the best business decisions to be made and facilitating the achievement of strategic goals.

Often in veterinary practice, veterinary owners do not allow managers to manage the practice; they have been designated to manage but are often stripped of those duties when it comes to daily activities. For example, managers would like to hold team members accountable for their poor performance, but the owner steps in and prevents the manager from enforcing accountability. Examples such as this prevent the owner from practicing great medicine (as they place their attention on the people aspect of the business) and making good business decisions, resulting in leadership fatigue for the manager.

Leadership fatigue can be experienced by both owners and managers and results from lack of communication, lack of delineation of job duties, and feeling that they are constantly haggling with the team to carry out policies and procedures. In situations such as this, culture is usually poor, the VMVs have not been created and/or implemented at every level (and with every role) within the practice, the VMVs may not align with the goals, and the goals have not been clearly communicated to the team members. When team members do not understand the goals, policies and procedures do not make sense and they resist the change. Therefore, leadership begins to experience the "haggling feeling."

To explore organizational design a bit further, consider how the team helps achieve the practice goals. Every team member contributes to the success of the practice in one way or another, but if they have not been trained effectively, engaged in the business, leveraged effectively, or developed a sense of purpose as a team member within the practice, then team morale drops and turnover and burnout increases. Ensure every team member is leveraged appropriately (Chapter 2), and that the organizational hierarchy does not interfere with the delivery of relationship-centered care. A relationship-centered practice is defined as utilizing empowered veterinary team members who share veterinary knowledge to develop long-lasting relationships with clients and patients (Dowdy, 2017). Clearly define job responsibilities, establish resonating VMVs, and consistently communicate goals to the team to carry out a successful organizational design.

Achieving strategic goals is a team sport. Everyone has to be on board and support the goals, but they cannot do that without having the tools, knowledge, and skills to do so. Build a superior culture that no team member wants to leave (encompass psychological safety, continuous coaching, and communication), develop an exceptional onboarding and mentoring program so no team member is left behind, establish team member loyalty early, and never stop providing educational growth opportunities for them. When allowed, CE brings excitement, knowledge sharing, and the practice of best medicine and service, all of which contribute to the development of a sense of purpose in every team member. Review Chapter 2, Leadership, for more details.

ORGANIZATIONAL DEVELOPMENT

Organizational development is different than organizational design in that development looks at the process of enhancing the effectiveness within the practice. An easy question to ask oneself in strategy development is "What can make our practice more effective and efficient?" There are several advantages to enhancing organizational development, including the building of diverse teams, the ability to act and make changes quickly, enhanced practice culture, speeding up the process of

KEY AREAS OF ORGANIZATIONAL DEVELOPMENT

Client Experience *(Chapter 11)*
- Are clients satisfied? Do appointments run on time?
- Are client communications clear?
- Does the practice use the most current technology?

Patient Care
- Are all patients receiving an elevated standard of care on every visit? *(Chapter 11)*
- Are low-stress handling techniques and Fear Free initiatives being utilized for every patient? *(Chapter 11 and 12)*

Team Member Development
- Are team members effectively trained from day one of hiring *(Chapter 4)*?
- Do team members receive continuous continuing education as it relates to the VMVs?
- Are employee communications handled quickly and in the best way possible?
- Are employees engaged and accountable for their actions?

Revenue Centers within the Practice*
- Client Experience *(Chapter 11)*
- Inventory *(Chapter 13)*
- Controlled Substance Management *(Chapter 14)*
- Financial Management *(Chapter 16)*

** List is only examples and is in no way complete.*

Fig. 17.3 Practice Areas to Evaluate for Organizational Development.

decision-making, and prioritizing decisions that elevate the achievement of strategic goals (Fig. 17.3).

Steps of Organizational Development

Defining the problem, designing a solution, implementing the solution, and following through with evaluation are the four components of organizational development.

Defining the problem includes collecting data and identifying gaps that exist with a particular inefficiency. As with all gap analyses, identify how the subject area is performing today and where it should be in the future. Identify any causes of the gap, and always consider the different stakeholders that could be involved (clients, patients, team members, vendors). See Chapter 2, Leadership, for a Gap Analysis example.

Designing a solution is often the most difficult part of organizational development. Be sure to involve the team when developing clearly defined objectives (allowing measurement in the evaluation phase) and identify the tools that will be needed to achieve those objectives. Will the team members need any additional knowledge, skills, and abilities (KSAs) to achieve the change? Consider how one efficiency affects another and how changes may affect another department, and always include a risk assessment (it is important to identify all risks associated with creating change. Some risks can be mitigated, and others will need to be managed throughout the change process). See Chapter 12, Marketing, for the use of written SMART goals that will identify objectives, measurables, and resources/tools needed to achieve (and measure) goals.

WHEN ORGANIZATIONAL DEVELOPMENT MIGHT FAIL

- Leadership did not support or commit to changes.
- The wrong message was delivered and/or the message did not resonate with the team.
- Changes were communicated forcefully upon the team versus introduced collaboratively.
- Lack of clear communication regarding change.
- Change(s) does not align with the VMVs.

Fig. 17.4 Common Reasons for Failure of Organizational Development.

When improving efficiencies and effectiveness within the practice, the team will be asked to change "the way we have always done things." Identify what resistance could occur with the changes, and who might resist the change. One last important question to consider: does the practice culture support change? Many times, managers have tried to implement change, but things eventually revert to the status quo. Therefore, the perception of the team is that the culture of the practice does not support change (see Chapter 2, Leadership, and review Change Resistance).

The implementation phase is critical because this is where team communication is vital. Host team meetings to discuss changes, coach team members daily, and tie changes to the VMVs and performance reviews. Leaders may also consider adding incentives or rewards for team members embracing and championing change. Evaluate the metrics as developed in the design stage and report successes to the team. Common reasons for the failure of organizational development are listed in Fig. 17.4.

LEARNING ORGANIZATIONS AND ORGANIZATIONAL LEARNING

A learning organization is characterized by the ability to adapt to change and respond quickly to environmental/consumer changes. Consider large companies such as Apple and Google. Although extremely large, they have personified learning, changing, and adaptation philosophy. The demanding consumer environment changes constantly. To compete, businesses need to deploy innovation that is attractive to consumers; the company must learn, change, and adapt to the needs of the consumer to survive.

Veterinary practices must also adopt learning, changing, and adapting philosophies. The veterinary consumer is no longer the loyal customer they once were. Their needs are changing, and they look for technology and innovation in the veterinary practice (Telemedicine, access to their pets' medical records, the ability to make appointments online, themselves, request refills medications for medications at any time, and have medications shipped directly to their home). They want simple, easy methods to communicate with the veterinary practice on a regular basis (two-way text messaging). They want relationships that exist throughout the year, not just during an annual examination, and they want immediate answers to their questions. What has your practice done to meet these needs?

LEADERSHIP POINT

Become a learning organization by responding and adapting to environmental, technological, and consumer demands that can change quickly.

In a learning organization, knowledge must be acquired by the whole organization; this means that every team member must receive continuing education (not just DVMs and credentialed veterinary technicians) in order to help the practice adapt to consumer needs (also known as organizational learning, discussed later in this chapter). Team members cannot be expected to create innovative solutions when they have never been exposed to methodologies outside of the existing practice.

Learning organizations must also employ "systems thinking," meaning that every team within the practice must generate ideas together and create solutions that are beneficial for all parties involved (Fig. 17.5). For example, practices and policies put in place by the receptionist team cannot adversely affect the technician team. Or policies and procedures put in place for boarding animals cannot have a negative impact on the kennel and reception teams.

To employ systems thinking in a learning organization, every team member must actively live and breathe the VMVs of the practice. This ensures that all team members contribute to achieving the goals of the practice.

Team members need to know that leadership embraces change and readily accepts recommendations. Team members should be encouraged (psychological safety) to propose innovative ideas to deliver better services to clients and enhance diagnostics for patients. Some recommendations and protocols may not produce the results expected, and that cannot be penalized. Failures create learning opportunities. Every organization must expect failures at some point and embrace them and move forward. Regardless of who made an unsuccessful recommendation (leadership or team members), everyone can learn from mistakes and overcome obstacles to get back on track. This creates a stronger, more dynamic team.

Organizational Learning is also known as training and development for team members. A learning organization (covered in the previous paragraph) values *organizational learning* for team members. When employing successful training and development, it is critical to understand the adult learning theory (ALT). ALT emphasizes that adults learn differently than children. Child students learn by having information "pushed" into their brains. Students listen to the teacher, read a book, and complete homework. The information learned is then banked for later use. For adults to retain new information, it must be used immediately; when information is banked for later use, it is not retained as well. Additionally, adults have three learning styles: visual, auditory, and kinesthetic. Adults must see, hear, and touch what they are learning for the best retention results. In veterinary practice, this means when training team members, procedures should be explained while completed (hearing and seeing), and then team members are allowed to do the procedure themselves (kinesthetic) (Fig. 17.6).

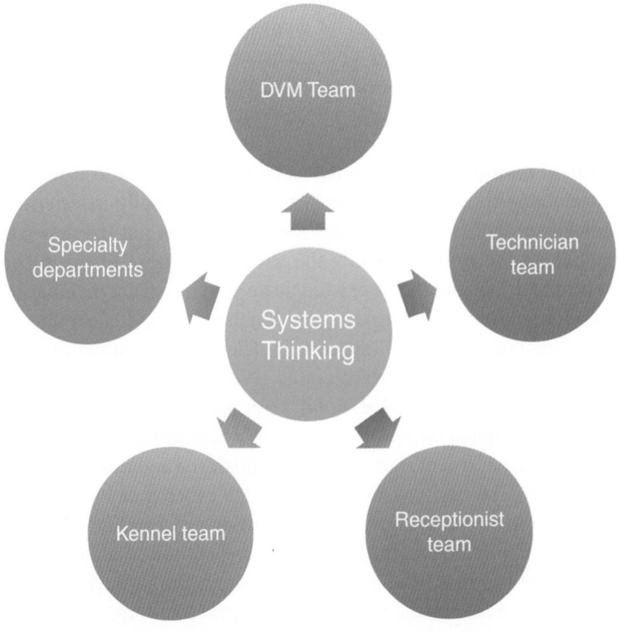

Fig. 17.5 Systems Thinking must be employed to understand how changes will impact each role in the veterinary practice.

There are also two forms of learning to consider. "Push" learning is defined as lecture-style delivery, where information is *pushed* to the team member. On the other hand, "pull" learning is defined as team members researching data and *pulling* the information to themselves. In adult learning theory, pull learning increases retention rates. Therefore, it is beneficial for practices to incorporate a combined learning style. Team members should be encouraged to research information online in addition to what they are taught in training sessions. And to take learning one step further, once the material has been learned by a team member it should be taught to others on the team. This additionally reinforces learning retention (review Chapter 4).

LEADERSHIP POINT

Incorporate adult learning theory into every training program.

Always tie all forms of learning back to the vision, mission, and values of the organization to achieve the goals set forth by the strategic plan. If there are team members who are resistant to further their education and knowledge base, leadership should explore the reasons why. Team members who don't feel education is beneficial can be toxic to the rest of the team and prevent the practice from growing (Fig. 17.7). See Chapter 2 (Leadership) and Chapter 4 (Human Resources) for potential reasons for CE resistance in team members.

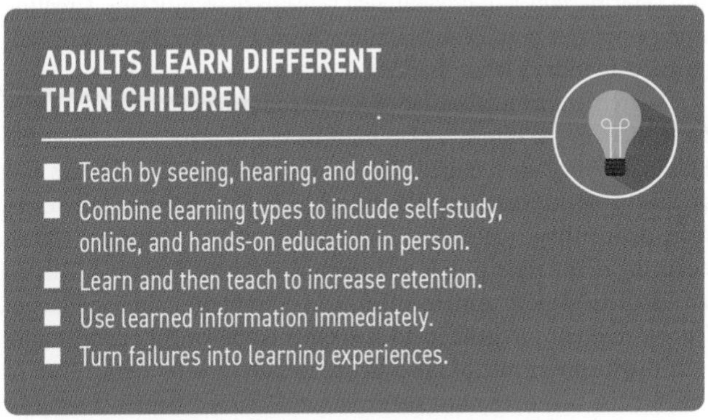
ADULTS LEARN DIFFERENT THAN CHILDREN
Teach by seeing, hearing, and doing.
Combine learning types to include self-study, online, and hands-on education in person.
Learn and then teach to increase retention.
Use learned information immediately.
Turn failures into learning experiences.

Fig. 17.6 Characteristics of Adult Learning Theory.

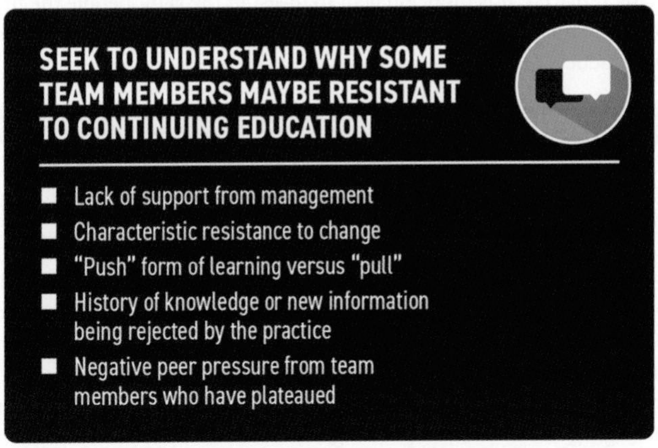
SEEK TO UNDERSTAND WHY SOME TEAM MEMBERS MAYBE RESISTANT TO CONTINUING EDUCATION
Lack of support from management
Characteristic resistance to change
"Push" form of learning versus "pull"
History of knowledge or new information being rejected by the practice
Negative peer pressure from team members who have plateaued

Fig. 17.7 Common Reasons for Resistance to Learning.

WORKFORCE PLANNING

Historically in veterinary medicine, practices do not plan well for developing team members (practices simply hire when a team member is terminated or leaves). Part of the strategic planning process is workforce planning, which is determining what team members will be needed to achieve the practice goals starting in the present day and for the next 1–3 years. By planning ahead, the right team members can be chosen and developed into valuable roles. In essence, the goal of workforce planning is to find, develop, and retain talented individuals to achieve strategic goals.

In addition to achieving strategic goals, workforce planning creates a strong employer brand. It is much more efficient, practical, and financially beneficial to develop existing team members into higher roles, and then hire and train new individuals for entry-level positions. Providing advancement opportunities creates longevity and loyalty from team members, which then supports the employer brand (or reputation). Clients also benefit from seeing the same team members year after year. It represents stability, security, and comfort for clients. Goal achievement is much easier when supported by having the right team members in the right seats on your bus.

Understanding Supply and Demand

When creating a workforce plan, identify positions that will be needed before they exist by considering future hiring needs. Develop plans for veterinarians, credentialed veterinary technicians, and support staff needed to achieve the long-term practice goals.

Supply refers to the employee workforce that is currently available to the veterinary practice. It is important to identify the capabilities of the team in place today, and where or what the team needs to deliver tomorrow's strategic goals. As identified in Chapter 1, the supply available in veterinary medicine is low, with the prediction of a shortage of both veterinarians and credentialed veterinary technicians. Creating a strong employer brand and planning ahead are critical to stay ahead of the game in today's labor market.

If current team members lack KSAs or competencies needed to deliver the services of the future, a plan must be put in place to build on these skills before they are required. This plan will make future changes easier for existing team members and should be built into future job descriptions, onboarding, mentoring, and phase training programs, allowing the hiring of the right people and training right the first time. This plan can also help identify team members that don't fit the culture of the practice and may encourage them to seek other employment opportunities.

If the turnover rate of the practice is high (greater than 13%), reasons for the turnover must be explored. Review Chapter 2 regarding culture, employee engagement, and employee motivation. Turnover is costly, averaging approximately 1.5 times the salary rate of the person being replaced. It is more efficient to invest in the right people the first time, creating a long-term career plan for every team member within the practice.

> **LEADERSHIP POINT**
>
> Determine future workforce needs today and plan accordingly to achieve strategic goals.

With a solid strategic plan in place, the practice will grow. There will occasionally be a natural loss of team members (attrition) as a result of nonemployment issues (team members moving out of the community, etc.). Leadership should estimate the number of team members needed in the future to deliver the procedures and services identified by the strategic goals while incorporating the attrition rate.

Information needed to determine future workforce needs includes the following:

1. Average number of current employees
2. Average practice growth in percent
3. Average attrition rate per year
4. Number of years the strategic plan encompasses

To determine the future employment number, take the current number of team members and multiply it by the average annual practice growth factor. This will provide an estimated number of team members needed for next year.

For example:

1. A practice currently has ten team members.
2. Historically, the practice grows business by 5% each year.
   Therefore, 10 team members × 5% growth = 0.5, therefore, one part-time person will be needed for the following year.
   Next, add in the average attrition rate (if the practice loses an average of one team member per year, the attrition rate = 1).
3. Therefore 1 + 0.5 = 1.5 (one full-time person and one part-time person will be needed).
   Next, multiply the total number of years the strategic plan encompasses (i.e., 1 for 1 year, 2, or 3). If the practice is planning for the next 2 years:
4. 1.5 × 2 = 3. Three full-time employees will be needed to meet the strategic goals for 2 years.

Demand considers the workforce needed to fill positions in the future. Will there be enough veterinarians and/or credentialed veterinary technicians to fulfill the need? What will the future workforce require to consider employment in your practice? Innovation, technology, flex scheduling, benefits, and career growth are all factors that should be considered when planning (see Chapters 1, 2, and 4 for review).

One last consideration is to evaluate the other employers within the community that are not veterinary-related). If Amazon has a warehouse in the community, they may be offering higher wages, improved benefits, career development, or flex scheduling to draw potential candidates. Veterinary practices can compete with employers such as this; however, plans must be put in place to do so.

Talent Acquisition and Management

The hiring of team members is covered in Chapter 4. Hiring the right team members is important to strategic goal achievement. The previous topic covered the supply and demand that should be considered when planning for team members. Ensure that accurate job descriptions are developed (knowledge, skills, abilities, core values, credentials, etc.) and that the right people are hired to fit the practice culture and help achieve strategic goals.

Talent management is defined as building the team to deliver the strategic goal that has been put in place. Traditionally in veterinary medicine, practices hire fast, train for 1 week, then put the new team member on the front line (only the strong survive!). When utilizing this protocol, leadership, the existing team, and new team members are set up for failure. Leadership has put valuable time and effort into hiring the right candidate and the team has taken time from their responsibilities to develop the new member. When an employee does not work out everyone has failed. Soon, both leadership and team members resent bringing on new employees that may not stay.

Talent management starts with the onboarding and training process (Chapter 4). The first days of an employee's experience builds loyalty and branding of the hospital. The onboarding process may take weeks to months, depending on the experience level of the new team member. Create a plan to make the onboarding process simple and successful. Use structured mentoring and training programs to improve retention rates and increase success rates for keeping new hires on the team.

Increase team member efficiency (Chapter 2) by providing skill development on a routine basis. The more skills obtained, the more valuable each employee becomes with problem solving and accountability. For example, team members can (and should!) learn how to manage a crisis versus leadership having to put out fires. Place continuing education and skill development into the strategic plan, and budget accordingly.

LEADERSHIP POINT

Tie the VMVs and expected behaviors into performance management systems. Both coaching and performance reviews should take place on a routine basis. When employees receive regular coaching, the team member grows exponentially.

Succession Planning

Succession planning is defined as identifying and fostering the growth of high-performing employees and preparing them to fill critical positions within the practice in the future. These high-performing team members will need more than just medical skill development; they will also need leadership, strategy, and personal development abilities. Succession planning takes into consideration the strategic goals in place, as well as team members that may be retiring in the future. When succession plans are made, essential positions are easy to fill, preventing practices from being negatively affected when a vacancy occurs. It can take 12 to 36 months to prepare a team member for a leadership position. This includes intense coaching and the sharing of knowledge with the person they may replace.

Effective succession planning requires open communications and dialogue between all individuals and assurance that succession planning is not about job replacement. Team members must understand that succession planning ensures the future success of the practice and supports the achievement of strategic goals. Fig. 17.8 lists the imperative positions that should be considered for succession planning in the veterinary hospital.

To create a succession plan, complete a gap analysis of team members and identify current KSAs to determine what will be required in the future to fulfill essential positions. Develop a plan that harnesses those KSAs along with leadership, strategy, and personal development training.

Employee Engagement

Managing and developing team members is imperative in achieving strategic goals. But those are only two pieces of the puzzle. *Employee engagement* is a third component that must be incorporated. Employee engagement is defined as ensuring team members are emotionally invested in the success of the practice and accountable for goal achievement. Without employee engagement, team members show up for their jobs with little regard for the practice VMVs. Employee engagement ensures team members come to work committed every day and understand how their role helps to achieve strategic goals. Review Chapters 2 and 4 for specific details.

THESE LEADERS SHOULD HAVE A SUCCESSION PLAN IN PLACE

- Veterinary medical director
- Practice manager
- Office manager
- Department head (specialty practices)
- Lead technician
- Boarding/kennel manager

Fig. 17.8 Critical Positions to Consider for Succession Planning.

Every position within the practice must have meaning and a sense of purpose. For every team member to gain that understanding, leadership must clearly communicate the goals and include team members in the decisions to help achieve those goals. In addition, team numbers must be able to work with autonomy and master their skills (Chapter 2, Understanding Motivation).

Cultures that support innovation, creative thinking, high-level and clear communication, and open-book management (Chapter 16, Finance), foster employee engagement. In addition to a positive culture, supporting team members' emotional well-being drives employee engagement. Emotional well-being is defined as the physical health, psychological health (ability to deal with stress, having confidence and resilience), and connectedness (relationships with coworkers, work/life balance, and respect for one another) of team members. Other factors that affect emotional welfare (practices may not be able to control but can influence) include technology, environmental culture, and the economy. The economic factor is often tied directly to wages paid by the practice. Wages play a large role in sustaining employees' happiness; however, practices often feel they cannot afford raises. To promote healthy profit margins, it is important to ensure that all services are being charged for, service prices are appropriate, inventory is managed well, products are priced competitively, and service offerings are maximized (see Chapter 16, Finance, for more tips). A practice can usually capture an additional 17% of net income when the criteria mentioned previously are achieved, allowing for investment into the team (increased wages), thus driving employee engagement and well-being (WMPB, 2017).

Review Chapter 2, Understanding Motivation and Maslow's Hierarchy of Needs. If the very basic levels of safety and security are not met, the team member will never become engaged nor be motivated to become engaged.

Leadership and management behavior also play a pivotal role in employee engagement and well-being. Team members want to know that leaders care about them. They appreciate having gratitude shown for hard work and recognition of accomplishments. Team members also cherish receiving coaching daily. Remember, team members follow in the footsteps of their leaders; illustrating positive characteristics will enable team members to become fully engaged in the practice.

Engaging, motivating, and retaining the team is a long-term investment and takes commitment from leadership. Measure turnover rates, team member absenteeism, and tardiness as they relate to employee engagement. If any of these factors is high, culture, leadership behavior, and management practices need to be evaluated.

INTEGRATING TECHNOLOGY

Technology is changing rapidly, not only within the scope of veterinary medicine itself but also in the ability to enhance staff efficiency, communicate with clients, and deliver improved services. Technology must be integrated into the strategic plan today to help the practice grow in the future.

Allow team members to contribute technology ideas that will advance efficiencies within the practice and the team. Review software applications such as Teams or Slack (Chapter 2, Internal Communication) to promote team member communications. Consider a customized practice app to improve communications with clients, making it easier for them to refill medications and make appointments (Chapter 12, Marketing). Consider online pet portals that allow clients to review their pet's medical records, diagnostic results, and medical history. Provide an online pharmacy (Chapter 15, Inventory Management) to meet the client's need for shopping after hours. Telehealth is rapidly emerging in veterinary medicine and became a necessity during the pandemic. Telehealth encompasses a broad variety of technologies and tactics to deliver virtual medical, health, and education services.

CONSIDER THE PRACTICE OF THE FUTURE

Developing a dream practice can become a reality with appropriate planning. Whether the veterinary practice is a brand-new start-up business or has been in business for several years, the dream can still be achieved. Start with a true assessment of what the practice of the future should look like, and for whom they will provide services. Always be a patient advocate first and foremost, and then develop methods that can produce profits to sustain the team over the long term.

Provide the team with the tools they need to achieve the practice goals. No one person can achieve the practice of the future alone, but by encouraging the team to help carry out the goals, the dream can be achieved.

Technology is constantly changing. Stay on top of advancements that may benefit the practice by meeting and exceeding client and patient needs. Research telehealth to understand how it can be integrated to make client and patient visits better. To some degree, telehealth is already practiced every time a client calls for advice over the phone. Telehealth will incorporate better diagnostics in the future.

Be a patient advocate by *always* considering patient welfare. The practice of the future should encompass low-stress handling techniques, Fear Free protocols, and a reduction in the separation of clients and patients. The Mayo Clinic experience models all care on keeping parents and children together whenever possible. You would never go to the Mayo Clinic and expect them to take your child to the "back" to draw blood; this is a model that should also be built into veterinary practices. Clients should be welcomed in extended areas within the practice to have the opportunity to see the care level you are proving while providing comfort for their pets.

PHASES OF STRATEGIC PLANNING

Strategic planning should be broken into two phases to enable easier implementation. When planning occurs in stages, processes can be better identified and created, allowing better outcomes. The following section will dive into strategic plan formulation, development, implementation, and evaluation.

Formulation

The formulation phase of strategic planning includes the development of the (VMVs) of the organization (Chapter 2); identifying the practice's *s*trengths, *w*eaknesses, *o*pportunities, and *t*hreats (SWOT) analysis (Chapter 12), and a gap analysis (Chapter 2) to determine how to get from point A to point B in a strategic plan.

The creation of the VMVs is absolutely critical in the development of a strategic plan because they represent the goals of the organization. Every decision made for the business, team members, clients, or patients must support the goals, or the MVVs. If the practice currently has VMVs, but they are irrelevant to where the practice wants to be in the future, they should be reevaluated and updated to bring alignment. In addition, if the team members cannot relate to the mission statement developed by leadership, it should be reevaluated [or the employee(s) need to be assessed to determine whether they are the right fit for the organization]. Every team member, including leadership, must live and breathe the MVVs. If leaders do not "walk the walk" of the MVVs, neither will the team, and strategic goals will not be achieved.

SWOT analyses are often seen in marketing plans, but they also need to be included in strategic planning. **Strengths** identify what the practice is particularly good at, just as weaknesses identify where improvements are needed. It is important to honestly assess both strengths and weaknesses. When the **weaknesses** are identified, a plan should be developed to address and overcome the issues, especially if they tie to the overall goal of the practice. For example, if the practice mission statement is "to provide advanced veterinary care for every patient," a strength may be the highly trained veterinarian(s) on staff, and a weakness may be the lack of credentialed veterinary technician(s) on staff. To deliver advanced veterinary care to every patient, credentialed veterinary technicians would need to be hired. Therefore a goal, objective, and action plan can be developed from the weakness identified. Strengths and weaknesses are evaluated from within the practice.

Opportunities are circumstances that can improve practice strength. For example, a practice may identify the opportunity to expand services to include rehabilitation which would increase the client and revenue base. Or a practice may see an opportunity to promote a stellar employee to a management position, offering leadership to the team and improving efficiency.

Threats are events or situations that could occur with a negative impact on the practice. It is important that the practice be aware of threats and mitigate the risk as much as possible. For example, if the practice is in a common hurricane zone, then the practice must develop a plan to alleviate the severity of this threat. The practice should ensure electronic medical records are backed up regularly (Chapter 9); equipment and supplies must be actively recorded (Chapter 13), and appropriate insurance coverage should be addressed. The practice has no control over the threat from Mother Nature, but it can reduce the risks associated with loss of data and medical records and can ensure business continuity. See Chapter 12 for more SWOT tips.

Once the VMVs have been developed (or updated), and the SWOT analysis has been completed, a gap analysis should be completed. A gap analysis involves the comparison of current performance with potential or desired performance. For a veterinary practice, this means evaluating how the practice is doing at present and where it would like to be in the future. A gap analysis creates the path into the development phase of strategic planning.

Questions to ask during a gap analysis include:

- What services and procedures does the practice deliver today?
- What services or procedures does the practice want to be able to deliver in the future?
- What KSAs (*k*nowledge, *s*kills, and *a*bilities) does the practice need to achieve the ability to deliver the services or procedures of the future?
- What kind of team members will be needed to deliver the services or procedures of the future?
- What competencies (attitude and behavior) does the team need to deliver the services or procedures of the future?
- What is the current retention rate of employees in the practice?
- Is there a succession plan in place for current team members?
- Can team members create a career out of their position, or is it just a job?

Development

During the development phase of the strategic planning process, the practice considers the VMVs, evaluates the SWOT and gap analyses, and creates a plan to achieve desired goals. How will this practice get from point A (now) to point B (the future)? Consider:

Team members:

- Assess the skill level. Will continuing education need to be factored in? If yes, how will that occur? When? Where?
- Where will the practice obtain these team members?
- How will the practice retain these team members (benefits and future payroll considerations)?

Clients

- Who is the target client?
- How will that client be found, and how will they be retained?

Patients

- What equipment/tools/inventory will be needed to provide the highest standard of care?
- Considering the progression of technology, what equipment/tools/inventory will be needed when point B is attained?

Budget

- How much money will be needed to get to point B? How will that money be obtained? Traditionally, veterinary practices have not created budgets and have lacked organization, planning, and strategy. This is not a sound business practice, and without a plan in place, a practice cannot grow. Strategic plans include funding to deploy initiatives and a budget must be created to support that plan.

Marketing: A strategic plan should be established before a marketing plan is even thought of. Why would a marketing plan be created if the goal of the organization is unknown? Marketing plans are designed to help achieve strategic goals.

Once the strategic plan is created, identify areas of the revenue process that can be positively affected through marketing plans. Advertising and marketing are two different things. Review every internal process, ensuring the team is ready to deliver what is being promised in advertising. Keep in mind, the team is always marketing through their everyday actions, intentionally or unintentionally. Review Chapter 12 for marketing ideas.

Numerous options may be considered in determining the highest potential for successfully reaching the goals. The outcome of the development phase is developing a strategy that has a "strategic fit." When a strategic fit exists, the practice's activities are consistent with the strategy, they interact with and reinforce each other, and they are optimized to reach the strategic goal.

Objectives that can be measured in the evaluation phase must be established in the development phase. Objectives are defined as specific results that a practice aims to achieve within a specified timeframe and with available resources. Examples of specific objectives could include minimizing expenses or expanding revenue centers. Objectives should be prioritized based on importance to achieve goals. See Chapter 12 for a complete SMART goal example that outlines objectives used to achieve specific goals.

Implementation

During the implementation phase of the strategy, strategic intent is translated into specific plans of action. The success of the strategy rests on allocating resources to the right initiatives, communicating them to team members, and managing plans effectively.

Consider the tools that will be needed to deliver the objectives. Education, team member knowledge, skills and abilities, and appropriate staffing are tools that are often overlooked. Goals cannot be achieved without the use of these tools.

Incorporate "systems thinking," in which one must consider how every department affects another. For example, IT will affect everything in the practice, from medical records and how the receptionist completes transactions to the veterinary medical team integrating and reading radiographs. Another example is employee benefits. By not having benefits, or benefits that are noncompetitive, the talent pool could be affected, and the practice may have to hire less qualified candidates instead of the right candidate(s). When highly skilled team members are not hired, it affects client service, patient care, practice revenue, and, ultimately, practice value.

LEADERSHIP POINT

When a strategic fit exists, the practice's activities are consistent with the strategy, they interact with and reinforce each other, and they are optimized to reach the strategic goal.

When creating a plan of action during the implementation phase, consider using the SMART acronym: **Specific, Measurable, Action Items/Accountability, Resources, and Timebound**.

Specific defines the specific goal that is to be achieved.

Measurable identifies how the success of the goal will be measured.

Action Items/Accountability defines who will carry out the action items/objective(s) of the goal.

Resources identifies what resources will be needed to achieve and implement the goal successfully.

Timebound identifies when the goal will be achieved by and establish check-in points between the practice manager and the person accountable for achieving the set objectives.

Managing the implementation of the strategy is important. Consider clearing away obstacles that will block progress. This may require identifying performance issues (such as conflicts, performance gaps, inadequate communications, or team morale problems) and taking steps to correct them. It is important to ensure that all expectations are clearly understood among team members and leadership, and that "check-in" points are established along the way. It is also important to monitor measurements (KPIs, or key performance indicators) throughout the initiative. Waiting to measure and monitor KPIs until the end of the initiative prevents adjustments from being made that could be used to achieve the goals.

Evaluation

During the evaluation phase, the objectives that were developed during the development phase must be evaluated. If check-in points were established during the implementation phase, and KPIs were monitored, all goals should be achievable. A practice may also consider tying in other measurements to the evaluation. A simple balanced scorecard can be created showing the "state of the state" of the practice (Fig. 17.9). A scorecard may have entries such as client satisfaction, team member satisfaction, the financial picture of the practice, and the learning and development that has occurred within the organization. These metrics often show the side effects of successful strategy implementation but can also show whether changes have affected other business parts.

Audits within the veterinary practice are relatively unheard of, but from a strategic point of view, they are a "must-have." Just as with a lack of proper budget planning, practices typically only plan audits of their infrastructure when required by the IRS, Department of Labor, or OSHA. Strategic planning ensures that *all* of the processes that protect a practice have been put in place.

Follow the audit processes listed in Fig. 17.10 to perform audits on a routine basis. In addition to the areas listed in Fig. 17.11, each chapter lists SOPs that must be audited, completed, or at minimum, reviewed.

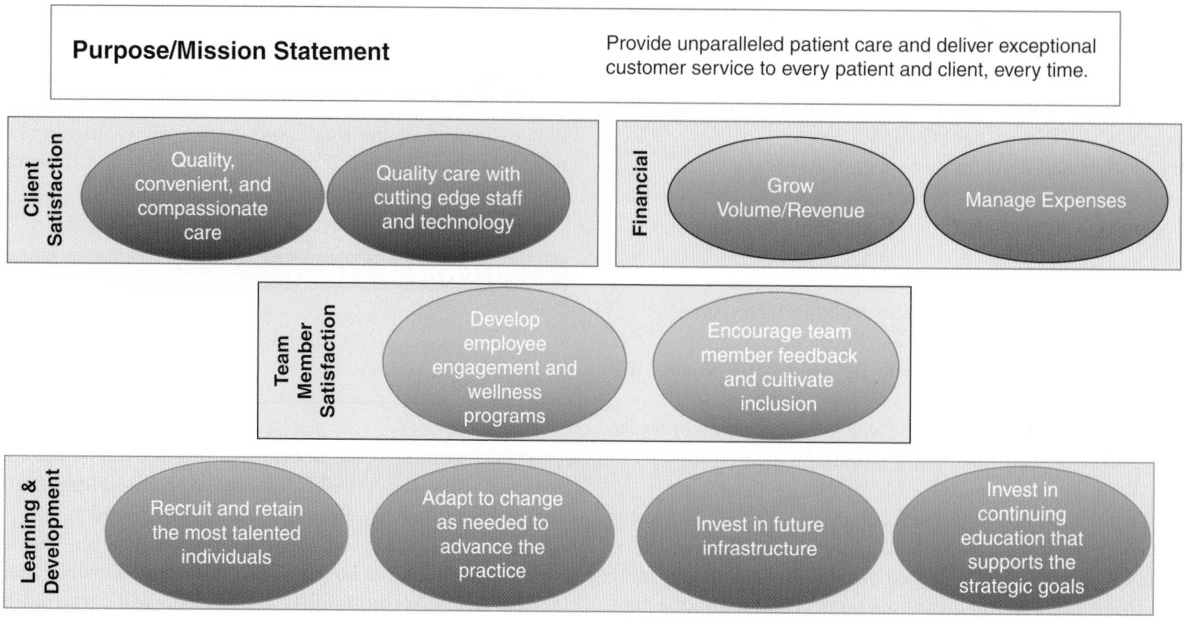

Fig. 17.9 Example of a Balanced Scorecard.

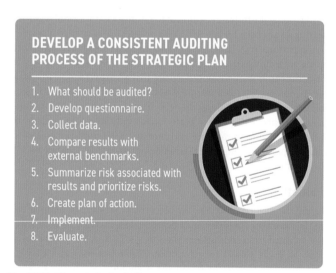

DEVELOP A CONSISTENT AUDITING PROCESS OF THE STRATEGIC PLAN

1. What should be audited?
2. Develop questionnaire.
3. Collect data.
4. Compare results with external benchmarks.
5. Summarize risk associated with results and prioritize risks.
6. Create plan of action.
7. Implement.
8. Evaluate.

Fig. 17.10 Steps to in Audit Process.

CRITICAL AUDIT POINTS IN THE VETERINARY PRACTICE

- Human resources (Employee law, records retention, and benefits)
- End-of-day reconciliation
- Controlled substances
- Financial
- Insurance (liability, property, building, employee health)
- Disaster response (OSHA, natural disasters)
- Data recovery (server failure, power loss)
- Safety (OSHA)
- Best practices (compare internal and external benchmarks)
- Strategic plans (do VMVs align with goals? Does leadership model the VMVs? Define the strengths and weaknesses of the practice: do they align with the strategic plan?)

Fig. 17.11 Practice Areas to Consider for Routine Audits.

PRACTICE MANAGER SURVIVAL CHECKLIST FOR STRATEGIC PLANNING

☐ Incorporate building maintenance into budget planning and strategic objectives.
☐ Develop a budget that achieves strategic goals.
☐ Develop a written strategic plan and share it with the team (and share monthly updates).
☐ Update the practice management system when applicable.
☐ Develop succession planning for team members.
☐ Implement equipment maintenance schedules (diagnostic and treatment equipment, refrigerators, heaters, coolers, etc.) and monitor frequently.
☐ Host strategic planning meetings annually (at minimum).
☐ Attend advanced leadership courses annually.
☐ Develop a business continuation plan and review it annually.
☐ Ensure adequate insurance coverage and review annually (fire, flood, general, liability, professional, etc.).

REVIEW QUESTIONS

1. Define a strategic plan.
2. Name the four phases of strategic planning
3. Name the four phases of a business life cycle.
4. Define organization design.
5. What are the four steps of organizational development?
6. Define a learning organization.
7. What is workforce planning?
8. Define talent management.
9. Define succession planning.
10. How far in advance should strategic plans be developed?
    a. 1 year
    b. 3 years
    c. 10 years
    d. All of the above
11. Which is NOT a phase of strategic management?
    a. Development
    b. Formulation
    c. Evaluation
    d. Communication
12. Which is NOT a phase of the business life cycle?
    a. Growth
    b. Acceleration
    c. Decline
    d. Maturity
13. MVVs should be developed during which phase of the business life cycle?
    a. Introductory
    b. Growth
    c. Maturity
    d. Decline
14. Which is NOT part of the formulation phase in strategic management?
    a. Developing MVVs
    b. Identifying strengths and weaknesses
    c. Creating SOPs
    d. Creating a gap analysis
15. What does the "S" stand for in the SWOT analysis?
    a. Standards
    b. Strengths
    c. Supplements
    d. Supportive

RECOMMENDED READING

Dowdy, T.: The #1 Problem Preventing Practices from Being Successsful. TracyDowdy Consulting. January 2019. https://tracydowdy.com/category/strategic-mission-and-vision/. Accessed June 8, 2023.

Tumblin, D., Tassava, B., Traub-Warner, M.: Well Managed Practice Benchmarks (WMPB) 2017. https://wellmp.com/2021-study-fees/. Accessed June 2018.

ABBREVIATIONS

Abbreviation	Definition
AD	right ear
ad-lib	freely as wanted
ARF	acute renal failure
AS	left ear
AU	both ears
BAR	bright, alert, responsive
BID	twice daily
BM	bowel movement
BP	blood pressure
BTT	blue-topped tube
BW	body weight
cc	cubic centimeter
CHF	congestive heart failure
CRF	chronic renal failure
d	day
d	diarrhea
D5W	5% dextrose in water
DIC	disseminated intravascular coagulation
DJD	degenerative joint disease
DM	diabetes mellitus
DOA	dead on arrival
Dx	diagnosis
ECG, EKG	electrocardiogram
ECHO	echocardiogram
EENT	eyes, ears, nose, throat
FB	foreign body
FeLV	feline leukemia virus
FIP	feline infectious peritonitis
FPV	feline panleukopenia virus
FUO	fever of unknown origin
FUS	feline urologic syndrome
FVR	feline viral rhinotracheitis
Fx	fracture
g, gm	gram
gal	gallon
GDV	gastric dilatation volvulus
gtt	drops
h	hour
HBC	hit by car
HR	heart rate
Hx	history
ICH	infectious canine hepatitis

Abbreviation	Definition
ID	intradermal
IM	intramuscular
IN	intranasal
IP	intraperitoneal
IT	intratracheal
IV	intravenous
IVD	intervertebral disk disease
IVP	intravenous pyelogram
kg	kilogram
L	liter
LN	lymph node
LRS	lactated Ringer solution
LTT	lavender-topped tube
MAP	mean arterial pressure
mcg, μg	microgram
mEq	milliequivalent
mg	milligram
MI	mitral insufficiency
mL	milliliter
MLV	modified live virus
mm	mucous membrane
NPO	nil per os
NSF	no significant findings
OCD	osteochondritis dissecans
OD	right eye
OFA	Orthopedic Foundation for Animals
OS	left eye
OTC	over-the-counter
OU	both eyes
OVH, OHE	ovariohysterectomy
PM	postmortem
PO	per os
ppm	parts per million
PPN	partial parenteral nutrition
prn	as necessary
PTS	put to sleep
PTT	purple-topped tube or lavender-topped tube
q	every
qd	every day
qh	every hour
qid	four times a day
qod	every other day

Abbreviation	Definition
R/I	rule ins
R/O	rule outs
RTT	red topped tube
Rv	rabies vaccination
S/R	suture or staple removal
SC, SQ	subcutaneous
sig	label
Sx	surgery
tab	tablet

Abbreviation	Definition
tid	three times a day
TPR	temperature, pulse, respiration
Tx	treatment
UA	urinalysis
URI	upper respiratory infection
UTI	urinary tract infection
v	vomiting
WNL	within normal limits

GLOSSARY

1099-MISC A year-end report that businesses provide independent contractors for services rendered in the preceding fiscal year. 1099-MISC forms are due to contractors no later than January 31, allowing contractors to report income on their own business taxes.

401(k) A retirement fund to which employees may contribute; employers are not required to contribute but may do so if they wish.

Accountability The ability of individuals to take responsibility for tasks and duties.

Accounts payable Amounts owed to suppliers that are payable in the future.

Accounts receivable Money owed to a practice for services rendered or products sold that are not paid at the time of service or when the product is dispensed.

Accrual-based accounting A system that recognizes income when it is earned and expenses when they are incurred rather than when the actual cash transaction occurs.

Active income Income produced by veterinarians through examinations, diagnostics, surgical procedures, and prescribing medication.

Administrative ethics Involves the action by administrative government bodies that regulate veterinary practice and activities in which veterinarians engage.

Allowance The maximum amount available for a specific diagnosis in pet health insurance.

Anesthetic release form A form signed by the client accepting risks associated with surgical and treatment procedures.

Anger A stage of grief that people experience.

Annual deductible An amount a client chooses to pay out before receiving benefits from pet health insurance.

Annual payout limit The maximum amount a pet health insurance company will pay out over the year for a pet's policy.

Appointment book template The outline of the appointment book.

Appointment cards Cards given to clients stating their scheduled appointment date, time, and patient name.

Appointment units The specified amount of time that correlates to 1 unit. For example, 15 minutes equals 1 unit, and 30 minutes equals 2 units.

Assets Any property owned by a business or individual. Cash, accounts receivable, inventory, land, buildings, leasehold improvements, and tangible property are examples of assets.

Average client transaction Revenue per client visit, calculated by dividing the income by the number of clients or patients seen.

AVMA The American Veterinary Medical Association: an organization developed to improve and set standards for veterinary medicine.

AVMA Model Practice Act A set of guiding principles for states that are, or will be, preparing to revise the state veterinary practice act.

Balance sheet A financial report detailing practice assets, liabilities, and owner's equity.

Barrier to patient care The block that clients face when trying to access care for their pets, is often due to the veterinary practice(s) being overbooked with current patients, not accepting new patients, or being understaffed.

Benchmarking The process by which a practice compares itself to others (especially those known for outstanding performance) in an attempt to improve performance.

Benefit The payment made for a specific diagnosis per an insurance plan.

Better Business Bureau Also known as the BBB; accepts complaints of unhealthy business practices from consumers.

Billing cycle The period between statements produced for clients.

Biohazard A needle, glass, or sharp object that is contaminated with vaccinations, pathogens, or human blood and must be disposed of in a leakproof container. The container must be incinerated by an approved company.

Blogging The practice of creating a "new" newsletter that must be linked to the practice's webpage; can detail the everyday happenings around the veterinary office.

Body language Posture, stance, and position that communicate messages to a listener.

Bookkeeper Generally, a self-taught accountant who maintains payroll and books.

Brand An identifying symbol, words, or mark that distinguishes a company from its competitors.

Break-even analysis The process used to determine how much money or service must be recovered or performed to cover the cost of purchasing equipment or adding a service to the practice.

Budget An estimate of revenues and expenses for a given period.

Bundled treatment plans A collective group of common codes used when developing a treatment plan to diagnose or treat a patient with a specific protocol. Bundled treatment plans decrease missed charges and increase the efficiency of the veterinary team.

Burnout Physical or emotional exhaustion, especially as a result of long-term stress or dissipation.

Business life cycle Similar to the life cycle of people and pets, businesses experience an introductory stage, growth stage, mature stage, and decline stage.

Capital inventory Equipment that is purchased for use in business.

Carcinogen A chemical or substance that is known to cause cancer.

Career planning The ongoing process of making career choices that are reviewed from time to time.

Cash-based accounting A system that recognizes income as it is received and expenses as they are paid, rather than when the income was earned, or the expense was acquired.

Cash flow statement Report on the sources of cash and its use during a specific period of time.

Central inventory location A central location within the practice where excess inventory is stored; often a locked location.

Change management The action of creating change in the veterinary practice. Change management involves identifying the problem, completing a gap analysis, presenting the findings to the team, creating a solution, implementing the solution, and following through with the solution.

Chronic condition A condition of a pet that progresses over time.

Civil law Relates to the duties between people and the government.

Claim A submission for a request for payment in pet health insurance.

Client communication Listening to and understanding client needs and then delivering the information needed to ensure complete understanding.

Client compliance A key performance indicator monitoring the level of clients' accepting recommendations made by the practice team.

Client discharge instructions Explicit instructions that are given to a client upon the release of a pet from the hospital for post-release care, including activity, food, and medication instructions.

Client grievances Client complaints.

Client patient information sheet A sheet that is filled out by the client, requesting client contact information, along with patient data.

Client retention A key performance indicator determining the number of clients who are retained in a practice between two set dates.

Client survey A survey asking clients of their thoughts and opinions of the services received in a practice.

Cloud-based server a centralized server that is hosted and delivered over a network, typically the internet, and accessed on demand by multiple users.

COBRA – Consolidated Omnibus Budget Reconciliation Act It requires employers to continue insurance coverage for a specified time. COBRA requires employers to continue coverage for former employees who have a medical condition that would prevent them from obtaining immediate coverage from a new employer.

Code of ethics Developed to help members of the veterinary profession achieve high levels of behavior through moral consciousness, decision making, and practice.

COGS – Cost of goods sold The expense incurred to purchase merchandise sold during a period.

Collections agency A business that has been hired to collect funds from nonpaid accounts.
Community service The donation of time to a nonprofit organization.
Company-supported website A website typically created by a design company; the practice may have little or no access to the content provided.
Compassion fatigue The cost of caring. To experience compassion fatigue, individuals must have an ability for empathy and be involved in a caregiving relationship.
Compliance rate The measure of whether pets actually receive the care that has been recommended by the veterinary team.
Computerized medical records Medical records that are kept on the computer; all images, signed consent forms, and blood work are stored in the computerized medical record.
Conflict management The use of processes and skills to find creative and respectful ways to manage disagreements.
Congenital condition Generally referred to as an abnormality present at birth, whether apparent or not, that can cause illness or disease.
Consent The voluntary acceptance or agreement to what is planned or is done by another person.
Contract employee An individual who has established a business for themselves and contracts out services to other businesses; relief veterinarians, groomers, and consultants can be contract employees.
Contract law Deals with duties established by individuals as a result of contractual agreement.
Controlled substance A drug that has been deemed by the DEA to have the potential to be abused.
Controlled Substance Act of 1970 An act passed to reduce drug abuse by identifying substances that have high abuse potential.
Controlled substance log A log or record used to manage all controlled substances dispensed.
Copay A specified dollar amount of covered services that is the policyholder's responsibility.
Core values See values.
Cost analysis Breaking down the costs of some operations and reporting on each factor separately.
Cover letter A letter placed with a resume showing interest in employment.
CPA – Certified public accountant A college-trained accountant professional who has attained certification in the state in which they reside, by passing a comprehensive examination and maintaining continuing education.
Cremation The incineration of a body.
Criminal law Prosecutes crimes committed against the public as a whole. Most criminal laws focus on acts that injure people or pets.
Culture The evolving set of collective beliefs, values, and attitudes of the veterinary practice. It is a key component of the business and has an impact on the achievement of strategic goals.
DEA – U.S. Drug Enforcement Administration Provides approved means for proper manufacturing, distribution, dispensing, and use of drugs through licensed handlers.
Debit transactions Transactions paid with a credit card that is linked to the customer's checking account.
Deductible The dollar amount an individual must pay for services before the insurance company's payment. Clients may have a choice of per incident deductible or annual deductible.
Delegation Authorizing subordinates to take assigned responsibilities and make decisions.
Deposit Placing or transferring funds into a savings or checking account.
Diagnoses code A code used in the Practice Integration Management Software (PIMS) that is used when a patient is diagnosed with a condition. Diagnoses codes allow specific reports to be generated to better manage patient care, client expectations, and practice goals.
Diagnosis The identification of an illness or issue by examination and diagnostic workup.
Direct deposit An automatic transaction that places money into an employee's checking account for payroll.
Direct expense An expense that can be directly related to a patient, client, or revenue center.
Direct marketing The most popular form of marketing and has been around for years. The Yellow Pages are a classic example of direct marketing.
Directive management Task-oriented style of management.
Distributor representative A representative of a company that sells products of larger manufacturing companies.
Domain name A name given to a web address that is recognizable because web addresses are provided in numeric format.
Effective communication Communication to both clients and team members that is clear, conceptual, and easy to follow.
Electrocardiogram A record of the heart's electrical activity.
Embezzlement The fraudulent appropriation of funds or property entrusted to your care when it is actually owned by someone else.
Emotional intelligence The ability to identify, assess, and control one's emotions.
Emotional well-being The ability to produce positive emotions, moods, thoughts, and feelings, and adapt when confronted with adversity and stressful situations.
Employee benefits A collection of perks provided by employers (in addition to wages) that may include health insurance, retirement plans, or incentive packages.
Employee engagement The state in which employees are involved in the veterinary practice, are committed to the goals and values, and are motivated to contribute to the success of the practice.
Employee manual A manual explaining the terms and conditions employees must operate under while working for a given business.
Employee Polygraph Protection Act The EPPA prohibits most employers from using lie detector tests for either preemployment screening or during the course of employment. Employers cannot discriminate against employees who refuse to take a lie detector test.
Employee procedural manual A manual explaining the procedures employees must follow while working for a given business.
Employment law Laws that govern the relationship and their employer, including the rights and responsibilities of each party.
Empower/empowerment The act of sharing managerial power with subordinates. It is the concept of encouraging and authorizing workers to take initiative to improve operations, reduce costs, and improve customer service.
EMRs – Electronic Medical Records Medical records that are recorded in an electronic PIMS platform, backed up on a local or cloud-based server, and can be accessed from multiple locations.
End-of-day reconciliation The process required to close the business books at the end of the day; cash, credit cards, and checks must balance with the computer-generated report.
Equity The rights or claims to properties. Assets = Equities + Liabilities
Equal Employment Opportunity Prevents discrimination against race, color, sex, religion, and national origin. Employers cannot deny a promotion, terminate, or not hire a potential employee because of any of the reasons just mentioned.
Ergonomics The science that studies the relationship between people and their work environments.
ERISA The Employee Retirement Income Security Act regulates retirement funds once established in a business.
Estimates A printed idea of the cost of services and products that clients will incur while their pet is treated.
Etiquette The rules that society has set for the proper way to behave in dealing with other people.
Euthanasia The induction of a painless death.
Euthanasia release form The owner's consent to perform euthanasia.
Evaluation A report provided to employees stating their work performance and any improvements that need to be made; generally performed on an annual basis.
Exclusion A condition that would be excluded from the coverage of a medical plan.
Exempt employee an employee who does not receive overtime pay or qualify for minimum wage. Exempt employees are paid by salary, rather than hourly, and work in a professional, administrative, or executive role.
External marketing A marketing technique that targets potential clients.
Fair Credit Reporting Act A federal law that regulates prescreening reports issued to employers by outside agencies called credit reporting agencies.

Fair Debt Collection Practices Act An act that was passed to protect the public from unethical collection procedures.

FDA – U.S. Food and Drug Administration An agency of the U.S. Department of Health and Human Services that is responsible for regulating and supervising the safety of foods, dietary supplements, drugs, vaccines, biological medical products, blood products, medical devices, radiation-emitting devices, veterinary products, and cosmetics.

Fear Free® Providing a veterinary practice environment that alleviates fear, anxiety, and stress in pets.

Finance charge Money charged for payments that extend beyond an agreed-upon time limit. The amount of the finance fee must be clearly indicated on the client's invoice.

First notice of accident The initial reporting of an accident to the owner or practice manager, as required by OSHA.

Fixed cost A cost that does not change with the variation of business. Rent, mortgage, and utility costs remain the same, regardless of how busy the practice is.

FLSA – Fair Labor Standards Act Federal law that sets minimum wage and overtime regulations.

FMLA – Family and Medical Leave Act Federal law that allows employees to take up to 12 weeks of unpaid leave to attend to a family member.

Form W-2 IRS form that reports income paid and taxes withheld by an employer for a particular company during a calendar year.

Form W-4 IRS form that determines the amount of federal taxes the employer will withhold from a person's paycheck each pay period.

Formalin A chemical that preserves tissue for histopathology. Formalin is a known carcinogen; therefore, caution must be used while handling it.

Forward booking Scheduling a client's next appointment before they leave the place of business.

Frictionless client experience Creating a client experience free of friction for clients, one that makes it easy for the clients to do business with the practice.

Frictionless employee experience Creating an employee experience that reduces the opportunity for friction with fellow colleagues, is a great place to work, and whole team utilization is employed.

FUTA – Federal Unemployment Tax Act Tax required to be paid by the employer.

Gap analysis A method of assessing the performance of a business unit to determine whether business requirements or objectives are being met, and if not, what steps should be taken to meet them.

Gas sterilization A chemical sterilization technique that uses ethylene oxide to sterilize products.

General administrative expenses All executive, organizational, and clerical expenses associated with the general management of and operations of a practice, rather than with the delivery of patient care.

General anesthesia Controllable and reversible loss of consciousness induced by the intoxication of the central nervous system.

Gingivitis The inflammation associated with gum disease.

Groomer A professional who bathes, clips, and styles the hair of pets.

Gross income Income resulting from all veterinary operations before any cost or expense deductions are made.

Gross profit A monetary amount computed by subtracting the total cost of professional services from gross income.

Herd health records Records that pertain to an entire herd; if one cow is treated for a disease, they may all be treated on the same record.

Hereditary conditions An abnormality that is transmitted by genes from the parent to the offspring, whether apparent or not, that can cause disease or illness.

Histopathology The study of tissue or cells.

Hospital safety manual A manual required by OSHA listing hazards associated with the job, training topics, and procedures in case of an emergency.

Host A computer that is connected to a network or the Internet. Each host has a unique IP address.

Human-animal bond A description of the emotion humans feel toward animals.

Human skill The ability to understand people and what motivates them and to be able to direct their behavior through effective leadership.

Hyperlinks a digital reference to data that the user can follow or be guided to by clicking the link.

Incident An individual accident, illness, or injury, including those that may require continual treatment until resolution.

Income statement Report on financial performance that covers a period of time and reports incomes and expenses during that period. Income statements are also known as profit and loss statements.

Indemnity insurance A system of pet health insurance in which the client is reimbursed for services after they have been provided.

Independent contractor A person hired to do temporary work in which they have complete control of their role and available hours and are responsible for paying their own taxes.

Indirect expense An expense that contributes to the delivery of patient care but cannot be tied directly to a patient, client, or revenue center.

Indirect marketing A marketing technique that is used by practices on a daily basis; clean facilities, genuine service, and excellent customer care are a few examples.

Informational brochure A marketing piece of material informing existing and potential clients of the services offered by the practice.

Informed consent A person's agreement to allow something to happen, such as a medical treatment or surgery that is based on full disclosure of the facts necessary to make an intelligent decision.

Intangible property Nonphysical property that has value; franchises, copyrights, client lists, goodwill, and covenants not to compete are examples of intangible property.

Interest The cost of borrowing money, assessed by the lender over time, usually expressed as a percentage of the principal amount borrowed.

Internal marketing A marketing technique that targets current or existing clients for services offered within the practice.

International health certificates An official letter stating that an animal appears healthy for international travel.

Intervention A process that helps a drug addict recognize the extent of their problem.

Intrastate health certificates An official letter that states a pet appears healthy for travel within the United States.

Intrinsic motivation the doing of an activity for its inherent satisfaction rather than for some separable consequence. When intrinsically motivated a person does something because they want to not because they are told to.

Inventory Extra merchandise or supplies that the practice keeps on hand to meet the demands of customers.

Inventory management software Veterinary software that produces reports and PO numbers and develops a list of needed items when requested.

Inventory turns per year The number of times an item must be reordered within a stated period. Eight to 12 turns per year should be a goal of each practice.

IRCA The Immigration Reform and Control Act prohibits employment discrimination against any employee or potential employee because of national origin.

Just-in-time ordering The process of ordering and receiving product just as it is needed rather than storing excess inventory.

Kennel assistant A team member who cleans kennels, aids in medical treatments, and observes hospitalized patients.

Key performance indicators Statistics that can be generated from client transaction data and reviewed for performance data.

Label printer Printers designed to produce labels for bottles, containers, or envelopes.

Laboratory log A log used to keep track of the tests performed in-house or samples submitted to an outside laboratory.

Lateral recumbency The placement of an animal on the side for an examination or completion of a procedure. Can be either right or left lateral recumbency.

Law Bodies of rules that are developed and enforced by the government to regulate human conduct.

Lead time The amount of time between placing an order and receiving the order.

Leadership The ability of a person to create followers who carry out the goals of the veterinary practice. Great leaders are usually visionaries who influence others in a positive, nonassertive manner.

Leadership fatigue A state that is often experienced when leaders are met with continuous resistance to change and growth from a team, and results when policy and procedures are implemented without practice goals in mind.

Leadership fatigue A common condition experienced by practice managers and/or owners who lack practice direction and goals; symptoms exhibited may include poor morale, inability to problem solve, create a vision, or move the practice in the upright direction.

Legibility The degree to which glyphs and vocabulary are understandable or readable based on appearance.

Lethargy Fatigue or exhaustion.

Liabilities Obligations resulting from past transactions that require the practice to pay money or provide service. Accounts payable and taxes are examples of current liabilities.

Lifetime limit The maximum dollar amount a company will pay out on one policy, for the lifetime of the pet.

Malpractice A limiting term specifically describing a professional's failure to practice the quality of medicine set by similarly situated veterinarians in a given geographic area if the accused is a general practitioner.

Manufacturer representative A representative of a large company that produces products for businesses. Manufacturers may have distributors distribute product for them.

Markup The amount or percentage added to a product or service to cover the cost of the product or service, including a percentage of overhead expenses, and produce a profit. Most products are marked up 150% to 200%.

Maslow's Hierarchy A model for understanding the motivations for human behavior.

Master problem list A list placed in the front of a client record indicating all of the diseases, conditions, medications, and vaccinations a patient has had.

Medical records Daily written reports by veterinarians and technicians on each animal that is treated. Records must be legible and complete.

MISC-1099 A form a company issues to independent contractors, citing all money paid to the individual on an untaxed basis.

Mission statement A statement of the role or purpose, by which a practice intends to serve its stakeholders. It can clarify the way in which a practice plans to achieve its goals.

Mobile media Mobile media implies that webpages are mobile (smartphone) friendly. Mobile media supports the immediate connection clients want to have with a practice.

Monthly statement A statement produced for those with outstanding accounts; may include finance charges and/or statement fees.

NAVTA – National Association of Veterinary Technicians in America A nonprofit organization dedicated to improving the knowledge and professionalism of veterinary technicians.

Negligence Performing an act that a person of ordinary prudence would not have done under similar circumstances, or the failure to do what a person of ordinary circumstances would.

Net income A calculation determined when the expenses are subtracted from the income, with the desire of having a positive number.

Net profit The funds available to an owner after all expenses have been met.

Noncompete agreement An agreement made between two professionals limiting the ability to practice medicine within the established area, for a specified time, if one should leave the practice.

Nonexempt team member Employees that are paid on an hourly basis and entitled to minimum wage, and overtime when they exceed more than 40 hours per week.

Normalize The ability to make difficult topics easier to talk about. Suicide and compassion fatigue can be difficult topics in the veterinary setting; therefore, to normalize the topics, the negative stigma associated with them is removed.

Normative ethics Refers to the search for correct principles of good and bad, right and wrong, justice or injustice.

NSF checks Checks that are returned to the business because of lack of funds or a closed client checking account.

Office manager A manager of a practice who oversees the reception area and possibly also accounts receivable.

On-hold messaging Messages that are played while clients are placed on hold, marketing products or services that the practice provides or recommends.

On-site hosting website A predesigned web page that allows practices to change information on-site.

Open house An event inviting clients to view the practice during nonworking hours. Tours, lectures, or the introduction of a new veterinarian may encourage this internal and external marketing technique.

Order book A book that provides distributor and manufacturer information as well as the order history for products purchased.

Organizational behavior The development, improvement, and effectiveness of an organization; it includes the culture, values, system, and behaviors of the practice.

Organizational design The methodology that identifies aspects of workflow, procedures, roles, and systems and aligns them to fit current business realities/goals.

Organizational development The process of enhancing the effectiveness within the practice.

Organizational learning The training and development of team members.

OSHA – Occupational Safety and Health Administration Developed in 1970 to protect the safety of employees. Every employee has the right to know all of the hazards associated with their employment.

OSHA Form 300 A form required by OSHA to be filled out and maintained that states the facts of an injury that has occurred. The form must be kept for several years.

OSHA Form 300A A form required by OSHA to be posted each year from February 1st to April 30th, summarizing all injuries that occurred while on job premises.

Owner equity Owner's interest or claim in the practice assets.

Paper medical records Handwritten medical records that are kept in a file folder and include all laboratory work results, consent forms, or correspondence with the owner.

Passive income Income generated by the veterinary team excluding the doctor's active income that is produced by exams, diagnostics, surgery, and the prescribing of prescription products. Examples include obtaining radiographs, completing dental prophies, and obtaining ultrasound scans.

Perimeter lighting The lighting on the outside of the practice; excess lighting provides a safer environment for team members and clients.

Per-incident deductible The dollar amount that the policyholder is responsible for before the insurance company will begin to pay out, for each incident that a claim form is submitted.

Per-incident limit The maximum dollar amount an insurance company will pay out, per incident filed.

Permissible exposure limits The maximum exposure amount listed as being safe before harmful side effects may occur.

Personal ethics Defines what is right or wrong on an individual basis.

Personal protection device A device used to protect oneself; may include mace, a Taser, or a personal gun.

Personal skills The skills or attributes an individual possesses; they are achieved through practical experience, education, and personal life lessons.

Pet Portals A pet management app (for clients) that is hosted by the practice and organizes all the pet's information in one place, including upcoming appointments, current medications, and when vaccinations are due.

Petty cash Cash that is held on the premises for purchasing miscellaneous items that may be needed for business; examples include pizza for the staff, special lunch meat for a meticulous patient, or cat litter.

Postdated checks Checks that are written by a client on the current date yet dated to be deposited on a future date.

PPE – Personal protective equipment Equipment provided by the practice that individuals must wear to provide protection from direct or indirect contact with hazardous substances. Examples include eyewash stations, lead gowns and thyroid collars, and safety goggles.

Practice Integration Management Software A software that automates and streamlines a veterinary practice's administrative and billing functions to increase the efficiency of the team. The software must integrate medical records, appointment calendars, invoicing for clients, treatment whiteboards, including reporting capabilities, and function with third-party vendors to have the most efficacious impact on a veterinary hospital.

Practice manager An administrative position that oversees the practice's financial condition, organization, and training.

Preexisting condition Injury or illness contracted, manifested, or incurred before the policy effective date.

Premium The amount paid annually or monthly for a policyholder to maintain an insurance policy.

Preoperative instructions Instructions for clients to follow before a patient's procedure.

Primary complaint The main reason a client visits the practice with their pet.

Principle cost Initial cost of equipment when purchased.

Privacy Act of 1974 An act that states, in part: No agency shall disclose any record which is contained in a system of records by any means of communication to any person, or to another agency, except pursuant to a written request by, or with the prior written consent of, the individual to whom the record pertains.

Professional ethics Developed by the professionals of a particular discipline. They include rules, codes, and conduct for the profession to follow.

Profit and loss statement Summary of the practice's income, expenses, and resulting profit or loss for a specified period of time. Also known as the income statement.

Prognosis The estimated result or condition of a patient.

Psychological safety The belief that employees will not be punished or humiliated for speaking up with ideas, questions, concerns, or mistakes. In the veterinary practice, it is a shared expectation held by members of the team that teammates will not embarrass, reject, or punish them for sharing ideas, taking risks, or soliciting feedback (Center for Creative Leadership; www.ccl.org).

Purging records The act of separating inactive clients from active clients and placing them in another location of the practice that can be easily accessed.

Purpose A sense of purpose is a driving force, self-motivation, and a guiding light that provides individuals with fulfillment as they work towards achieving goals. Purpose helps team members plan career goals effectively, and aligns with values, beliefs, and behaviors that are expected of an individual's surrounding circle.

Push notifications Small pop-up messages sent to a user's device by a mobile app that appears even when the app isn't open.

Rabies certificate A certificate that provides proof of vaccination for rabies.

Rabies neutralizing antibody titer Titer levels in response to a rabies vaccination.

Recalls The process of making phone calls to follow up with clients regarding procedures that were performed in the practice.

Reception area The area of the practice that welcomes clients and provides a comfortable seating area while they wait to be seen by the veterinarian.

Receptionist A team member who greets clients, answers phones, makes appointments, and provides excellent customer service to clients.

Recombinant vaccine A vaccine that inserts a microorganism or engineered protein into a nonpathogenic vector to induce an immune response.

Record retention The number of years a specific record is required to be kept by a federal, state, or local government agency, all of which can vary in length by state.

References People listed within a resume who can provide feedback on the performance of the applicant.

Reminders The generation of cards or letters reminding clients that their pet is due for a procedure.

Remote patient monitoring A healthcare delivery method that utilizes technology to monitor patient health outside of the traditional veterinary practice.

Reorder point The inventory level at which additional product is ordered.

Reorder quantity A set amount of product that is reordered.

Resume A marketing tool that sells the applicant to the potential employer; it should be tailored to the specific job in which the applicant has an interest.

Return on investment The income that investment generates, return on investment is a measure of how effectively a firm uses capital to generate profit.

Revenue centers The areas of the practice that generate revenue: dentistry, pharmacy, laboratory, etc.

Rider An extension of coverage that can be purchased and added to a base medical policy.

Role-playing A training technique that simulates situations and allows the proper response to be practiced.

Scavenger system A system designed to scavenge excess anesthetic gases to increase the safety of the team members. Active, passive, and adsorbent scavengers are examples.

SDS – Safety data sheet Detailed explanations about each drug or chemical providing all important information regarding the use of a substance or chemical.

Search Engine Optimization The process of improving the quality and quantity of website traffic through strategic practices that align with the search engine algorithm.

Secondary traumatic stress The emotional duress that results when an individual hears about the firsthand trauma experiences of another.

Security system A system designed to protect the practice from theft after hours. Alarms, video surveillance, and pager systems are examples that may be used.

SEPs – Simplified Employee Pension Plans These plans are similar to a profit-sharing plan and are appropriate for small organizations. They are funded by tax-deductible employer contributions, and employees are not allowed to contribute.

Server A server stores information on the computers it connects to. When users connect to a server, they can access programs, files, and other information from the server.

sIRA – SIMPLE IRA – Savings Incentive Match Plan for Employees, Individual Retirement Plan A retirement plan in which employees and employers contribute pre-taxed money to an established account.

Situational leadership Using various leadership techniques, depending on what situation is present at the time. One leadership technique may not work in all situations.

SMART Goals SMART goals define needed elements to successfully implement goals. **(S): Specific** defines the specific goal that is to be achieved **(M): Measurable** identifies how the success of the goal will be measured. **(A): Action Items** identify what tasks will need to be completed to achieve the goal. **(R): Resources** identify what resources will be needed to achieve and implement the goal successfully. **(T): Timeline** identifies when the goal will be achieved by and establish check-in points with the responsible individuals.

SOAP medical record An acronym that identifies the most common data entry formats used by veterinary practices (subjective, objective, assessment, and plan).

Social ethics The consensus principles adopted by or accepted by society at large and codified into laws and regulations.

Spam Information including emails that are not considered useful and can be damaging to the user.

Spam filter A device that filters spam, preventing it from infiltrating the user's computer.

Species A basic unit of biological classification and a taxonomic rank.

Standard of care Statements of what a practice believes in and recommends for its patients for wellness testing, pain management, nutrition, senior pet care, and other aspects of patient care.

Standard operating protocol A step-by-step guide that is developed for routine tasks that when repeated, creates consistency and efficiency.

Statement A document that advises clients of their balance and indicates charges, payments, and the balance of their account for the month that has just concluded. Also, a request for money.

Steam sterilization The use of heat and moisture to sterilize objects.

Strategic planning The process of setting goals for the veterinary practice to achieve and creating a plan of action to achieve such goals.

Stress The reaction(s) of people and animals to deleterious forces that disturb homeostasis initially provided in nature.

Stressors Produced as a result of stress and may be internal, external, or environmental.

Substance abuse The use of drugs or alcohol that violates social standards or is self-destructive by nature.

Succession planning Creating an individual development/educational plan for an employee to prepare them for future promotion.

Supportive management Management theory that supports discussion, opinions, and delegation.

System backup Recording the computer data nightly onto another disk or system off premises.

SWOT analysis An internal analysis of a company's strengths, weaknesses, opportunities, and threats.

Tangible property Physical property such as desks, chairs, equipment, computers, software, and vehicles that have value.

Target marketing A type of marketing in which a particular segment is picked to receive a specific marketing plan.

Teleconsult Established when the veterinarian (that has a VCPR) consults with a veterinary specialist regarding a specific case.

Telehealth The use of telecommunication and digital technologies to deliver and enhance veterinary services, including veterinary health information, medical care, and veterinary and client education.

Telemedicine The communication between a veterinary team and a client that has established a veterinary-client-patient relationship (VCPR).

Teletriage Teletriage and teleadvice are often given by the veterinary healthcare team, with careful navigation of not providing a diagnosis or prognosis, but rather scheduling an appointment to be seen (for those without a VCPR) or to create a telehealth appointment with a DVM.

The right to know OSHA's standard that every employee has the right to know the hazards associated with their job.

Tort A civil offense to an opposing party in which harm has occurred.

Transaction A purchase that must be recorded.

Transferable skills Skills that have been gathered through various jobs, volunteering, work, hobbies, sports, or other life experiences that can be used for career changes.

Travel sheet A sheet that is always kept with (travels with) a client record and lists all of the transactions a patient is to be charged for.

USERRA The Uniformed Services Employment and Reemployment Rights Act was created to protect individuals who are enrolled in any branch of the military service; employers cannot discriminate against past, present, or potential duties that an employee or potential employee serves with the armed forces.

Values Guiding principles that are not to be compromised during change; they provide ethical guidance and will not be violated.

Variable cost Any cost that varies with the volume of business for the practice. Medical supplies and drugs increase or decrease, depending on the volume of business.

Verbal image The professional image that a person portrays while educating clients. Knowledge of the procedure, clarity of communication, and correct pronunciation contribute to verbal image.

Veterinarian A professional who has attended a 4-year AVMA-accredited program to receive the DVM degree.

Veterinary assistant A team member who assists the veterinarian and technician with animal restraint, procedures, and client education.

Veterinary ethics Four branches of veterinary ethics exist: descriptive, official, administrative, and normative ethics.

Veterinary Practice Act Law established within each state outlining veterinary medicine.

Veterinary technician A team member who has attended a 2- or 4-year AVMA-accredited program and obtains licensure. This team member assists the veterinarian and may provide client education as needed.

Vision The desired future of the practice.

Voice recognition Technology that allows a computer to input information from spoken commands.

VSPN – Veterinary Support Personnel Network An online veterinary support staff working with, for, or in the field of veterinary medicine, under the direction of a licensed veterinarian.

VTNE – Veterinary Technician National Examination The national examination is administered to those that have graduated from an AVMA-accredited school and who wish to receive credentials within the state they wish to practice in.

WAG – Waste anesthetic gases Anesthetic gases that are eliminated from a patient that should be expelled into an anesthetic machine for scavenging.

Waiting period The time between when an application for health insurance has been accepted and the date when the plan goes into effect.

Want list A list developed of needed inventory items.

Website A site developed on the Internet to market the services available for the practice.

Workers' compensation insurance Insurance required by many states to cover accidents that may occur on the job site. Some states do not require workers' compensation insurance but must contribute to a state fund that pays out for accidents that occurred while working.

Workforce Employees.

Note: Page numbers followed by "*f*" indicate figures, "*t*" indicate tables, "*b*" indicate boxes.

A

D

G

H

O

P

Q

R

S

T

U

V

W

Y

Z